Assistive Technologies and Environmental Interventions in Healthcare

Assistive Technologies and Environmental Interventions in Healthcare

An Integrated Approach

Edited by

Lynn Gitlow, PhD., OTR/L, ATP, FAOTA
Associate Professor
Department of Occupational Therapy
Ithaca College, Ithaca, NY, USA

Kathleen Flecky, OTD, OTR/L
Associate Professor
Department of Occupational Therapy
School of Pharmacy and Health Professions
Creighton University
Omaha, NE, USA

WILEY Blackwell

This edition first published 2020

Registered Office(s)
John Wiley & Sons, Inc., 111 River Street, Hoboken, NJ 07030, USA
John Wiley & Sons Ltd, The Atrium, Southern Gate, Chichester, West Sussex, PO19 8SQ, UK

Editorial Office
9600 Garsington Road, Oxford, OX4 2DQ, UK

For details of our global editorial offices, customer services, and more information about Wiley products visit us at www.wiley.com.

Wiley also publishes its books in a variety of electronic formats and by print-on-demand. Some content that appears in standard print versions of this book may not be available in other formats.

Library of Congress Cataloging-in-Publication Data
Names: Gitlow, Lynn, editor. | Flecky, Kathleen, editor.
Title: Assistive technologies and environmental interventions in healthcare : an integrated approach / edited by Lynn Gitlow, Kathleen Flecky.
Description: Hoboken, NJ : Wiley-Blackwell, [2020] | Includes bibliographical references and index. |
Identifiers: LCCN 2019015586 (print) | LCCN 2019017025 (ebook) | ISBN 9781119483236 (Adobe PDF) | ISBN 9781119483267 (ePub) | ISBN 9781119483229 (pbk.)
Subjects: | MESH: Self-Help Devices | Rehabilitation Research | Social Environment | Needs Assessment | Disability Studies | Models, Theoretical | United States
Classification: LCC R858 (ebook) | LCC R858 (print) | NLM WB 320.5 | DDC 610.285–dc23
LC record available at https://lccn.loc.gov/2019015586

Cover Design: Wiley
Cover Image: © filo/DigitalVision Vectors/Getty Images

Set in 10.5/12.5pt Minion by SPi Global, Pondicherry, India
Printed and bound in Singapore by Markono Print Media Pte Ltd

10 9 8 7 6 5 4 3 2 1

Contents

List of contributors

Baxter, Amy, PT, DPT, ATP/SMS
Seating and Mobility Specialist
Baldwinsville, NY, USA

Behnke, Kirk, M.Ed., ATP
Former Lead for the Texas Assistive Technology Network (TATN)
Houston, TX, USA
CEO, Behnke Consulting, LLC
Meadowbrook, PA, USA

Bowser, M. Gayl, M.Ed.
Independent Consultant, Assistive Technology Collaborations
Camas Valley, OR, USA

Bryden, Anne, MA, OTR/L
Director of Clinical Trials and Research
Institute for Functional Restoration
Case Western Reserve University
Cleveland, OH, USA

Camp, Susan, MFA
Adjunct Assistant Professor of Art,
University of Maine
Orono, ME, USA

Caswell, Tina N., MS, CCC-SLP
AAC/AT Clinical Specialist, Clinical Assistant Professor, Department of Speech-Language Pathology and Audiology, Ithaca College
Ithaca, NY, USA

Cook, LaWanda, PhD
CRC Extension Faculty,
Yang-Tan Institute on Employment and Disability
Cornell University, Ithaca New York
Ithaca, NY, USA

Dunn, Jennifer, PhD, PT
Research Fellow, Department of Orthopaedic Surgery and Musculoskeletal Medicine
University of Otago
Christchurch, New Zealand

Eiten, Leisha R., Au.D., CCC-A
Associate Director of Audiology,
Boys Town National Research Hospital
Omaha, NE, USA

Feathers, David Joseph, PhD
Assistant Professor, College of Human Ecology,
Department of Design and Environmental Analysis
Cornell University
Ithaca, NY, USA

Ferguson, Robert C., MHS, OTR/L
Stroke Rehabilitation Program Manager,
Neurorehabilitation & Therapeutic Technology Clinical Specialist, University of Michigan Health System Department of Physical Medicine & Rehabilitation Occupational Therapy Division
Ann Arbor, MI, USA

Flecky, Kathleen, OTD, OTR/L
Associate Professor, Department of Occupational Therapy, School of Pharmacy and Health Professions
Creighton University
Omaha, NE, USA

Gentry, Tony, PhD, OTR/L, FAOTA
Associate Professor, Department of Occupational Therapy, College of Health Professions, Virginia Commonwealth University
Richmond, VA, USA

Gitlow, Lynn, PhD, OTR/L, ATP, FAOTA
Associate Professor, Department of Occupational Therapy, Ithaca College
Ithaca, NY, USA

Golinker, Lewis, Esq.
Director, Assistive Technology Law Center
Ithaca, NY, USA

Goodman, Glenn, PhD, OTR/L
Professor Emeritus, School of Health Sciences
Master of Occupational Therapy Program
Cleveland State University
Cleveland, OH, USA

Herz, Nathan "Ben," OTd, MBA, OTR/L, CEAS
Founding Director, OTD Program
Presbyterian College
Clinton, SC, USA

Jacobs, Steve
President, Apps4Android, Inc., IDEAL Group, Inc.
West Jefferson, OH, USA

Phillips, BevVan, OTR/L, CAPS
Key Complete Therapies
Omaha, NE, USA

Rakoski, Douglas, OTD, OTR/L, ATP
Assistant Professor, Occupational Therapy, School of Allied Health Professions, Loma Linda University
Loma Linda, CA, USA

Ripat, Jacquie, PhD, MSc, BMR(OT)
Associate Professor, Department of Occupational Therapy, Rady Faculty of Health Sciences
University of Winnipeg, MB, Canada

Rominger, Amy, AuD, CCC-A, FAAA
Clinical Associate Professor, Department of Speech-Language Pathology and Audiology, Ithaca College
Ithaca, NY, USA

Schoonover, Judith, MEd, OTR/L, ATP, FAOTA
Occupational Therapist/Assistive Technology Professional, Loudoun County Public Schools
Loudoun County, VA, USA

Smallfield, Stacy, DrOT, MSOT, OTR/L, BCG, FAOTA
Associate Professor, Occupational Therapy and Medicine, Assistant Director, Entry-Level Professional Programs, Program in Occupational Therapy
Washington University School of Medicine in St. Louis
St. Louis, MO, USA

Strobel Gower, Wendy
Director, Northeast ADA Center
Ithaca, NY, USA; and
Yang-Tan Institute on Employment and Disability
Cornell University
Ithaca, NY, USA

Veety, Lindsey, PT, DPT, ATP/SMS
Seating and Mobility Specialist
Sparrowbush, NY, USA

Verdonck, Michèle, PhD, BSc
Occupational Therapy, School of Health and Sport Sciences, University of the Sunshine Coast
Queensland, Australia

About the companion website

This book is accompanied by a companion website:

www.wiley.com/go/gitlow/assitivetechnologies

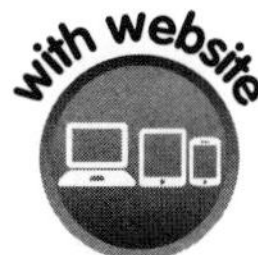

The website includes
interactive MCQs for each chapter

1

The person, the environment, and technology: Introduction to the human-tech ladder

Lynn Gitlow and Kathleen Flecky

Outline

Learning outcomes

After reading this chapter, you should be able to:

1. Describe human technology as a complex interaction between a person and the environment.
2. Delineate distinguishing features of the Human-Tech Ladder and a client-centered approach.
3. Describe the relationship between the Human-Tech Ladder and assistive technology.
4. Identify the components of the assistive technology continuum.
5. Compare medical and social models of disability in relationship to a client-centered focus on the Human-Tech Ladder and assistive technology.
6. Define assistive technology and environmental intervention.

Assistive Technologies and Environmental Interventions in Healthcare: An Integrated Approach, First Edition.
Edited by Lynn Gitlow and Kathleen Flecky.

Companion website: www.wiley.com/go/gitlow/assitivetechnologies

Active learning prompts

Before you read this chapter:

1. Describe the role that technology plays in your life in terms of how you interact with the environment on a daily basis to meet needed and desired tasks and goals.
2. Complete a brief literature search using the keywords, client-centered, health, disability and assistive technology, medical models of disability, and social models of disability.
3. Using the website, www.resna.org, define assistive technology and locate the eligibility requirements for Rehabilitation Engineering and Assistive Technology Society of North America (RESNA) certification as an Assistive Technology Professional.
4. Define assistive technology using two or more sources.
5. Compare and contrast three definitions of assistive technology.
6. Classify assistive technology in three different ways.

Key terms

Assistive technology
Assistive technology continuum
Client-centered
Contextual factors
Disability
Disability models
Environmental factors
Environmental intervention (EI)
Human-Tech Ladder
Technology
Technology and environmental intervention (TEI)

The person, the environment, and technology: Introduction to the human-tech ladder

The changes we have all seen in technology and correspondingly with assistive technology in the past 10 years are mind-boggling. Futurist and inventor Ray Kurzweil (2000) stated early in the twenty-first century that computers are 100 million times more powerful than they were 50 years ago. The exponential growth of computer capacity that Kurzweil and others predicted in the late 1990s continues to advance and has the potential for improving all aspects of life (Diamandis and Kotler 2014). These exponential changes in technology make it hard to keep up with the latest innovations. For example, one of the chapter authors worked in an assistive technology laboratory in which serial port add-ons to computers evolved into Universal Serial Bus (USB) ports rendering the former connections and their attachments obsolete within in less than five years. Currently, computers no longer come with disk drives and all of the software one needs to load on the computer comes from the cloud. Vicente (2006) stated, "... more and more technology is being foisted upon us at a faster and faster pace" (p. 13).

In addition, technology is clearly a necessary part of our lives. For many of us, it is difficult to remember a time when cell phones, laptops, or navigation devices were not available to those who could afford it. Furthermore, the convergence of multiple technologies into a single, small, handheld device such as a smartphone is common as part of our work and personal experiences.

Medical technology has evolved to intervene when the body fails. For example, you may know someone who has a heart pacemaker to pick up the pace when the heart lags. Moreover, as older adults live longer in many countries, these family members or neighbors may likely experience a joint replacement or utilize assistive or medical devices to recover or make daily tasks easier on either a short-term or a long-term basis.

Given the pervasiveness of technology in our lives, it is not surprising that the words "human" and "technology" are conceptualized in new ways to describe the link between our humanness and the non-humanness of technology. The "Human-Tech Ladder" is a unique concept developed by Vicente (2006) to merge the humanistic view of social sciences with the mechanistic and reductionist views of basic sciences and technological sciences. It is a systems approach that considers how to holistically match humans and technology. Rather than coming up with a new conceptual model, this book will use Vicente's Human-Tech Ladder to provide a systematic way of structuring the text to consider all of the factors, which interact to make a match between humans and technology. The Human-Tech Ladder is a five-level visual model which can be used to conceptualize human factors, such as personal and environmental factors that interact with technology.

According to Vicente (2006), a bad fit or match occurs if human factors are not at the center of the technology design process. Knowing how the human mind and body react to multiple stimuli and situations with technology, and understanding the complexity of human interaction with both the physical and the social environment, can lead to better use of technology (Vicente 2006). This multifactorial approach mirrors development in the field of matching those who have disabilities with technology interventions. Moreover, a multifactorial approach is considered to be critical to making a successful human technology match (National Academies of Sciences, Engineering, and Medicine 2017). This interactive approach in using technology as an intervention for people with disabilities has not occurred in a vacuum, and changes in ways of thinking about people with disabilities are important to review as an introduction to this text.

Models of disability

With the primary chapter author having practiced in the area of assistive technology for over 20 years, there have been many changes in the field, which influence the things one needs to consider when using assistive technology as an intervention. One critical change is the way that disability is viewed. *Disability* is "the dynamic interaction between an individual (with a health condition) and that individual's contextual factors (personal and environmental factors)" (World Health Organization [WHO] 2001, p. 190). This change in thinking about disability parallels the shift in thinking about disability from viewing it as strictly a medical problem to viewing it more as an interactive social problem (Charlton 2000). *Disability models* are conceptual frameworks that delineate how disability has been regarded by society over the centuries.

For example, within the medical model, disability is viewed as being a personal problem – one that lies within an individual and must be fixed by a practitioner's intervention. This model is aligned with a mechanistic or reductionist view of human life (Vicente 2006). In this view, the practitioner is the expert and the client or person with a disability has little to add to the relationship.

In the 1950s, Carl Rogers used the term *client-centered* to describe the active and directive role of the client in collaboration with the therapist to problem-solve issues uniquely related to each client's care (Rogers 1951). Building on the work of Rogers and others, terms such as client-centered care, client-centered counseling, and person-centered practice are used to describe a focus on the client or patient as central to all decision-making about care, emphasizing client strengths and unique cultural and environmental contexts and capacities (Fearing and Clark 2000; Institute of Medicine [IOM] 2001, 2003; Morgan and Yoder 2012). In rehabilitation therapies, client-centered care respects the client as an active partner whose choices and participation in care are valued and facilitated with dignity and respect (Law 1998; Sumsion 2006).

Vicente's concept of human technology as noted earlier highlights the importance of the person as the center of the technology process in a similar way to that in which client-centered concepts view the client as person in the center of the therapeutic process (Vicente 2006). Following this client-centered focus and in concert with the human rights movements of the 1960s and 1970s, people with disabilities advanced a social model of disability which emphasized that disability results from a mismatched and therefore unsuccessful interaction between an individual and the environment (WHO 2001).

This interactive relationship, exemplified in the International Classification of Functioning, Disability and Health (ICF) (WHO 2001), moves the notion of disability from an individual issue to a societal issue, increasing the complex causality of disability. Disability is viewed as the interaction of a person with factors external to that person. Thus, it is critically important that practitioners consider environment, often also called context, when making technological intervention recommendations for clients. According to the WHO (2001), *contextual factors* "represent the complete background of an individual's life and living. They include two components: Environmental Factors and Personal Factors, which may have an impact on the individual with a health condition and that individual's health and health-related states" (p. 22). For example, if a healthcare practitioner recommends that a client use a wheelchair, then one must simultaneously consider that some home modifications or workplace modifications may be required. *Environmental factors* are organized in relationship to the individual's immediate environment, in which one interfaces with physical or material aspects of daily life, or the societal environment, in which one engages at a community, institutional, attitudinal, and policy level (WHO 2001). Practitioners using assistive technology with clients must have an awareness and knowledge of the key contextual and environmental factors impacting a client's daily life when making any assistive technology recommendations.

Assistive technology and the environment

As will be presented later in this textbook, the conceptual practice models that guide thinking about assistive technology (AT) and environmental interventions (EIs) recognize the influence of environment or context as well as technology or AT when providing interventions for clients. In general, *AT* is conceptualized as services and products that aim to support and aid an individual's ability to engage with the environment, regardless of disability. Later in this chapter, AT will be defined from a legal perspective. Since AT is utilized in a variety of settings, its definition takes on complexity and specificity based on setting, service, product, and client. *Environmental intervention* or *EI* is a term frequently used in combination with AT. It refers to how the environment can be changed or modified as part of the AT process and is occasionally used synonymously with the term AT. For example, with the emergence of smart home technology, the Internet, and remote caregiving, technology interventions may be the same as or part of EI.

While AT and environment interventions have commonly been regarded to impact disability and the disabling process, over the past few decades there has been a shift from viewing AT and EI as separate entities to a unified whole. Environment is such an integral part of the disabling process that an environmental task force was created by the World Health Organization (WHO) to inform the development of the ICF (Schneider et al. 2003). The ICF acknowledges the impact that environment has on creating disability (WHO 2001). "The environment may be changed to improve health conditions, prevent impairments, and improve outcomes for people with disabilities. Such changes can be brought about by legislation, policy changes, capacity building or technological developments" (WHO and World Bank 2011, p. 4).

In 2010, The American Occupational Therapy Association (AOTA) updated the document *Assistive Technology within Occupational Therapy Practice* (AOTA 2004) with the revised document *Specialized Knowledge and Skills in Technology and Environmental Interventions for Occupational Therapy Practice* (AOTA 2010). This document reflected a change from thinking about AT and the environment as separate to recognizing they are vital to each other. This is consistent with what was discussed earlier in this chapter in terms of conceptual models of disability changing over time and how the environment, both physical and social, is now considered as part of disability and the disabling process. Thus, in this book both AT and EI will be considered together as *technology and environmental intervention* (TEI). Use of this term reflects the interactive relationship between technology and environmental factors in the AT process.

It is important to state from the outset of the book that, when thinking about TEI, the editors do not just consider and provide recipes for providing assistive device(s) or EIs. Consistent with a client-centered approach and conceptual models which guide practice, TEI must be considered with a person in mind who functions in an environment or context and wants to do something that he or she cannot do without the intervention.

Ladner (2010) would assert that this is no different for able bodied people than for people with disabilities and states "'(a)ssistive technology' is a really redundant term because, in some sense, all technology is assistive, making tasks possible or easier to do" (p. 25). Conceptual practice models that guide TEI practice, presented in more depth in Chapter 2, have also resulted from shifts in the way disability is perceived by society (from a medical to a social model). Inherent in these models are the outcomes one expects from use of AT for people with disabilities. These outcomes are influenced by a variety of factors that go beyond the person. For example, in the medical model the outcomes expected for people with disabilities are that they will be fixed and return to "normal" (Silvers 2010). The technology aligned with this model is that which enables a person to be as close to fixed or normal as possible, for example, through the recommendation of prosthetics for an impaired limb.

Alternately, if disability is regarded from a social model, people with disabilities do not need to be fixed as their disability is part of who they are and should be accepted as part of our human differences and diverse social fabric. Finally, if disability is viewed from a legal model, then people with disabilities are protected by certain laws and have rights. Therefore, technology provision and environmental access are mandated by legislation (Ladner 2010).

Successful implementation of TEI is a complex issue, which involves creating change at multiple levels, including at the level of individual, the healthcare provider, the healthcare organization and also at the levels of policy and legislation. For example, according to Gritzer and Arluke (1986), "Before World War II, disability was not considered a medical or social problem in America" (p. 8). As previously mentioned, sociocultural views related to disability have changed over time due to a variety of social influences. Changes in persons with disabilities are now regarded and the notion of disability impacts policy and legislation, which, in turn, influences services and outcomes that service providers recommend for their client.

Thus, even though we as practitioners may see ourselves as providing services for a given client whom we serve in our practice, there is a complex set of issues which influence this one-to-one interaction. In day-to-day practice, for example, a service provider may make a recommendation for a client to use a mobility device such as a wheelchair to increase the client's ability to participate in daily activities. Anyone who has made a similar recommendation is aware of numerous other factors which must be considered, such as funding, training, environmental assessment, and the costs and considerations that go along with that recommendation. In addition, what if the client does not want to use a mobility device? We hope you understand by now that the provision of TEI is a complex issue. Whenever change is being made at the level of an individual or beyond, many factors must be considered.

Because there are so many considerations that impact the use of TEI, the editors have chosen Vicente's (2006) Human-Tech Ladder as a roadmap to guide the writing of this book. Additionally, the road map is suggested as a systematic framework, which can be used in practice to help practitioners consider many factors, which interrelate to make a successful human-tech interaction when using technology as a therapeutic intervention. Using this road map will help the reader reflect on complex issues that impact our delivery of TEI.

Moreover, readers will be challenged to expand current notions of TEI by exploring a full range of simple to more complex options in each section. In a research study by Gitlow et al. (2011), results indicated that practitioners who utilize AT in mental health settings reported their reluctance to recommend a range of low and high technology because they perceive themselves as having a lack of AT competency and knowledge.

The editors of this book hope that, as a reader, you will be empowered to realize that, as healthcare professionals, all of us use technological or adaptive strategies in our work with others. Why professionals often do not realize this fact is that we don't perceive this technology as TEI. It may be that healthcare practitioners do not really understand the definition of TEI. Once the definition is elucidated, the reader will quickly understand that the no tech or low-tech solution is often the best option yielding the most successful outcome for the client (Carlson and Ehrlich 2006; Norman 2013).

Choosing the human-tech ladder

Contemporary approaches to the way that the disabling process is conceptualized did not evolve in a vacuum. Vicente (2006) describes new ways of viewing the nature of knowledge (epistemology) that parallel what underlies healthcare professionals' changing notions of disability. As stated above in the section "The Person, the Environment, and Technology: Introduction to the Human-Tech Ladder," underlying the medical model is a reductionist or mechanistic approach to the nature of knowledge (Kielhofner 2009). In this approach, knowledge is divided up into parts and different disciplines are experts in each part. According to Vicente, those who take a mechanistic approach focus solely on technology. In contrast are the humanists who focus on the human or people aspect of the world (Vicente 2006). This may parallel with a more social model of disability where people with disabilities no longer need to have their parts fixed but may need TEI options to function optimally.

Vicente (2006) stated that both views need to be considered and presents his human-tech approach. This approach reflects a systems approach, which guides us to think about the relationship between humans and technology. It is this human-tech approach that Vicente (2006) refers to as the Human-Tech Ladder. The human-tech approach helps us to "... organize our knowledge of people systematically, in a multi-faceted way ..." (Vicente 2006, p. 53). This approach in turn helps us to view the complexities we described above in a systematic way. While using different frameworks and approaches to understand complex issues is not new, we have chosen Vicente's approach for a variety of reasons.

One way of making sense out of complexity is to use a conceptual model to guide one's thinking. Some authors (Cook and Polgar 2015) have chosen one conceptual model, the Human Activity Assistive Technology (HAAT) model, to guide their presentation of AT-related information. The editors have decided not to do so here because there are numerous conceptual models that are available for the reader to explore and make your own. You will be introduced to them in Chapter 2. Other authors have used a three-dimensional analysis at macro, meso, and micro levels to consider environmental impact on the disabling process (Fougeyrollas and Gray 1998). More recently, Sanford (2012) employed the principles of universal design, which will be discussed in more depth in Chapter 2, to structure an approach to rehabilitation intervention.

One reason the editors of this book find Vicente's Human-Tech Ladder useful as a road map for this text is that one of the levels of the ladder considers the team. It is the only road map that we know of that gives recognition to the importance of the team of people who work together to provide TEI. There are numerous people who make up a TEI team, including the client, therapists, educators, building contractors, architects, engineers, and the list goes on. TEI requires collaboration and teamwork in order for changes to occur. When teams work well, change can happen (Fullan 2015).

However, literature has also revealed that working successfully as part of a team is challenging and often can present barriers to successful implementation of TEI (Decoste et al. 2005; Vicente 2006). Because the team is so important to the TEI process the topic, this book will contain two chapters devoted to best practice of teams. The importance of teamwork will also be presented throughout other chapters in this book. Finally, Vicente's Human-Tech Ladder considers multiple factors that impact the complexity described above.

Human-tech ladder

Vicente places equal value on all levels of the ladder and emphasizes that not all levels are integral in every individual case. Yet we will begin our discussion on the Human-Tech Ladder by taking a top-down approach to honor the importance of all levels of the ladder in learning to apply this model for the first time (Vicente 2006). As displayed in Figure 1.1, the Human-Tech Ladder, the top rung of the ladder is the political rung. Here different laws and policies will be listed as they influence TEI.

These will include laws that protect people with disabilities form discrimination, laws that provide services for people with disabilities, laws that regulate the built environment, and more. The chapter describes important laws as well as the funding policies that result from these laws and how these policies influence the provision of services in the area of AT and EI intervention. An example of how this level of the Human-Tech Ladder impacts practice can be seen in the way technological innovation interacts with policies, laws, and funding decisions.

Within the past five years, tablets and smartphones have become very important additions to the toolbox of interventions that practitioners can use with their clients. Reimbursement of these devices is very controversial, being paid for in certain settings and not funded in others. Many practitioners are involved at a political level trying to change the funding requirements to enable people who could benefit from these new technologies to obtain them. As the pace of technological innovation continues, this will be an ongoing consideration for those who work in the field.

A review of the *World Report on Disability* (WHO and World Bank 2011) provides a stunning example of how the political rung of the road map influences

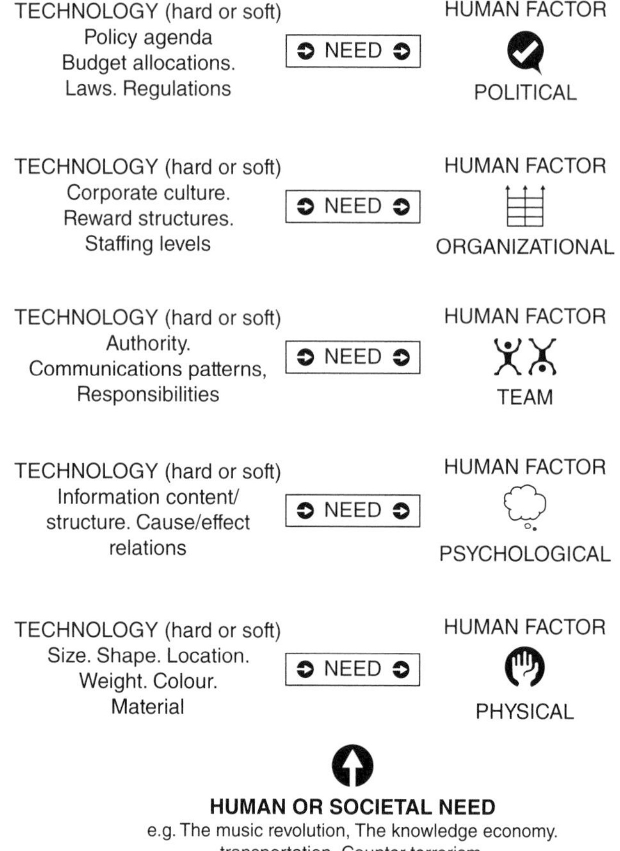

Figure 1.1 The human-tech ladder. Source: Reproduced with permission of Taylor & Francis.

treatment and policy regarding people with disabilities worldwide. It discusses policies and practices that are necessary to provide people with disabilities the services and responses that will enable them to participate in society on an equal par with their non-disabled counterparts. Best practices based on scientific evidence are illuminated in the report to promote accessibility of health and wellness for all people as a human right. Reviewing and updating legislation and policies, and funding mechanisms, which relate to people with disabilities is one of the first recommendations described in this important report (WHO and World Bank 2011). For example, the report states, "United States surveys report considerable unmet needs – often caused by funding problems – for assistive technologies" (WHO and World Bank 2011, p. 103).

Next on the Human-Tech Ladder is the organizational level (Vicente 2006). TEI is provided in a variety of organizations each with its own rules, regulations, and requirements. Medical, educational, and vocational organizations, and the Veterans Administration, have a great deal of variety in the way they define, regulate, and view TEI. For example, in medical environments, Medicare does not use the term assistive technology in its reimbursement vocabulary. Devices that are considered AT are called durable medical equipment and have to have qualifying attributes to be considered for a client (Centers for Medicare and Medicaid Services 2015). This is just one example of the difference between a medical organization and the numerous other organizations where AT and EI interventions are provided. In this section of the book, authors who work in the wide variety of organizations that provide TEI will describe the considerations specific to each venue.

The next step on the ladder is the team. TEIs are provided by an interdisciplinary group of practitioners. Members of Rehabilitation Engineering and Assistive Technology Society of North America (RESNA) encompass a wide variety of practitioners including rehabilitation engineers, educators, occupational therapists, physical therapists, speech-language pathologists, and manufacturers and suppliers of assistive devices (RESNA 2011). While it is often taken for granted that teams work together successfully, this is not always the case, as shown by literature gathered by the Institute of Medicine (IOM 2001).

Moreover, in a report entitled *Health Professions Education: A Bridge to Quality* (2003), the Interprofessional Education Collaborative Expert Panel noted the need for educational programs to prepare preservice healthcare providers to work as team members and it was cited as one of the most important needs for improving the future of healthcare delivery. Making sure that team members communicate and collaborate as well as understand and respect the variety of perspectives that come together to provide successful TEI outcomes is a complex task and one that can make or break successful interventions. In Chapters 9 and 10, best practices related to teams will be described.

The next rung on the ladder, the psychological rung, considers cognitive as well as psychosocial factors that are part of the human experience (Vicente 2006). The classic story of the therapist trying to explain to someone that they must remove their beloved scatter rugs from the floor to prevent falling only to meet with absolute resistance is an example of the psychological impact practitioners face. In this section, cognitive factors such as memory, problem-solving, and expectations of technology are considered. These are critical considerations for matching a person to a TEI.

At the bottom of the ladder are the physical attributes of people as a human factor (Vicente 2006). Strength, size, capabilities, and limitations are considered here. In this section, physical factors are targeted in providing TEI services. While factors such as strength, range of motion, and sensory factors such as touch, hearing, and vision to name a few are important to assess, research shows that technology considerations beyond merely the physical factors are essential to investigate in order to have a successful match between a human, a technology, and/or an EI (Polgar 2010; Scherer et al. 2005; Scherer and Bodine 2006).

The human-tech approach adds a systematic breadth and depth to the relationship between technology and human factors in a way that enriches the area of AT and EI with insights into human behavior. The next part of this chapter will introduce legislative and professional policy statements that present various definitions of AT, and environment/context interventions.

In the definition section of this chapter the hard and soft attributes of technology are described as they relate to the human experience. The hard attributes are the technology itself, while the soft attributes are things like information that relate to the technology (Rogers 2003). Both of these aspects of TEI vary from organization to organization, further complicating the situation. Vicente (2006) states that these subtle factors at the organizational level can certainly impact the human-tech fit.

Why are definitions important?

A variety of professionals have long been involved in promoting everyday engagement in valued activities by matching a person with environmental demands. This match often involves the use of adaptive equipment, AT, and/or EI.

If you have looked at the certification requirements listed on the RESNA website (https://www.resna.org/certification) you will have learned about the wide variety of professionals listed under the term rehab science. Rehab Science, for the purposes of this book, is defined as one of the following: medicine, nursing, low vision rehabilitation, occupational therapy, physical therapy, speech-language pathology, audiology, special education, vocational rehabilitation, engineering (biomedical, clinical, or rehabilitation), prosthetics and orthotics, recreation therapy, and rehabilitation technology.

Despite the group of qualified professionals who provide TEI, research suggests that many practitioners from a variety of rehabilitation fields perceive themselves as not having the skills and knowledge necessary to provide technology-related or EIs to those who might need them (Gitlow and Sanford 2003; Gitlow et al. 2007; Long and Perry 2008). Please review Box 1.1 for an evidence-based practice application activity.

Box 1.1 Here's the evidence

Gitlow, L., Hofmaster, P., and Wade, J. (2007). Investigating the assistive technology skill and need for knowledge of CPRPs. *International Journal of Psychosocial Rehabilitation* 11 (2): 61–73.

Key Words: psychiatric rehabilitation practitioners, assistive technology

Purpose: Investigate the knowledge and skills of certified psychiatric rehabilitation practitioners in the area of AT.

Sample/Setting: Convenience sample of certified psychiatric rehabilitation practitioners.

Method: Survey design.

Findings: Surveyed practitioners reported having a basic knowledge in technologies related to activities of daily living (ADLs) learning disabilities and team collaboration. Areas reported as having a need for training and education included: medication management, enhanced vocational activities, self-advocacy, time management skills, memory skills for clients, and funding of devices.

Critical Thinking Questions:

1. After reading this research article, what do you understand to be the limitations of this research? Are there any limitations not stated?
2. If you were to replicate this study using a different method or design, what designs would you use to increase the rigor and why?
3. Based on the findings of this study, what additional research is needed that is not addressed in the discussion section?

Once you have reviewed Box 1.1, this lack of perceived competence may appear to stem from confusion about what exactly the terms assistive technology and environmental intervention mean. Definitions and understanding of terms help us to be clear. Confusion in defining terms can result in misunderstandings about concepts that we are trying to communicate to others. It may be that this is the case when trying to define the terms technology, AT, and EI. Demystifying the definitions of technology and AT may help to understand where some of the confusion is coming from.

Defining technology

Refer to Box 1.2 and investigate definitions of AT from credible resources.

Let's see how your findings compare with what is presented below. As stated in the preface to the book, the authors feel that it is important for students to engage in active learning so that they will expand their notion of what these definitions mean by doing their own research and then comparing it to the text. A Bing browser search engine retrieval for definitions of "technology" came up with 17 900 000 entries while a Google search engine query for AT yielded over 8 420 000 entries for the definition of "assistive technology." Research demonstrates how most practitioners tend to narrowly define technology and AT (Gitlow and Sanford 2003; Gitlow et al. 2007; Long and Perry 2008). Examining how laws, policies, and leaders in the field define these terms can help to broaden what we really mean by these definitions.

Box 1.2 Active learning: definitions of AT

Define AT using two credible resources or references	
Definition 1:	Resource:
Definition 2:	Resource:

A definition of *technology* that the authors find useful is "any tool – physical, virtual conceptual, or cultural – that helps people make decisions, act, and achieve their goals is technology" (Vicente 2006, p. 20). Further, Rogers (2003) stated, "A *technology* usually has two components: (1) a *hardware* aspect consisting of the tool that embodies the technology as a material or physical object, and (2) a *software* aspect consisting of the information base for the tool" (p. 13). With these two definitions, we begin to broaden our idea of technology to include any tool that helps us to achieve a goal and begin to consider that technology is more than just the physical or material tool.

In practice, clinicians need to provide information about a technology tool and how to use it in order for it to be useful. This is important to remember because we must always think of technology as part of a system that involves multiple factors. As will be presented later in Chapter 11, which focuses on psychological factors related to TEI use, failure to think of technology in a systematic fashion is one of the biggest reasons for its lack of use. Remember, no matter how simple a tool a practitioner provides to a client, failure to consider where the tool will be used and how the client feels about using the tool can result in lack of its use.

Let's return to the technology definitions. How did these two definitions fit with what you investigated? Were there differences? Similarities? Hopefully the definitions you found have expanded your thinking about what technology is.

Defining AT

Now let us go on to define AT in a specific way. In the search for definitions of AT, examples include legal, organization, or setting-based definitions. Furthermore, there are also insurance-based definitions of AT which further complicate our understandings. One definition stated that the term AT is used to describe a wide variety of technologies that are helpful for people with disabilities to gain independence. It is a general term that covers everything from wheelchairs to alternative keyboard computers (Coombs 2005).

The Assistive Technology Act of 2004, which amends the previous act of 1998, defined the term AT as "technology designed to be utilized in an assistive technology device or assistive technology service" (Assistive Technology Act of 2004 2004). Important in this definition is that AT is not conceived as merely a device. This mirrors Roger's definition earlier in the chapter, that technology, and thus AT, is more than just a device. The law also defines an AT device as "any item, piece of equipment, or product system, whether acquired commercially or off the shelf, modified, or customized, that is used to increase, maintain, or improve functional capabilities of individuals with disabilities" (Assistive Technology Act of 2004 2004).

In addition, AT services are defined as, "any service that directly assists an individual with a disability in the selection, acquisition, or use of an assistive technology device" (Assistive Technology Act of 2004 2004).

These services include AT evaluation, selecting and obtaining AT, fitting and fabricating service coordination, training, advocacy, etc. The Individuals with Disabilities Education Improvement Act (IDEIA) of 2004 (IDEIA of 2004 2004) incorporated essentially the same definition within its document. More information regarding this definition will be discussed later on in this book in the chapter on educational organizations in Chapter 6.

Returning to initial definitions of technology in this chapter, take time to review hard and soft aspects of technology, which may include more than just the device. Refer to Box 1.3 and fill in these definitions as part of your resource investigation active learning exercise. What did you find?

The practitioner must think about legislation, and there is more than just the technology itself to consider when matching a device to a person. Devices (hard) and services (soft) correlate to these dual aspects of technology, and under the law both are mandated.

Box 1.3 Active learning: Definitions of hard and soft technology

Define hard and soft technology using two credible resources or references

Hard technology Definition 1:	Resource:
Hard technology Definition 2:	Resource:
Soft technology Definition 1:	Resource:
Soft technology Definition 2:	Resource:

Environmental interventions

Another useful definition for AT is based on Gitlin (2002) and relates to EI: AT is viewed as including the following items: (i) structural alterations (changes to the original structure of a physical environment, e.g. widening doors in a house); (ii) special equipment (attachments to the original structure of the physical environment, e.g. handrails, grab bars, and stair glides in the home); (iii) assistive devices (applied to or directly manipulated by a person, e.g. wheelchairs, reachers, voice output communication aids, and hearing or vision aids); (iv) material adjustment (alterations to non-permanent features of the physical environment, e.g. clearing pathways, removing throw rugs, and adjusting lighting in the home); (v) environmentally based behavioral modification (changes to a person's interaction with the physical environment, e.g. conserving energy in particular activities and segmenting tasks to facilitate their execution). This begins to broaden the definition even more by including a consideration of the environment within the definition of AT.

Further, broadening of the term AT to include the concept of environmental adaptation follows an historical change in the way disability is defined. This change was previously noted in this chapter, when it was stated that when notions or models of disability changed from a medical model view to a more inclusive social model of disability, the environment became a critical part of the disablement process. In the medical model, disability is viewed as being a personal problem that lies within an individual and must be fixed by a practitioner's intervention. In a social model, disability occurs from an interaction between an individual and the environment in which he or she chooses to function (Longmore and Umansky 2001). Disability occurs as an imbalance between the two. Thus, it is not possible to consider an AT intervention without considering the environment as well.

So, let's return to focus on definitions again. Although there is certainly a range of variability within these definitions, most include some mention of a device and most make reference to these devices impacting access or independence for people with disabilities. More specifically, if we look at Coomb's definition, we see that it

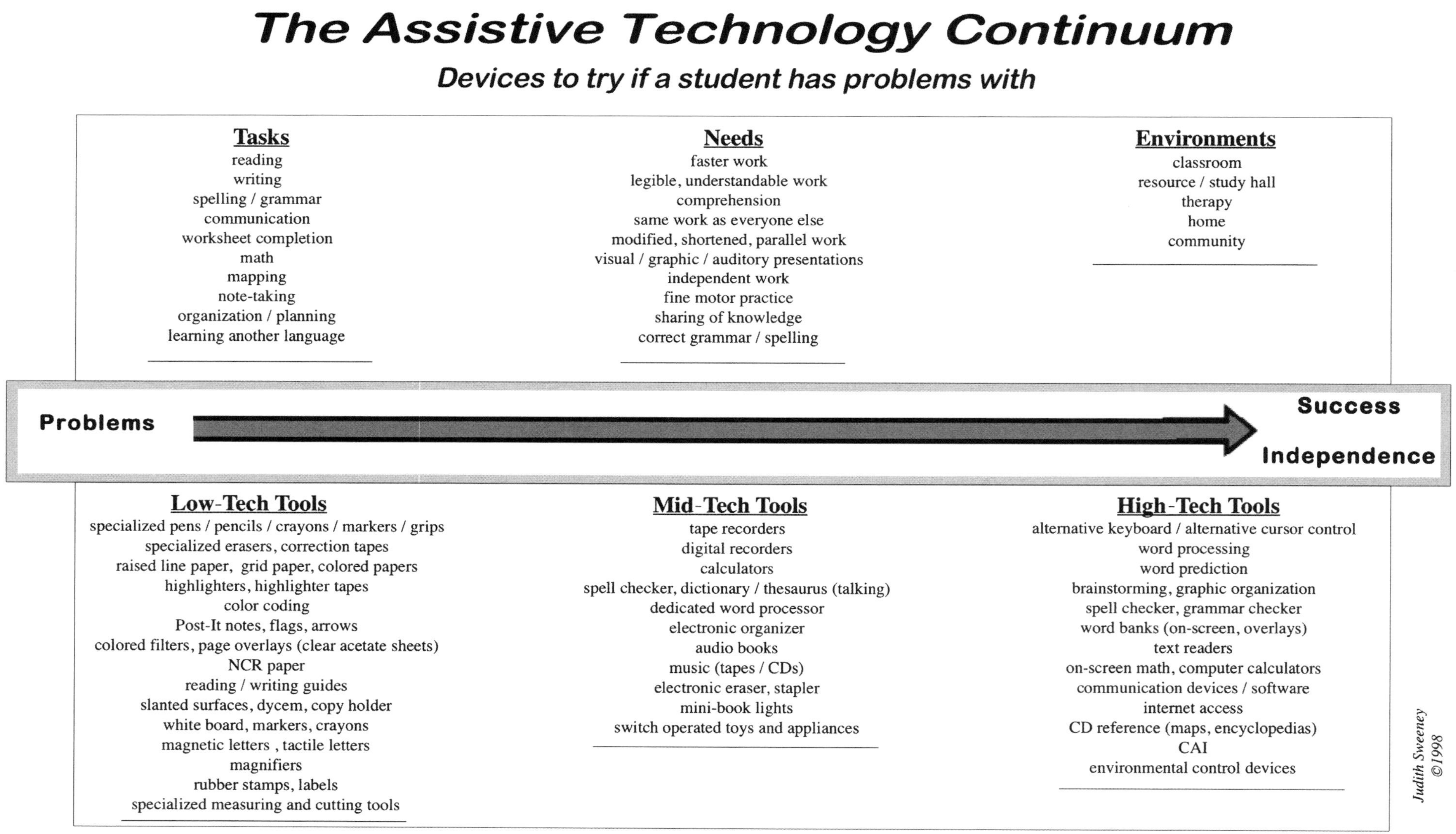

The Assistive Technology Continuum

Devices to try if a student has problems with

Tasks

reading
writing
spelling / grammar
communication
worksheet completion
math
mapping
note-taking
organization / planning
learning another language

Needs

faster work
legible, understandable work
comprehension
same work as everyone else
modified, shortened, parallel work
visual / graphic / auditory presentations
independent work
fine motor practice
sharing of knowledge
correct grammar / spelling

Environments

classroom
resource / study hall
therapy
home
community

Problems → **Success** / **Independence**

Low-Tech Tools

specialized pens / pencils / crayons / markers / grips
specialized erasers, correction tapes
raised line paper, grid paper, colored papers
highlighters, highlighter tapes
color coding
Post-It notes, flags, arrows
colored filters, page overlays (clear acetate sheets)
NCR paper
reading / writing guides
slanted surfaces, dycem, copy holder
white board, markers, crayons
magnetic letters , tactile letters
magnifiers
rubber stamps, labels
specialized measuring and cutting tools

Mid-Tech Tools

tape recorders
digital recorders
calculators
spell checker, dictionary / thesaurus (talking)
dedicated word processor
electronic organizer
audio books
music (tapes / CDs)
electronic eraser, stapler
mini-book lights
switch operated toys and appliances

High-Tech Tools

alternative keyboard / alternative cursor control
word processing
word prediction
brainstorming, graphic organization
spell checker, grammar checker
word banks (on-screen, overlays)
text readers
on-screen math, computer calculators
communication devices / software
internet access
CD reference (maps, encyclopedias)
CAI
environmental control devices

Figure 1.2 Assistive technology continuum. Source: Retrieved from http://opsb.us/wp-content/uploads/2014/01/AT_Continuum.pdf.

stated that AT includes a wide variety of devices (Coombs 2005). The AT law (Assistive Technology Act of 1998) states that it is *any* device and Gitlin's (2002) definition includes a range of devices from reachers to voice output communication aids. Therefore, our notion of AT continues to expand: it can be simple device such as an adapted pencil or an extremely high-tech device such as a robotically controlled prosthetic. Figure 1.2 shows a continuum of technology considerations that might be useful in thinking about solutions for a client or user. While this figure relates to school-based settings, it provides us with a visual of the *AT continuum*, which is a range of various TEI options categorized as low technology to mid technology to high technology.

Additionally, it is important to remember that technology intervention is more than providing just a device. Providing service related to the device and its use is equally as important, and both the device and the service depend on the environment and context of the user. Use of a cane is different if the individual is using it to kneel in church versus walking down a long hospital hallway. This is a point the authors will reinforce over and over in this book. Additionally, environmental modification has a variety of options. It range from something as simple as removing a rug to prevent falling to more complex interventions such as installing elevators.

Categories of AT

Table 1.1 displays two ways of categorizing AT using disability models. Based on Table 1.2, sample differences show a data collection tool that organizations receiving funds through the AT Act use to collect program outcomes data. The other is from abledata.acl.gov, an online database that categorizes over 45 000 products (make sure to visit this website often). Included in both you will notice environmental adaptations along with specific product categories and a very wide variety of things included in the categories of AT.

Please review differences in how AT is categorized in Table 1.2. In addition to these types of categorization, we also find AT classified as being no-tech, low-tech, or high-tech. No-tech or low-tech devices are inexpensive and easy to obtain. High-tech devices tend to be more expensive and more complicated to obtain (Cook and Polgar 2015). Examples of no-tech or low-tech AT solutions are built-up handles for utensils, or pencil grips. High-tech solutions may include computer technologies, robotics, and smart home technology. It is important to remember, when considering AT solutions, to systematically begin investigation at the no-tech end of the spectrum and move up rather than starting

Table 1.2 Sample Differences in How AT is Categorized.

Assistive Technology Act of 2004 Data collection categories	AbleData AT product database
Speech communication	Aids for daily living
Vision	Blind and low-vision products
Hearing	Communication products
Computers and related daily living learning	Computer products
Cognition and developmental	Control products: environmental controls, control switches
Environmental adaptations	Deaf and hard-of-hearing products
Mobility	Deaf–blind products
Seating and positioning	Education products
Vehicle modification and transportation	Environmental adaptations products
Recreation, sports, and leisure	Housekeeping products
Other	Orthotics braces and other products to support and supplement joints or limbs
	Prosthetics products for amputees
	Recreation
	Safety and security products
	Seating products
	Therapeutic aids products
	Transportation products
	Walking products
	Wheeled mobility products
	Workplace products

Table 1.1 Disability Models.

Features	Religious model	Medical model	Social model
Views of disability	Either afflictions due to sinfulness and deviancy, or impairments that indicated a special relationship with higher powers	Impairments and disability are a result of disease, illness, injury, and other abnormal health conditions; impairments are the cause of disability	Social, economic, and political factors create disability along with individual characteristics

Source: Adapted from: Flecky and Goertz (2014).

right at the high-tech end of possible solutions. We will discuss this more in later chapters in the book.

How did these categories compare to the ones you found? Has this changed your understanding of the full range of possibilities included in the definitions we have presented in this chapter?

At this point, the authors hope that you have expanded your notion of what solutions are available to you when you use AT and environmental adaptations as interventions. The range is quite inclusive, and if you understand the full range of low-tech to high-tech options available to increase independence for those who need it, maybe you will feel less intimidated and more empowered to use these interventions in your everyday or future practice. Our goal in requesting that you investigate definitions and categories of AT and then compare them with the book's definitions is to help you to expand your awareness and understanding of these important definitions within this book.

In conclusion, there are common elements that recur in the definitions discussed in this chapter. In all of the definitions, there is a device to think about as well as a user of the device or a person. Then there is a goal or task or an increase in independence that the person wants to accomplish, which must be considered, as well as the context or environment in which the person wants to do the task or increase their independence. Finally, when targeting a potential device, there are more than just the physical attributes or the hard aspects of the device that must be considered. There is relevant information, training, psychological impact, etc. or the soft attributes to inform the thinking process. Finally, we summarize the chapter with these elements within our definitions to build the foundation for the next chapter, which will discuss conceptual models that guide thinking processes about TEI.

Summary

In this introductory chapter, a conceptual road map for visualizing technology and the human experience has been presented. The roadmap is derived from Dr. Kim Vicente's (2006) work exemplified in the book *The Human Factor: Revolutionizing the Way People Live with Technology*. As an engineer, Dr. Vicente provides a fresh perspective of the interaction of technology with human physical, psychological, organizational, and sociopolitical dimensions. His professional engineering expertise and work with engineering students as described in this book uncovers a way of thinking that integrates mechanistic and humanistic philosophies to focus on human needs and behaviors foremost and technology adjunctively to meet needs, or human-tech (Vicente 2006). Various definitions and ways of categorizing technology, AT, and EIs were presented. Multiple elements, which underlie TEI, have been described and in the next chapter will be related in the theories that guide TEI practice.

References

American Occupational Therapy Association (2004). Assistive technology within occupational therapy practice. *American Journal of Occupational Therapy* 58: 678–680. https://doi.org/10.5014/ajot.58.6.678.

American Occupational Therapy Association (2010). Specialized knowledge and skills in technology and environmental interventions for occupational therapy practice. *American Journal of Occupational Therapy* 64: S44–S56. https://doi.org/10.5014/ajot.2010.64S44.

Assistive Technology Act of 1998 (1998). Pub. L. No. 105-394 Sec (3) (a) 3–4. Retrieved from https://www.congress.gov/105/plaws/publ394/PLAW-105publ394.pdf.

Assistive Technology Act of 2004 (2004). Pub. L. No.108-364, § 29 U.S.C. 3001. Retrieved from http://www.gpo.gov/fdsys/pkg/PLAW-108publ364/content-detail.html.

Carlson, D. and Ehrlich, N. (2006). Sources of payment for assistive technology: findings from a national survey of persons with disabilities. *Assistive Technology* 18: 77–86.

Centers for Medicare and Medicaid Services (2015). *Medicare Claims Processing Manual*. Chapter 20: Durable medical equipment, prosthetics, orthotics, and supplies (DMEPOS). Section 10.1.1: Definition of durable medical equipment. Retrieved from https://www.cms.gov/manuals/downloads/clm104c20.pdf.

Charlton, J. (2000). *Nothing About Us Without Us: Disability, Oppression and Empowerment*. Berkley, CA: University of California Press.

Cook, A. and Polgar, J. (2015). *Cook and Hussey's Assistive Technologies: Principles and Practice*, 4e. St. Louis, MO: Mosby.

Coombs, N. (2005). EASI: equal access to software and information. Retrieved from http://easi.cc/index.htm.

Decoste, D., Reed, P., and Kaplan, D. (2005). *Assistive Technology Teams: Many Ways to Do it Well*. Roseburg, OR: National Assistive Technology Education Network.

Diamandis, P. and Kotler, S. (2014). *Abundance: The Future Is Better than You Think*. New York: The Free Press.

Fearing, V.G. and Clark, J. (2000). *Individuals in Context: A Practical Guide to Client Centered Practice*. Thorofare, NJ: Slack.

Flecky, K. and Goertz, H. (2014). Occupational performance and health. In: *Occupational Therapy Essentials for Clinical Competence*, 2e (ed. K. Jacobs, N. MacRae and K. Sladyk), 75. Thorofare, NJ: Slack.

Fougeyrollas, P. and Gray, D. (1998). Classification systems, environmental factors and social change: the importance of technology. In: *Designing and Using Assistive Technology: The Human Perspective* (ed. D. Gray, L. Quatrano and M. Leiberman), 13–28. Baltimore, MD: Paul H. Brookes.

Fullan, M. (2015). *The New Meaning of Educational Change*, 5e. New York: Teachers College Press.

Gitlin, L.N. (2002). Assistive technology in the home and community for older people: psychological and social considerations. In: *Assistive Technology: Matching Device and Consumer for Successful Rehabilitation* (ed. M.J. Scherer), 109–122. Washington, DC: American Psychological Association.

Gitlow, L., Dininno, D., Choate, L. et al. (2011). The provision of assistive technology by occupational therapists that practice in mental health. *Occupational Therapy in Mental Health* 27: 178–190.

Gitlow, L. and Sanford, T. (2003). Assistive technology education needs of allied health practitioners in a rural state. *Journal of Allied Health* 32: 46–51.

Gritzer, G. and Arluke, A. (1986). *The Making of Rehabilitation: A Political Economy of Medical Specialization*. Los Angeles, CA: University of California Press.

Individuals with Disabilities Education Improvement Act of 2004 (2004). Pub. L. No. 08-446 § 20 U.S.C. 1400. Retrieved from http://www.gpo.gov/fdsys/pkg/PLAW-108publ446/pdf/PLAW-108publ446.pdf.

Institute of Medicine (2001). *Crossing the Quality Chasm: A New Health System for the 21st Century*. Washington, DC: National Academy Press.

Institute of Medicine (2003). *Health Professions Education: A Bridge to Quality*. Washington, DC: National Academy Press.

Kielhofner, G. (2009). *Conceptual Foundations of Occupational Therapy Practice*, 4e. Philadelphia, PA: F.A. Davis.

Kurzweil, R. (2000). *The Age of Spiritual Machines: When Computers Exceed Human Intelligence*. New York: Penguin Books.

Ladner, R. (2010). Accessible technology and models of disability. In: *Design and Use of Assistive Technology: Social, Technical, Ethical, and Economic Challenges* (ed. M.M.K. Oishi, I.M. Mitchell and H.F.M. Van der Loos), 25–32. New York: Springer.

Law, M. (1998). *Client-Centered Occupational Therapy*. Thorofare, NJ: Slack.

Long, T. and Perry, A. (2008). Pediatric physical therapists' perceptions of their training in assistive technology. *Physical Therapy* 88: 629–639.

Longmore, P. and Umansky, L. (2001). *The New Disability History: American Perspectives (History of Disability)*. New York: New York University Press.

Morgan, S. and Yoder, L.H. (2012). A concept analysis of person-centered care. *Journal of Holistic Nursing* 30 (1): 6–15.

National Academies of Sciences, Engineering, and Medicine (2017). *The Promise of Assistive Technology to Enhance Activity and Work Participation*. Washington, DC: The National Academies Press https://doi.org/10.17226/24740.

Norman, D. (2013). *The Design of Everyday Things: Revised and Expanded Edition*. New York: Basic Books.

Polgar, J. (2010). The myth of neutral AT. In: *Design and Use of Assistive Technology: Social, Technical, Ethical, and Economic Challenges* (ed. M.M.K. Oishi, I.M. Mitchell and H.F.M. Van der Loos), 17–24. New York: Springer.

Rehabilitation and Engineering Society of North America (RESNA) (2011). Professional specialty groups. Retrieved from https://www.resna.org/professional-development/volunteer-and-leadership-opportunities/special-interest-groups/professional.

Rogers, C.R. (1951). *Client-Centred Therapy*. Boston, MA: Houghton-Mifflin.

Rogers, E. (2003). *Diffusion of Innovations*, 5e. New York: Free Press.

Sanford, J. (2012). *Universal Design as a Rehabilitation Strategy: Design for the Ages*. New York, NY: Springer Publishing Company.

Scherer, M.J. and Bodine, C. (2006). Technology for improving cognitive function: report on a workshop sponsored by the U.S. Interagency Committee on Disability Research. *Disability and Rehabilitation: Assistive Technology* 1 (4): 257–261.

Scherer, M.J., Sax, C., Vanbeirvliet, A. et al. (2005). Predictors of assistive technology use: the importance of personal and psychosocial factors. *Disability and Rehabilitation* 27: 1321–1331.

Schneider, M., Hurst, R., Miller, J., and Ustün, B. (2003). The role of environment in the International Classification of Functioning, Disability and Health (ICF). *Disability and Rehabilitation* 25: 588–595.

Silvers, A. (2010). Better than new! Ethics for assistive technology. In: *Design and Use of Assistive Technology: Social, Technical, Ethical, and Economic Challenges* (ed. M.M.K. Oishi, I.M. Mitchell and H.F.M. Van der Loos), 3–16. New York, NY: Springer.

Sumsion, T. (2006). *Client-Centred Practice in Occupational Therapy. A Guide to Implementation*, 2e. New York: Churchill Livingstone.

Vicente, K. (2006). *The Human Factor: Revolutionizing the Way We Live with Technology*. New York: Routledge, Taylor & Francis Group.

World Health Organization (2001). *International Classification of Functioning, Disability and Health*. Geneva, Switzerland: World Health Organization.

World Health Organization & World Bank (2011). *World Report on Disability*. Geneva, Switzerland: World Health Organization.

2

Conceptual practice models and clinical reasoning

Lynn Gitlow, Douglas Rakoski, and Robert C. Ferguson

Outline

Assistive Technologies and Environmental Interventions in Healthcare: An Integrated Approach, First Edition.
Edited by Lynn Gitlow and Kathleen Flecky.

Companion website: www.wiley.com/go/gitlow/assitivetechnologies

Learning outcomes

After reading this chapter, you should be able to:

1. Describe the importance of conceptual practice models for TEI.
2. Define what is meant by a conceptual model in assistive technology and TEI practice.
3. Identify key components of the following conceptual practice models: ICF, HAAT, CMOP-E, SETT, and TUT.
4. Describe strategies to assess the assistive technology needs of a client and potential TEI based on conceptual models.
5. Identify models of clinical reasoning and therapeutic use of technology to enhance decision-making and client care in TEI practice.

Active learning prompts

Before you read this chapter:

1. What is the value of using a conceptual practice model to guide your clinical work?
2. Research conceptual models that guide assistive technology and environmental intervention (TEI) practice.
3. Look up definitions of clinical reasoning and identify the steps involved in a clinical reasoning process.
4. Reflect upon the relationship of therapeutic use of technology to other conceptual models you might use in your professional practice.

Key terms

Canadian Model of Occupational Performance and Engagement (CMOP-E)
Clinical reasoning
Conceptual practice models
Human-Tech Ladder
International Classification of Functioning, Disability and Health (ICF)
Matching Person and Technology Model (MPTM)
Student, Environments, Tasks, and Tools (SETT) Model
Technology and environmental intervention practitioner (TEIp)
Therapeutic Use of Technology (TUT)

Introduction

This chapter begins with the importance of conceptual practice models to guide decision-making and clinical reasoning in technology and environmental intervention (TEI) followed by a brief overview of several of these models used in practice. Various conceptual frameworks relevant to TEI will be highlighted including: the International Classification of Functioning, Disability and Health (ICF), the Human Activity Assistive Technology (HAAT) Model, the Canadian Model of Occupational Performance and Engagement (CMOP-E), the Matching Person and Technology Model (MPTM), and the Student, Environments, Tasks, and Tools (SETT) Model. Within each model, strategies to assess the assistive technology needs of a client will be delineated. Additionally, TEIs will be discussed in relationship to conceptual practice models and a case study. Finally, the clinical reasoning process and decision-making in TEI will be presented through a discussion of modes of clinical reasoning and Therapeutic Use of Technology (TUT) as part of thinking and action processes of TEI practice.

Chapter 1 reviewed historical changes that have influenced current views of disability and how practitioners work with people with disabilities. For example, the notion of disability has evolved from an individually located, binary situation (you are disabled or you are not) to a complex interaction between an individual, an activity in which the person wants to participate, and the environment, which is composed of both physical and social attributes. Additionally, the Human-Tech Ladder, which guides the structure of the text, informs us that there are many factors that influence service delivery in the area of TEI. Practitioners must consider not only the client who drives the TEI process but a variety of other factors which surround the client, including the team and multiple organizational and legislative factors. This chapter highlights several conceptual practice models, which guide our clinical practice thinking and insights as well as how practitioners apply these conceptual practice models through clinical reasoning.

What are conceptual practice models?

"*Conceptual practice models* provide special professional lenses through which the therapist sees the client and the therapy process, develops plans, and solves problems" (Kielhofner 2009, p. 13). In order to operationalize multiple constructs such as "person, environment, technology and participation/performance" into clinically meaningful guidelines, one can look for conceptual practice models to provide a blueprint for organizing our thoughts. To solve clinical problems, the *technology and environmental intervention practitioner* (TEIp) begins with a client evaluation, then proceeds with interventions that produce outcomes. This term is used to denote the professional who engages in TEI with a client.

Conceptual practice models provide a systematic way of progressing through the TEI process. For example, when deciding how to structure this textbook, the editors used a framework provided by Vicente (2006), The Human-Tech Ladder, to provide a structure and guide for the outcome of the book. This was done for several reasons. First, the editors believed in the values that underpinned Vicente's writing, which emphasized that there is a complex relationship between humans and technology and that in order to understand this relationship we must use a systematic approach. Review the rungs on the Human-Tech Ladder in Figure 2.1.

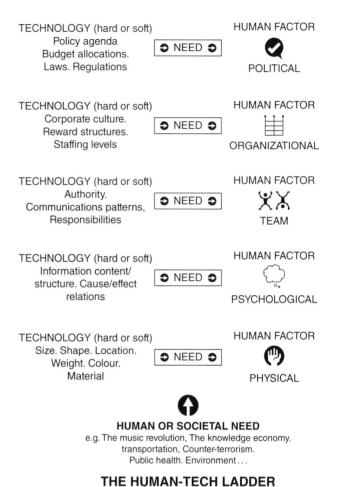

Figure 2.1 Human-tech ladder. Source: Reproduced with permission of Taylor & Francis.

The client and solving human problems are a critical part of the TEI approach. Finally, multiple factors must be considered from the level of the individual, team, and policy perspectives to ensure a good fit when solving TEI-related problems. Vicente provided the editors with a road map that ensured they would consider the complex relationships among numerous factors to include in our text. In this same way, TEI practitioners select theories, conceptual practice models, and frameworks to guide their day-to-day practice.

Edyburn and Smith (2004) highlight the importance of using a theoretical framework supporting the relationship of variables involved in AT outcomes, for example, satisfaction, performance, use, and quality of life. This is consistent with Kielhofner's (2009) use of the term conceptual practice model, which organizes diverse concepts into theory. The authors will use the term conceptual practice model to describe the models presented in this chapter in order to guide TEI practice.

Although there are numerous other models applicable to TEI practice which are discussed in other chapters in the text, the models presented in this chapter adhere to Kielhofner's definition of a conceptual practice model to focus your attention on the theoretical rationale, research, assessment, and intervention within each model for the following reasons: (i) "once organized, theoretical concepts help practitioners identify areas for assessment and intervention" (Mitcham 2003, p. 73), (ii) conceptual practice models provide us with tools for assessment and intervention, and (iii) conceptual practice models provide research and evidence to support practice (Kielhofner 2009, p. 11).

In reviewing the definitions section of Chapter 1, one will recall that common but diverse concepts recur in the definitions that were considered. In all the definitions reviewed, both an assistive technology device and a user of that device are mentioned. Then there is an outcome, activity, or increase in participation that the person wants to accomplish that must be considered, as well as the context or environment in which the person wants to participate or increase their independence. All of these concepts relate to one another and underlie the theories that guide our practice.

Box 2.1 Case study

A TEIp has just returned from a conference where the latest and greatest new technology developments are presented in the exhibit hall. One of the products that the practitioner discovers is a computer with an interface designed to be "senior friendly." Visualize a large touch screen monitor with large simple buttons that allow the user to touch one onscreen button to access email or touch another button to access the Internet, another button to access the news, and so on. To the practitioner, the interface is intuitive, easy to use, and she can't wait to find someone to recommend it to upon returning home.

When the practitioner gets home, a colleague refers a client to her. Jake is 86 years old, has macular degeneration, and wants to use his computer again. Yes! "This is perfect," thinks the practitioner, "I have just seen the perfect technology solution for this client." The practitioner visits the client and sees that his current computer has an old operating system with few accessibility features built in and the monitor is very small, especially for someone who has macular degeneration and needs magnification. The practitioner recommends that the family buy Jake a "senior friendly" computer like the one she saw at the conference based on the Windows operating system. She chooses the Windows OS because she knows that it has the Ease of Access Center where she can make changes to the computer to meet Jake's visual needs.

To make a long story short, the computer was purchased with a 30-day trial period and sent back at the end of the trial period because: (i) Jake needed much more magnification than was available through the Windows operating system accessibility features, (ii) Jake was only interested in doing email and reading a family blog, rendering all the other buttons useless, (iii) he had an old copy of Zoomtext (Ai Squared 2009), which turned out to be the option that worked on a regular computer with a large monitor, and (iv) his family was familiar with Zoomtext and able to provide him with support to learn that program and make it work with what he wanted to do.

What happened here and what can we learn from this case? The practitioner started the process with the technology and tried to fit the person to the technology rather than taking into account all the factors that need to be considered to make the right person-technology match. She forgot to ask Jake (the person) what he wanted to do with the technology (participation/performance). She did not sufficiently assess his vision, cognition, or fine motor control and did not consider his social and physical context. She neglected to do a systematic evaluation of the whole situation, instead focusing on the technology and what she thought it could do for Jake. The technology was abandoned: a term we will hear much more about as we proceed through the book. Technology abandonment occurs when the consumer is not involved in its selection and does not see the relative advantage of using the device (Reimer-Reiss and Wacker 2000; Scherer 2012). As the chapter proceeds, Jake will be a recurring case study used to demonstrate how using a conceptual practice model could have helped to avoid the situation above.

Finally, when thinking about the device/intervention, there are more than just the physical attributes or the hard aspects of the device that must be considered. One must also consider information, training, psychological impact, etc. or the soft attributes that were described in Chapter 1 which also influence practice outcomes. Again, these terms, which emerge from the definitions, are the constructs which underlie the conceptual practice models that will be talked about next in this chapter.

Need for conceptual practice models

As mentioned above, the Human-Tech Ladder (Vicente 2006) was used by the authors to guide the structure of this book. We used this framework so we would consider all of the aspects of the ladder when writing a book about TEI practice. All of the rungs of the ladder interact to provide a good fit between a human and technology. Without this structure to guide us in writing this book, we may have been remiss in excluding some of the factors that are critical to making this match. This is the same reason that practitioners are encouraged to use conceptual practice models to guide their practice. The case study in Box 2.1 helps to illustrate this point.

Conceptual practice models that guide TEI

International Classification of Functioning, Disability and Health

The *ICF* is a useful model to consider the relationship between all of the diverse constructs practitioners must consider when providing TEI. Although the ICF is technically a classification system, rather than a conceptual practice model, what it does is similar to what a conceptual practice model does, for example, it is a means to focus on the outcome or goal of TEI that reflects current thinking on disability (Palmer and Harley 2012; World Health Organization [WHO] 2013). Additionally, it is designed for a diverse group of professional users and is beneficial, providing a common language or taxonomy within interdisciplinary research (WHO 2001, 2013). Given that TEI is an interdisciplinary field, we find the ICF useful, as do other authors (Frederici and Scherer 2012; Sanford 2012; WHO 2013) to encourage a common language among many disciplines. The following

ICF Applications
Service Provision

At the individual level...

- For the assessment of individuals: *What is the person's level of functioning?*
- For individual treatment planning: *What treatments or interventions can maximize functioning?*
- For the evaluation of treatment and other interventions: *What are the outcomes of the treatment? How useful were the interventions?*
- For communication among physicians, nurses, physiotherapists, occupational therapists and other health works, social service works and community agencies
- For self-evaluation by consumers: *How would I rate my capacity in mobility or communication?*

At the institutional level...

- For educational and training purposes
- For resource planning and development: *What health care and other services will be needed?*
- For quality improvement: *How well do we serve our clients? What basic indicators for quality assurance are valid and reliable?*
- For management and outcome evaluation: *How useful are the services we are providing?*
- For managed care models of health care delivery: *How cost-effective are the services we provide? How can the service be improved for better outcomes at a lower cost?*

At the social level...

- For eligibility criteria for state entitlements such as social security benefits, disability pensions, workers' compensation and insurance: *Are the criteria for eligibility for disability benefits evidence based, appropriate to social goals and justifiable?*
- For social policy development, including legislative reviews, model legislation, regulations and guidelines, and definitions for anti-discrimination legislation: *Will guaranteeing rights improve functioning at the societal level? Can we measure this improvement and adjust our policy and law accordingly?*
- For needs assessments: *What are the needs of persons with various levels of disability - impairments, activity limitations and participation restrictions?*
- For environmental assessment for universal design, implementation of mandated accessibility, identification of environmental facilitators and barriers, and changes to social policy: *How can we make the social and built environment more accessible for all person those with and those without disabilities? Can we assess and measure improvement?*

Figure 2.2 Use of international classification of functioning, disability and health (ICF) model for service provision.

Figure 2.2 illustrates some of the uses of the ICF model for service provision recommendations.

As previously noted in Chapter 1, the view of disability presented in the ICF reveals a complex construction of disability with a combination of both the medical model and the social model of disability. The ICF asserted that one model alone is inadequate to describe the phenomena of disability (Palmer and Harley 2012; WHO 2001, 2013). It classifies the personal or body structure and function aspects of disability as well as the contextual (environmental and situational) aspects, as seen in Figure 2.3.

The outcome of therapeutic intervention is not a fix or a cure (as in the medical model) but participation and health (WHO 2001, 2013). It is important to recognize that both activity, defined as "the execution of a task or action by an individual" (WHO 2001, p. 10), and participation, "involvement in a life situation" (WHO 2002, p. 10), are equally important outcomes of the ICF.

Why are these definitions important to practice? Let's envision TEI practice in a rehabilitation setting in which a client is discharged as independent in washing and dressing (activity). However, when the client returns to his or her home setting, there are environmental barriers, such as a bathroom that cannot be accessed. There may be situational factors at home, such as a fear of falling, that interfere with the client's ability to participate in this activity. In the ICF, as well as analogous conceptual practice models, the focus of intervention is more than just performance of an activity: it is the ability to participate and engage in needed or desired activities. The first part of the ICF focuses on functioning and disability and is comprised of: (i) body component factors including the structure and function of the individual and, (ii) participation and activities factors relating to the roles and activities in which the individual participates. The second part of the ICF considers factors such as environment and personal factors (WHO 2001), which influence the individual and impact participation and health as noted in Figure 2.4.

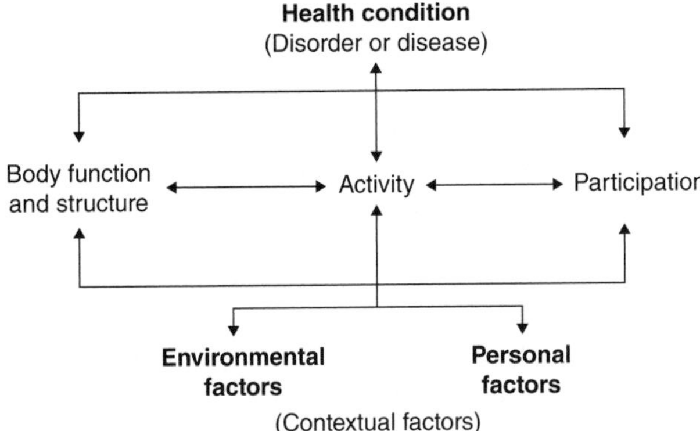

Figure 2.3 International classification of functioning, disability and health (ICF) representation of a model of disability. Source: Used with permission by World Health Organization.

Through use of the ICF in the evaluation process of TEI, factors related to body components and participation and activity impact clinical reasoning and decision-making. This is the value of using the ICF – it gives us a blueprint to ensure that we don't miss critical considerations, which may impact the effectiveness of our intervention planning. Of particular value to TEIp in the ICF (2001) plan is that within the environmental factors section, products and

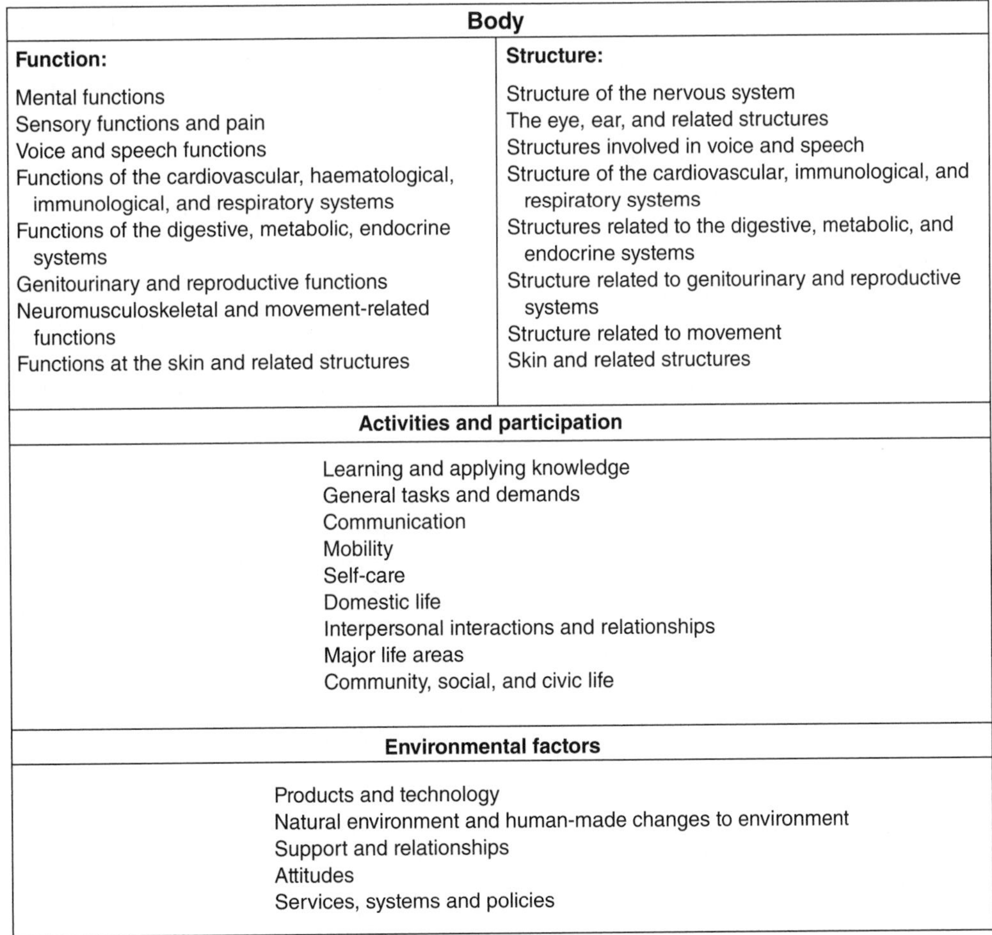

Body	
Function:	**Structure:**
Mental functions Sensory functions and pain Voice and speech functions Functions of the cardiovascular, haematological, immunological, and respiratory systems Functions of the digestive, metabolic, endocrine systems Genitourinary and reproductive functions Neuromusculoskeletal and movement-related functions Functions at the skin and related structures	Structure of the nervous system The eye, ear, and related structures Structures involved in voice and speech Structure of the cardiovascular, immunological, and respiratory systems Structures related to the digestive, metabolic, and endocrine systems Structure related to genitourinary and reproductive systems Structure related to movement Skin and related structures
Activities and participation	
Learning and applying knowledge General tasks and demands Communication Mobility Self-care Domestic life Interpersonal interactions and relationships Major life areas Community, social, and civic life	
Environmental factors	
Products and technology Natural environment and human-made changes to environment Support and relationships Attitudes Services, systems and policies	

Figure 2.4 International classification of functioning, disability and health (ICF) components: domains and chapters. Source: Used with permission by World Health Organization.

technology as well as other aspects of the environment, such as support, relationships, attitudes and services, systems and policies, are examined (Scherer and Glueckauf 2005). Because these features are included in this framework, when the TEIp uses it to guide client assessment, she or he will consider these issues as part of the evaluation process (WHO 2002, p. 16). Overall, use of the ICF lends support to the dynamic relationship between assistive technology, technology interventions, and the environment in working with a client. An example of the ICF as a conceptual model for assessment and intervention with the previous case of Jake is noted in Table 2.1.

The ICF provides a variety of practice assessment resources for TEIp. As suggested by others in the field (Frederici et al. 2012), assessment tools should be both objective and subjective, and the ICF offers both types of tools. The ICF Checklist "is a checklist of major categories of the International Classification of Functioning, Disability and Health (ICF) of the World Health Organization" (WHO 2003a, p. 1). The ICF Checklist is used to record information related to the functioning and disability of an individual. The checklist should be used along with the ICF or ICF pocket version (WHO 2003a, p. 1). This checklist, completed by the clinician, provides an objective assessment tool to guide TEI.

Table 2.1 International Classification of Functioning, Disability and Health (ICF) model and case of Jake.

Body structures and function	Assess Jake's vision, cognition, and fine motor capacity
Activity and participation	Use the computer to stay in touch with family via email and the family blog.
Environment	Physical access to the space where the computer stays is adequate; family support available to help with computer access.
Products and technology	Has Zoomtext; needs a larger computer screen and an updated OS.

Source: Used with permission: World Health Organization.

A second assessment tool is the *WHODAS 2.0: The World Health Organization Disability Assessment Schedule* (WHO 2003b). There are several versions, including a 12-, 24-, or 36-item version, which can be completed by the client, a proxy for the client, or through a client interview. The introduction to the self-administered 12-item form states, "This questionnaire asks about difficulties due to health conditions. Health conditions include diseases or illnesses, other health problems that may be short or long lasting, injuries, mental or emotional problems, and problems with alcohol or drugs" (WHO 2003b, p. 1).

In summary, the ICF provides a conceptual framework and assessment tool, which inform assessment, intervention, and research. A variety of international centers actively involved in research using the ICF can be reviewed at the following website: http://cirrie.buffalo.edu/icf/resources.php. Several authors also note the value of using the ICF and associated tools in TEI (Lenker and Paquet 2003; Manoj et al. 2014). Refer to Box 2.2 for an in-depth look at the use of a conceptual model to support TEI using evidence-based practice.

The Canadian Model of Occupational Performance-Engagement

The next conceptual practice model is the *CMOP-E*. This model, originally the Canadian Model of Occupational Performance, now in its eighth edition, was developed in the late 1990s and early 2000s (Polatajko et al. 2007). It describes the relationship of a

Box 2.2 Here's the evidence

Manoj, S., Gallagher, J., Holt, R. et al. (2014). Investigating the International Classification of Functioning, Disability and Health (ICF) framework to capture user needs in the concept stage of rehabilitation technology development. *Assistive Technology* 26(3): 164–173.

Key Words: robot, stroke, user involvement, user-centered design

Purpose: To investigate the usefulness of the ICF Core Set for Stroke in investigating user needs in developing rehabilitation technology.

Sample/Setting: Convenience sample of persons who have experienced stroke and professionals who work with those who have experienced stroke.

Method: Qualitative interview.

Findings: Results indicated that the ICF framework (in this case core set for stroke) is a tool that can be used in research to understand user needs that can guide the development of technology interventions relevant to this group. Most concepts covered in the ICF framework were relevant to user need.

Critical Thinking Questions:

1. After reading this research article, what do you understand to be the limitations of this research? Are there any limitations not stated?
2. If you were to replicate this study using a different method or design, what designs would you use to increase the rigor and why?
3. Based on the findings of this study, what additional research is needed that is not addressed in the discussion section?

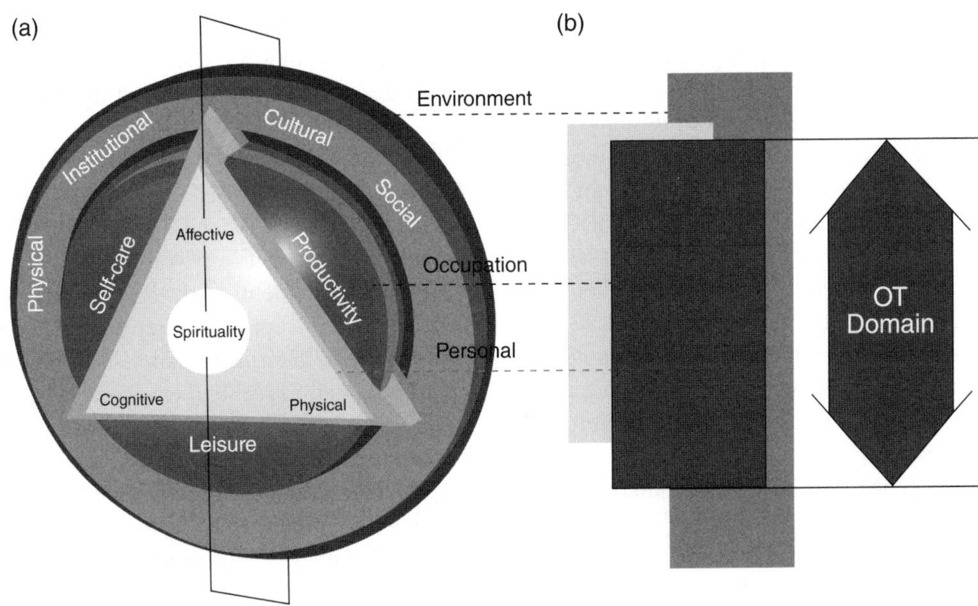

Figure 2.5 Canadian model of occupational performance-engagement (CMOP-E). Source: https://commons.wikimedia.org/wiki/File:CMOP-E.jpg.

person, the environment, and occupations (Letts et al. 2003; Sanford 2012). The conceptual practice model was chosen for this chapter because it has relevant tools for TEI and has been used to investigate outcomes of AT intervention. "The CMOP-E: An extension of the 1997/2002 conceptual framework … describes occupational therapy's view of the dynamic, interwoven relationship between persons, environments and occupations; engagement signals occupational therapy interests that include and extend beyond occupational performance over a person's life span and in diverse environments" (Polatajko et al. 2007). Refer to Figure 2.5 for a visual representation of the CMOP-E.

Using this conceptual practice model, the TEIp would investigate and collect information on human, environmental, and occupational factors that impact Jake's occupational performance. When there is a mismatch between the client, the environment, and their occupations, TEI should be considered as a model to guide evaluation, intervention, and outcomes. The diagram in Figure 2.5, section A, notes relevant factors, such as environmental, occupational, and personal, which are important to investigate when the TEIp is analyzing a compatible fit between attributes of the client, occupations, and the environment. The use of the CMOP-E model enhances the process of inclusion of multiple factors, which influence a person's ability to participate in meaningful life roles as part of the TEI process.

As part of the CMOP-E evaluation process, the client assists in identifying what goals and outcomes of intervention are personally important to him/her, which is a central aspect of a client-centered process. Based on the client's strengths, interests, and concerns, the TEIp incorporates this information along with other key enabling and hindering factors of this conceptual model to focus on AT assessment and intervention. Later in this chapter, clinical reasoning, which is a thinking and action process through which a TEIp organizes and analyzes information to generate goals, outcomes, and AT strategies for intervention, will be described in more detail. Review Table 2.2 for details on how this conceptual practice model would inform the TEI evaluation process for Jake.

Table 2.2 Case of Jake and the Canadian Model of Occupational Performance-engagement (CMOP-E) Model.

Occupational performance	Identify his areas of concern, which in this case would be to keep in touch with family using email and reading a family blog. We would rate his performance and satisfaction with his ability to do this occupation before and after out TEI intervention. The Canadian Occupational Performance Measure (COPM) discussed below would be used for this.
Person	Identify his physical, cognitive, and affective areas using appropriate assessment tools.
Environment	Describe relevant aspects of the environment that would also be considered in this model, including physical and social aspects of the environment which promote or interfere with occupational performance in the areas which Jake identified in the COPM.

The CMOP-E is a potent client-centered practice tool, which guides the clinician in key areas of strength and concern to the client in terms of occupational performance and participation. Additionally, the assessment tool based on the CMOP-E, the *Canadian Occupational Performance Measure* (COPM), is an outcome measure that, while not exclusively a tool dedicated to TEI outcomes, has been reported in the literature in relationship to TEI (Bernd et al. 2009; Lenker and Paquet 2003; Petty n.d.; Petty et al. 2005). The chapter in this text on outcomes-based assessment (Chapter 5) will expand on the importance of the incorporation of outcome measures as part of the evaluation and intervention process.

Moreover, the COPM tool is a client-centered, individualized, outcome measure (Law et al. 2005) that denotes occupational performance in the areas of self-care, productivity, and play and leisure. Areas of performance as defined by the client are highlighted for assessment and intervention, which is consistent with a user-centered approach that is relevant to current models of disability, such as a social model of disability (American Occupational Therapy Association 2014; WHO 2001). The COPM detects change in a client's satisfaction with occupational performance in meaningful occupations over time. It is a standardized, reliable, and valid assessment tool and has been used in over 35 countries worldwide and is available in 12 languages. For more information, the website, http://www.caot.ca/copm/description.html, has a listing of relevant research.

Matching Person and Technology Model

The *MPTM* (Scherer 2005), unlike the two models discussed previously, is specific to the area of assistive technology and the client's environment. However, this model has common elements to the ICF (Scherer and Glueckauf 2005). This conceptual framework incorporates aspects of the person, the milieu, and assistive technology. It is a client-centered model and emphasizes the importance of team involvement (Corradi et al. 2012). The model was derived from qualitative research and is concerned with factors that predict use or non-use of assistive technology (Lenker and Paquet 2003; Scherer 2005).

Key elements of the model are the milieu/environment, which contain both physical and societal considerations, characteristics of the person's needs and preference, as they relate to the TEI, and characteristics of function and attributes of the technology to be used (Scherer and Craddock 2002). Please refer to the conceptual model in Figure 2.6 to see the areas which must be taken into consideration when using this conceptual practice model.

The aim of the MPTM is to improve the participation and quality of life of an individual (Corradi et al. 2012).

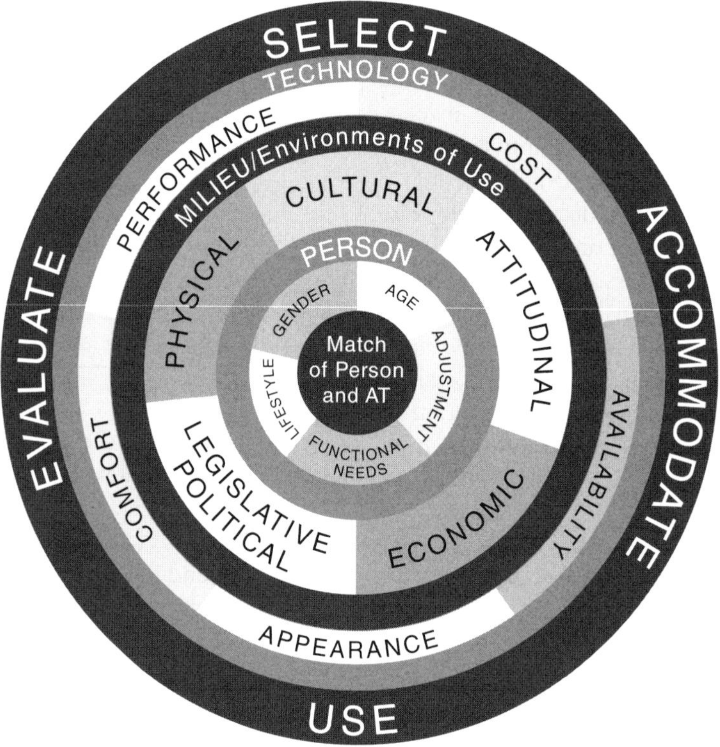

Figure 2.6 Matching person and technology model (MPTM). Source: Courtesy of IMPT.

According to the MPTM conceptual practice model, the extent to which TEI can do this can only be determined by the client and his or her predisposition to consider clinician recommendations. At the center of the model is the person, and considerations at this level are prior use of technology, functional needs, adjustment, mood, and lifestyle. The next level of the model contains the milieu or environmental concerns that the TEIp must consider in assessment and evaluation. These include physical, political/legislative, cultural, attitudinal, and economic factors.

The next level of the model reflects the technology factors. These include affordability, availability, cost, performance, and comfort. The final level of the model is a depiction of an AT service delivery model, which includes the following steps: (i) evaluate, (ii) select, (iii) accommodate, and (iv) use. There are numerous assessment process guidelines and forms based on this conceptual practice model that are available for use (Scherer and Glueckauf 2005). They are available for a wide variety of practice settings and age groups. The tools have reported reliability and validity and are extensively used in national and international research (Scherer 2008). Please refer to Table 2.3 to see how the MPTM would be applied to Jake's case.

Research validating the MPTM assessment tools is ongoing and Dr. Scherer and her collaborators both nationally and internationally present their research at a wide variety of venues. For example, in 2012 at the Rehabilitation Engineering and Assistive Technology Society of North America (RESNA) Annual Conference, Scherer (2012) presented findings of research devoted to developing an assessment tool based on the MPTM to match persons with cognitive disabilities with AT. Furthermore, Scherer et al. (2005) investigated the validation of MPTM-based tools with a sample of vocational rehabilitation counselors. The findings of the study support the use of the MPTM-based tools in carrying out evidence-based practice. More information on this model and related assessment tools and research can be reviewed via the following website: www.matchingpersonandtechnology.com. Review Table 2.3 for details on how this conceptual practice model would inform the TEI evaluation process for Jake.

Table 2.3 Case of Jake and the Matching Person and Technology Model (MPTM).

Characteristics of the person	What are Jakes needs, capabilities, and supports? What prior use of technology and environmental intervention (TEI) does he have? Is he motivated to use TEI to engage in his lifestyle choices?
Characteristics of the milieu/ environment	What physical, cultural, economic, attitudinal, and legislative considerations must be looked at?
Characteristics of the technology	Is the technology available and acceptable to Jake? How does it perform and is it affordable?

Student, Environments, Tasks, and Tools model

The *SETT* conceptual practice model is "a four-part model intended to promote collaborative decision-making in all phases of assistive technology service design and delivery from consideration through implementation and evaluation of effectiveness" (Zabala 2012; Zabala et al. 2005).

In the SETT Framework (Figure 2.7), the student, the environment, the task, and the tools are the elements, which interact to yield the outcome of inclusion in educational settings.

The team is emphasized in this conceptual practice model, and consideration of the student, environment, and tasks occur before recommending tools. As stated in the beginning of the chapter, the models included here provide us with assessment and intervention practice tools. The SETT practice tools consist of a series of scaffolds which can be obtained from the website http://www.joyzabala.com/Documents.html. The tools provide the practitioner with a systematic way of thinking about evaluation and intervention planning that ensures that all of the elements of the framework will be considered. The scaffolds guide the TEIp as part of the team to ask questions about the student, the tasks the student needs to do, the environment in which she or he needs to do these tasks, and then the tools that would

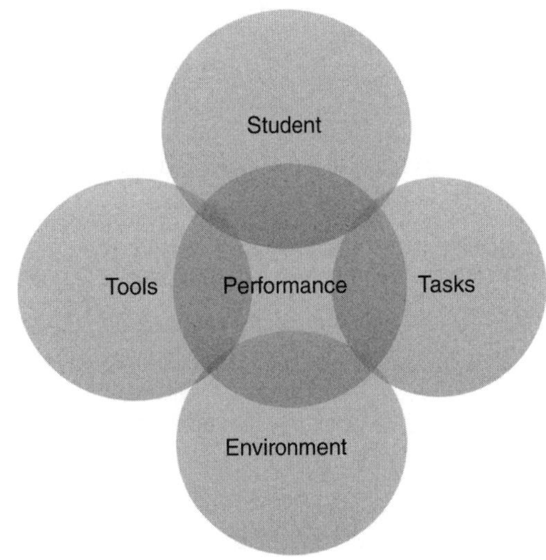

Figure 2.7 Student, environment, tasks, and tools SETT model.

be appropriate for the student to use to accomplish these tasks in the most inclusive way. For example, when assessing the student one might ask the following questions:

- What are the student's current abilities?
- What are the student's special needs?
- What are the functional areas of concern?
- How is the student performing compared to peers?
- What does the student need to independently perform in a way that is currently difficult or impossible?

Finally, the model has been recognized in numerous federally and state-funded grant and training projects. (Assistive Technology Training Online Project 2005; North Dakota Department of Special Education 2015).

While originally developed for use in a school-based setting, SETT has potential in other settings in which assistive technology is used with clients. Review Table 2.4 for details on how this conceptual practice model would inform the TEI evaluation process for Jake.

In summary, there are many conceptual practice models that can be used to guide clinicians thinking about TEI. Those presented here come from many disciplines. As you read though the remaining chapters you will find numerous other models and guidelines presented by contributing authors that have not been mentioned here. The model that one uses to guide one's day-to-day practice is a personal choice that develops over time and depends on a variety of factors presented in the Human-Tech Ladder. Where one works, in what setting, who makes up the team, what legislation and funding streams are available all impact the choice of the approach one uses to guide one's practice. The important point conveyed in this chapter is that, regardless of the choice one makes to guide practice, it should be systematic and align with the values that one hopes to deliver when providing services. There is an extensive list of assessment tools for TEI called the Informational Database of Assistive Technology Assessments (ID-AT-Assessments) at the following website: http://www.r2d2.uwm.edu/atoms/idata.

Table 2.4 Case of Jake and the Student, Environments, Tasks, and Tools (SETT) Model.

Person/student	What cognitive, sensory, physical, and communicative needs does Jake have?
Tasks	What specific concerns with the ability to carry out tasks do Jake and his team have? What barriers are encountered when trying to do the tasks?
Tools	What tools is Jake using? Are they adequate? Are new ones needed?
Environment	What is the customary environment where the task is done?

The next section of the chapter provides insight into the clinical reasoning process that practitioners in the field use to match a user with the features of the technology or the environment to promote participation in meaningful life roles. Feature matching is a term you will hear throughout the book and it reminds us that there is no one technology or environmental intervention that is the magic bullet for a given situation. The process of matching a person to a TEI is unique and multifaceted and one size does not fit all.

Clinical reasoning I

TEI practitioners have the challenge of matching the features of new technologies to a dynamic client who varies in abilities, goals, and roles. Each client requires a personalized evaluation that explores the goals of the individual and features of the technology system to create the perfect match. However, there is currently limited research explicitly on the clinical reasoning involved in selection of assistive technology or software for client-centered therapeutic intervention. A better appreciation of this process can provide a better understanding of the clinical reasoning process that integrates clinician knowledge and the need to advance toward client-centered goals.

On a clinician level, this improved understanding and a potential model of how it is done can assist therapists to efficiently select appropriate TEI. On a more global level, improved understanding and the creation of a TEIp clinical reasoning model can be used to educate students and new therapists to use technology to efficiently meet client-centered goals. The importance of understanding the clinical reasoning process, which is used to match a person with a technology, is often the hardest thing to clarify for the TEI novice.

Similar to the case study presented in the first part of the chapter, trying to provide a TEI to a person without using a conceptual model and a clinical reasoning strategy leads us down the wrong path and can result in abandonment or discontinuance of the device or recommended interventions.

Therapeutic use of technology

In this section of the chapter, Rakoski and Ferguson introduce a clinical reasoning process for TEI practice entitled *TUT*. TUT is a complex, dynamic, interconnected process that involves the person, practitioner, and technology for performance enhancement.

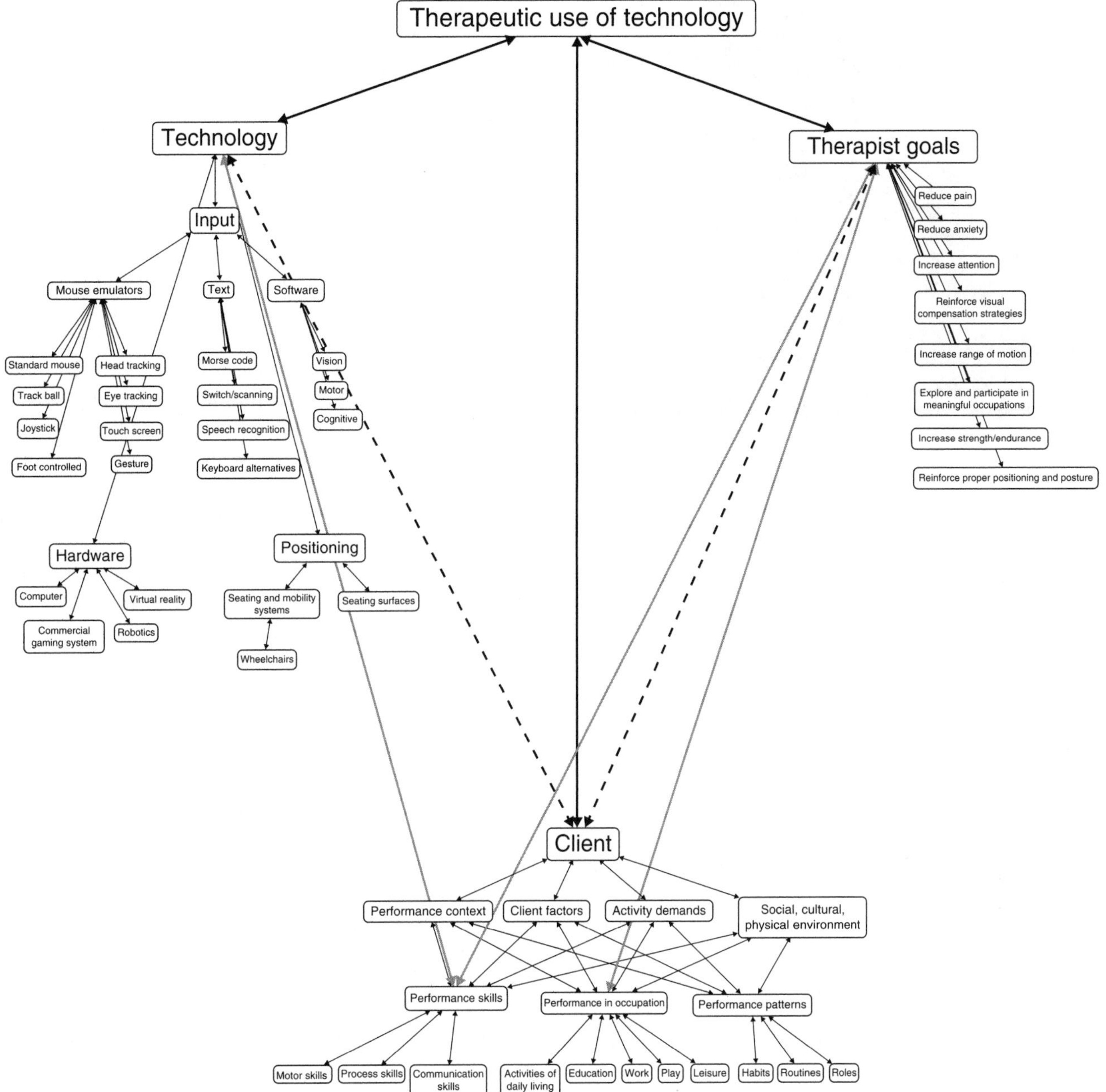

Figure 2.8 Therapeutic use of technology (TUT).

The person drives the process through selecting an occupation or activity that they desire to achieve. This initiates the process where the practitioner identifies skill components, interests, and technology features that will assist in developing the skills necessary for performance. In Figure 2.8 this process is illustrated through a brainstorming, interconnecting web that is dynamic and consistently changing to meet the needs of the person and also providing the "just right" challenge for skill growth.

Client dynamics

TUT is a cyclical process that is initiated by the client's need for skill obtainment in an activity or occupation, driven by their interests, and evolves as their skills emerge and grow. An example is the case of Denise, a 47-year-old female who was involved in a motor vehicle accident resulting in multiple lower-extremity fractures (Figure 2.9).

Her desire was to participate in a bear-hunting trip that was scheduled for six weeks post her discharge from

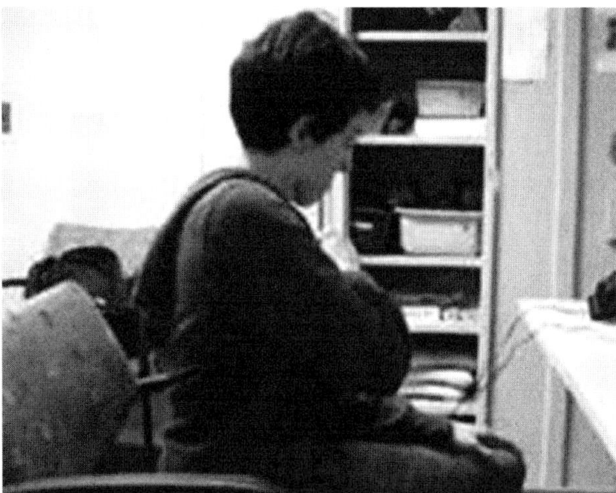

Figure 2.9 Case study photo of Denise.

the hospital. Denise feared that she would not be able to participate in the hunt due to her mobility status and impaired ability to hold, aim, and fire a rifle. Exploring this activity was limited in the hospital setting due to the organization's (Vicente's second rung on the Human-Tech Ladder) restriction on bears and firearms on the premises. Denise was extremely disappointed that she would be missing this trip and wondered if she would ever return to this activity again. Through this example, we can see the psychosocial (Vicente's fourth rung on the Human-Tech Ladder) importance of Denise's role of a hunter which fueled her desire to achieve the skills necessary for the hunt. Additionally, we can see the psychosocial impact or disappointment that could result from not being able to participate in this role.

Practitioner dynamics

The practitioner's role in utilizing technology to assist Denise in skill obtainment can be used to illustrate the clinical reasoning process, which drives matching technology features with the performance components required for hunting. The clinician's thinking process begins with the identification of bear hunting as the desired occupation to be addressed, an evaluation of Denise's current physical abilities and the skills that are required for bear hunting, and an exploration of technologies that will be utilized in treatments to assist with skill development required for the occupation. Through this evaluation, we are able to see that Denise will be hunting at wheelchair level due to her lower-extremity fractures and needs to address upper extremity strength to hold a rifle, sitting balance to aim a rifle, and postural control to maintain an upright seated position following the recoil when she fires the rifle. The practitioner then needs to examine technologies and their features, to ascertain which will best facilitate Denise's ability to engage in the hunting process.

Technology

In the TUT process, a technology is selected based upon the ability of the technology features to facilitate client motivation, develop skills necessary for an occupation, and assist the client in seeing future performance. This is the skilled role of the practitioner, to blend the client's interest with technology features to facilitate the emergence of new skills. In the example of Denise, the Nintendo Wii and the game Deer Drive were selected for the intervention. These technologies were selected due to their features of holding out in space a plastic firearm that had to be aimed on the screen. The software was selected for moving targets, target acquisition, and the motivation/anticipation of shooting a bear that is moving toward the player.

The role of the practitioner is also to grade the complexities of the intervention, and this was done by having Denise play the game in a variety of situations including both a supported seated position and an unsupported seated position, by adding weight to the plastic firearm to simulate rifle weight, and having the practitioner induce recoil when she fired the rifle during game play. Through the example with Denise, we are able to see that she drives the process but it is facilitated by the practitioner's clinical reasoning process, which blends the person's interest, performance goals, and technology features. Further exploring the blending of the TUT process and the skilled clinical reasoning that is required by a practitioner to facilitate that process is discussed next.

Clinical reasoning II

Professionals differ in the way that they critically think to solve problems related to their roles or functions within their professions. Novice practitioners of a profession tend to think linearly and use algorithmic approaches to solve practice-related problems. Although algorithmic thinking is used in practice, practitioners must utilize a great deal of non-linear heuristic strategies due to the variability of client and practitioner experiences. Understanding how to use the various modes of clinical reasoning in practice allows practitioners to develop their ability to heuristically approach the fluid changes occurring during and between treatment sessions with their clientele. Clinical reasoning also enables practitioners to better understand and utilize best evidence as well as allow them to maintain their intuitive processes to stimulate innovation.

The dynamic relationships between client dynamics, practitioner dynamics, and technology in the TUT process are facilitated and guided by a practitioner's clinical reasoning. Clinical reasoning bridges the various concepts and considerations for using technology in a therapeutic versus an assistive perspective. There are many models and definitions of clinical reasoning. Throughout this chapter, we will be using modified and expanded definitions related to the aspects or modes of clinical and professional reasoning described by Schell and Schell (2008) and Unsworth (2011).

Defining clinical reasoning

Mattingly (1991) characterized *clinical reasoning* as a form of complex interpretive thinking used by therapists to examine various aspects of the lived experience of clients and engage in creative problem-solving about clients' strengths and needs. Moreover, Fleming (1989, 1991) described the clinical reasoning used by occupational therapists as thinking with a three-track mind using four kinds of reasoning: narrative, procedural, interactive, and conditional. Clinical reasoning uses logical thinking to plan, direct, provide, influence, and reflect on patient care. It helps us learn from the treatment process and can be influenced by our attitudes, education, and experience. Clinical reasoning has many modes and while each mode is presented in this chapter as a separate and distinct concept, it is important to remember that clinical reasoning is a dynamic process and practitioners move between or combine several modes of reasoning during the treatment process. All modes of reasoning should be considered before making final clinical assumptions during treatment.

Modes of clinical reasoning

Scientific reasoning

Scientific reasoning uses a logical and systematic approach to help practitioners make decisions in practice. It is impersonal and doesn't take into account client-specific information. Practitioners reflect on the facts, information, and research related to the diagnosis or condition of the client and how the condition will most likely progress (Schell and Schell 2008; Unsworth 2011). The focus is on understanding the condition and its typical consequences on client function.

When considering the condition, practitioners think about the available knowledge in order to understand the characteristics of the condition better, hypothesize cause and effect, test their hypotheses, and facilitate innovation of new knowledge or understanding. Scientific reasoning provides a way for practitioners to balance their use of experience, professional dogma, or intuition often utilized in practice. Its use is critical in analyzing and synthesizing research findings into practice.

Diagnostic reasoning

Diagnostic reasoning is considered a component of scientific reasoning. A key factor that differentiates diagnostic reasoning from scientific reasoning is that diagnostic reasoning begins to personalize information to a specific client's condition (Schell and Schell 2008; Unsworth 2011). Practitioners consider a client's motives, wishes, goals, and values and compare the client's actual condition with a typical presentation of the condition. They collect and analyze information to establish relevant relationships and make inferences and predictions about the why and how of a client's performance in order to develop and test treatment hypotheses and apply practice theory. This kind of thinking is crucial when designing, reflecting on, and modifying therapeutic interventions that promote participation.

Pragmatic reasoning

Pragmatic reasoning is the kind of thinking related to the real-world issues of a practitioner's practice context. It is used to fit therapy possibilities with the realities of practice. This includes the practitioner's organizational and political environment as well as economic influences such as resources and reimbursement issues. It also includes practitioner's personal contexts that can include the practitioner's own motivation, knowledge, assumptions, competency and skills, and ability to understand their environment's effect on practice culture. Pragmatic effects on a practitioners reasoning can be both positive and negative, depending on how it influences clinical decision-making condition (Schell and Schell 2008; Unsworth 2011).

Ethical reasoning

Ethical reasoning relates to the thinking associated with the analysis of a moral situation, conflict, or dilemma and the subsequent problem-solving and resolution process condition (Schell and Schell 2008; Unsworth 2011). It comes into play when balancing conflicting information noted between personal and professional values as well as between the various modes of clinical reasoning. The focus is on doing the right think. A few examples include how a practitioner thinks about and determines what to do when facing decisions regarding dogmatic practice versus research evidence, productivity and billing practices, treatment needs/desires of the client versus the knowledge and skill of the practitioner.

Narrative reasoning

"Narrative reasoning is the process through which practitioners make sense of people's particular circumstances; prospectively imagine the effect of illness, disability, or occupational performance problems on their daily lives and create a collaborative story that is enacted with clients and families through intervention" (Schell and Schell 2008).

Our client's narrative establishes the meaning of the client's condition in relation to their life story. We take into consideration the person's past, present, and future contexts. This is where as a practitioner you obtain and reflect on the person's occupational profile and determine how it has been changed due to their current circumstances. This is a critical first step in thinking about and determining how we will collaborate with our clientele during our interactions with them along their personal journey.

It is important to remember that the narrative belongs to the client you are working with. Although we have our own perspective on how their circumstances are affecting their narrative, we must ensure that we view it from the perspective of the client. We need to know, understand, and give due consideration to their preferences and their motivations. Finally, consideration of your client's narrative is pervasive throughout each of the modes of professional and clinical reasoning. We must learn their perspective on their condition/situation as this will greatly determine how we use other modes of professional and clinical reasoning in our practice.

In this new chapter of their narrative, we need to discover if they are in a time and place where they are either an agent of change in their personal story or if they view themselves as a victim of their circumstances. How do you proceed with a client who sees themselves in a victimic role in their personal life story? Can they see the connection between the TUT and their narrative? How do you facilitate the next chapters of their personal narrative?

Procedural reasoning

Procedural reasoning is the thinking associated with planning, using, and reflecting on treatment process including diagnostically related information from evaluations and interventions, strategies, activities, and protocols related to the client's condition and the client's occupational performance condition (Schell and Schell 2008; Unsworth 2011). Practitioners use this information to develop, select, and modify an appropriate treatment plan. It is important to ensure that procedural reasoning considers personal, contextual, and environmental constraints on performance.

Interactive reasoning

Interactive reasoning guides practitioner interactions with the client. It means being "present" in all aspects of the client interaction in order to create a collaborative relationship (Schell and Schell 2008; Unsworth 2011). It is pervasive in all areas of professional reasoning. It involves considering the best approach to communicate with the client and to engage the client in therapy. It focuses on better understanding the client as a person and understanding their situation from their perspective to individualize therapy, including their occupations, their performance, potential treatment solutions, and the treatment plan.

Interactive reasoning is a collaborative process that features shared problem identification and problem-solving as identified through scientific, diagnostic, and procedural reasoning condition (Schell and Schell 2008; Unsworth 2011). It is also used when thinking about the interaction and relationship with the person regarding their condition and intervention.

Generalization reasoning

Generalization reasoning is used within the context of the other modes of clinical reasoning. With generalized reasoning, the practitioner reflects on past experience or knowledge to assist them to better understand a client's current situation or circumstance as well as their own performance as a practitioner (Schell and Schell 2008; Unsworth 2011). The more experience or information a practitioner has, the better the accuracy with their generalizations.

When considering the use of generalization reasoning, it is important to remember a few things. As beneficial as generalizations can be, they can also be wrong or even harmful. Don't rely solely on generalization reasoning. Balance generalizations with scientific, diagnostic, and ethical reasoning. Practitioners should also consider anecdotal experience against an evidence background. Generalization should be used to help fill in the gaps in the reasoning process.

Conditional reasoning

Conditional reasoning is a logical process whereby a practitioner integrates multiple modes of professional reasoning in collaboration with their client to understand the multi-variable factors of their current state of function and the fluid nature of change within the therapeutic process, in order to develop a prospective view of performance skills and patterns. This prospective view develops throughout individual treatment, during episodes of care, post-episodic care, and personal, organizational, and population-level participation condition (Schell and Schell 2008; Unsworth 2011).

The focus of conditional reasoning is on collaborative reflection and envisioning the client's future potential and progressing the client toward that potential. It is an inherently imaginative and integrative reasoning about the client's past, present, and potential future conditions within a broader social, temporal, cultural, and virtual narrative. Think of it as taking a view of the client's life "in process."

With all the variables involved in a client's situation and the multiple types of reasoning occurring during the therapeutic process, there is a greater difficulty in accurately imagining a future state for the client. This may be the thinking behind why this type of reasoning is seen more frequently and more fluently with an experienced practitioner than a novice practitioner. A great deal of skill is used in integrating multiple modes of reasoning and marrying them with past therapeutic experiences, and examples are required to fully imagine all the potential future states for a particular patient (Box 2.3).

Clinical reasoning: The TUT process

Note: Clinical reasoning used to guide each component of the TUT process is in parentheses.

The technology to be used in treatment needs to approximate the abilities required to don Susan's jacket as well as meet her emergent motivational interests in technology. The practitioner collaborated with Susan to determine what performance components needed to be developed and then matched that with the aspects of the available technologies. Let's look at the clinical reasoning used in the TUT and Schell process as Susan and her practitioner selected the technology to match her goal, as described in Table 2.5.

Client Dynamics: Susan and her practitioner had to answer some basic questions about her goals and abilities to help them decide on a treatment activity and technology choices. (Diagnostic, Pragmatic, Narrative, Interactive, Procedural, Conditional, Generalization)

1. What client factors and activity demands were required in order to put the jacket on? In order for Susan to put her jacket on, she needed to be able to grasp her jacket, thread it over her left arm, and pull it up to her shoulder. She then needed to extend, abduct, and internally rotate her shoulder past her right hip and further flex her elbow in order to thread the jacket over her right hand behind her. Finally, she needed to extend her elbow and bring her arm forward to get her arm through the sleeve. Once in this position, Susan was satisfied with fastening her jacket using her left hand. (Scientific, Diagnostic, Pragmatic, Interactive, Procedural, Generalization)
2. What strengths did she have already and what skills did she need to further develop (performance skills, performance patterns)? It was noted that she could position her hand for grasp, complete basic grasp, and then relax her grasp for release of small objects. She could bring her right hand to her left forearm, but not above the left elbow. She could partially raise her arm at the shoulder and partially internally rotate her shoulder to bring her hand toward but not past her right hip. When her hand was placed in the small of her back, she was able to extend her elbow and bring her hand back to her lap. (Scientific, Diagnostic, Interactive, Procedural, Conditional, Generalization)

Box 2.3 Clinical reasoning with TUT: A case study

Susan is a 34-year-old PhD researcher. She and her family enjoy outdoor activities, working out, and playing mini-golf. Immediately after giving birth to her son, Susan suffered a left middle cerebral artery stroke. As a result of the stroke, Susan demonstrated right hemiplegia, non-fluent aphasia, apraxia, right hemianopsia, impaired right hemi-body sensation, and a lack of right-sided proprioception. During her inpatient rehabilitation stay, she was introduced to the TUT as a means of improving her function. She requested to continue using technology to assist with her recovery. After five weeks of intensive inpatient rehabilitation, Susan began outpatient treatment with a 28% recovery of right upper extremity motor function as identified by the *Fugl-Meyer Assessment of Motor Recovery*. After an additional three months of outpatient therapy at another facility, she demonstrated no additional motor recovery.

Susan returned to her original facility for additional evaluation and treatment recommendations. Susan's outpatient occupational therapy assessment revealed that she was modified independent with completing her basic self-care needs, but that she identified the desire to improve her right upper extremity function and advance beyond using one-handed strategies for bathing and dressing herself. As winter was approaching, she stated that she wanted to use her right arm to put her jacket on like she did before her stroke.

The practitioner and Susan agreed that it was impractical and frustrating for her to repeatedly practice donning her jacket. They also agreed that by using the clinic's available technology, she might be able to achieve sufficient repetition to develop the necessary skills to enable her to re-learn to put her jacket on.

Table 2.5 Clinical Reasoning and Technology Considerations with Therapeutic Use of Technology (TUT) Model.

Reasoning	Key reasoning features	Example: Technology considerations
Scientific	• Is impersonal. • Use of logical and scientific methods. • Reflect on diagnosis, condition, and research findings to understand client condition and progression.	• Effect of technology on condition. (e.g. damage to right posterior thalamus causing sensory misperception of graviceptional vertical/midline and the effect of vibration on sensory perception) Does the technology have the potential to affect the condition? • Medical devices that would affect the decision to use certain technologies (e.g. pacemakers with electrical stimulation). • Conditions that commonly require assistive technology or rehabilitation technology (weakness, spasticity, cognitive, visual motor, or perceptual impairment, etc.).
Diagnostic	• Begin to personalize client condition. • Using subjective and objective information from assessment/evaluation, evidence-based practice, practice-based evidence to explain the client's experience. • Goes into the why and how In order to develop and test treatment hypothesis and apply practice theory.	• Common tangible assessment tools (e.g. cognitive, perceptual, and sensorimotor assessments). • Computerized and virtual assessments. Telehealth applications. • Occupational profile to help determine occupation-based intervention. • Consider how personal, contextual, and environmental constraints exist to determine appropriate technology.
Pragmatic	• Looks at personal and Practice context that constrains actions in therapy. Includes: o personal and organizational culture o practitioner's skills/competency training o time o cost, supplies, equipment o management, team dynamics o reimbursement, legal issues.	• Practitioner knowledge and competency of specific technology applications and modifications. • Is the work culture accepting of the use of the technology or technophobic? • Does the work environment allow space and time for technology use? • What levels of technology can the organization afford? • Can the technology cost be recovered? • Is the use of technology reimbursable? • What are the safety considerations for the use of the technology? • How much money and time is required for technology training? • What is the cost–benefit of using technology in your own environment?
Ethical	• Focuses on doing the right thing. • Resolving ethical dilemmas. • Balance conflict between the types of reasoning? (e.g. pragmatics vs. evidence).	• How engaged are practitioners when using high tech? Are they busy doing other things when the technology seems to do much of the work? • Do you rely on the "app" providing the therapy vs. using intervention strategies? • Does using a tablet "app" to work on "fine motor" activities really provide fine motor activity when clients don't actually manipulate anything? • If the evidence shows the effectiveness of a specific technological tool or intervention, what responsibility does a practitioner or an organization have in providing that technology? How do they plan for obtaining future technology? • If a practitioner is technophobic or is under productivity constraints, what do they do when the technology is available? • Evidence-based research hasn't been conducted on a specific technology, but practice-based evidence shows potential.

Table 2.5 (*Continued*)

Reasoning	Key reasoning features	Example: Technology considerations
Narrative	• Establishes meaning of the client's condition on their life story (past, present, and future contexts). • Learn the client's perspective on their condition/situation, their preferences and their motives. • Is the client in a time-place where they are an agent of change or a victim of their circumstances? • How do you facilitate the next chapters of their personal narrative?	• What is a client's experience with and how do they feel about various levels of technology? • Provides a tangible anchor to functional activities when using a virtual context with technology. • Can the client see the connection between technology and occupation? ○ Can you? Can you facilitate the connection? • Recognize when clients are at an appropriate stage in their current narrative for the use of various levels of technology.
Interactive	• Collaborative process that shares problem-solving as identified through scientific, diagnostic, and procedural reasoning. • Thinking about the interaction and relationship with the client regarding their condition and the assessment/intervention. • Process used to obtain client perspective on their situation, occupations, performance, and potential solutions for the treatment plan.	• Constantly engage the client for their perspective on their situation, the task, their performance, potential solutions, and the technology. • Blend client's goals and roles with the device and application features. • Trial appropriate technologies, making feature adjustments or changing the device while gaining client's feedback.
Procedural	• Using and reflecting on treatment processes, strategies, activities, and protocols related to the client's condition. • Considers occupational, task, activity constraints (personal, contextual, environmental).	• Use the technology yourself first. Learn the device and/or software features in order to determine which technology choices best match the client's factors, performance skills, and patterns. • Determine what traditional treatment models can be used with the technology. • How can you provide treatment facilitations, strategies, techniques, and activities while using the chosen technology?
Conditional	• Used to holistically integrate the different types of reasoning used in the treatment process to monitor a client's changing condition. • The focus is on collaborative reflection and envisioning the client's future potential and progressing the client toward that potential. • Is an imaginative and integrative reasoning about the client's past, present, and potential future conditions within a broader social, temporal, and virtual narrative. • It takes a view of the client's life "in process." • Facilitates a new perspective or view of the future and the potential for change.	• Use interactive strategies to reflect on past and current treatment successes and failures with technology in order to modify interventions that utilize technology. • Matching technology with client's goals. • Will the technology be able to continue to be a part of the client's narrative? • Consider whether a client will be able to access the technology at home.

Source: Adapted from Schell and Schell (2008).

3. What activities does she enjoy when using technology? Through her previous experience with technology during her inpatient rehabilitation, Susan developed an emergent motivation for virtual mini-golf and online card games. She expressed that she hoped to return to playing "real" mini-golf in the future. (Pragmatic, Narrative, Interactive, Procedural, Conditional, Generalization)

Practitioner Dynamics: Susan and her practitioner needed to determine what they wanted to achieve during the treatment session based on Susan's client dynamics and technology considerations. (Pragmatic, Interactive, Procedural, Generalization)

1. Reinforce visual compensation strategies. Based on Susan's loss of her right visual field and her impaired proprioception, she needed to watch her right arm whenever she reached toward her right side. (Procedural, Generalization)
2. Increase range of motion, strength, and coordination. Susan needed to increase her right elbow flexion and horizontal adduction to reach her right shoulder. She needed to improve her shoulder extension and internal rotation to position her hand behind her. Finally, Susan needed to further flex her elbow in order to reach her jacket sleeve hole. (Diagnostic, Procedural, Conditional, Generalization)
3. Explore/participate in meaningful occupation. Since Susan expressed her enjoyment of virtual mini-golf and online card games, these activities were selected as they were meaningful to her. (Pragmatic, Narrative, Interactive, Procedural, Conditional, Generalization)
4. Simulate/reinforce functional movement patterns. Susan needed repeated practice of the correct movements required to put her coat on. (Pragmatic, Procedural, Conditional, Generalization)

Technology: Susan and her practitioner needed to determine how their own dynamics were going to influence the selection of technology and vice versa? (Scientific, Diagnostic, Pragmatic, Ethical, Narrative, Interactive, Procedural, Conditional, Generalization)

Input – The use of a touch screen provided a simple and quick way to relocate the cursor during the activity. Susan's identified virtual mini-golf and online card games were selected due to their meaningfulness to her as well as the static visual environments and simple rules they provided to maximize visual search strategies while maintaining simplicity. Jelly Bean and large Joggle switches were utilized as the left click mouse function and were placed at key target points to simulate desired movement patterns. (Scientific, Diagnostic, Pragmatic, Interactive, Procedural, Generalization)

Hardware – The games utilized were free online games that enabled a motivational virtual context for activities that Susan looked forward to completing in the future. Universal mounts were utilized to provide stable key target points and to facilitate quick and easily adaptable target relocation to modify the challenge. (Scientific, Diagnostic, Pragmatic, Ethical, Narrative, Interactive, Procedural, Conditional, Generalization)

Susan alternated back and forth between activating the left shoulder switch and the right hip switch to practice the missing components of the desired goal of donning her jacket. She progressed to having the hip switch placed posteriorly to practice the movement required to place her hand into the jacket sleeve. She completed over 200 repetitions for each movement during this particular treatment session. The chair with armrests was used to guide and restrain extraneous arm movements during the activity. After several interventions, Susan was able to put her jacket on successfully and to her satisfaction.

Summary

TUT is a creative process driven by clinical reasoning. This process brings together the interests of the client and the creativity of the clinician to create an experience where skills are built and reinforced. It is important to have a systematic approach for determining the performance skills to be addressed, technology selection, and client engagement. Outcomes for this process can be measured by gains in occupational performance. As technology evolves and new equipment becomes available, this process can continue to be applied to maximize client performance. TUT will allow clients to explore their roles and maximize their goals well into the future.

In closing this chapter, the most important point is to emphasize that providing TEI involves a process of systematic thinking and clinical reasoning. A conceptual model provides a systematic process for evaluation, intervention, and outcomes identification and assessment. Clinical reasoning, which is continually adapted according the changing needs of the client, delineates the thinking processes that underlie the steps along the way from evaluation to outcome achievement. Regardless of the technology options available to be used as interventions, it is the systematic thinking and reasoning that the TEIp uses that ensures a good match between the user and the technology. While readers of this text may be wondering when am I going to learn about the technology, the authors of this chapter hope you realize that while a text can never keep up with rapidly changing technological innovation, it can present conceptual practice models and clinical reasoning strategies which will provide you with tools to know how to implement technology in practice.

References

Ai Squared (2009). Zoomtext v.10. Retrieved from http://www.aisquared.com/products/zoomtext.

American Occupational Therapy Association (2014). Occupational therapy practice framework: domain and process (3rd ed.). *American Journal of Occupational Therapy* 68 (Suppl 1): S1–S48.

Assistive Technology Training Online Project (2005). Retrieved from http://sphhp.buffalo.edu/cat/client-services/projects.html.

Bernd, T., Van der Pijl, D., and De Witte, L.P. (2009). Existing models and instruments for the selection of assistive technology in rehabilitation practice. *Scandinavian Journal of Occupational Therapy* 16 (3): 146–158.

Corradi, F., Scherer, M.J., and Lo Presti, A. (2012). Measuring the assistive technology match. In: *Assistive Technology Assessment Handbook* (ed. S.N. Federici and M. Scherer), 49–66. Boca Raton, FL: CRC Press.

Edyburn, D.L. and Smith, R.O. (2004). Creating an assistive technology outcomes measurement system: validating the components. *Assistive Technology Outcomes and Benefits* 1 (1): 8–15.

Fleming, M.H. (1989). The therapist with the three-track mind. In: *The AOTA Practice Symposium Program Guide* (ed. American Occupational Therapy Association), 70–75. Rockville, MD: American Occupational Therapy Association.

Fleming, M.H. (1991). The therapist with the three-track mind. *American Journal of Occupational Therapy* 45: 1007–1014. https://doi.org/10.5014/ajot.45.11.1007.

Frederici, S. and Scherer, M. (2012). The assistive technology assessment model and basic definitions. In: *Assistive Technology Assessment Handbook* (ed. S. Federici and M. Scherer), 1–10. Boca Raton, FL: CRC Press.

Frederici, S., Meloni, F., and Corradi, F. (2012). Measuring individual functioning. In: *Assistive Technology Assessment Handbook* (ed. S. Federici and M. Scherer), 25–48. Boca Raton, FL: CRC Press.

Kielhofner, G. (2009). *Conceptual Foundations of Occupational Therapy Practice*, 4e. Philadelphia: F. A. Davis.

Law, M., Baptiste, S., Carswell, A. et al. (2005). *Canadian Occupational Performance Measure*, 4e. Ottawa, ON: CAOT Publications ACE.

Lenker, J. and Paquet, V. (2003). A review of conceptual models for assistive technology outcomes: research and practice. *Assistive Technology* 15 (1): 1–15.

Letts, L., Rigby, P., and Stewart, D.W. (2003). *Using Environments to Enable Occupational Performance*. Thorofare, NJ: Slack.

Manoj, S., Gallagher, J., Holt, R. et al. (2014). Investigating the International Classification of Functioning, Disability and Health (ICF) framework to capture user needs in the concept stage of rehabilitation technology development. *Assistive Technology* 26 (3): 164–173. https://doi.org/10.1080/10400435.2014.903315.

Mattingly, C. (1991). What is clinical reasoning? *American Journal of Occupational Therapy* 45: 979–986. https://doi.org/10.5014/ajot.45.11.979.

Mitcham, M. (2003). Integrating theory and practice: Using theory creatively to enhance professional practice. In: *Becoming an Advanced Healthcare Practitioner* (ed. G. Brown, S. Esdaile, S. Ryan and O. Adams), 64–89. New York: Butterworth Heinemann.

North Dakota Department of Special Education (2015). Guidelines for the provision of assistive technology to students with disabilities under IDEA Part B. Retrieved from https://www.nd.gov/dpi/uploads/60/ATGuidelines.pdf.

Palmer, M. and Harley, D. (2012). Models and measurement in disability: an international review. *Health Policy and Planning* 27 (5): 357–364.

Petty, L.S. (n.d.). Client centered outcome measures. Inclusive Design Research Centre, OCAD University. Retrieved from http://idrc.ocad.ca/index.php/resources/idrc-online/23-conference-slides/233-client-centered-outcome-measures.

Petty, L.S., McArthur, L., and Treviranus, J. (2005). Clinical report: use of the Canadian Occupational Performance Measure in vision technology. *Canadian Journal of Occupational Therapy* 72: 309–312.

Polatajko, H.J., Townsend, E.A., and Craik, J. (2007). *Canadian Model of Occupational Performance and Engagement (CMOP- E)*. In: *Enabling Occupation II: Advancing an Occupational Therapy Vision for Health, Well-Being & Justice through Occupation* (ed. E.A. Townsend and H.J. Polatajko), 27–33. Ottawa, ON: CAOT Publications ACE.

Reimer-Reiss, M. and Wacker, R. (2000). Factors associated with assistive technology discontinuance among individuals with disabilities. *Journal of Rehabilitation* 66: 44–50.

Sanford, J. (2012). *Universal Design as a Rehabilitation Strategy: Design for the Ages*. New York: Springer.

Schell, B.A. and Schell, J.W. (2008). *Clinical and Professional Reasoning in Occupational Therapy*. Philadelphia, PA: Wolters Kluwer Health/Lippincott Williams & Wilkins.

Scherer, M.J. (2005). *Living in the State of Stuck: How Assistive Technology Impacts the Lives of People with Disabilities*, 4e. Brookline, MA: Brookline Books.

Scherer, M.J. (2008). Matching person and technology: validation studies. Retrieved from http://www.matchingpersonandtechnology.com/validation.html.

Scherer, M.J. (2012). Assessing the match of person and cognitive support technology. Paper presented at the Annual Rehabilitation and Engineering Society of North America [RESNA] Conference, Baltimore, MD (28 June–3 July).

Scherer, M.J. and Craddock, G. (2002). Matching Person & Technology (MPT) assessment process. *Technology and Disability* 14: 125–131.

Scherer, M.J. and Glueckauf, R. (2005). Assessing the benefits of assistive technologies for activities and participation. *Rehabilitation Psychology* 50: 132–141.

Scherer, M.J., Sax, C., Vanbiervliet, A. et al. (2005). Predictors of assistive technology use: the importance of personal and psychosocial factors. *Disability and Rehabilitation* 27 (21): 1321–1331.

Unsworth, C. (2011). The evolving theory of clinical reasoning. In: *Foundations for Practice in Occupational Therapy* (ed. E. Duncan), 209–232. Edinburgh: Churchill Livingstone Elsevier.

Vicente, K. (2006). *The Human Factor: Revolutionizing the Way People Live with Technology*. New York: Routledge, Taylor & Francis Group.

World Health Organization (2001). *International Classification of Functioning, Disability and Health*. Geneva, Switzerland: World Health Organization.

World Health Organization (2002). *Towards a Common Language for Functioning, Disability and Health: ICF*. Geneva, Switzerland: World Health Organization Retrieved from http://www.who.int/classifications/icf/training/icfbeginnersguide.pdf.

World Health Organization (2003a). ICF Checklist, Version 2.1a, clinician form for International Classification of Functioning, Disability and Health. Retrieved from http://www.who.int/classifications/icf/training/icfchecklist.pdf.

World Health Organization (2003b). WHODAS 2.0 World Health Organization disability assessment schedule 2.0: 12-item version, self-administered. Retrieved from http://www.who.int/classifications/icf/WHODAS2.0_12itemsSELF.pdf.

World Health Organization (2013). *How to Use the ICF: A Practical Manual for Using the International Classification of Functioning, Disability and Health (ICF). Exposure draft for comment.* Geneva, Switzerland: WHO. Retrieved from http://www.who.int/classifications/drafticfpracticalmanual2.pdf?ua=1.

Zabala, J. (2012). Sharing the SETT Framework. Retrieved from http://www.joyzabala.com/Home.php.

Zabala, J., Bowser, G., and Korsten, J. (2005). SETT and ReSETT: concepts for AT implementation. *Closing the Gap* 23 (5): 1–4.

Additional resources

ATOMS Project Technical Report: Models and taxonomies relating to assistive technology. This report available on line at http://www.r2d2.uwm.edu/atoms/archive/technicalreports/fieldscans/tr-fs-taxonomiesmodels.html is the result of a literature review which lists a variety of models and taxonomies related to assistive technology.

MPT website where you can obtain the MPT assessment tools http://matchingpersonandtechnology.com.

3

The design process: Solving human-tech problems

Susan Camp

Outline

Assistive Technologies and Environmental Interventions in Healthcare: An Integrated Approach, First Edition.
Edited by Lynn Gitlow and Kathleen Flecky.

Companion website: www.wiley.com/go/gitlow/assitivetechnologies

Learning outcomes

After reading this chapter, you should be able to:

1. Gain a basic understanding of principles of design and how they can contribute to developing technology and environmental interventions.
2. Develop an appreciation for open-ended exploration and group brainstorming.
3. Learn about the application of the design process through a case study.
4. Gain a basic understanding of how materials and aesthetics impact user understanding and satisfaction.
5. Identify resources for "making" TEI solutions.

Active learning prompts

Before you read this chapter:

1. Do you or someone you know wear glasses or use contact lenses? How did you or the person you know make decisions about whether or not to use these devices? How did you or the person choose the pair that they use?
2. Now think about your own experience with adaptive equipment. Have you ever used crutches or a wheelchair? How did you feel about the experience?
3. Do you have older family members who could benefit from using adaptive equipment? Why do they accept or resist using this equipment?
4. How does the decision to use glasses or contacts compare and contrast to the decision to use adaptive equipment. What thoughts do you have about this?

Key terms

Affordance
Balance
Conceptual model
Emphasis
Hue
Materiality
Proportion
Prototype
Rhythm
Saturation
Scale
Unity
Value

Part one: Asking questions, getting started

> Always the beautiful answer who asks a more beautiful question.
>
> E.E. Cummings

At the beginning of the semester, a professor writes this quote on the blackboard in the studio where he teaches three-dimensional design. On the first day of class, he initiates a conversation about the quote in the following way:

> I tell my students that when I Googled this quote, I was surprised to find all sorts of articles where the writers insisted on adding "correct" punctuation and grammar, and as a result were obviously missing the boat. I use this quote as a springboard to encourage the incoming students to accept uncertainty; and to engage unfamiliar ideas and materials without having to make them appear to be something familiar; something with "correct" punctuation.
>
> (W. Hall, personal communication, November 14, 2012)

Because Cummings has provided us with ambiguity by omitting the anticipated punctuation, this quote can be read in both directions. The beautiful answer can be had, by asking the beautiful question, and also a beautiful answer can lead to the next beautiful question. Both these approaches are incredibly useful to the artist and to the designer. Embracing push and pull, and the resulting possibilities, is inherent in the creative process. Non-linear thinking, rephrasing or reconstructing the question, thinking about problems in multiple ways and from myriad directions can offer us the most intriguing solutions. Viewing previous solutions and asking more questions is also a fruitful part of the process.

This may seem a departure from the way that most assistive technology (AT) is designed, chosen, and put to use. But perhaps it should not be. In earlier chapters, the necessity of considering context for providing technology and environmental intervention (TEI) for clients has been introduced. The importance of teamwork and a client-centered approach has also been broached. This author believes that artists and designers are vital parts of any well-functioning team, and important contributors to this field of endeavor. Artists and designers are good at asking questions – with less concern than many for political correctness, appropriateness, or even answerability. Some of the questions that an artist or designer on a TEI team might ask include: What are the best materials for this project? How can this device be designed so the user will know how to use it? Want to use it? Feel it is part of them? Visual practitioner designers and artists are trained to have an understanding of color and form for more than strictly functional uses, in fact sometimes in opposition to their potential functionality. We are inculcated to see intrigue and even beauty in things not normally thought of as having these attributes. Infusing the study of TEI with these perspectives can help to frame a question in a new way, lead to an unpredicted answer, or perhaps an unexpected subsequent question; and that is where innovative design begins.

The nine-dot exercise, which follows, is a classic exercise to encourage thinking outside the box:

In Figure 3.1, nine dots are arranged in a set of three rows. Try to “connect” 9 dots with four lines, *without lifting your pencil from the paper*. Each line must start where the last line finished (Dewey 2017). If you are not familiar with this problem, Google the answer when you are finished.

What did you discover about your thinking while doing this exercise?

Part two: What is design and why should we care?

When teaching a course on design to second year occupational therapy students, the author noticed that the topic itself elicited anxious glances, dismissive looks, or occasional yawns. What, after all, could design possibly have to do with their future professional lives? And more to the point, what exactly were they going to be doing in this course? A good deal of the disconnect may have been caused by approaching these students as the professor would have approached a group of art students, and they were of a very different mindset. Their education, up to this point, had been primarily practical and linear. Action x elicits response y. Many predicted that in their roles as future therapists they would be assessing clients and essentially dispensing appropriate existing solutions. They assumed that other people designed things. *Designers* (those strange and foreign elves) developed new products that medical professionals would simply put to use.

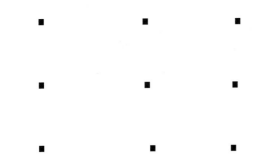
Figure 3.1 Nine dots.

Once the rationale for learning about art and design was presented in a methodical fashion, connections to their professional development started to clarify. The following is some of what we discussed.

Aesthetics matter

We like things that we perceive as attractive. The reasons for this are far beyond the scope of this chapter, but it is important to recognize that we value objects we perceive as beautiful. Ellen Dissanayake (1988) is a scholar and researcher who argues convincingly that the making and enjoying of art (or more precisely for Dissanayake, making an object, act, or event *special*) is a biological phenomenon. Dissanayake (1988) contends that the arts have biological as well as cultural and social relevance, and that it has been evolutionarily beneficial for us to engage in the practice of art.

> In neo-Darwinian terms, “What is art for?” means “Does art have selective value?” and “If so, what is (or was) this selective value?” Three characteristics of art suggest that art has had selective value.
>
> The first characteristic is that the arts are ubiquitous. Although no one art is found in every society, or to the same degree in every society, there is found universally in every human group that exists today, or is known to have existed, the tendency to the arts: dancing, singing, carving, dramatizing, decorating, poeticizing speech, image making. In evolutionary theory it is a generally accepted postulate that if a characteristic such as an anatomical feature of behavioral tendency is widely found in an animal population, there is an evolutionary reason for its persistence: it has contributed in some way to the evolutionary fitness of the members of that species.
>
> Second, we observe that in most human societies the arts are integral to many activities by individuals or groups; this also suggests that these are activities that have survival value in a Darwinian sense.
>
> Third, the arts are sources of pleasure. Nature does not generally leave advantageous behavior to chance; instead, it makes many kinds of advantageous behavior pleasurable.
>
> (Dissanayake 1988, p. 6)

Even if one doesn't recognize the evolutionary advantages of participating in the arts, we can easily recognize the desire most people have for their clothes, accessories, and the places they live and work to be attractive. People invest a lot of time, energy, and money revamping and decorating their physical and virtual contexts, including homes and yards and even their computers' desktop. Economic statistics support the idea that Americans enjoy and value decorating and dressing up their homes. According to data from the National Retail Federation (NRF), in 2011 the average person was expected to spend nearly \$47 on holiday decorations and an additional \$18 on seasonal flowers such as poinsettias (StreetStaff 2011).

Alternately, if the appearance and aesthetic value of a space is neglected, research suggests that degradation may lead to problems with morale. For example, the broken windows theory, first introduced by George L. Kelling and James Q. Wilson (1982), postulates that if an environment is in disrepair (hence the broken windows) it can increase the level of disrespect people have for the environment, leading to more broken windows and eventually a potential rise in crime. Though the demonstrable correlation between broken windows and increased criminal behavior is illusive and has been contested (Levitt and Dubner 2005), a lot of anecdotal experience pertaining to disrepair in college art studios can be offered by art faculty. If the studio is well organized, well lit, and clean at the start of the semester, it is much easier to get those using the studio to maintain it over the course of the term than if the space is a mess at the start of the semester!

When we look specifically at the use of assistive devices, it is immediately apparent that aesthetics is exceptionally important to the user. One of the most important reasons devices are abandoned is because their users perceive them as ugly or stigmatizing (Holloway and Dawes 2016; Kintsch and DePaula n.d.; Lupton 2014; Scherer 2005). (This will be discussed in greater depth in Chapters 2 and 11). Aesthetic choices are closely tied to our personal identities and are identified in the psychological rung of the Human-Tech Ladder (Vicente 2006), which is important to examine when matching a person with a TEI (Shinohara and Wobbrock 2016). (See Chapter 11 for further discussion.)

Important terminology

In order to understand some of the ways we evaluate the attractiveness or aesthetic value of an object or environment, it is important to investigate some of the terms important to artists and designers. The information in this next section is taken from the author's personal notes and the reference books cited in the Toolbox at the end of the chapter.

Unity

Unity is one of those terms that is so broad it can seem meaningless. For our purposes the term is used to mean the coordination of all parts of an object, or piece of art. A unified piece appears coherent and complete. The parts feel like they belong together. In three-dimensional work this means that you should be able to look at the piece from any angle and it will somehow feel "right."

Rhythm *(repetition, variety, proximity)*

In the piece (Figure 3.2) "Good Morning" by artist Linda Stillman, the repetition and even spacing (proximity) of coffee filters creates a dynamic image that transforms this everyday material into a dynamic composition of rhythm.

Dimensions: 28 × 28 in.
Medium: coffee filters and acrylic medium
Date: 2008
© Linda Stillman

Repetition and *variety* in forms tends to create visual rhythm. Most of us first encounter rhythm in music. For artists and designers, rhythm refers to the way forms are organized in space. *Repetition* is the use of a similar design feature or features again and again. This does not mean that everything is the same, but rather that there are some elements that are recurring in the design of the

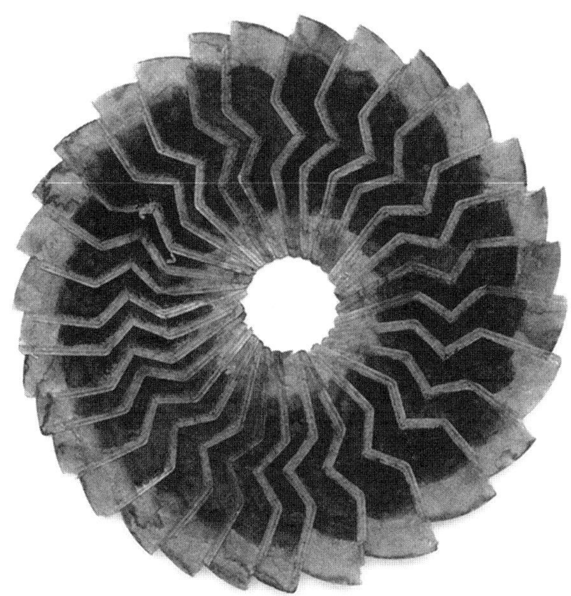

Figure 3.2 Good morning.

object. Repetition of elements tends to tie things together whether they are touching or not. *Proximity,* or how close various features are to each other, also impacts how we read the rhythm of the piece. *Variety* allows for divergence in parts of the piece. Variety can be established by creating variations in similar repeated elements, or it may be achieved by the addition of an unexpected element.

Balance *(visual weight, materiality)*

When talking about visual balance we are not assessing the physical ability of an object to stay in one place, but rather the perception that the piece is stable. A visually balanced piece is not necessarily symmetrical, but does not make us feel it is too "heavy" in any one area. Pieces exhibit a certain *visual weight*, which may or may not correspond to actual weight. Factors such as value, texture, form, size, and color effect our perception of visual weight. Materials used to construct a piece also influence our understanding of visual weight. *Materiality* is a term that can be used to help explain the way we understand the nature of materials from previous exposure and experience. If we see something that looks like granite, it is assumed to be strong, resistant to weather, and heavy. This may or may not be true, but because we have experienced these qualities in materials with similar appearances, we assume the same for our present granite-like substance. Some materials elicit positive emotional responses, others are neutral, and some are offensive and troubling to look at. This can be used to the artist's or designer's advantage. This will be discussed in greater detail later in the chapter.

The walnut table (Figure 3.3) created by artist Wayne Hall exhibits a strong sense of balance, even though the supporting legs are not identical or evenly spaced.

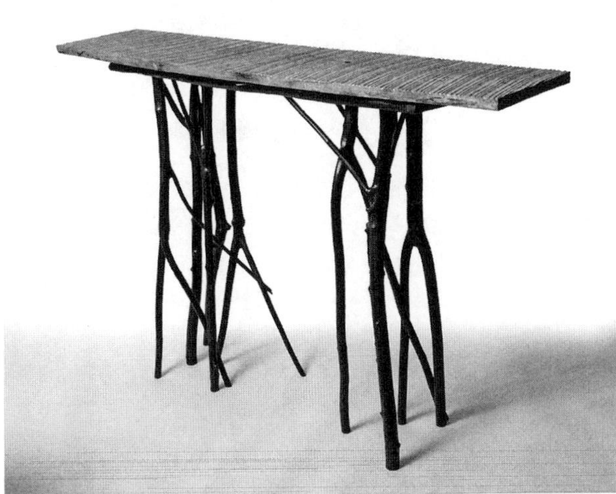

Figure 3.3 Walnut table. Source: https://upload.wikimedia.org/wikipedia/commons/c/c1/Washington_Monument_Dusk_Jan_2006.jpg. Licensed under CC BY SA 4.0.

Emphasis *(economy)*

Emphasis stresses a particular area or characteristic. One method of achieving emphasis is to make one area or quality dominant, or most important visually, with other areas contributing but subordinate. Another way to create emphasis is to employ economy. When we talk about *economy* in art or design we are usually referring to a simplification of the form or forms, limiting the viewer's focus to only a few elements.

The Washington Monument (Figure 3.4) is an example of a design that relies on the principle of *economy.*

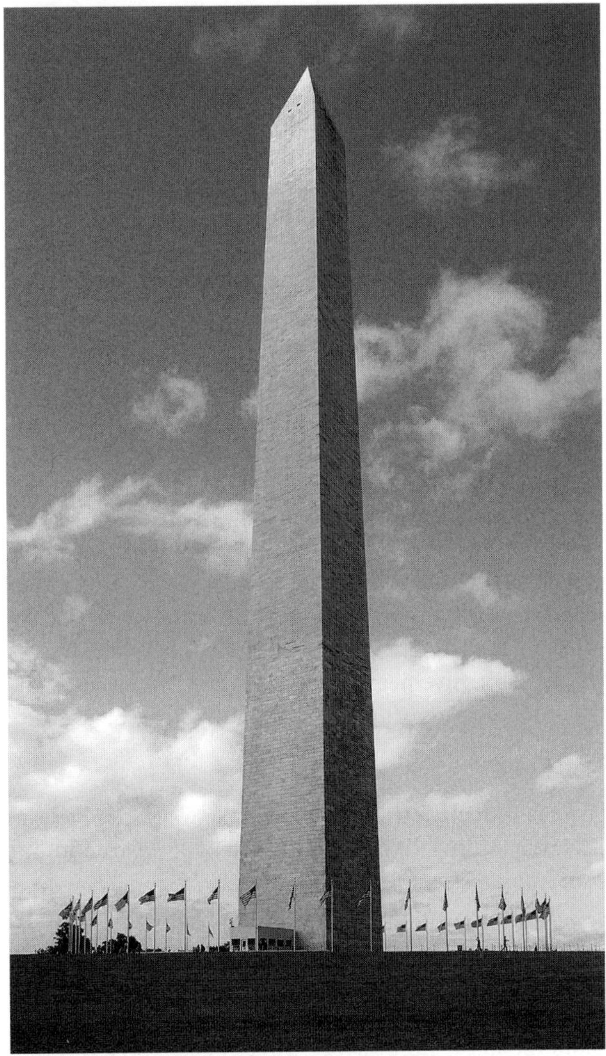

Figure 3.4 Washington Monument.

Proportion and scale

Proportion and scale are easy to confuse, but each has a distinct definition and place in our discussion of design. Proportion refers to the size relationships among parts

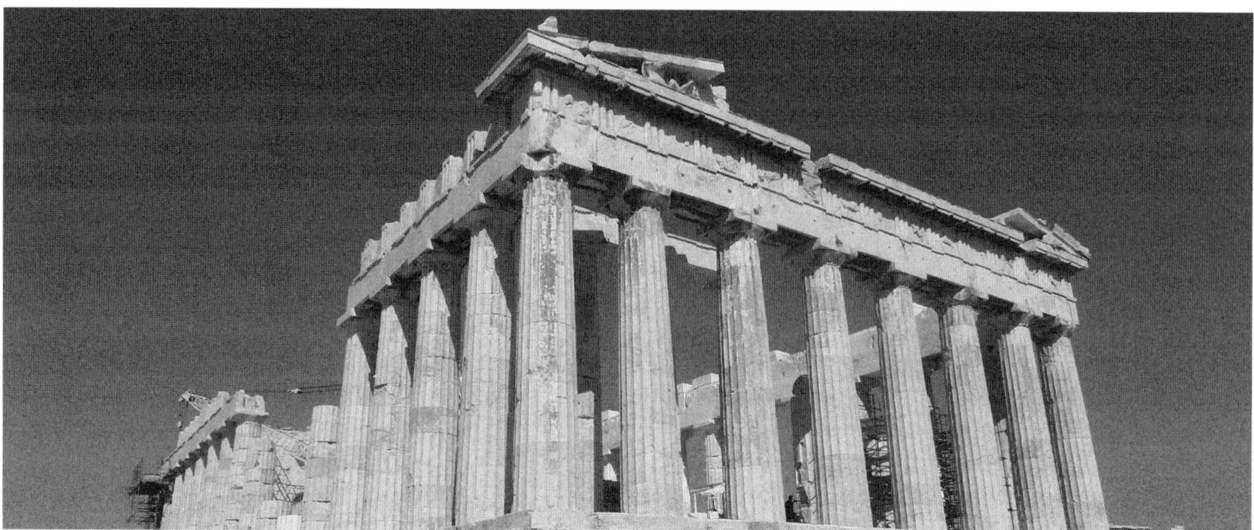

Figure 3.5 Parthenon. Source: https://en.wikipedia.org/wiki/Golden_ratio#/media/File:7234014_Parthenonas_(cropped).jpg. Licensed under CC0.

of a work. When proportions are correct, they feel right and seem satisfying to the viewer. The ancient Greeks believed that the most aesthetically perfect size relationship between two unequal parts of a whole was 1:1.61803 (Elam 2001). This ratio is called the golden section, and these proportions were thought to be the epitome of beauty.

This ratio can be found in many natural growth patterns. The golden section was used in the designing of buildings such as the Parthenon (Figure 3.5).

Proportion

Perhaps proportion is most easily understood relative to the human form. When seeing a body or face that is proportionate, one finds it attractive. If, however, the proportions seem extreme in any one element (nose, ears, eyes, etc.) it can be perceived as being humorous or disconcerting. This is why cartoonists use disproportion when rendering characters, and horror movie characters often have distinctive and disproportionate features. A clunky, obtrusive hearing aid might be perceived by the user to be disproportionate and unattractive (Figure 3.6).

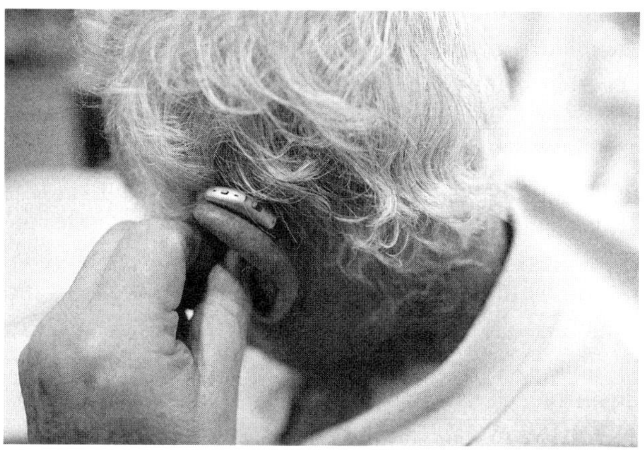

Figure 3.6 Person using hearing aid.

Scale

Scale is the relationship of the whole designed object to its surroundings. We base our idea of scale around our own human size – we judge sizes relative to our own.

Things that are much smaller than us, we deem to be miniature. Often, we think of miniature objects as being precious or childlike. Things larger than human scale are thought to be monumental. You have probably seen monumental sculptural pieces in city centers, celebrating founders or war heroes.

Color *(hue, saturation, value, texture, light)*

Artists and designers spend years studying color, learning how colors relate or interact and how to mix pigments or light to create the colors they want. Even without delving into the complex study of color, there are many things to be aware of when assessing color in design. First, it is important to understand that we all perceive color slightly differently. Not everyone sees the same intensity of color or the same range of hues (blues, greens, reds, etc.) Our ability to perceive color also changes as we age (Hooper and Dal Bello-Haas 2009).

In order to better understand how designers and artists use color in three-dimensional work, one needs to examine the three basic attributes of color: hue, saturation, and value. A truncated explanation of these characteristics is included immediately below. For additional information, please consult one or more of the sources listed in the Toolbox.

Hue is the characteristic one identifies by color names, i.e. yellow, blue, orange, etc. Variations between hues are almost infinite; a model of their relationships can be seen on the color wheel. Complimentary colors are those lying opposite each other on the color wheel: red and green, blue and orange, yellow and purple. The term complementary does not mean these colors necessarily work well together, but rather that the pigments of compliments mixed together neutralize each other. (If you mix blue and orange together, you should get a gray.) In fact, when complementary colors are paired, they usually increase the vibrancy of each other. Have you ever noticed how a red bow changes the look of a Christmas wreath? Analogous colors are close together on the color wheel, and usually can be paired harmoniously (for instance, greens and blues, yellows and oranges). With just a rudimentary awareness of how colors interact, one can begin to make more informed choices about how to use color combinations. If you want to tone down the appearance of a color it would be a mistake to pair it with its compliment!

Saturation is the most difficult attribute of color to really see and understand, since it is heavily influenced by both hue and value (definition follows). Saturation is a measure of the purity or brightness of a color, how intense a color looks.

Colors are said to be highly saturated when they are very bright. Colors of low saturation, those closer to the grays, are sometimes called neutrals. Neutral colors are often used in office and home decoration since these colors can be used with a wide variety of saturated colors without undesired clashes and contrasts. When putting their property up for sale, homeowners are often advised to paint their walls white in order to create a "clean" palette. This neutral background allows prospective buyers to imagine their furnishings in the home, no matter what color couch they may have!

Value is the third attribute, and is defined as the relative lightness or darkness of a color. If you removed all the color from an object you would be left with the value of that object. Consider how an object would look if you were to desaturate it in Photoshop (this effectively removes its hue and saturation). Value is the result of the inherent value of the object (how light or dark it actually is) combined with the available light source.

Texture can also impact our perception of value. A rough or highly textured surface will create more shadows and reflect less light than a smooth polished surface, so a polished surface will appear to have a lighter value when it is well lit. A highly textured object such as the pottery shown in (Figure 3.7a) reflects less light than an object with a smooth, shiny surface (Figure 3.7b).

The quality and direction of *light* also influences how we perceive objects and spaces. Bright, overhead fluorescent lights tend to reduce saturation and value, making forms look washed out and less texturally intriguing (Figure 3.8).

Lighting from lower angles increases drama and interest in forms, though it can reduce clarity. Natural lighting shifts with time of year, time of day, and weather patterns, and can shift the perception of colors with each of these changes.

Sometimes materials are chosen for use in a specific product or piece in part because of their inherent color. For instance, furniture makers consider the attributes of different types of wood when constructing their wares, and color is one of those factors. Color is an important

(a)

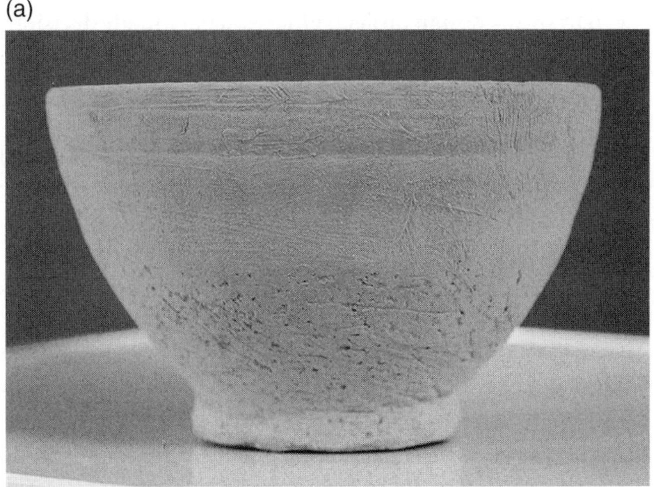

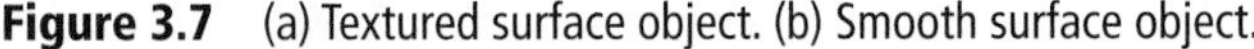

(b)

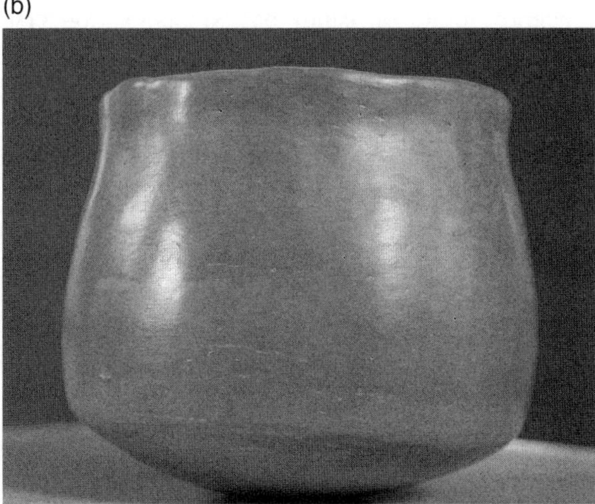

Figure 3.7 (a) Textured surface object. (b) Smooth surface object.

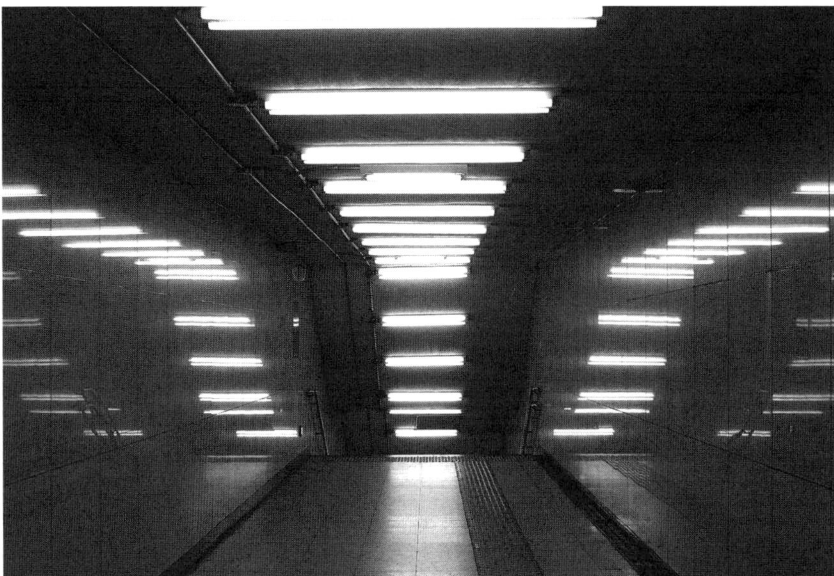

Figure 3.8 Objects under florescent lighting. Source: https://en.wikipedia.org/wiki/Fluorescent_lamp#/media/File:Fluorescent_lamps_artistic.jpg. Licensed under CCBY 2.0.

part of the materiality of a chosen medium, and it can run the gamut from beautiful and luxurious to off-putting and sterile-feeling.

Different cultures have specific associations with different colors. White is used in the west to denote purity but in China is associated with death. Colors can also be age and gender associated. Highly saturated bright colors are often used in children's toys, or in instances where the idea of youth is being marketed; bright red sports cars become oversized toys for single drivers. More subdued colors are often used for minivans and station wagons, the assumption being that owners of these vehicles are not attempting to draw attention to their identity through their vehicle (Stewart 2002).

Bright colors, perceived as being playful and fun, are frequently found on candy bar wrappers. Conversely, subdued, desaturated colors are often used to market "natural" products. Apply design concepts to your life by answering the series of questions in Box 3.1.

Apply environmental concepts to your life by answering the series of questions in Box 3.2.

Review resources in Box 3.3 to expand your knowledge about color as an element of design.

Reflect upon the various responses and "fixes" offered for the space with another classmate. At this point you can start to assess how practical these changes would be in this environment. For instance, if a classmate suggests replacing all the overhead lights with lower-wattage lamps, consider the impact on the work being done there and on a varied client population with different visual acuity. Work with fellow classmates in small groups and try to come to some kind of consensus about what changes are really important to make the environment more aesthetically pleasing and still allow for functionality. Group consensus is always difficult, but is a major part of any design project! Once you have made decisions about changes in the space that you think clients would appreciate, consider and discuss changes to the environment that would make it pleasant for them to work there.

Even if you are not designing new products, you will most likely have to help people make choices about the products they will use. For example, color is often discussed by TEI practitioners to help cue clients to pay attention to certain environmental changes such as stairs or operational buttons on devices.

There is also a good chance you will have to modify a device, or communicate with someone who will be modifying a device. Understanding some basics about aesthetics and materials and having the language to communicate with fabricators can be extremely useful. As mentioned in other Chapters (8 and 9), you can also

Box 3.1 Active learning prompt: Your environment, your decisions

Given these design concepts, we now ask you, the reader, to think about how you make decisions about what is attractive or unattractive. How does your environment impact your mood and behavior? For example, is your bedroom the same color as your other living spaces? How does your mood impact your wardrobe choices for the day?

Box 3.2 Active learning prompt: Space assessment from a visceral standpoint

Visit a facility or office where people working in their field are employed. Try not to think about working in the environment, or how equipment is set up relative to function, but rather to imagine the space as if they are a potential client who is somewhat unsure about what to expect from their experience in this place. Assess the environment in terms of color, form, and materials used. How do you feel about the space? Is it welcoming? Do you feel safe here? What kinds of materials are used in this space? Discuss the associations you have with these materials. What is the lighting like? What colors are the walls, floors, and any furnishings? Are there images (paintings, photographs, prints) on the walls? If so, what is the subject matter and what is the color palette used in these images? Do you like them? Do they feel original or mass produced? If there is a waiting area for clients, look at how the furniture is placed. Where is it facing? Are seats in rows or clusters? Try to use the terms you have learned and write an assessment of this environment.

Now make specific suggestions for how you would change the environment if it were yours to rework. Would you change the colors, lighting, or layout? Furniture? Materials? Artwork on the walls? The beautiful thing about this part of the exercise is you are not constrained by budget! You can spend as much as you want on your imaginary workspace. Bring in specific colors (gathered from magazines, paint chips, or other readily available sources) and present your ideas to the group.

Box 3.3 Additional resources for design and color elements

Banks, A., and Fraser, T. (2004). *Designer's Color Manual: A Complete Guide to Color Theory and Application.* San Francisco: Chronicle Books LLC.

Barrett, T. (2011). *Making Art: Form & Meaning.* New York: McGraw-Hill Companies, Inc.

Hornung, D. (2005). *Color: A Workshop Approach.* New York: McGraw-Hill.

discuss the concepts of universal design with fabricators and team members as you work to design products that will promote inclusion rather than stigmatize the user.

At the very least, you will be working in a space with other people. An awareness of design can help to organize this space so it is more inviting to clients and coworkers. A more comfortable client is more likely to communicate readily (Okken et al. 2013). It is important for work environments to be pleasant – especially in stressful job situations – to allow direct care workers to work comfortably. This can help prevent burnout (Gallagher 1993).

Part three: The design process – who can do it?

> To me, product design is the process of identifying, defining, solving, inventing and shaping physical solutions to the problems of living.
>
> (P. Dressler, as cited in Hannah 2004, p. 3)

This quote, from a product designer, bears similarities to descriptions TEI practitioners offer when explaining their role in the healthcare field. However, because the term *design* is often associated with the production of visual art, students in rehabilitation fields can feel inadequate, believing that they need to have special training in order to succeed in designing products or environments.

There are many examples of individuals designing incredible products, without specific training. These innovators do possess several qualities that are necessary for producing successful products: First, they have a clear understanding of the need they are addressing. As you might imagine, this means that people who need a specific piece of equipment or an environmental adaptation for their own use are often the best assessors of the design (Lupton 2014; Pullin 2009). Second, it is necessary to be conversant with materials and fabrication methods. Third, the designer must be tenacious in working through design flaws and failures, and possess a willingness to rethink and rework the product. And finally, the designer needs to understand and consider the user and their priorities both in terms of function and aesthetics.

An example of a "non-designer" creating a powerful product is John Rackley, the creator of Renegade Wheelchairs. John's story is one of innovation and perseverance to figure out how to get back to doing what he loved after a spinal cord injury: hunting. He writes on his website:

> As a wheelchair user who loves the Maine outdoors, I struggled pushing my wheelchair down paths and tote roads to get to my favorite spots. There were many times I couldn't get to where I wanted and would have to turn back.
>
> Even after a light snow, when deer hunting is at its best, I would be stuck in the house because of my inability to push the snow-filled wheels. While fishing or just going off-road, onto soft terrain would all but make it impossible for me to enjoy the outdoors.
>
> Now, after developing the Renegade All-Terrain Wheelchair (Figure 3.9), I can wheel off-road trails, through soft terrain or several inches of fluffy snow with relative ease. My hands never touch muddy or wet wheels, keeping them warm and dry.
>
> (Rackley n.d.)

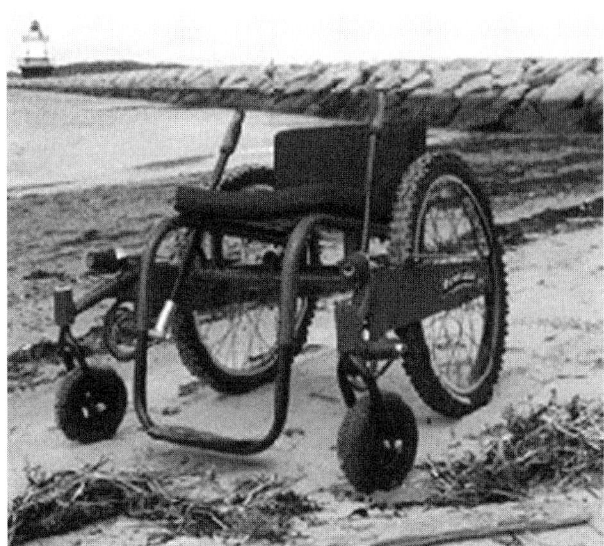

Figure 3.9 Renegade wheelchair.

John has all the attributes listed at the beginning of this section. He knew the need he wanted to address, because it was his own. He knew the terrain he would have to move through as an experienced hunter, and he had first-hand experience of the drawbacks of a conventional wheelchair in this landscape. He was already a skilled welder, familiar with bicycle construction, and clearly a tenacious and dedicated worker. He also knew the hunting culture in Maine, aesthetic preferences of his peers, and the most important functional aspects of his Renegade Chair.

Fortunately for the rest of us, we don't need to possess all these qualities. Designers often work in teams, and with good reason. (See Chapters 8 and 9 for more about the team process.) Each member of the team can bring important insights to the project. Even if there is only one designer actively working on a project, consultations should always be part of the design process. Vicente (2006) highlights the importance of teams in his Human-Tech Ladder. This author would encourage all teams looking at issues of accessibility to include at least one artist in their process.

Graham Pullin (2009) devotes much of his book *Design Meets Disability* to advocating a shift in the current paradigm used for product design, specifically the inclusion of designers.

> Traditionally, design for disability has paid more attention to the clinical than the cultural diversity within any group. The same prosthesis, wheelchairs and communication devices are often offered to people with a particular disability, whether they are seventeen or seventy years old, and regardless of their attitudes, toward their disability or otherwise. And does inclusive design, in its aspiration to be universal, risk stereotyping everybody? Meanwhile, mainstream design, whatever its other shortcomings, is devoting more effort to a richer understanding of people.
>
> (Pullin 2009, pp. 89–90)

Part four: The design process – getting started

If you have never designed anything before, it can be difficult to know where to begin. In her guide for studio foundations courses, Stewart (2002) outlined four questions to ask when beginning a new project:

1. What is required?
2. What existing designs are similar to the required design?
3. What is the difference between these designs and the required design?
4. How can we transform, combine, or expand these existing designs?

(Pullin 2009)

Asking questions is a potent way to start the process. Following the logic of E.E. Cummings, one sees they may not lead us in a straight line, but rather backwards and forward, and most likely to a whole slew of new questions. It is important to note that these questions and steps can also be utilized by people who are assessing designed objects or who may need to adapt already existing products or environments.

Based on our collective experience teaching design, a colleague and the author compiled the following sections for navigating the process of product design.

Identification of need/creation of the team

At this phase, the specific need is identified and researched, through investigating both published information and interviews. This is a very open and fluid part of the process. Ask the question, rephrase the question; ask others to rephrase the question. Look at existing solutions for this particular need or similar needs. It is important to be open to input from a variety of sources, and not to latch onto one potential solution too quickly.

At this time a team of people should be established, ideally including a potential consumer and a designer. In the case of AT or TEI, other team members can be rehabilitation therapists, other health professionals, engineers, caregivers, and equipment vendors, to name a few. Potential consultants should be lined up.

Goals and directions

In response to the research, specific goals are outlined and refined. Roles and responsibilities are divided

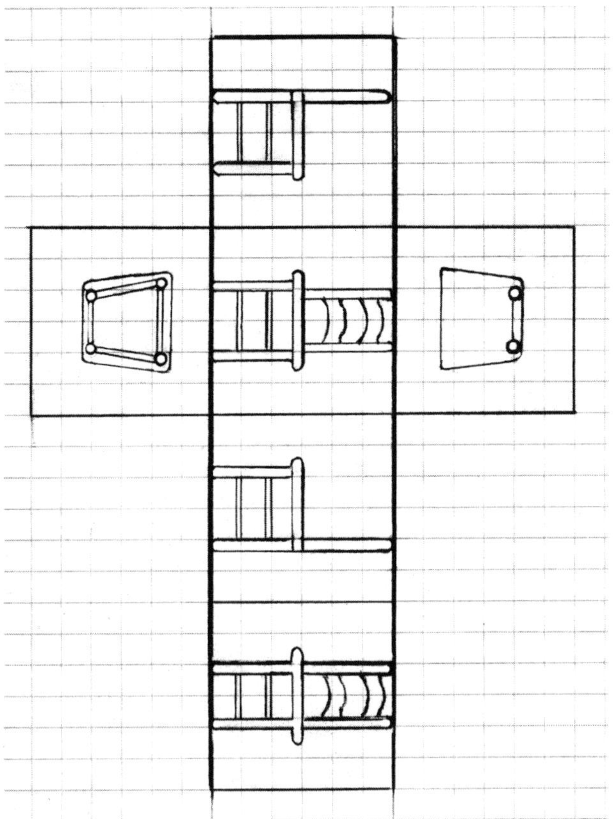

Figure 3.10 Orthographic drawing.

among the team. It is never a bad idea to have some duplication if your team is large enough! Sketches and orthographic drawings should be made at this point. Orthographic drawings (Figure 3.10) are a set of related views of a proposed object.

If you imagine your object enclosed in a transparent box and draw the views that you would see from the top, bottom, and each of the four sides, you will have created a complete set of orthographic drawings. These drawings are plans that do not attempt to create an illusion of depth, as one might do with sketches. Instead they accurately depict to scale a plan for each portion of the object. For this reason, orthographic projections are frequently done on graph paper. Ching (1998) has provided an in-depth explanation of this pictorial system, which can help to elucidate the process for those interested in communicating design ideas.

Try to make specific lists that itemize each task that lies ahead.

Experimentation/exploration with materials and methods

This is a part of the process where you need someone familiar with a wide range of materials, methods of fabrication, and *materiality*. Remember the term *materiality* is being used as the way we assess and understand materials – whether or not that understanding is based in fact.

Donald A. Norman (1988), who has written pivotal texts on how we understand the designed world, uses the term *affordance* when he discusses our perceptions of materials and our expectations of how particular common design forms function. He offers a potent illustration of our perception of materials in the following case where the British Rail system attempted to reduce graffiti on the walls of shelters where patrons waited for the train. They attempted to decrease defacing of the shelters by putting up glass panels:

> In one case the reinforced glass used to panel shelters (for railroad passengers) erected by British Rail was smashed by vandals as fast as it was renewed. When the reinforced glass was replaced by plywood boarding, however, little further damage occurred, although no extra force would have been required to produce it … Glass is for seeing through and for breaking. Wood is normally used for solidity, opacity, support or carving. Flat, porous, smooth surfaces are for writing on. So wood is also for writing on. Hence the problem for British Rail: when the shelters had glass, vandals smashed it; when they had plywood, vandals wrote on and carved it. The planners were trapped by the affordances of the materials.
>
> (Norman 1988, p. 9)

Norman also discusses how we as designers can use affordances to our advantage.

> Affordances provide strong clues to the operation of things. Plates are for pushing. Knobs are for turning. Slots are for inserting things into. Balls are for throwing or bouncing. When affordances are taken advantage of, the user knows what to do just by looking: no picture, label, or instruction is required. Complex things may require explanation, but simple things should not. When simple things need pictures, labels or instructions, the design has failed.
>
> (Norman 1988, p. 9)

Based on the goals and directions established by your team, the experiments with materials and production methods can begin. It may be that you can use any materials or processes you choose, but often there are financial restrictions as well as limits on the complexity of the production process.

It is important to remember at the initial stage that high-tech solutions are not always the best. It is tempting to believe that science and technology can solve our problems, and indeed there have been a lot of wonderful developments, especially in the area of communications. However, high tech often means that when something fails there is a far more specialized process needed for repairs or revisions.

> Christopher Frayling, rector of the Royal College of Art, says that one big issue with design students is that technical constraints and technical possibilities can all too often be allowed to dominate. We should be as skeptical about doing things just because they are possible as we are ambitious about achieving difficult but desirable ends. It is time to stop letting the technology "push us around," observes Frayling, "Let's bring the users in and let's bring delight back into everyday products, because it seems to have gone."
>
> (Pullin 2009, p. 75)

Prototype development

This phase is closely linked to the previous process of material and methods investigation, and the two often overlap as designers make changes and revisions. It is helpful at this point to create a scale model of the object. The materials used should approximate those that are being considered for the final project. This portion of the planning phase can reveal problems with the design that are not apparent in two dimensions. Competent designers and architects have long understood the value of this practice, as Leon Battista Alberti indicated in 1452 in the fundamental architectural treatise *De re aedificatoria*:

> As far as I'm concerned, I must say that very frequently I conceived a project which, at first, seemed to me full of merit, but which once sketched proved to contain errors, serious errors, in the very sections that I liked best; rethinking what I had conceived, and measuring again the proportions, I would now recognize and deplore my carelessness; finally, after building a model, I would often find, upon examining the different elements, that I had even made a mistake in their number.
>
> (Alberti cited in Manguel 2000, p. 228)

After responses to the scale model have been evaluated, a full-scale prototype should be constructed, using the intended material. At this point, fabrication methods may be reconsidered, and materials adopted or abandoned. It is not uncommon to have to revisit an earlier part of the process at this point.

Testing the prototype

Once a prototype has been successfully constructed, it is time to show it around! It is important to make sure at this point that you have a variety of people use the product and that you listen carefully to their feedback. More modifications are likely to be needed at this point. It is critical to include people with the need that inspired the design and others in situations that might also appreciate the design. It is important to get feedback from people of different age, gender, financial status, and cultural background whenever possible. Pullin (2009) describes his vision for approaching a product that not only takes these variables into consideration, but also embraces them.

> I would like to propose the term *resonant design* for a design intended to address the needs of some people with a particular disability and other people without that disability but perhaps finding themselves in particular circumstances. So, this is neither design just for able-bodied people nor design for the whole population; nor even does it assume that everyone with a particular disability will have the same needs. It is something between these extremes, not as a compromise, but as a fundamental aspiration. To appeal to both groups, such design would also need to embody the design quality which mainstream market demands.
>
> (Pullin 2009, p. 93)

It is also vital that you conduct durability tests if the product is intended to last for a specific period of time. We have all seen the car commercials where the sports car is driven at high speeds down steep mountainous roads, or where a truck pulls a heavy object up an unfathomably steep incline. Though one suspects the creators of these commercials took liberties with the imagery they show us, it does bring home the point that you need to test your new product in harsher environments than those in which you imagine it will be used.

Investigating the assumptions users make and the actions they take when dealing with the prototype is also an important step in this process. Norman (1988) called our assumptions about how a product works the *conceptual model*. Conceptual models are developed by our observations of visual cues and reading of cause and effect. We press a button and a door opens, so we understand that the button causes the door to open. This may or may not be true. Perhaps the door opened coincidentally; nevertheless, we have a conceptual model that has been established, until it fails to work. It is important that the designer's conceptual model (the way he or she understands the object to function) is made easily understandable for the user. If the user has a different (inaccurate) conceptual model of the way a device functions, it may result in difficulty using the object.

> A good conceptual model allows us to predict the effects of our actions. Without a good model we operate by rote, blindly; we do operations as we were told to do them; we

> can't fully appreciate why, what effects to expect, or what to do if things go wrong. As long as things work properly, we can manage. When things go wrong, however, or when we come upon a novel situation, then we need a deeper understanding, a good model.
>
> (Norman 1988, pp. 13–14)

Norman believes that by keeping things simple and providing good feedback the user's actions can make design much better. (For more on conceptual models in this context it is beneficial to read the complete text of the *Design of Everyday Things*; Norman 1988).

Dissemination/marketing

If you are making or adapting a single product for an individual, the process is complete after your testing, consultations, and final revisions have been made. Marketing a product is beyond the scope of this text, but would certainly require that members of your team be experienced with this type of process.

Part five: A design case study

A professor and practicing occupational therapist returned from Ecuador, where she worked as a volunteer for a non-profit organization focused on getting people with disabilities the assistive devices that they need to be able to engage in their communities. One of the things she found frustrating was the lack of good seating and positioning devices for individuals who use wheelchairs who would benefit from them. The expensive adaptations used in the United States were not available or affordable options for the people with whom she was working. She saw people using foam cut out of abandoned car seats and some adaptations that were made from cardboard or melted PVC pipe for seating and positioning devices, but no solutions that were particularly successful, local, sustainable, or cost-effective.

While we discussed the situation, the therapist showed me some of the treasures she and her husband had brought back from their trip. One of these objects was a felted poncho. It seemed to me, as an artist with a strong materials background, that this felted garment offered a potential solution.

Felting is an ancient practice of matting together animal fibers (usually wool) to form an unwoven fabric that can be weather resistant and strong (Laufer 1930). Created by subjecting the fibers to water, heat, and agitation, this material has been used by many cultures for clothing, footwear, and even yurts or tents. Some of you may have accidentally replicated parts of this process by allowing a woolen sweater to go through the washing machine with warm water. Felt is commercially produced and used for a wide variety of products, particularly for sound deadening, wall covering, or padding (New World Encyclopedia 2013). Automotive manufacturers use felt in various parts of vehicles to minimize noise. Rug pads, wall padding, or any other area that needs physical softening are places where you might see felt used.

I declared the use of felt an easy solution to the issue, but soon learned there was nothing easy about it and in the course of this project came to hold a much greater appreciation for the practice of product development. Despite the hubris exhibited in my assertion, that felt was the solution, I knew from the start that I did not have all the skills or experience to complete this project on my own. I needed to form a team. I needed someone in the group to help me understand what was necessary from a therapeutic point of view, and also to give me insight into the local culture where the product would ideally be used. I also wanted to bring someone skilled in felting into the project, and I found such a collaborator in a fiber artist.

The team decided that since none of us had ever approached a project quite like this, we would map out the process as we thought it should unfold and set specific guidelines and deadlines. This is when we created the sections outlined in "Identification of Need/ Creation of the Team" through "Dissemination/ Marketing," above. I have included some of our experiences with the process in order to try to offer a picture of what can happen in the design process.

Identification of need

This was the impetus for the project, as outlined by the occupational therapist after her trips to Ecuador. We wanted to address the need for affordable, functional, local, and sustainable seating/positioning devices that ideally could be made on site by local individuals, perhaps even by the individuals who needed the devices. We were also concerned with the impact of any processes on the health of the fabricators and the quality of the environment – their current method of fabricating with melted PVC can be quite toxic. One of the things we were immediately cognizant of was the choice of materials that were currently in use, and the message sent by these materials. Not only were they unsatisfactory in terms of functionality, they were materially off-putting. What kind of message do you convey to a person who needs an assistive device if you make it out of something unattractive like PVC or an obvious, unconcealed waste product like an old automobile seat? As mentioned earlier in the chapter, aesthetics needed to be a part of the conversation. The core team lined up consultations with local suppliers and fabricators of seating devices.

Goals and directions

These are the goals we outlined:

1. The general exploration of low-tech processes that could be mirrored using various naturally occurring or common indigenous materials, with an emphasis on developing one prototype or series of devices that meet a range of medical needs.
   More specifically, we want to start by researching current hi-tech medical positioning devices, and then designing similar devices that combine up-to-date medical technology with indigenous materials and skills. We are aiming to develop a versatile and well-targeted prototype device that could be replicated and adapted to individual and regional needs.
2. We would like to support social entrepreneurship, involving an internal economic structure that would allow indigenous communities to utilize these technologies.
3. We would like to support the use of recyclable, non-toxic, and sustainable materials and processes. Through efficiency of design, and economy of materials, we aim to develop devices that will allow individuals to live well without harming their environment or themselves.
4. We would like our product to be attractive, and able to be personalized with various colors and patterns.
5. We would like to emphasize collaboration and flexibility across fields of research, in order to achieve the necessary expertise.
6. The product of this research would ideally be a prototype package developed for a case study region.

In looking back on these goals now, a member of the team observed:

> It was important to have a big picture to start with. We needed these goals to be lofty in order to understand the specific things we were making, because we needed to understand the context within which we were working. I feel like those things all came into play as we were manifesting this device in the world. This is in line with any art making I have done, whether the goal was to make a functional object or not. You start out with a concept and you know it's going to be significantly transformed. That's what keeps it interesting.

Experimentation/exploration with materials and methods

Through our meetings with consultants and research into existing seating devices we decided to base our design on the ROHO® cushion. (See https://permobilus.com for information about these devices.)

The ROHO cushion is designed with rows of pods that can be independently inflated creating individualized support. It is a comfortable, effective seating device. The cost of these cushions is more than £300 and so out of reach for people in Ecuador. In retrospect we probably limited our thinking to some degree by trying to replicate the design with other materials, but it gave us a good springboard. At this point we decided that we would pursue a cushion, like the ROHO, made of rows of pod-like forms. Though, when first introduced to the challenge, I had proclaimed felted material to be the obvious solution, we realized that we should not limit our investigation to one material at an early phase of the project. We began our research by looking at many different kinds of products already being manufactured or already accessible to the local population. We were especially intrigued with the idea of using by-products, so looked at local manufacturing and what could be found in the waste stream.

Our most promising experiment was using plastic bags from the waste stream as potential filling for the pods of our cushioning device. We discovered that by crocheting the plastic it could create a stronger more supportive substance, though it ultimately proved too easy to compress when we tested it. (Yes, we sat on it for long periods of time.)

After a good deal of testing and experiments with materials, we concluded that felting would likely be our best avenue of exploration. Wool is readily available in much of Ecuador; it has natural antimicrobial properties and can be washed if it gets soiled. Importantly, the people in this region were already skilled in the felting process and had the ability to make aesthetically pleasing things from this material. An example of the ROHO cushion is provided in Figure 3.11.

We hoped to develop a method of creating dense, buoyant pods out of felt that would then be adhered to,

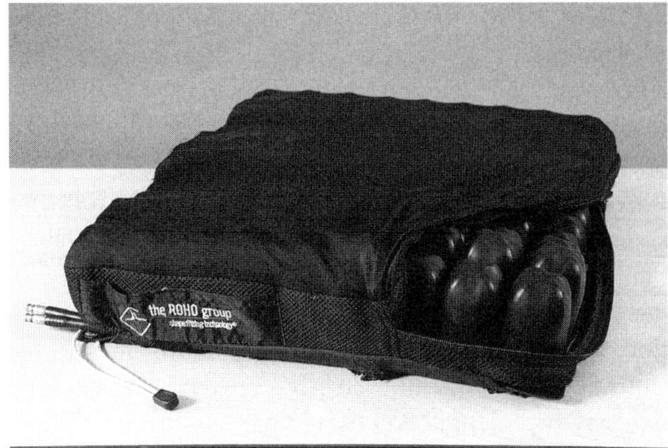

Figure 3.11 ROHO cushion.

or inserted into, the cushion support. It was important for the individual pods to be removable and modifiable so that wear, change in need, or accidental damage would not necessitate the replacement of the entire cushion. What we thought would be a simple transformation of the ROHO-style cushion to a felted design was not working well.

We spent a lot of time on the fabrication process, because ultimately, we did not want to produce cushions, but rather a prototype and process to be examined and then, we hoped, adopted and improved upon by the people in Ecuador. We looked to traditional felting procedures and learned from them. Our fiber artist made a simple tumbler from a plastic bucket to reduce some of the physical work of the felting and to enable the creation of multiple pods at one time. Our experiments were enjoyable, but failed to produce a pod that was dense enough to remain firm when we sat on it for long periods of time.

Having tried all of the low-tech ways to make pods we could conceive of, we realized that pods were not really what we needed. We were making the process more difficult than it should be! We decided to simplify the process and make felt in the most basic form – a sheet – and then cut and roll portions of the sheet into cylinders. These could be needle felted together and the surfaces cut to contour the body of the individual user. Needle felting is a process that uses dry fiber. Handheld needles or tools with multiple needles are repeatedly jabbed into the fiber. This action tangles and compacts the fibers and allows the formation of three-dimensional felted forms (Davis 2009). With this method we could produce the individual pieces more quickly and achieve a denser material. This process is very simple and has an easy learning curve, so could be applicable to people without previous felting experience, or with some limits in dexterity. Examples of the felting process are provided in Figures 3.12a–c.

Figures 3.12a and b show the process of placing alternating layers of wool in a large sheet. The felting process begins by agitating the fibers between sheets of burlap, using hot water and soap.

Figures 3.13a–c show rolled sheets of felted material. These were subjected to hot water and agitation in a conventional washing machine. This step can also be done by hand. Figure 3.14 displays additional steps in felting.

Prototype development

In many ways this step was integrated into the previous step with this particular project. The actual making of the cushion was quite simple, even for a novice felter such as myself, and seemed exceptionally quick after all our time spent experimenting.

Testing the prototype

Two of the team members have been using our cushion for some time now and find it to hold up well in our initial tests. We have also discussed the fact that this process could be valuable for creating cushions for home use and perhaps contoured pads for things like baby changing tables. We are at the point in the process where we need to make two or three more prototypes and send them off to Ecuador in order to solicit feedback, and make potential improvements in both the process and product. We are hopeful that will happen this upcoming summer.

Dissemination/marketing

Though we have no plans to market this procedure as a product in a traditional sense, we would like to have our research disseminated to others who might find it useful. Thus it's inclusion in this text.

The core team members were surprised by all the failures we endured before we got back to the rule of thumb: use the simplest process you can. It was not a linear execution of the idea, but the creative process never is.

Summary

In summary there are several key points to review.

- How things are designed affects us every day. Choices are made for us about our designed environment without us really taking notice. When we do start to pay attention, it is amazing how much good and bad design we can see. As therapists it is important to try to understand how assistive devices function and how they look to each of your clients.
- Aesthetics matter! Our feelings about the technology we use are influenced by how those things look. Client preferences may be very different and a lack of nuanced attention to their preferences may lead to abandoning of assistive devices.
- Communication and teamwork are essential in assessing needs for individuals, and creating viable solutions. The design process, which includes choosing and adapting existing designed objects, should be a group process.
- Hopefully, by learning about some of the key elements considered in any design, and glimpsing how a new product might be developed, you will be more attuned to the environment around you and assistive devices you encounter. Most importantly, when considering design, be sure to ask questions, ask your clients, ask your friends, and ask people in other fields, it can lead to a beautiful answer, or a beautiful question.

Medical Assistive Cushion

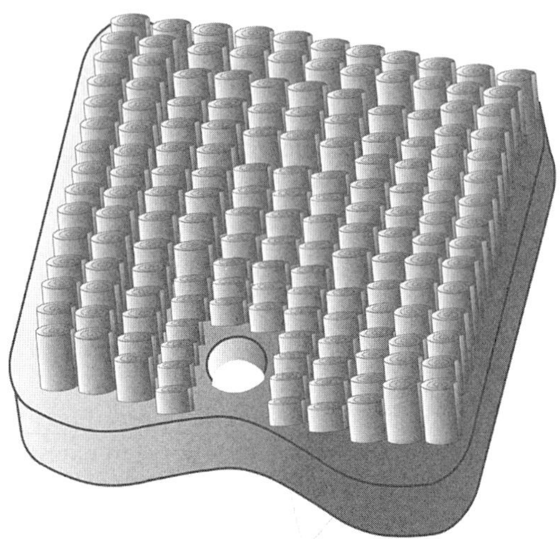

varying, interchangeable units allow for customization of cushion contours

high-density felt cylinders provide continuous, long-lasting support

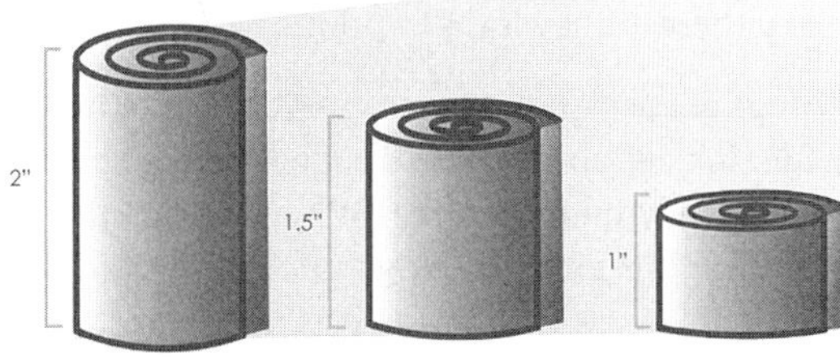

Cylinders are made from cutting a sheet of handmade, high-density felt into strips, then binding or needle-felting the strips into spiraled cylinders.

Cover

Dimensions:
Approx. 24"L x 24"-30"W x 6" thick

Purpose: Containment of interior structures, skin comfort

Materials: Soft, sturdy fabric that does not irritate skin, but is easily cleaned/semi moisture/mold resistant- wool, cotton, silk, linen, or possibly moisture-sealed paper yarn

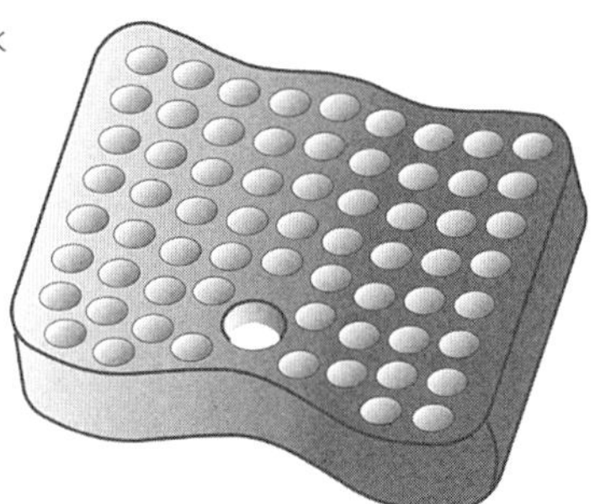

Felt Cylinders

Dimensions:
Units range between 1-2"h x 1.5"diam.

Purpose:
Interchangeable/adjustable to individual needs. Each unit can be arranged or replaced to support or relieve specific pressure points.

Materials: Various felted fibers, according to availability.

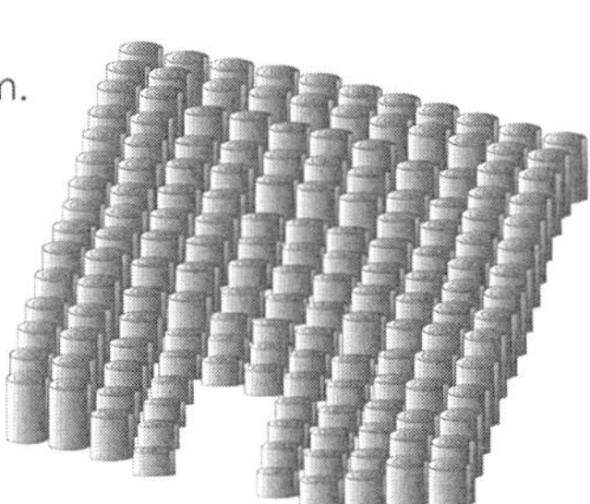

Cushion Blanket

Dimensions:
24"L x 24"-30"W x 1/2-1" thick

Purpose: additional cushioning, but also a matrix to help hold units in place

Possible Materials:
Wool felt, recycled denim felt, or soft woven or knit fabric with high pile/loft, crocheted paper yarn.

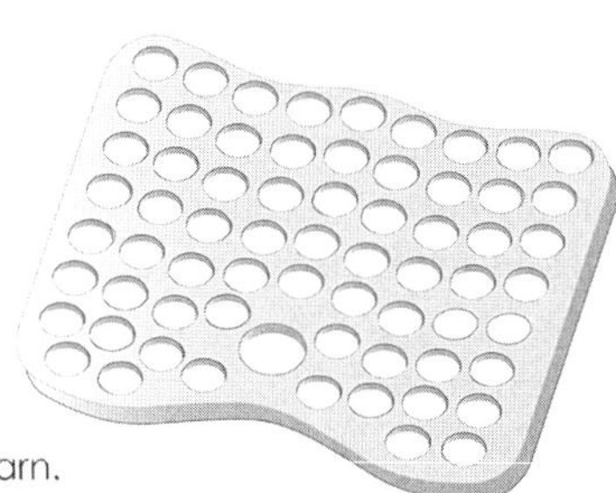

Base Structure

Dimensions:
Approx. 24"L x 24"-30"W x 3" thick

Purpose: Semi-rigid base support, holds cushion in place.

Possible Materials:
sealed paper mache or cardboard, papercrete, woven hemp, reeds, bamboo, lacqured wool

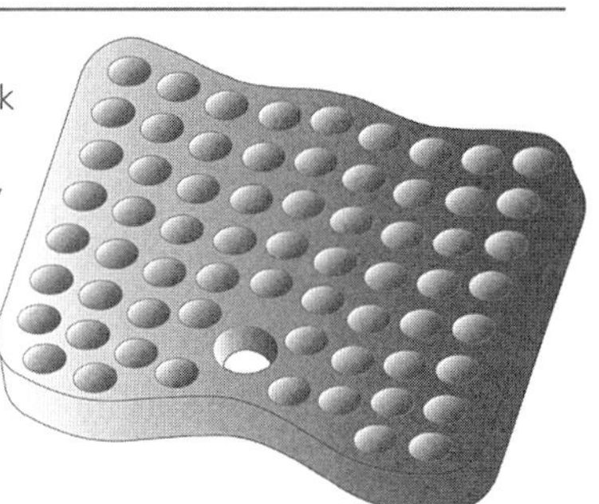

Figure 3.12 Cushion prototype.

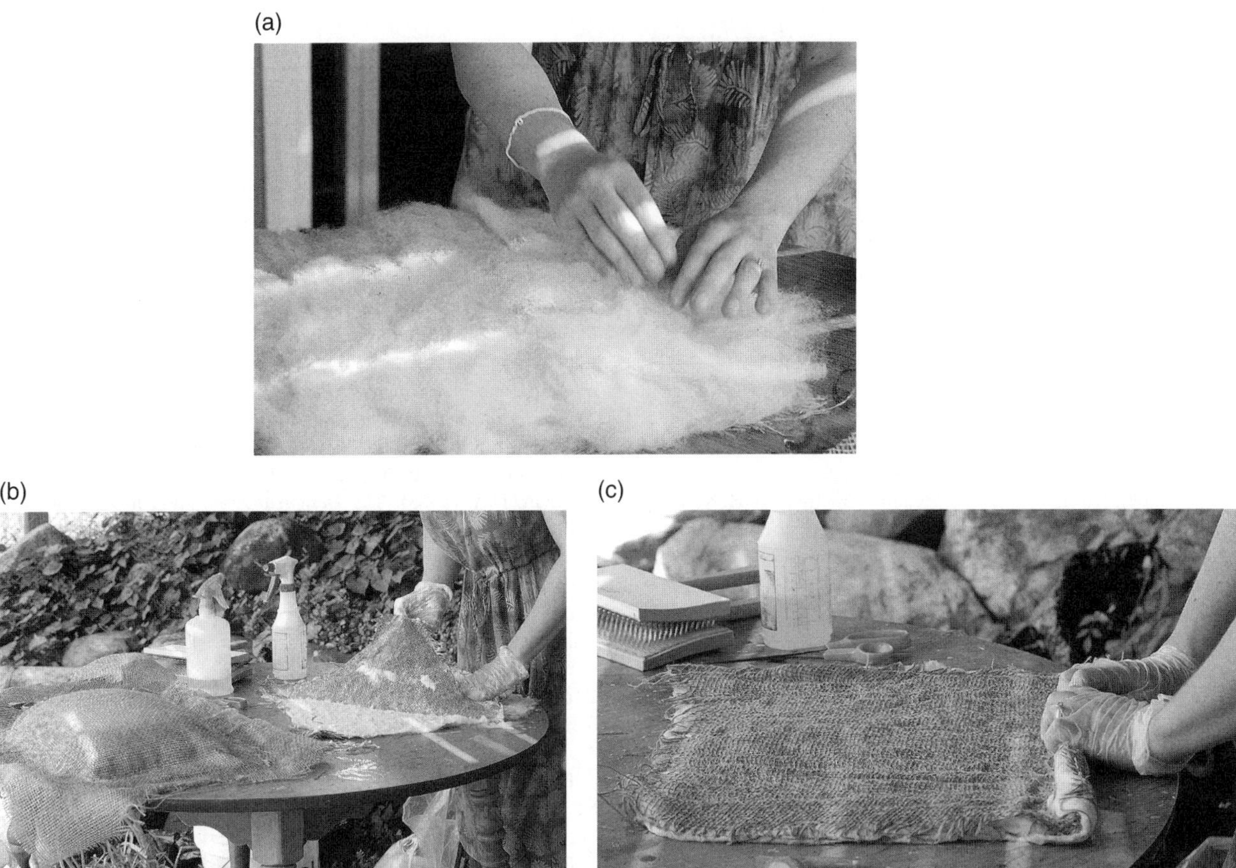

Figure 3.13 (a) The felting process. (b) The felting process continued. (c) Felting through agitation.

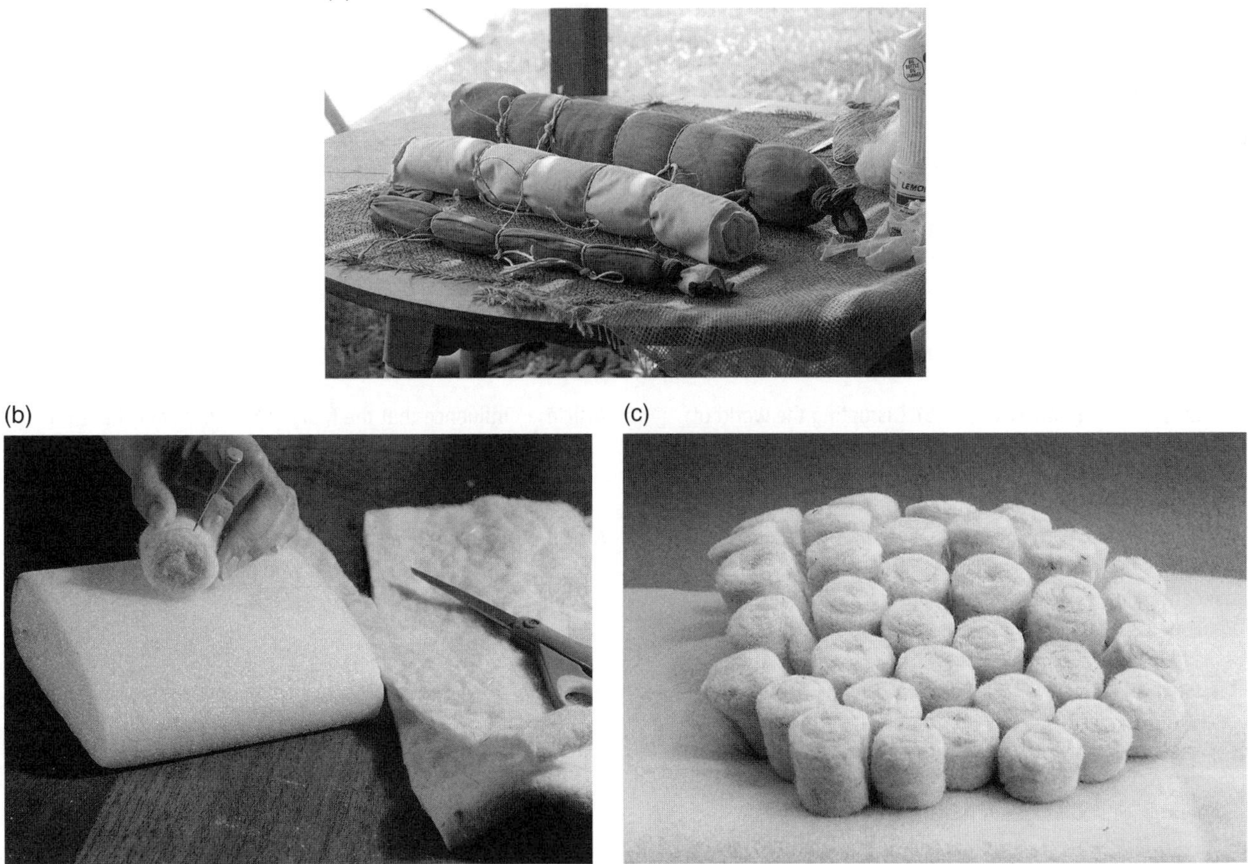

Figure 3.14 (a) Rolled sheets of felted material. (b) Needle used to create a cylindrical shape. (c) Completed conical forms cut to various heights to create the cushion.

- Finally, as rapid prototyping technologies (e.g. 3D printers, CAD programs, open-source hardware and software, and more) become more ubiquitous, interdisciplinary teams of users, practitioners, and others are coming up with AT solutions that meet the needs of individuals. Please refer to the Toolbox for information about the AT Maker Movement.

References

Ching, F. (1998). *Design Drawing*. New York: Wiley.

Davis, J. (2009). *Felting: The Complete Guide*. Cincinnati, OH: Krause.

Dewey, R. (2017). Problem solving in psychology: an introduction. Retrieved from http://www.psywww.com/intropsych/ch07-cognition/problem-solving.html.

Dissanayake, E. (1988). *What is Art for?* Seattle, WA: University of Washington Press.

Elam, K. (2001). *Geometry of Design*. New York: Princeton Architectural Press.

Gallagher, W. (1993). *The Power of Place: How Our Surroundings Shape Our Thoughts, Emotions, and Actions*. New York: Poseidon Press.

Hannah, B. (2004). *Becoming a Product Designer: A Guide to Careers in Design*. Hoboken, NJ: Wiley.

Holloway, C. and Dawes, H. (2016). Disrupting the world of disability: the next generation of assistive technologies and rehabilitation practices. *Healthcare Technology Letters* 3 (4): 254–256. https://doi.org/10.1049/htl.2016.0087.

Hooper, C.R. and Dal Bello-Haas, V. (2009). Sensory function. In: *Functional Performance in Older Adults*, 3e (ed. B. Bonder and V.D. Bello-Haas), 101–121. Philadelphia: F. A. Davis.

Kelling, G.L. and Wilson, J.Q. (1982). Broken windows: the police and neighborhood safety. *The Atlantic* (March). Retrieved from http://www.theatlantic.com/magazine/archive/1982/03/broken-windows/304465.

Kintsch, A. and DePaula, R. (n.d.). A framework for the adoption of assistive technology. Retrieved from http://citeseerx.ist.psu.edu/viewdoc/download?doi=10.1.1.124.3726&rep=rep1&type=pdf.

Laufer, B. (1930). The early history of felt. *American Anthropologist* 32 (1): 1–18.

Levitt, S.D. and Dubner, S.J. (2005). *Freakonomics: A Rogue Economist Explores the Hidden Side of Everything*. New York: Harper Perennial.

Lupton, E. (2014). *Beautiful Users: Designing for People*. New York: Princeton Architectural Press.

Manguel, A. (2000). *Reading Pictures: What We Think About When We Look at Art*. New York: Random House.

New World Encyclopedia (2013). Felt. Retrieved from http://www.newworldencyclopedia.org/entry/Felt#Uses_of_felt.

Norman, D.A. (1988). *The Design of Everyday Things*. New York: Perseus Press.

Okken, V., Rompay, T.V., and Pruyn, A. (2013). Room to move: on spatial constraints and self-disclosure during intimate conversations. *Environment and Behavior* 4 (6): 737–760.

Pullin, G. (2009). *Design Meets Disability*. Cambridge, MA: MIT Press.

Rackley, J.W. (n.d.). The story of renegade. No longer available.

Scherer, M. (2005). *Living in a State of Stuck: How Assistive Technology Impacts the Lives of People with Disabilities*, 4e. Cambridge, MA: Brookline Books.

Scinto, M. (2011). Americans are spending a whopping $6 billion on christmas decorations this year. *Business Insider* (7 December). Retrieved from https://www.businessinsider.com/americans-are-spending-a-record-6-billion-on-christmas-decorations-2011-12.

Shinohara, K. and Wobbrock, J.O. (2016). Self-conscious or self-confident? A diary study conceptualizing the social accessibility of assistive technology. Retrieved from https://faculty.washington.edu/wobbrock/pubs/taccess-16.pdf.

Stewart, M. (2002). *Launching the Imagination: Three-Dimensional Design*. New York: McGraw-Hill.

Vicente, K. (2006). *The Human Factor: Revolutionizing the Way People Live with Technology*. New York: Routledge, Taylor & Francis Group.

Toolbox: AT maker movement

Buehler, E., Branham, E., Ali, A., Chang, J., Hofmann, M., Hurst, A., and Kane, S. (2015). Sharing is caring: assistive technology designs on Thingiverse. *CHI 2015: Extended abstracts publication of the 33rd Annual CHI Conference on Human Factors in Computing Systems*: April 18–23, 2015, Seoul, Republic of Korea.	Article	Describes the variety of AT designs on Thingiverse since 2008.
Holloway, C., and Dawes, H. (2016). Disrupting the world of disability: the next generation of assistive technologies and rehabilitation practices. *Healthcare Technology Letters* 3(4): 254–256. doi:10.1049/htl.2016.0087	Article	Influence that the Maker Movement may have on increasing access to AT – good references.
Hook, J., Verbann, S., Durrant, A., Oliver, P., and Wright, P. (2014). A study of the challenges related to DIY assistive technology in the context of children with disabilities. *DIS '14*, June 21–26, Vancouver, BC, Canada. Retrieved from http://eprints.whiterose.ac.uk/87615/1/p597_hook.pdf	Article	A qualitative study investigating challenges of getting AT to children who need it, including DIY AT.
Meissner, J. L., Vines, J., McLaughlin. J., Nappe, T., Maksimova, J., and Wright, P. (2017). Do-it-yourself empowerment as experienced by novice makers with disabilities. *Proceedings of the 2017 Conference on Designing Interactive Systems*, Edinburgh, United Kingdom: ACM.	Article	Discusses the importance of empowerment

Willkomm, T. (2013). *Assistive Technology Solutions in Minutes, Book II: Ordinary Items, Extraordinary Solutions.* Durham, NH: University of New Hampshire, Institute on Disability.	Book	Described as the MacGyver of AT, Dr. Willkomm's books are a must-have for any DIY ATer.
Willkomm, T. (2005). *Assistive Technology Solutions in Minutes: Make a Difference.* Durham, NH: ATTech Services.	Book	The first Dr. Willkomm book.
Smith, B.A. (2012). *The Recycling Therapist: Hundreds of Simple Therapy Materials You Can Make*, 2e. Framingham, MA: Therapro.	Book	Excellent resource for low-tech items.
Press, M. (2005). *PVC Project Book*, 2e. Short Hills, NJ: Burford Books.	Book	DIY projects made from PVC.
Packer, B. (1989). *Digitised 2013. Appropriate Paper-Based Technology (APT): A Manual.* Harare, Zimbabwe: Practical Action Publishing Ltd.	Book	Using paper-based materials to make AT.
Campbell, M., and Truesdell, A. (2000). *Creative Constructions: Technologies that Make Adaptive Design Accessible, Affordable, Inclusive, and Fun.* Cambridge, MA: Creative Constructions.	Book	Paper and other materials to make custom designed AT solutions.
http://atmakers.org	website	This website introduces Makers and AT users and gives these two communities the tools they need to collaborate.
www.DIYAbility.org	website	The goal of DIYAbility is to create a community for people who believe that technology is world opening. The tools and software available today can let anyone implement and make their own devices and make almost anything else. It is not just about AT and all that orthopedic-looking stuff – it is about acting on an idea whether it is for personal fun or assistance.
http://enablingthefuture.org	website	The e-NABLE Community is a group of global volunteers who are using their 3D printers to create free 3D printed hands and arms for those in need of an upper limb assistive device.
https://www.neilsquire.ca	website	Developed over 30 years ago by Bill Cameron for his relative Neil Squire, this group's mission is to empower people with disabilities to be able to participate in life through AT.
https://makezine.com/tag/assistive-technology	website	*Make* magazine's AT site.
https://www.youtube.com/user/ATinNH	website	Here is one website on YouTube with DIY info. But search the YouTube site and you will find tons more.
http://www.instructables.com/id/Assistive-Technology-Projects	website	Tons of AT projects to share here.
www.demand.org.uk	website	Full of creative AT projects.
http://www.adaptivedesign.org	website	Excellent resources at this website to help you make your own creative AT solutions.
https://www.pinterest.com/explore/assistive-technology/?lp=true	website	This is only one example of the numerous AT solutions available on Pinterest.
https://www.google.org/impactchallenge/disabilities/grants.html	website	Check out these projects funded by Google.

4

Funding in the United States

Lewis Golinker

Outline

Learning outcomes

After reading this chapter, you should be able to:

1. Introduce rehabilitation therapy providers (e.g. occupational therapists, physical therapists, speech-language pathologists, special educators, and vocational rehabilitation counselors) to "third-party" funding for assistive devices.
2. Identify the rehabilitation therapy providers' role in the "third-party" funding process.
3. Describe the importance of using program-specific vocabulary to explain and support assistive device funding requests.
4. Identify the most common sources of funding for assistive devices.
5. Describe the common substantive requirements of health benefits programs, the largest source of funding for assistive devices.
6. Describe how assistive devices are covered by health benefits programs.
7. Describe how assistive devices meet the "medical necessity" requirement of health benefits programs.
8. Describe the characteristics of the therapeutic treatment plan, a required element of any funding request to a health benefits program for an assistive device.
9. List legislation relevant to funding for assistive devices.

Assistive Technologies and Environmental Interventions in Healthcare: An Integrated Approach, First Edition.
Edited by Lynn Gitlow and Kathleen Flecky.

Companion website: www.wiley.com/go/gitlow/assitivetechnologies

Active learning prompts

Before you read this chapter:

1. Look up definitions of assistive devices in programs that fund them.
2. Explore insurance company policy manuals to see what information is provided about the funding of assistive technology.
3. Identify three laws that mandate the provision of assistive technology.
4. Identify online resources that could help you with writing a letter of medical necessity.

Key terms

Ameliorate
Assistive technology devices and services
Durable medical equipment
Durable
Medical purpose
Dual use
Not useful vs. can use
Prosthetic devices
Medically necessary
Least costly equally effective alternative
Least costly alternative
Treatment plan
Waivers
Exclusions and limitations

Introduction

Assistive devices are tools used to help individuals achieve therapeutic treatment goals. As time has passed, the range of equipment items and their sophistication have both increased. For many items, so too has their cost. Presently, many assistive devices that provide extremely important functional benefits are quite expensive and are beyond the financial reach of the individuals who need them. For this reason, access to these devices will be dependent on practitioners' (rehabilitation therapy providers, such as occupational and physical therapists, speech-language pathologists, special educators, and vocational rehabilitation counselors) skill and commitment to securing funding from *third-party* funding sources.[1] Among their required tasks is understanding the legislation, rules, and policies that control access to this funding.

The roles of the practitioner

The practitioner will be the key figure in securing third-party funding for assistive devices[2] for individuals with disabilities. The practitioner's roles may include any – or all – of the following: conducting a needs assessment; coordinating or supervising a trial use period with equipment being considered; recommending an assistive device; preparing a written report describing the evaluation, trial, recommendation, and plan for treatment; advocating with funding source staff for acceptance of the recommendation; providing initial setup of the equipment upon delivery; and training the client and possibly the client's family and other services providers on device use.

Why me? The practitioners' role arises from their:

- unique knowledge of and obligation to implement the current standards of their profession;
- unique knowledge of the professional literature supporting the range of interventions, including assistive devices, that will treat specific functional limitations arising from illness, injury, or disease;
- unique ability to conduct a functional evaluation based on current professional standards and professional literature; and
- unique skill and experience to make a recommendation for a specific assistive device and, as needed, associated equipment items, and prepare a written report and treatment plan explaining why this equipment a specific assistive device is the most appropriate way for the client to meet his or her functional goals.

This scope of responsibilities is broad but practitioners do not have to perform them by themselves. Instead, they will be performed in collaboration with the client and, frequently, the client's family members; with representatives of the equipment supplier; and with the individual's physician. In some cases, other practitioners also may be involved, depending on the challenges presented by the client's abilities and needs.

Funding sources for assistive devices

There are many public and private programs in the United States that provide direct services or funding assistance to reduce the impacts of disability on daily life. Please review Table 4.1 for examples of federal funding.

Table 4.1 Federal Laws Related to Funding for Assistive Devices and Services.

Subject and brief description of laws	United States Code Citation
Education	
Individuals with Disabilities Education Act (IDEA)	20 U.S.C. 1400 et seq.
The IDEA was initially enacted in 1975 as the Education for All Handicapped Children Act. It states that all students with disabilities between the ages of 3 and 21 have a right to a "free appropriate public education" (FAPE), including necessary special education and related services, that will be provided in the "least restrictive environment" (LRE). The IDEA specifically identifies assistive technology devices and services as covered benefits to be provided when necessary to support students' FAPE and LRE. The IDEA provides funding for public schools to meet the costs of educating students with disabilities.	
Vocational rehabilitation	
Rehabilitation Act	29 U.S.C. 701 et seq.
Title I of the Rehabilitation Act authorizes funding for state vocational rehabilitation services programs. These programs support individuals with disabilities to develop the skills needed to seek, obtain, and retain their vocational goals, including employment. VR programs are authorized to provide funding for necessary assistive technology devices and services as part of the rehabilitation technology benefit.	
Health care	
Medicare	Vol. 42 Code of Federal Regulations (CFR) Sect. 414.202. Medicare Claims Processing Manual, Medicare Publication No. 100–04, Chapter 20: Durable Medical Equipment, Prosthetics, Orthotics, and Supplier (DMEPOS), at Section 10.1.2, *posted for review at* http://www.cms.gov/Regulations-and-Guidance/Guidance/Manuals/Internet-Only-Manuals-IOMs.html Public Law 89-97 (July 30, 1965) Health Insurance for the Aged Act, *codified at* Vol. 42 United States Code (U.S.C.) Sect. 1395 et seq. (Medicare).
Medicare is the nation's largest health benefits program. It provides benefits to individuals aged 65 and older and certain younger individuals with disabilities. Medicare provides payment for inpatient hospital and outpatient treatment services and prescription drugs. It covers and provides payment for assistive devices under its "durable medical equipment" and "prosthetic device" benefits.	
Medicaid	Public Law 89-97 (July 30, 1965) Health Insurance for the Aged Act, *codified at* Vol. 42 United States Code (U.S.C.) Sect. 1396 et seq. (Medicaid).
Medicaid is a health benefits program jointly funded and administered by the federal and state governments. It is a voluntary program all states have elected to join. Medicaid provides benefits to individuals who are poor, especially poor children, and people with disabilities. Medicaid provides payment for assistive devices under several benefits categories, including home healthcare (medical equipment); prosthetic devices; eyeglasses and other aids to vision; as necessary equipment under the physical, occupational, and speech-language pathology benefits; rehabilitation services; nursing facility services; and intermediate care facility for individuals with mental retardation or developmental disabilities. States also are allowed to expand the scope of their Medicaid programs through "waivers" that offer services not otherwise covered by the program. Among the benefits that can be provided as waiver services are "assistive technology" and "home modifications."	

Table 4.1 (*Continued*)

Subject and brief description of laws	United States Code Citation
Tricare Tricare, formerly known as the Civilian Health and Medical Program of the Uniformed Services (CHAMPUS), is a health program provided to active duty military service personnel and their dependents, and to military retirees and their dependents. Tricare provides coverage and payment for assistive devices under both its durable medical equipment (DME) and its prosthetic device benefits categories.	10 U.S.C. 1076 et seq.
Patient Protection and Affordable Care Act The Affordable Care Act, also known as the ACA and Obamacare, does not *provide* healthcare benefits directly, in contrast to Medicare or Medicaid. Instead, as originally enacted, it expands healthcare funding opportunities by requiring individuals to have health benefits coverage through a publicly funding benefits program or an insurance policy or employer-sponsored health benefits plan. It also set minimum standards for the content or scope of benefits that insurance policies subject to the ACA must offer. The mandatory services are called "essential health benefits," one category of which is "rehabilitative and habilitative services and devices." This benefit category is broad enough to include rehabilitative therapy services, such as OT, PT and SLP services, and both DME and prosthetic devices. The ACA also has a non-discrimination provision that allows individuals to challenge coverage limitations and exclusions for assistive devices. In this way, the ACA provides broader non-discrimination protections than does the ADA or Section 504.	Pub. L. No. 111-148 (March 23, 2010)
Americans with Disabilities Act; Section 504 of the Rehabilitation Act The ADA and Section 504 are statutes prohibiting disability-based discrimination. They are not health benefits programs. Both programs protect clients from disability-based discrimination in publicly funded programs, but they are of far more limited value in providing protections against benefits limitations and exclusions found in insurance policies and health benefits plans.	42 U.S.C. 12101 et seq.; 29 U.S.C. 704
Technology Related Assistance for Individuals with Disabilities Act The "Tech Act," initially passed in 1988, is not a health benefits program and does not provide funding for assistive devices. Instead, it supplies definitions of "assistive technology devices" and "assistive technology services" which have been copied into the scope of benefits offered by the IDEA and Rehabilitation Act. The Tech Act also provides funding to the states. Some use these funds in part to support low-interest loan programs for people with disabilities to purchase assistive devices.	29 U.S.C. 2201 et seq.

These programs were established to address specific social issues such as health care, special education, and vocational rehabilitation (Box 4.1). The greatest number of programs and those that serve the greatest number of people are related to health care. They include publicly funded programs – Medicare, Medicaid, Tricare, the Veterans Administration – and privately funded commercial health insurance and employer-sponsored health benefits plans. Complementing these programs are a broad array of charitable organizations with similar goals and purposes.

Assistive devices (or funding to assist their purchase) are among the benefits provided by many of these programs and by many charities.[3] Their inclusion – called coverage – reflects the importance of these devices to help clients meet these programs' goals and purposes. For example, an assistive device to improve functional performance, such as for mobility or communication, will ameliorate (lessen) the effects of physical impairment – a positive health outcome. That outcome also will aid independence as well as participation and substantive performance in school and work – positive educational and vocational outcomes.

For a particular client, accessing needed assistive devices requires the identification of *which* programs

Box 4.1 Case study: Assistive technology evaluation

Active Learning Questions:

1. How would you describe your role in the "third-party" funding process in this case?
2. What program-specific vocabulary would you use to explain and support assistive device funding requests in this case?
3. Describe how the assistive device that is recommended meets the "medical necessity" requirement of health benefits programs.
4. Describe the characteristics of the therapeutic treatment plan, a required element of any funding request to a health benefits program for the assistive device/s that would be recommended in this case if within your role.

Name	Carly
Age	91
Date of service	July 21, 2018 1–2:30 p.m.
Evaluators	Evaluators: OT, SLP
Diagnosis	Left Cerebrovascular accident (CVA) with right side hemiparesis, hypertension (HTN), congestive heart failure (CHF), and central hearing loss.
Introduction	Carly is a 91-year-old female who was seen at Shady Acres Nursing Home where she now lives. Also attending the evaluation were two facility-based occupational therapists, an SLP, and Carly's son and daughter-in-law. Carly is non-verbal at present due to severe Broca's aphasia resulting from her stroke. She was referred by her physician for an AT evaluation focused on increasing her ability to communicate her medical needs.
History	Carly presently lives at Shady Acres Nursing Home. Her family states that she will continue to reside at Shady Acres as they are not able to meet her current needs for care at home.
Evaluation	The Lowenstein Occupational Therapy Cognitive Assessment– Geriatric (LOTCA – G) and observation of task performance were used for this evaluation. The LOTCA–G is an assessment tool designed with subtests that identify a client's abilities and limitations in areas of cognitive processing.
Affect and appearance	Carly was alert and was dressed appropriately by caregivers for the setting where we met her. She is quite friendly and responded to all of the things that we asked her to do. She wears glasses and has bilateral hearing aids.
Physical functioning	Carly uses an Invacare 9000 XT manual wheelchair for her mobility. She has a seating cushion in the wheelchair. Caregivers move the wheelchair for her presently. She is unable to transfer or stand independently and requires max assist for all transfers. She has right-sided hemiparesis. Her range of motion (RUE) is non-functional with subluxation noted in the R shoulder. She was wearing a soft splint for positioning on her R hand during this evaluation. Her Lower upper extremity (LUE) is functional. She has an ankle foot orthotic (AFO) on her RLE. Dyspraxia was noted in her ability to identify objects correctly and identify directions on her body.
ADL and IADL functioning	Carly requires max assist for all of her ADL's. She is able to independently drink from a cup but requires supervision when eating due to swallowing problems resulting from her stroke. She seems motivated to increase her independence in ADLs; however, that was not the focus of this evaluation.
Hearing and vision	Carly wears bilateral hearing aids and glasses. It is reported that she has R visual neglect.
Cognition	Carly knows that she is in a nursing home and that it is summer. She was not as clearly oriented to her location prior to being admitted to the nursing home. As noted, praxis is impaired. Carly was able to attend to and participate in an evaluation, which lasted over an hour, trying to complete everything we asked her to do. She was able to correctly visually identify objects and visually distinguish black and white outlined pictures of objects. Spatial relations and distinguishing overlapping figures were difficult. She was able to complete a puzzle and complete a pegboard construction task, but construction of a three-dimensional pattern was impaired. These skills have implications for selection of communication symbols and will be discussed in the recommendations section of this report. Carly's memory seems to be adequate to remember pictures and items for 20 minutes. She is able to follow one-step directions; however, dyspraxia is noted.
Current assistive technology	Presently, Carolyn uses a wheelchair for mobility.

can be asked to provide funding and a determination *whether* the program will do so. It will be common for clients to be eligible for multiple programs. For example, a family in which both spouses work may have health benefits coverage from each employer. A child with a disability in that family can be covered by both health benefits sources and also may be eligible for special education services and for vocational rehabilitation services as well. On the other hand, because eligibility for each program is purpose-based, some clients will "fall through the cracks" and will not be eligible for any of them. For example, adults will not be eligible for public education; individuals not interested in working or otherwise unable to work may not be eligible for vocational rehabilitation; and there are many reasons why individuals have no access to a health benefits program. Thus, one of the first tasks of the practitioner is to identify all the funding programs the client is or may be eligible for.

Identifying *all* programs also is necessary because even though a program has the authority to provide funding for an assistive device, it does not mean it will do so. Application may have to be made to all available sources to identify one that will approve and provide access to the needed device. Also, funding programs have a priority or sequencing procedure that controls the order in which they will pay when clients are eligible for more than one.

Another reason to be alert to all possible sources of funding is that there are clear distinctions among them in the vocabulary used to describe assistive devices. In general, health-based funding programs use the phrase "durable medical equipment" or "prosthetic devices." By contrast, education and vocational rehabilitation programs use the phrase "assistive technology" or "rehabilitation technology" devices. In reports and all other communication with funding source staff, use of vocabulary applicable to another program creates wholly preventable risk of a denial. It will be safest to avoid "categorical" descriptions and instead to call a device or equipment item by its more specific label, such as "wheelchair," "standing device," or "speech-generating device."

Answering the *whether* question: on what basis will a funding source approve a request for an assistive device, is the subject of the rest of this chapter. Because health benefits programs reach more people and provide more funding for more assistive devices than any others, this chapter will describe their structure and function.

Health benefits program funding for assistive devices

Funding for health benefits may come from one or more sources or from none at all. In 2016, approximately 91% of Americans were enrolled in publicly funded health benefits programs, including Medicare, Medicaid, Tricare, and the Department of Veterans Affairs, or privately funded benefits sources, including health insurance policies and health benefits plans. Approximately 9% – 27 million people – were covered by none of these programs.[4]

Medicare and Medicaid were created in 1965. Medicare was created to assist individuals aged 65 and older in meeting the costs of their healthcare needs. It was later expanded to include younger individuals who had worked but had become disabled through injury or illness. By contrast, Medicaid was created to assist specific populations of individuals who were presumed to be too poor to meet the costs of their healthcare needs. Tricare is a program that provides health benefits funding to active duty military personnel and their families and to military retirees and their families. The Department of Veterans Affairs provides health benefits directly to military veterans.

Private benefits sources

Health insurance policies and health benefits plans provide funding for healthcare services. They are most commonly offered as a fringe benefit of employment. Individuals also may purchase insurance policies on their own behalf.[5]

Benefits request – funding process: Four questions

All health benefits programs serve the same purpose: their common goal is to help eligible individuals meet the medical needs that arise in the course of their daily lives. Also, all follow a standard protocol or outline to determine whether the program must provide funding for a specific equipment item or service. This protocol asks four questions:

- Is the individual seeking the device eligible for the program?
- Is the device "covered" by the program, i.e. does it fit within at least one of the program's covered benefits categories?
- Is the device "medically necessary"?
- Is the request unaffected by any program limitations or exclusions that bar or limit access to the device?

If the answer to all four questions is "yes," then the program must provide funding for the requested device.

Question 1: Individual eligibility: is the individual a beneficiary, participant, or recipient of the benefits program?

Because there is no uniform source of health benefits, the practitioner must identify the health benefits program or programs for which the client currently is eligible.

To do this, clients should be directed to present the identification card or similar proof for each health benefits program to which they are eligible. It is important to ask clients to identify *all* programs to which they are eligible: eligibility for more than one health benefits program is common.

This is an *information gathering* and not an advocacy task. Practitioners are not responsible to establish eligibility *for* clients.

Question 2: Is the device "covered" by the program, i.e. does it fit within at least one of the program's covered benefits categories?

Eligibility means the client can *ask* the health benefits program to provide funding for any assistive devices identified as needed. But no program covers *everything*. Just as there is no one source of health benefits, no health benefits program will provide funding for every healthcare intervention. Instead, each will identify the health benefits they cover. For a health benefits program to offer funding, clients' needs must match the scope of health benefits the program covers (offers).

Health benefits programs generally rely on *descriptive* statements of coverage: they identify broad categories of health care from which specific types of care will be provided. They also will provide definitions, examples, or descriptions of the types of benefits that "fit" within each category. Examples of typically covered benefits categories include "physician services," "inpatient and outpatient hospital services," "durable medical equipment," "home health services," "rehabilitative services," "prescription drugs," and "prosthetic devices."

The covered health benefits categories of public benefits programs will be identified in the statutes that created the programs and they may be defined or described further in regulations and in policy manuals or other guidance. Many benefits programs post this information for review at their web page. For insurance policies and health benefits plans, identification, definition, and description of covered benefits will be stated in a "certificate of coverage" (insurance policies) or in a "summary plan description" (SPD) (health benefits plans). These documents will be provided to clients by their employer or directly from an insurer. They may be provided in hard copy or be posted online.[6] Among all health benefits programs, the most common categories that offer coverage for assistive devices are "durable medical equipment" (DME) and "prosthetic devices" or "prosthetic appliances."[7] A DME benefit is provided by all publicly funded health benefits programs and almost all insurance policies and health benefits plans.

Durable medical equipment

There is no uniform definition of DME. However, because of its status as the largest health benefits program in the United States, Medicare's rules and policies often are copied by other health benefits programs for their own use. One example is the Medicare DME definition which is widely copied by Medicaid programs and insurers and health plans. Medicare defines DME as follows:

DME is equipment which:

- is able to withstand repeated use;
- is primarily and customarily used to serve a medical purpose;
- generally is not useful to an individual in the absence of an illness or injury; and
- is appropriate for use in the home.[8]

To be eligible for coverage as DME, an equipment item being recommended for a client must be able to establish that it has all of these characteristics. For many assistive devices this will not be the practitioner's burden: they already have been accepted as DME.[9] But for rarely needed devices, and some others such as those that support standing, and for certain types of wheelchairs, such as power chairs with integrated standing features, the practitioner may have to establish that each element of the DME definition is satisfied.

Is able to withstand repeated use

According to Medicare, an item that is *durable* is one that can "withstand repeated use." The common meaning of "durable" is something that is "long-lasting" and "able to exist for a long time without significant deterioration." The characteristics of typically sought equipment items will easily meet this criterion. They are intended for everyday use for a period of years.[10]

Some insurers and health plans use different vocabulary to describe this characteristic of DME items: they state that items of DME are "not consumable or disposable." These terms should be considered synonymous.

A "disposable" item is the polar opposite of a *durable* equipment item. A disposable item is designed to be used once and then thrown away. "Disposable" does not describe the characteristics of typically sought equipment items. Also, the prices of many equipment items will be a significant fact to establish they are not disposable. That these equipment items cost hundreds or thousands of dollars will rebut any suggestion they are intended to be used once and thrown away.

Likewise, *durable* equipment items are not "consumable," something that is used up or destroyed. Equipment items such as oxygen tanks, which are emptied through use, and power wheelchairs or speech-generating devices, whose batteries are depleted through use, are not "consumable." A Medicare administrative law judge found that a speech-generating device was durable *because* it ran on rechargeable batteries.[11] Oxygen tanks are designed to be refilled and battery-powered equipment items are designed to be recharged on a repeated basis. They are not "destroyed" through use.

Typically, it will not be difficult to establish or be a matter of controversy that equipment items are "durable," because they can "withstand repeated use," and are "not disposable" and "not consumable."

Primarily and customarily used to serve a medical purpose

The second element of the DME definition requires that an equipment item be "primarily and customarily used to serve a medical purpose." As with the "durability" element, some benefits programs use synonyms for the phrase "medical purpose," such as "treatment," or "therapeutic" purpose. All three share a common meaning. The words "medical" and "therapeutic" both include "treatment" as part of their definition.

To establish an equipment item will be used to serve a *medical* purpose, the practitioner must show in his or her report that the item is being sought and will be used as part of a program or plan of *treatment*. The terms medical purpose and treatment are synonyms.[12]

When thinking about "treatment," outcomes other than "cure" and "correct" are equally valid. Treatment may be directed to those goals, but also to prevention, to amelioration (to lessen the severity of the adverse effects of a condition, rather than to affect the condition directly), and to palliation. Most assistive devices are preventive or ameliorative forms of treatment:

- A wheelchair will ameliorate the adverse functional impacts of spinal cord injury or amyotrophic lateral sclerosis (ALS) to enable clients to move from point A to point B, but will have no direct impact (and need not have any direct impact) on the underlying condition.
- A standing device will help prevent the onset of contractures and spasticity for clients with conditions that impede their ability to stand and bear weight, but will have no direct impact (and need not have any direct impact) on the underlying condition.

The following tasks related to assistive devices: assessment and recommendation for, necessary fabrication of, and services to support their use, all serve a *medical purpose* because all are recognized as within the scope of occupational therapy (OT), physical therapy (PT), and speech-language pathology (SLP) treatment.[13] OT, PT, and SLP services generally are accepted as serving a medical purpose because almost all funding sources (all the public benefits programs and almost all insurance policies and health plans) cover and provide funding for OT, PT, and SLP services. Services related to assistive devices involve the use of these tools, but both the goals and the purpose of the clinical services remain the same. The following framework explains this point:

- OT, PT, and SLP services are covered; therefore, they are recognized by the funding source as serving a *medical purpose*.
- All OT, PT, and SLP services are focused on the same functional goal: to enable clients to meet daily functional needs, such as seating and positioning, performing activities of daily living (ADLs) and instrumental activities of daily living (IADLs), ambulation and mobility, standing, and expressive communication.
- Clients present a very wide range of abilities, based on the complexity and severity of their impairments and correspondingly a wide range of OT, PT, and SLP treatment methodologies will be recommended as treatment.
- Among the long accepted OT, PT, and SLP treatment methodologies is the use of assistive devices.
- Assistive devices are recommended when clients are unable, using natural methods of performing functional tasks, such as standing, ambulation, or speaking, to meet daily functional needs; regardless of the treatment methodology recommended, the treatment goal remains the same.
- Thus, if services *serve a medical purpose* when directed to improve a client's natural ability to stand, to walk, or to speak, an assistive device will serve the same *medical purpose* when services directed to improving natural functional abilities will not be sufficient for daily needs to be met.

This discussion or explanation will be *required* for equipment items where coverage as DME is not clear, but it should also be included even where the item is accepted as DME. It will serve an additional purpose: to aid the establishment of *medical necessity* for the device. There is a substantial overlap between the facts that establish an equipment item serves a medical purpose and those that establish it will address a medical need.

A "continuum" of client abilities and needs (Figure 4.1) and of treatment methods to address those needs is a useful alternative way framework to explain that an equipment item serves a medical purpose.

For clients with less complex or severe impairments, treatment can be directed to improving the function of natural means of accomplishing functional goals, such

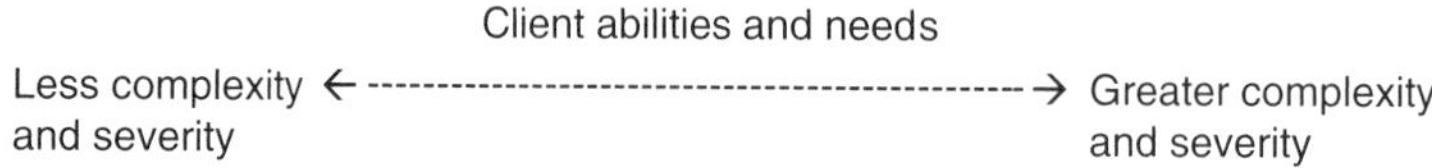

Figure 4.1 Client abilities and needs.

as strengthening balance, endurance, gait, and other functional elements of ambulation. But as the complexity and severity of clients' impairments increase, these efforts may not be sufficient. When that judgment is made, the focus of the assessment process turns to assistive devices that can assist or be a substitute method for the client to achieve the same functional goals.

A continuum linking impairment complexity and severity to a variety of treatment methods exists for many healthcare issues: mild cardiac impairments may be satisfactorily addressed by lifestyle changes such as change of diet, elimination of smoking, and increased exercise, but as the severity of the impairment increases, other means of treatment will have to be considered. At some point, consideration of an angioplasty with stent, and devices such as a pacemaker, defibrillator, or ventricular assist device becomes appropriate, as may heart bypass surgery, or a transplant. Regardless of their specific differences, all of these interventions serve the same medical purpose and seek to achieve the same functional goal. This metaphor is equally useful to describe the medical purposes of OT, PT, or SLP treatment in the form of standing frames, wheelchairs, or speech-generating devices, or other equipment items.

In general, including the following rhetorical question in the practitioner's report will help establish that the device being recommended serves a *medical purpose:*

> if there was a form of surgery or a pill that will improve the client's functioning to the same level that can be achieved with the recommended device, will providing that drug or performing that surgery be recognized as serving a medical purpose?

The point being made here is that surgery and use of medication are accepted as *medical* interventions, serving *medical* purposes. That no surgery or pill may exist to achieve this outcome for a particular client's functional needs, and instead, an item of DME is being recommended to serve the same purpose and achieve the same goal, should not raise any question that the equipment is serving a *medical* purpose.

Another metaphor to explain the medical purpose of various assistive devices is that they will serve as a *functional bypass* or *functional substitute* for body parts or systems that are non- or malfunctioning, due to injury, illness, or disability. Wheelchairs, communication devices, and standing devices all serve these purposes: when an individual wishes to move from point A to point B but cannot due to a spinal cord injury, the brain can issue motor instructions to the hands and arms to propel a manual wheelchair or to direct a power wheelchair joystick to accomplish this purpose. An individual whose speech cannot be understood due to severe dysarthria secondary to cerebral palsy or ALS can have motor instructions redirected to the hands or another body part that will instruct an SGD to produce the intended message. A person with advanced ALS, Duchenne muscular dystrophy, or spinal cord injury still can obtain a range of benefits through the use of a standing device. When used to accomplish these goals, each of these devices will be serving a medical purpose.

A final note on this point: the equipment recommendation always should be described as *the most appropriate form of treatment available to enable the client to meet the client's daily functional (ambulation, standing, mobility, speech, respiration,* etc.*) needs.*

In some cases, practitioners may be asked or required to provide professional literature to support the "medical purpose" of a requested equipment item. Organizations such as the American Occupational Therapy Association (AOTA), the American Physical Therapy Association (APTA), the American Speech–Language–Hearing Association (ASHA), and the Rehabilitation Engineering and Assistive Technology Society of North America (RESNA) should develop, keep updated, and make widely available to practitioners and advocates, reference lists identifying professional literature that supports the effectiveness of various assistive devices, and update these lists regularly as new resources become available.

In addition to establishing a medical equipment item serves a medical purpose, this DME criterion requires that the device be "primarily and customarily used" to serve that medical purpose. To address this requirement, the practitioner can report for most DME items that they are used *solely* for medical purposes: that they have no other use and serve no other purpose. A wheelchair serves only to overcome impairments to ambulation or mobility. A standing device serves only to overcome the many adverse functional effects associated with an inability to stand or bear weight.

For speech-generating devices (SGDs), which are using off-the-shelf tablet computers as hardware with increasing frequency, the same statement can be made about their purpose: that their *sole* purpose is as speech-language pathology treatment to overcome the adverse effects of severe expressive communication impairments.[14] But more of an explanation is required. To meet this DME characteristic the SGD model being recommended must be modified (locked or made dedicated) so that its *only* use will be as an SGD. These modifications will disable the general computer features of the device. (These models generally are described as "Medicare-compliant," because Medicare was the first funding source to require these modifications.)

When modified in this way, the speech generating functions will not compete with other features such as word-processing, internet access, entertainment, or games, eliminating the need to find ways to explain which of these "purposes" are "primary and customary" and which are "ancillary." Because dedicated SGDs can only generate speech, *only* a person unable to meet daily communication needs using speech or other natural communication methods such as writing, gesture, or sign will be evaluated for, be recommended, want, use, or benefit from the device the client seeks.

Generally is not useful to a person in the absence of an illness or injury

The third element of the DME definition states that the item "generally is not useful to a person in the absence of an illness or injury." As a general rule, any individual able to meet a specific functional goal through natural means, e.g. standing, walking, or speaking, will not be evaluated for, recommended, prescribed, seek funding for, need, or use an assistive device to accomplish the same functional outcome. For something to be "useful," it must fill a need and be cost-effective. The latter consideration focuses on the cost of the item, and how burdensome it may be to acquire it and to use it. It must be likely the individual *will* use the item to accomplish the functional goal.

This element of the DME definition asks, "will the device be used"; it does not ask, "*can* an individual use the item for that purpose?" That phrasing is unworkable as a practical matter: almost everyone *can* use a wheelchair for mobility; almost anyone *can* use an SGD to speak. But when mobility or speech is not impaired by illness, injury, or disability, no one will want to or need to use a wheelchair or communication device. Walking and speaking are far more efficient and in many instances more effective means to accomplish these goals.

Likewise, when clients are able to stand, walk, or talk, the accomplishment of these tasks and the benefits they convey are achieved for free. No one will spend thousands of dollars for equipment items that will accomplish the same goals. In other words, if no one will buy one of these devices when the same goal can be accomplished without charge, then they will not "generally be useful" to anyone without specific need for them.

One class of equipment does *not* easily satisfy this criterion: "dual-use equipment." These devices are of value – sometimes great value – to members of the public, but they also will provide unique health benefits to clients with certain types of impairments. Because this equipment will be "generally of use to persons in the absence of illness or injury" it typically will *not* be covered as DME. An example is an air conditioner. Even though this item may enable a person with a temperature- or humidity-sensitive condition to avoid hospitalization, they will be identified as not covered because they generally *are* useful to everyone. Other examples include devices that aid clients' ability to reach for items; remote controls; and whirlpool baths. Most recently, transcutaneous electrical nerve stimulation (TENS) units, historically a covered item to address pain, have been advertised in a holiday gift catalog for general public use. If they become generally accepted consumer items, they too will cease to be recognized as DME.[15]

Off-the-shelf tablet computer-based SGDs also are often the focus of attention under this criterion. An off-the-shelf tablet computer obviously is "generally useful" to the general public. To satisfy this criterion, these and other computer-based SGDs are modified to disable or lock out their general computer functions, leaving only their ability to generate speech. Funding sources accept that "dedicated" computer-based SGDs will provide no benefit to, and therefore are not "generally of use" to individuals without severe speech impairment.[16]

Is appropriate for use in the home

The final element of the DME definition is that the item must be "appropriate for use in the home." Another phrasing of this element is that the item has been "designed for outpatient use."

This criterion has two parts: one related to device design; the other to the client's home. First, many equipment items, such as wheelchairs and other ambulation and mobility devices and communication devices, are designed and intended to come and go with the individual when and wherever she or he wants to move or speak. Their appropriateness is setting independent. Thus, that they may be "used" in places other than the client's home is not important. The criterion asks if the device is "appropriate for" use in the home. A device that satisfies this requirement is not disqualified because it *also* is appropriate for use or is used elsewhere.

Other items, such as standing devices, may be used in formal therapy sessions and settings, such as clinics, and professionals' offices. But a typical rationale for seeking funding for one of these devices *at home* is to allow clients to increase their time using the device and therefore obtain more benefit than is possible from use only in formal therapy sessions. The device itself is *as appropriate for* home use as in a formal therapy setting. In general, that Medicare will cover the same item as DME also helps to satisfy this element of the DME definition of any funding source. Medicare does not provide DME to residents in institutional settings such as hospitals or nursing facilities.[17]

If ever a question arises about the suitability of a specific equipment item for home use, the proposed DME supplier or the item's manufacturer can relate the history of sales of the item to establish they went to individuals residing at home and were not designed or intended primarily for use by residents of institutions.

Looking at the alternative phrasing of this criterion, few DME items can be said to have been "designed" for institutional use (the opposite of equipment designed for "outpatient" use). Even equipment items with life-saving roles such as iron lungs and ventilators were recognized by Congress more than 50 years ago as appropriate for use in the home and were identified as DME when Medicare was created.[18]

The second focal point of this criterion is practical. To be appropriate for use in the home, it must "fit" within the client's living space. A home visit will provide confirmation this requirement is satisfied.

Prosthetic devices or prosthetic appliances

It is most likely coverage for a needed equipment item will "fit" within a funding source's DME benefit. If so, there is no need to consider other benefits categories for the purposes of coverage. However, in some circumstances, an equipment item needed by an individual will not fit an insurance policy or health benefits plan's DME definition, or they may not include DME at all (all the public health benefits programs cover DME). In this circumstance, an alternative source of coverage must be found. "Prosthetic devices" or "prosthetic appliances" is the next place to look.

As with DME, there is no uniform definition of prosthetic devices or prosthetic appliances, but once again, the Medicare definition is widely copied by other funding sources. Medicare defines prosthetic devices in two ways. First:

> Devices that replace all or part of an internal body organ ...[19]

Alternately, Medicare states that prosthetic devices are:

> Devices which replace all or part of the *function of the permanently inoperative or malfunctioning internal body organ.*[20]

The second, "function-related" definition serves as the basis for Medicare coverage as prosthetic devices of equipment like the artificial larynx and cardiac pacemaker. Neither device replaces all or part of an internal body organ. Instead, each provides a functional substitute for a surgically removed or non-functioning larynx or for malfunctioning nerve impulses regulating the heartbeat. Similarly, cochlear implants are covered as Medicare prosthetic devices. They do not replace any part of the inner ear; instead, they provide a functional substitute for the normal transmission of sound to the cochlea. Thus, to cover devices of this kind, Medicare acknowledges that *functional* substitution or restoration, rather than *actual* substitution of the body part itself, is a characteristic of prosthetic devices.

Even when a funding program's prosthetic device definition does not reference "functional replacement," it is possible devices serving this purpose will be covered. Practitioners should ask about the specific equipment items the program acknowledges to be prosthetics to see whether any serve as functional rather than actual substitutes for non- or malfunctioning body parts. Coverage of the artificial larynx is a useful example to search for. It is both routinely covered and generally accepted as a prosthetic device.

Medical necessity

Medical necessity represents the "purpose" for which health benefits programs exist. They provide funding to enable eligible individuals to receive covered services *necessary* to meet the eligible individuals' *medical needs.*

No uniform definition of medical necessity is used by all health benefits programs, but there are four common elements in all their definitions. Each requires proof of the following:

- an injury, illness, condition, or disability;
- that the injury, illness, or condition causes an adverse health effect;
- that some form of treatment is required to cure, correct, alleviate, or ameliorate the adverse health effect; and
- that the treatment selected is the least costly equally effective alternative that will achieve that goal.

Practitioners will be required to establish in their reports that all recommended equipment items are medically necessary. For almost all assistive devices, the practitioner will be the key person to establish medical need as compared to the client's doctor. The physician's role will be to review the practitioner's recommendation and to confirm it with a prescription.

The concept of medical necessity or medical need can be viewed as having two elements. The first is generic to the equipment item. Is it recognized as "treatment"; for what conditions and circumstances is it "effective;"; is it "duplicative" of other forms of treatment that are equally effective and less costly? The second element of medical need directs these questions to the specific client and the client's facts and circumstances.

The "generic" element of medical need mirrors to a substantial degree the concept of "medical purpose" discussed in the context of the definition of "durable medical equipment." As stated in that discussion, for most assistive devices, the medical purposes served by equipment items have been acknowledged by the funding sources, so practitioners can focus their reports exclusively on how the device is medically necessary for the specific client.

Many funding sources have device-specific coverage criteria that outline the evaluation and practitioner's report required to establish medical necessity. If no device-specific coverage criteria exist, practitioners must conduct evaluations and produce reports that address all of the specific elements of the funding source's medical need definition. In general, medical need definitions will require the four elements previously stated (impairment; adverse effect; effective treatment; recommended treatment is the least costly equally effective alternative).

To address these points, practitioners often conduct a four step inquiry:

- What is the client's current condition; is it stable, improving, or progressing; how severe is it?
- What are the adverse effects of the current condition: what is the client's current level of functioning; how does the condition adversely affect the client's ability to meet daily functional needs?
- What interventions, if any, have been tried in the past, and what interventions currently are being implemented to address those adverse effects? Also, what adverse effects remained notwithstanding those past and current efforts? What daily functional needs continue not to be met?
- What is the least costly equally effective intervention to address those residual adverse effects, i.e. to augment the individual's natural functional abilities or to serve as an alternative or functional substitute, so that the individual will meet daily functional needs?

For example:

What is the client's current condition?

Based on examination, a practitioner learns a client has Duchenne muscular dystrophy (DMD). This is a progressive condition, with no effective treatment for the underlying physiological impairment. For individuals with DMD, the overall therapy goal is to maintain the individual's functional abilities and independence.

What are the adverse effects of the current condition?

The evaluation reveals the individual has lost the functional use of his legs to stand or bear weight,[21] and as a result of extended sitting has shown signs or symptoms of or is at risk of developing contractures, loss of bone density, and bladder and bowel malfunction.

What interventions, if any, currently are being implemented to address those adverse effects?

The individual may have begun a course of therapeutic (supported) standing for one hour, once per week in a clinic-based therapy session.

Do adverse effects remain notwithstanding current efforts?

The occupational or physical therapist concludes the opportunity to stand while in therapy is not enough time to maximize the benefits of standing (weight bearing) and to minimize the risks to the client of e.g., contractures; spasms; impairments to bowel and bladder function; and skin ulcers. The practitioner therefore recommends the client obtain and use a standing device at home to increase the client's time standing to one hour per *day* rather than per *week* so that the benefits of standing can be increased as well.

What is the least costly equally effective intervention to address those residual adverse effects?

The practitioner's obligation here is to identify alternate forms of treatment (if any) as well as alternate models of standing devices that may provide the same effects (benefits as well as risk reduction) as the specific type of standing device being recommended. These alternatives must be described as inappropriate and therefore ruled out because they will not provide the same amount of benefit, or because they may provide the same benefits but they cost more than the recommended device. (Cost is considered only among solutions that provide equal benefit.)

In this example, a standing wheelchair may be considered as an alternative for the client, because it can be described as offering equal benefits, but it would be ruled out because it is much more costly than a standing frame. However, if the client required assistance to transfer to a standing frame but that assistance was not available, a standing wheelchair might be recommended. In this circumstance the standing frame would have been ruled out as not equally effective because in the wheelchair the client can move to and from sitting to standing independently, while this is impossible with a standing frame.

Finally, all of these observations will be written into an evaluation report to be sent to the individual's physician for review.

Establishing medical need is essential to a successful funding request to a health benefits program for any intervention. In regard to assistive devices, establishing medical need is a critical responsibility of the occupational or physical therapist, speech-language pathologist, or other practitioner.

One question related to medical need is "how much" treatment is necessary? As a general rule, the starting point for consideration of medical need is the standard of practice of the professional responsible for identification of need. For physicians, or medicine in general, the goal is *cure* or *correct* illness, injury, or disease. In regard to "how much" treatment, these goals translate into sufficient treatment to enable the client to return to functioning within recognized normal limits.

Cure or correct goals may not be possible for chronic conditions that cause functional impairments, such as autism, ALS, cerebral palsy, muscular dystrophy, spinal cord injury, stroke, or traumatic brain injury. And aiding development of abilities or restoration of them to recognized normal limits also may not be possible. For clients with these conditions, the treatment goal may be amelioration of the adverse effects of these conditions. But that leaves unanswered the question of *how much* functional development- or restoration-related treatment must be provided.

Looking to standards of practice will provide an answer. Occupational therapy will be used here to illustrate this point, but any practitioner can use the same strategies to justify their intervention recommendations. The definition of occupational therapy states that it is "the use of purposeful activity or interventions to promote health and achieve functional outcomes. Achieving functional outcomes means to develop, improve, or restore *the highest possible level of independence* of any individual who is limited by" illness, injury, or disability. This is the standard that *all* occupational therapy treatment seeks to achieve, and this also should be the level of performance to be achieved by the provision of equipment as treatment.

A note of caution: reference to superlatives such as "highest possible" or "best" may be viewed by funding sources as beyond what constitutes "medically necessary" care. An alternative way to phrase the goal of treatment is to say that the goal is to *enable clients to meet daily ______________ needs*, with the blank representing the specific functional goal (e.g. ambulation; standing; communication; prevention) that is the treatment focus of the device. This phrasing may be said to be *better than "best."*

Another point to consider is the broad range of benefits that will flow from the treatment. All should be considered as *medical* needs. While it is hardly arguable that a skin protection cushion will serve a medical purpose if it will prevent development of decubitus ulcers, a standing device also will be serving a *medical* need because it aids the client's ability to perform activities of daily living and aids psychosocial status by permitting face-to-face and thus more normal interaction with peers. These are ordinary goals, purposes, or outcomes of providing occupational therapy services, and use of a standing device may be the most appropriate form of OT treatment for a client. Treatments directed to these goals are just another way to help the client achieve his or her "highest possible level of independence" or, alternatively, to help the client meet daily needs related to interaction and community participation.

Quality of life

Does medical need exist to improve "quality of life?" One might think this is a trick question: all medical interventions will be recommended and prescribed for the specific purpose of improving or maintaining health status and correspondingly improving or maintaining clients' quality of life. It is hardly possible to envision a recommendation or prescription for any intervention intended to make a client's health status *worse*: that will cause a *reduction* in quality of life.

The concept of "quality of life" raises a reporting issue, not one of substance. Improved quality of life obviously is an acceptable and desired outcome but it is *not appropriate* for practitioners to report quality of life improvement as an intended goal of a recommended intervention. It is neither necessary nor appropriate for practitioners to refer to this phrase in their reports. Rather, treatment goals and outcomes should be stated with greater precision: they should identify the type of treatment to be provided and the specific *functional* outcomes to be achieved. The types of treatment may be prevention, amelioration, rehabilitation (restoration of function; arresting or slowing the progression of functional loss), or habilitation (aiding development of function delayed or impeded by disability). The functional outcomes can be mobility, speech, or any other functional benefit the equipment will provide. All of these are appropriate ways to describe treatment types and treatment outcomes, while improved quality of life is not.

A final point to consider about medical need is that not all treatment options are equal alternatives. Increased exercise, smoking cessation, change of diet, a daily aspirin, bypass surgery, and transplants are all interventions for cardiac impairments but they are not *equally appropriate* or *equally effective* alternatives. Practitioners should consider alternative methods of treatment or alternative device choices in three steps: first, identify alternatives that will yield equal outcomes, i.e. the degree of positive effects to be achieved. Then, consider the cost of the alternatives that offer equal benefits. Finally, select the least costly option among the equally effective alternatives.

An example of alternatives that are not equally effective are communication devices that generate digitized speech and those that generate synthesized speech. Both produce speech, but digitized speech devices will not be appropriate for someone who can produce novel messages, as compared to selecting only from a roster of pre-prepared messages. Typically, a digitized speech output device will be ruled out as not appropriate for an individual who is able to spell and to read or is learning either task. Also, factors related to physical abilities will support ruling out digitized speech output devices. If a client requires a device with more than one page of messages but lacks the physical ability to remove and replace message pages, then digitized speech output SGDs are not appropriate, regardless of the client's linguistic skills. The client will require a touch screen that will allow display (message) pages to be changed electronically, which is a characteristic found only on synthesized speech output devices.

In this example, digitized speech output SGDs are less costly alternatives, but they are not equally effective. They won't provide access to speech that matches the client's expressive language skills. This fact justifies ruling them out for functional reasons; their cost is not relevant. Rather than looking first at cost, the proper analysis of medical need is to consider the level of benefit to be provided and to then examine the least costly way to achieve that level of benefit.

Practitioners also must note that comparison of cost among treatment alternatives includes *operational* costs, not acquisition costs alone. For example, a sit-to-stand standing device may provide the same functional benefits as a power wheelchair with a standing feature. The latter, however, will be far more costly in terms of acquisition costs. However, the client may not be able to transfer independently from a wheelchair to the sit-to-stand device. To accomplish this transfer safely may require a two-person assist. The practical availability of these aides as well as their cost must be included in the practitioner's comparison of alternatives in regard to both effectiveness and cost. In this example, family members, friends, or neighbors may be identified as potential sources of voluntary transfer assistance. But practitioners cannot count on their service and instead should consider the operational costs if paid aides provided the transfer assistance. In general, the cost of a human services provider will be greater than the cost of a device that provides the same function.

Limitations or exclusions

Health benefits programs may include a wide range of limitations or exclusions that affect access to an equipment item. Exclusions may be listed in text describing the scope of DME or prosthetic devices coverage or may be in separate section titled "What We Do Not Cover" or "Exclusions and Limitations."

Coverage limitations may apply to age (coverage for children but not adults); diagnosis (exclusions for autism); place of residence (coverage for people residing at home but not in nursing facilities); periods of time (coverage of one device within a specific time span); purpose (no coverage if to meet educational or vocational needs); type of device (covering only one type of device in a device category); or many other reasons. Coverage exclusions may be explicit (naming the specific item not covered) or may be based on some specific reason such as "experimental or investigational" care or "personal convenience."

Practitioners will most likely learn of coverage limitations or exclusions after a funding request for an equipment item is denied. The limitation or exclusion will be identified as the basis for the denial.

Although denials based on limitations and exclusions may *appear* to be impenetrable barriers to equipment access, many can be challenged successfully, leading to approval of the requested device. Whenever a denial is issued, for any reason, the practitioner should help the client find an advocate to assist with an appeal.[22]

The assistive device treatment plan

The treatment plan is an essential component of the practitioner's report. Without a treatment plan, a report should be considered incomplete. There are no generally recognized templates for treatment plans.

In lieu of a generally accepted model, it is suggested here that a treatment plan should be viewed as a stand-alone "executive summary" of the practitioner's report as a whole. It should include at least the following three elements:

- A plan of implementation that describes all aspects of how the recommended assistive device is to be used (frequency; duration; positions; activities);
- Identification or description of the professionals who will provide supervision, instruction, support, and reinforcement to the client, and training to be provided to family members and others, when necessary and appropriate. These services – to be called *treatment* – may be provided by the practitioner who conducted the evaluation and is making the recommendation, or by others;
- A set of measurable goals that these services will hope to achieve, including the anticipated or predicted time required for achievement. In setting goals, practitioners should be wary of measurement points far in the future. As time passes, the risk of changed circumstances that can affect the client's ability to achieve specific outcomes goals increases, making projections more guesses than goals. It is recommended that the time horizon for treatment plans should be no longer than six months after device delivery.

Basically, a treatment plan will identify what will happen upon device delivery: how the client will use it; what services will be provided to help the client; and what benefits the client is anticipated to receive from device use within the reasonably foreseeable future.

Summary

This chapter offered an overview of the largest source of funding for assistive devices: health benefits programs. It explained the two tasks practitioners must complete before health benefits programs will provide assistive device funding. Because these programs identify broad categories of health benefits as covered rather than identifying specific interventions or devices they will approve, practitioners' first task is *interpretive*: to review the definitions and scope of covered services to identify at least one category into which the recommended equipment item will fit.

Practitioners' second task is *descriptive* and is divided into three parts: to describe the client's illness, injury, or disability and unmet medical needs; to describe how the recommended device will serve as treatment for the client's condition and will improve function; and to describe why the recommended device is the least costly equally effective alternative to achieve those functional goals. Please check your learning from this chapter by reviewing Table 4.2.

Table 4.2 Review Your Learning.

1. Briefly describe at least three laws which are relevant to assistive devices?
2. Describe three different ways assistive devices are described based on different legislation and cite the legislation that uses each description.
3. List and briefly describe the common funding sources for assistive devices.
4. List the common substantive requirements of health benefits programs, the largest source of funding for assistive devices.
5. Describe your role in the funding process. What would you be required to do?
6. Using the case study in Box 4.1, recommend an assistive device for this client and document its medical necessity.

Notes

1 "Third-party" funding occurs when a third person or party becomes part of a transaction between a client and a supplier or provider of a needed service, such as a medical device supplier. The third party's role is to supply the funds necessary for the client to acquire the item or service from the provider or supplier. The third party can be a public source, such as one that provides government funds or a private source, such as a health insurance provider.

2 *Assistive devices* is a generic phrase used as a substitute for the inconsistent vocabulary found in the several sources of third-party funding discussed in this chapter. Individual programs will classify these devices most often as "assistive technology devices," "durable medical equipment," or "prosthetic devices."

3 The funding programs discussed here have legal duties and enforceable obligations to respond to client needs when their standards are met and procedures followed. For this reason it is essential practitioners know how they operate. Funding assistance also may be available from charities, but they have no "duty" or obligation to respond to client needs. For this reason, charities will not be further discussed here. They may be of help to some people, for some things, some of the time, but they can't and shouldn't be thought of as substitutes for the funding programs discussed in this chapter. Because they may provide essential help for some clients, practitioners should investigate possible funding assistance available from charities as well as their ability to serve as sources of equipment for trial use periods or as sources of no- or low-cost equipment loans.

4 Barnett, J.C. and Berchick, E.R. (2017). Health insurance coverage in the United States: 2016. United States Census Bureau. Report Number: P60-260. Retrieved from https://www.census.gov/library/publications/2017/demo/p60-260.html.

5 Publicly funded sources of health benefits are appropriately described as "programs." By contrast, health insurance and health benefits plans are assistive device funding sources, but are not "programs." For simplicity purposes, "programs" will be used throughout this chapter to describe all sources of health benefits.

6 For an example, you can visit https://www.opm.gov/healthcare-insurance/healthcare/plan-information/plan-codes/2018/brochures/71-005.pdf.

7 Medicaid is a partial exception. Medicaid does not offer "durable medical equipment" as a distinct benefits category. Instead, "medical equipment" is a benefit within the Medicaid home healthcare benefit category. Vol. 42 United States Code (U.S.C.) Sect §1396d(a)(7); Vol 42 Code of Federal Regulations (CFR) § 440.70(b)(3). Medicaid does cover "prosthetic devices" as a distinct benefits category. 42 U.S.C. § 1396d(a)(12); 42 CFR § 440.120(c). Medicaid also covers assistive devices within several other benefits categories including: nursing facility services; occupational, physical, or speech therapy services; rehabilitation services; intermediate care facility services for individuals with mental retardation or developmental disabilities; and through Medicaid "waiver" services.

8 Vol. 42 CFR Sect. 414.202. The current Medicare DME regulation includes a fifth criterion: that "items classified (by Medicare) as DME after Jan. 1, 2012, has an expected life of at least 3 years." Insurers and health plans often include one or two additional criteria that do not materially change the requirements of the Medicare definition. One common addition is the requirement that DME items be "ordered by a physician." This is a procedural requirement, not a characteristic of DME, and a physician prescription is a prerequisite of all health benefits programs for access to any covered service. Most often, it is not part of the DME definition. A second common addition to the DME definition is that DME items must not be "consumable or disposable." As discussed in the main text, demanding that equipment not be "consumable or disposable" is not meaningfully different from the requirement that they be "able to withstand repeated use."

9 To determine whether an equipment item already has been accepted as DME by a particular funding source, practitioners can search for the funding program's coverage guidelines to see if one exists for the specific item being recommended. These guidelines are commonly posted at funding program web pages. Second, practitioners can identify the "code" to which the specific DME item belongs, and then search the funding program's DME "fee schedule" to see if there is a code for that item. The presence of this code in the fee schedule can be used as an indicator of coverage. Third, practitioners can ask peers, suppliers, and manufacturers whether this funding source ever has paid for this item. Prior payment also can be used as an indicator of coverage.

10 Medicare also states that "an item is considered durable if it can withstand repeated use, i.e. the type of item which could normally be rented." This characteristic can be cited when applicable, i.e. when the practitioner can establish the equipment item sought is able to be rented. The ability of a device to be rented can be determined by review of the funding program's DME fee schedule. If the relevant code for the device is present, and there is a line for this code with the prefix "RR," the equipment in that code can be rented. Also, suppliers and manufacturers of the device can report whether the device is available on a rental basis.

11 *In re: Martin B.,* slip op. at 3, Social Security Admin. Office of Hearing & Appeals (29 November, 2001) posted at http://aacfundinghelp.com/funding_programs/MedicareAACDecisions/17.pdf.

12 *Blue v. Bonta,* 99 Cal. App. 4th 980, 121 Cal. Rptr. 2d 483 (1st Dist. 2002) ("We however must give the word 'medical' its ordinary sense, as referring more usually and broadly to the treatment, cure, or alleviation of any health condition, ...").

13 *See* e.g. American Occupational Therapy Association (2016). Assistive technology and occupational performance. *American Journal of Occupational Therapy* 70: 7012410030. http://dx.doi.org/10.5014/ajot.2016.706S02; American Physical Therapy Association (2014). Assistive technology: prescription, application and, as appropriate, fabrication or modification. In: *Guide to Physical Therapy Practice*; American Speech-Language-Hearing Association (1981). Nonspeech communication position statement. *ASHA* 23: 577–581; Am. Speech-Lang.-Hearing Assoc. (1989). Competencies for speech-language-pathologists providing services in augmentative communication. *ASHA* 31: 107–110; Am. Speech-Lang.-Hearing Assoc. (1991). Augmentative and alternative communication: position statement. *ASHA* 33 (Suppl. 5): 8; Am. Speech-Lang.-Hearing Assoc. (1992). Preferred practice patterns for speech-language pathology. § 30.3 Augmentative and alternative communication assessment, § 31.1 Augmentative and alternative communication system fitting/orientation (61–62, 87–88); Am. Speech-Lang.-Hearing Assoc. (1997). Preferred practice patterns for the profession of speech-language pathology. § 12.3 Augmentative and alternative communication assessment, § 15.2 Augmentative and alternative communication system and/or device treatment/orientation (141–142; 165–166); Am. Speech-Lang.-Hearing Assoc. (2001). Scope of practice in speech-language pathology, 1–28, 30; Am. Speech-Lang.-Hearing Assoc. (2002) Augmentative and alternative communication: knowledge and skills for service delivery; Am. Speech-Lang.-Hearing Assoc. (2004). Roles and responsibilities of speech-language pathologists with respect to augmentative and alternative communication: technical report; Am. Speech-Lang.-Hearing Assoc. (2004). Preferred practice patterns for the profession of speech-language pathology. § 26 Augmentative and alternative communication assessment, § 27 Augmentative and alternative communication intervention, § 28 prosthetic/adaptive device assessment, § 29 Prosthetic/adaptive device intervention (75–88). Retrieved from https://www.asha.org/policy/pp2004-00191/; Am. Speech-Lang.-Hearing Assoc. (2007). Scope of practice in speech-language pathology. Retrieved from https://www.asha.org/policy/sp2016-00343/.

14 D. Beukelman, D. and P. Mirenda, P. (1998). *Augmentative and Alternative Communication,* 2e, 73. (2nd Ed.) Baltimore, MD: Paul H. Brookes (comparing rate of speech production using natural speech and with SGDs). SGDs also present an additional issue: exception may be taken to one or more of the device's *ancillary* features. For example, some SGDs have environmental control ability, calculator functions, capability to store files in MP3 format, and a camera. Funding sources may argue that these or other device features do not serve a "medical purpose" and therefore their presence makes the device ineligible for funding. This analysis is incorrect. First, some of these features can be justified on a medical basis (e.g., MP3 file storage and a camera were included to aid the device's speech speech-generating device functions). Second, each of these features by itself and all of them together are no more than ancillary features. The "primary and customary" if not the exclusive use of this device will be as a communication aid. By definition, use of an ancillary feature will not and cannot be the "primary and customary" use of the device. Third, it is wholly unnecessary and inappropriate for an evaluation report supporting SGD funding to discuss any of these features (except perhaps the camera) as one the individual needs or will use or from which the individual will benefit. Practitioners should not equate a funding report with assessment or treatment notes. Reports should address only what funding sources require. No funding sources require discussion of any of these device capabilities or features.

15 Even if *not-covered* is the expected response based on application of this criterion, practitioners always should consider and, where appropriate, report that there is a cost to saying "no." Any equipment item will have an identifiable cost. But that amount may be significantly less than the cost to the funding program if the device is denied. If that occurs, the client's health may

deteriorate, necessitating different forms of care, such as inpatient hospital care for a client with a temperature- or humidity-sensitive condition. The best room air conditioner will cost far less than one day of inpatient hospital care. Equally true, a pressure relief surface or standing device will be significantly less costly than treatment for a skin ulcer, which may require hospital and/or nursing care to aid wound healing. In both instances there also will be significant yet wholly avoidable client suffering and/or pain. When these cost comparisons show significant benefits by providing the equipment, funding sources may recognize the cost savings of the requested device and will approve it.

16 Because these devices may be sold in either their "dedicated" configuration or "open," allowing access to all their computer- and speech-generating functions, it is essential practitioners always recommend that the "dedicated" models of these devices be provided.

17 42 U.S.C. § 1395x(n) (defining DME as equipment items "used in the patient's home" but excluding nursing facilities and hospitals).

18 42 U.S.C. § 1395x(n) (defining DME and citing as examples "iron lungs, oxygen tents, hospital beds and wheelchairs" as examples of covered items).

19 Vol. 42 Code of Federal Regulations (CFR) Sect. 414.202.

20 Medicare Claims Processing Manual, Medicare Publication No. 100–04, Chapter [20]: Durable Medical Equipment, Prosthetics, Orthotics, and Supplier (DMEPOS), at Section 10.1.2. http://www.cms.gov/Regulations-and-Guidance/Guidance/Manuals/Internet-Only-Manuals-IOMs.html.

21 It is important to note that therapy services, including use of assistive devices, can "augment" existing or residual function to achieve a level of function sufficient to meet all daily needs, or, an equipment item can provide a complete "alternative" way for the individual to achieve a specific functional outcome. In practical terms, this means that an individual will be appropriately considered for an assistive device when occupational therapy services cannot develop or restore natural functional abilities to enable the individual to meet the daily needs that arise in the course of daily activities. The individual may be able to stand for a very short time; walk a short distance; or speak and be understood to some extent – but none of these functional abilities is sufficient to meet all of the individual's daily needs. The individual's residual function or functional starting point may be, but does not have to be, zero for an assistive device recommendation to be appropriate.

22 A list of advocacy resources to help with appeals is attached to this chapter as Toolbox: Advocacy Resources.

Toolbox: Advocacy resources

Assistance for assistive device funding request appeals

National Disability Rights Network (NDRN): http://ndrn.org/en/ndrn-member-agencies.html	This web page provides contact information for a nationwide (state-by-state) network of "Protection & Advocacy Programs," which employ advocates and attorneys funded by the federal government to provide legal assistance to individuals with disabilities who seek assistive technology devices and services.
http://AACfundinghelp.com *or* www.aacfundinghelp.com	This web page offers a "contact us" link that will allow practitioners to ask assistive device funding questions and to refer funding request denials for speech-generating devices for individual review and possible appeal.

5

Outcomes, assessment, and research in assistive technology

Glenn Goodman, Jennifer Dunn, and Anne Bryden

Outline

Assistive Technologies and Environmental Interventions in Healthcare: An Integrated Approach, First Edition.
Edited by Lynn Gitlow and Kathleen Flecky.

Companion website: www.wiley.com/go/gitlow/assitivetechnologies

Learning outcomes

After reading this chapter, you should be able to:

1. Characterize conceptual practice models that inform high-quality outcomes, assessment, and research in assistive technology.
2. Examine and utilize existing resources, experts, and organizations that subscribe to excellence in outcomes research in assistive technology.
3. Describe and critique a variety of research designs currently used in outcomes research in assistive technology.
4. Identify aspects of the Human-Tech Ladder related to outcomes in assistive technology.

Active learning prompts

Before you read this chapter:

1. Define assistive technology by visiting the Resources page of the Rehabilitation Engineering and Assistive Technology Society of North America (RESNA) website (http://www.resna.org/resources). Explore existing resources to support outcomes research by consulting the Frameworks/Outcome Measurement page of the RESNA website (https://www.resna.org/frameworksoutcome-measurements). Additionally, investigate literature that portrays current and future visions of best practice in outcomes research for assistive technology, for example, the article by Fuhrer et al. (2003).
2. Describe potential team members capable of designing and implementing high-quality outcomes research in assistive technology, for example, visit Project DO-IT communities of practice (http://www.washington.edu/doit/Resources/cops.html).
3. Identify stakeholders and goals for outcomes research in assistive technology (AT) that would answer a research question related to the effectiveness of AT products or services.
4. Examine literature that analyzes existing efforts in the way of systematic literature reviews, meta-analysis, critical appraisals, randomized control trials, and high-quality quasi-experimental, descriptive, and qualitative research to replicate or improve upon existing knowledge, for example, *Assistive Technology Effects on the Employment Outcomes for People with Cognitive Disabilities: A Systematic Review* by Sauer et al. (2010).

Key terms

Assistive technology device (ATD)
Conceptual model
Experimental-type design (Quantitative)
Human Activity-Assistive Technology (HAAT) model
International Classification of Functioning, Disability and Health (ICF)
Matching Person and Technology Model (MPTM)
Naturalistic design (Qualitative)
Outcomes
Social cognition models

Outcomes, assessment, and research in assistive technology

This chapter begins with a review and expansion of conceptual models for assistive technology (AT) outcomes and practice presented in Chapter 2 to encourage readers to engage in outcomes research built upon existing theories and models of practice. It is the authors' belief that research based on theory and AT practice is superior to studies that lack a theoretical foundation. Next, research designs and methodology particularly relevant to the study of AT assessment and outcomes are examined. A brief review of various research designs and methods are described with examples of current or past studies to implement these designs. Finally, this chapter presents a Toolbox to identify resources, individuals, and organizations dedicated to the advancement of outcomes research in AT.

Conceptual models for AT Outcomes and Practice

Conceptual models provide a theoretical base for improvement and advancement of knowledge and practice. Using a conceptual model structures current knowledge, offers a perspective for examining new problems, and provides a means for planning and evaluating of services and intervention (Lenker and Paquet 2003). The AT field has long sought a single conceptual model that would serve the wide range of stakeholders involved in this field. The field of AT is one that historically faces rapid advancements, particularly in the past two decades, with the increased use of personal computers, mobile phones, and mobile computing by the public (Schulz et al. 2015). This has also expanded the options available to individuals with disabilities. Consequently, one of the critical responsibilities for all the stakeholders, such as clients, practitioners, manufacturers, funders, and policy makers, in the provision of AT is measuring the impact of the technology, particularly as interventions become more complex and costlier (Fuhrer 2001).

This section will provide a brief perspective on conceptual models used for AT selection and service delivery. All models denote the major factors in interaction of a person, technology, and external contexts (such as legislation and funding). These multiple factors align with the rungs on Vincent's Human-Tech Ladder. The Consortium on Assistive Technology Outcomes Research (CATOR) proposed measures from its taxonomy and hierarchical classification of outcome measures that are needed to adhere to the International Classification of Functioning, Disability and Health (ICF), one of the important conceptual models for AT (Jutai et al. 2005).

In addition to the ICF, other conceptual practice models relevant to the AT field include: the Human Activity-Assistive Technology (HAAT) model, the Matching Person and Technology Model (MPTM), and social cognition models. Each of these conceptual models will be depicted in relationship to measures and outcomes in AT.

International Classification of Functioning, Disability and Health

The ICF is part of the World Health Organization's (WHO) taxonomy of classifications developed to provide a common language for described functional states associated with health conditions (Gray and Hendershot 2000). The ICF provides a holistic, biopsychosocial framework for identifying and understanding rehabilitation needs and developing comprehensive service and treatment plans to address the identified needs. A visual depiction of the ICF is shown in Figure 5.1.

Beyond an individual level, the ICF has the capacity to facilitate understanding of the needs of communities, nations, and the world by leading to the development of strategies and policies to address rehabilitation and health-related needs (WHO 2001). The ICF components address the elements inherent in AT assessment and intervention. In addition, it speaks a common language, which is important due to the multitude of disciplines and researchers involved in the AT field. The ICF provides a unified and standard language and framework for the description of health and health-related states (WHO 2001).

The ICF describes individuals in terms of function rather than levels of deficit or dysfunction (WHO 2001). The de-emphasis on pathology and diagnosis in the ICF can enhance a view of rehabilitation centered on current and future functional performance outcomes. It provides a framework for assessment through use of the ICF Checklist (WHO 2001).

The aim of the ICF is to provide a scientific basis for the consequences of health conditions, to establish a common language to improve communications, and to permit comparison of data across countries, disciplines, services, and time (WHO 2001). Its goals are to move the origin and consequences of health conditions from a medical model to a social model of health (WHO 2001). By dividing the consequences of injury or illness into separate domains, the ICF provides a framework to describe the consequences of a health condition.

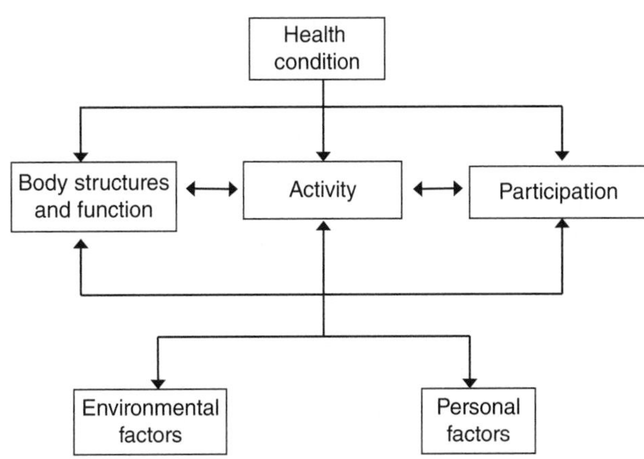

Figure 5.1 International classification of functioning, disability and health – (ICF) Source: World health organization 2001, p. 11.

Additionally, built into the ICF model are interactions and reciprocal influences between the domains, for example environmental and activity, as represented by the arrows in Figure 5.1. These arrows represent the interactive dimensions of health, and each domain is acknowledged as an influence on another domain (WHO 2001). Duggan and colleagues postulated that these interactions "breathe life into the ICF model" through reference to real life experiences or phenomena that defy being fit into the taxonomic scheme (Duggan et al. 2008, p. 986).

ICF components

The key ICF components are: body structures and function, activities and participation, environmental factors, and personal factors, as noted in Figure 5.1.

Body structures are anatomical parts such as organs or limbs. Body functions are the physiological functions of body systems. In the body structures and function component, an impairment occurs when there is any significant deviation or loss in body function or structure (WHO 2001). These impairments may include mental, sensory, speed and voice, cardiovascular, hematologic, immunologic, respiration, metabolic, neuromuscular, and movement (WHO 2001).

Activity is the execution of a task or action by an individual (WHO 2001). Gray and Hendershot (2000) noted that this task execution is not considered in the results of controlled clinical tests that examine the capacity or aptitude to perform specified activities. Along with activity, participation is described in this model. It is an individual's involvement in life situations in relation to health conditions, body functions and structures, activities, and contextual factors (WHO 2001). Participation restrictions are "problems an individual may experience in involvement in life situations" because of their disability (WHO 2001, p. 14). The measurement of participation restrictions is considered essential to understand the social impact of a chronic illness or disability on a person's life (Cardol et al. 2002).

Environmental factors refer to all aspects of the external or intrinsic world that form the context of an individual's life and, as such, have an impact of the person's functioning (WHO 2001). These include the physical world and its features, other people in different roles and relationships, attitudes and values, social systems, policies, rules, and laws (WHO 2001). Environmental factors are either facilitators or barriers to functioning. Facilitators are defined as "environmental factors in a person's environment that, through their absence or presence, improve functioning and reduce disability" (WHO 2001, pp. 213, 214). Conversely, barriers are described as the factors that limit function and create disability through their presence or absence (WHO 2001).

Within the ICF model, *assistive technology devices* (ATDs) are classified as environmental factors that are used to overcome health state impairments and activity and participation limitations and restrictions. The ICF is also appropriate for AT practice because environmental factors include: access to services, products, and funding for these interventions, which can be major barriers for many clients. An important limitation of the ICF in relation to AT is the imprecision of coding of assistive devices within the ICF (Smith et al. 2006). The ICF classifies AT devices according to the functional domains; it does not include details on function or features for the diversity of equipment.

Finally, personal factors include socioeconomic status, age, education, employment, and previous experience (WHO 2001). Many of these personal factors can have a profound impact on the potential user of AT, such as personal expectations and previous experiences (Scherer et al. 2007). While the environmental and personal factors are acknowledged by the WHO as being important, currently there is no way of measuring these factors or their impact on the three domains.

Studies have shown that while there is interaction between the components of the ICF, these are distinct, and a change in one component does not necessarily result in a direct change in any of the others (Cardol et al. 1999; Jette et al. 2003). There are differing opinions regarding the effect of an individual's impairment and limitation of activities on their life satisfaction or quality of life (QoL) or other outcomes measures that might be assessed that are relevant to AT intervention (Samsa and Matchar 2004).

Strengths and limitations of the ICF in clinical rehabilitation settings

Readers will recall from Chapter 2 and the beginning of this chapter that the ICF was developed as a classification system or taxonomy and not an assessment tool. The goals of assessment within rehabilitation and health are to evaluate the health status-related qualities within domains of functioning. Rehabilitation interventions are intended to maintain functioning, prevent loss of functioning, and enhance recovery and independence (Stucki et al. 2005). Thus, accurate classification of functioning will inform assessment within the domains of functioning and related interventions. The strength of the ICF is its use for clarifying and distinguishing between different areas of practice which tend to be domain specific. The ICF uses a universal, culturally responsive, interactive model of health and functioning that covers the entire life span of an individual (Ustun et al. 2003; WHO 2001).

The lack of temporal and causal components has been documented as a key limitation of the ICF model because they are particularly important when assessing outcomes in such areas as participation, cost, satisfaction, or QoL, as time and cause-effect may impact these domains. (Gray and Hendershot 2000).

Using the ICF in clinical rehabilitation settings

The ICF is comprised of over 1500 categories and is often too cumbersome for professional practitioners to incorporate into everyday clinical rehabilitation setting. To enhance the utility of the ICF, the ICF Core Sets have been developed for specific health conditions (Biering-Sorensen et al. 2006). These core sets have been developed through a rigorous, international consultation process that has identified the categories that are most clinically relevant to the rehabilitation needs of people with a health condition (Cieza et al. 2004). These aim to identify the common consequences of functioning for each health condition with the goal of valid and globally agreed tools that can be used in clinical practice, research, and health statistics (Biering-Sorensen et al. 2006; Cieza et al. 2004; Lenker and Jutai 1996; Ruof et al. 2004; Stucki and Cieza 2004; Stucki et al. 2003).

Human Activity-Assistive Technology model

The HAAT model was adapted from the Human Performance Model (Bailey 1989) and described comprehensively by Cook and Hussey (2002; Cook and Polgar 2008, 2014). In its seemingly concise and simple presentation, it considers an individual's use of AT for the goal of completing an activity. All three elements of the model – human, AT, and activity – can be impacted by contextual factors such as the social and physical aspects of one's environment or setting (Cook and Polgar 2014). According to Lenker and Paquet (2003), the descriptive traits of the HAAT model are relevant to AT use. The human aspect of the model is defined by the combination of a person's innate abilities and acquired skills or developed proficiency. AT is denoted as a device with a human interface and a processor to achieve the desired output to achieve an activity (Cook and Polgar 2014). The activities are viewed according to the broad domains described by the American Occupational Therapy Association's Uniform Terminology for Occupational Therapy (now replaced by the Occupational Therapy Practice Framework) – self-care, work/school, and play/leisure (Lenker and Paquet 2003).

Despite the strength of the descriptive qualities of this model, the predictive qualities have not been systematically tested. The benefit of the HAAT model is its consideration of factors related to the individual from the perspective of innate and learned abilities as well as the environment, including interactions of the social and physical settings.

Matching Person and Technology model

The *Matching Person and Technology Model (MPT)* (Scherer 1998) is another conceptual model that incorporates the interactions of the environment or milieu, the person, and AT. The interaction of these elements – (i) the environment in which the technology is used; (ii) preferences and needs of the user, and (iii) features of the AT itself – results in a continuum of outcomes ranging from positive to negative (Scherer 1998). Positive outcomes are associated with use of the technology whereas negative outcomes are associated with low use or abandonment of the technology (Scherer 1998).

A unique aspect of the MPT model is the set of instruments developed to characterize the three domains of the model. These instruments consist of self-report checklists designed to understand the needs and preferences of the consumer as well as technology-specific forms designed to aid consumers and practitioners in the selection of AT. Each instrument collects information from the consumer or prospective user of technology as well as the practitioner providing the technology (Scherer 2008).

Like the HAAT model, the descriptive traits of the MPT model are relevant to the AT process. The model provides excellent structure for prospectively studying and potentially predicting usage and user satisfaction of AT (Lenker and Paquet 2003). The MPT provides a practical approach for both consumers and practitioners to identify the broad range of factors associated with the selection and provision of AT to ensure the best match between the user and the technology.

Social Cognition models

The HAAT and MPT models both represent person–environment interactions and specifically include AT as a component of the model. Some studies of AT have incorporated *social cognition models*, adopted from the field of psychology, as a conceptual practice model. Examples of use of these models are evident in AT-related literature by various authors (Gitlin 1998; Roelands et al. 2002; Rogers 2003).

The premise behind social cognition theories is that a person has a natural tendency to engage in behavior that results in a personal expected positive benefit. An individual will balance their own attitudes and perceived sense of control against expectations of others, resulting in the choice of action that offers the most favorable outcome (Lenker and Paquet 2003). The benefits of using social cognition theories in measuring AT outcomes is limited, as they may not necessarily be specific to AT, or may focus only on usage of AT and not on the technology selection process (Bernd et al. 2009).

In sum, the conceptual models presented in this chapter provide foundational principles for the AT process, but continued theoretical development is needed as technology evolves. According to Gelderblom and deWitte (2002), the field of AT outcomes measurement is still developing and facing challenges including: (i) further development of instruments, (ii) standardization of the instruments and their application, and (iii) international collaboration.

Applied fields of AT practice benefit from conceptual models that provide a common theoretical framework and language for researchers and clinicians. Assessment is more accurate and useful when it is applied with clearly defined domains of disability, health, and functioning. Despite some limitations to application in outcomes research in AT, the ICF provides such a classification system as well as providing a common language that enhances rehabilitation within multidisciplinary teams. It is a model with strengths in international application (Jutai et al. 2004).

Outcomes

What is outcomes research?

Outcomes research seeks to understand the end results of healthcare practices and interventions. End results include effects that people experience and care about, such as change in the ability to function. For individuals with chronic conditions – where cure is not always possible – end results include QoL as well as mortality. By linking the care people get to the outcomes they experience, outcomes research has become the key to developing better ways to monitor and improve the quality of care.

> Outcomes research helps us understand whether and why AT interventions are meeting their intended purpose for users. The paucity of outcomes data affects many stakeholders in the assistive technology (AT) field, including clinicians, researchers, manufacturers, and consumers. This adversely influences funding decisions for consumers, hampers clinicians who need to demonstrate the value of their service delivery programs, and makes it difficult for manufacturers to demonstrate the cost-effectiveness of their products.
>
> (RESNA 2017)

A collection of patient- or client-reported outcomes is not necessarily tied to outcome research. Patient-reported outcomes (PROs) are any reports coming directly from patients about their appraisal of functioning or thoughts in relation to a health condition and therapy, without interpretation of the patient's responses by a clinician (Higgins and Green 2011). Most healthcare agencies are mandated to report outcomes and to include the stakeholders in the process. Often this form of outcome is neglected or disrespected by the medical and research community as unscientific and subjective. However, data collection on how clients feel or think regarding AT products and services is an important component of an AT outcomes research project (Clayback et al. 2015).

Outcomes research in AT should focus on consumer goals, adoption of the technology, employment or other forms of productive participation in activities of daily living, models of practice or practice settings, the external physical, social, cultural, institutional, and political environments, and QoL (Higgins and Green 2011). However, development of an outcomes-related study that addresses many of the above issues is challenging.

AT *outcomes* refers to what happens because of using an AT device or service. "The 'outcome' from the use of AT can cover a wide range of issues and goals, and could include whether: 1) technology was used or abandoned; 2) AT led to efficient completion of specific tasks/activities; 3) AT played a role in gainful employment; 4) cost savings were realized; 5) decreased family or caregiver support was realized; 5) increased independence resulted; or 6) the individual's quality of life was enhanced" (Lenker et al. 2002, p. 1).

Who are the important stakeholders? These are persons, agencies, or institutions who have a contributing interest or influence on AT provision and services. This is an important question that should be addressed in outcomes research. Additionally, the development of research questions, choice of assessment methods and instruments, type of data collected and format, data analysis methods, and formatting of results are other issues that should be carefully considered regarding the stakeholder question. Rust and Smith (2006) presented issues of importance to the developers of AT that may significantly differ from outcomes sought by service providers, third-party payers, politicians, or consumers. Pertinent questions are presented in Table 5.1.

Table 5.1 Questions related to AT.

- Estimated retail price
- Is the product unique?
- Does it provide a clear benefit for users?
- Can it be manufactured by the company?
- Who are the expected users?
- What is the market size?
- What is the competition?
- Is it safe to use?
- What is the manufacturing cost?
- Is tooling required and what is the cost of it?
- What is the estimated profit/year?
- Is it aesthetically pleasing?
- Is it patented?
- What is the "hunch" factor?
- What is the level of potential "ownership"? (Rust and Smith 2006, p. 36)

AT outcome measures

There are a variety of approaches to measurement of the impact of AT on consumers. Since AT is used primarily for persons with disabilities, several existing rehabilitation outcome measures are relevant to measure the impact of a given intervention. Unfortunately, existing rehabilitation outcome measures are often inadequate in characterizing the contributions of AT in the achievement of the user's goals at both an activity and a participation level.

A significant challenge is in the lack of one uniform definition and set of characteristics in which AT is regarded in the large body of existing outcome measures. Rust and Smith (2005) reviewed rehabilitation literature and identified 100 potential rehabilitation outcome instruments related to AT provision and services. There were three categories in which the use of AT was regarded or scored: (i) AT is not acknowledged or considered at all in the scoring, (ii) using AT discounted the functional outcome score, or (iii) AT was allowed and enhanced the functional score (Rust and Smith 2005). Out of the outcome instruments reviewed, most fell into categories (i) and (ii) above, with only 22 instruments within the (iii) category (Rust and Smith 2005).

Moreover, Jutai and Day (2002) identified two limitations in using existing health-related QoL measures in gauging the impact of AT: (i) they are too medically oriented and are not designed to measure the restoration of functional capacities that is provided by AT, and (ii) they are designed to measure health status, not the impact of an intervention using AT (Jutai and Day 2002).

These studies underline a significant flaw in the use of general measures for assessing AT's impact rooted in the lack of a uniform conceptual model on which to base outcome measures. Consequently, a growing number of AT-specific measures are needed and are emerging in the literature. Just as it is important to seek a uniform conceptual model to structure outcomes measurement, it is equally important to develop the evaluative and psychometric properties of existing measures. It is not practical to suggest that one measure would serve the needs for measuring all AT interventions; however, there are several general measures available for determining the impact of a wide variety of AT interventions across various populations. Researchers and AT professionals should take advantage of the strengths of existing measures and contribute to their further development for application in outcome measures. The next section will review some of the most promising AT-specific instruments that can reduce some of the challenges faced while development of outcome measures and a strong base of evidence to support the positive impact of AT evolves.

AT-specific assessment tools

The matching person and technology (MPT) assessment process

The MPT assessment process consists of a series of assessments designed to facilitate both the practitioner and the consumer to identify the best match between their personal characteristics and needs and the features of a prospective technology (Scherer 1998, 2008). The process consists of a suite of assessments that are environment or activity specific and presented in Table 5.2.

Each instrument consists of two components, one designed for the practitioner or provider and one targeted at the consumer of AT. Strengths of the MPT process include its focus on the needs of the consumer and its consideration of the person's QoL while accounting for all relevant influences on technology use (Scherer 2008). The by-product of this process is the identification of appropriate strategies to ensure the consumer's optimal use of technology as well as a reduction of wasted time and resources secondary to the prospective identification of a mismatch between the person and technology. Much work has been done developing the psychometric properties of the Assistive

Table 5.2 Matching person with technology (MPT) assessment tools.

- Survey of Technology Use (SOTU)
- Assistive Technology Device Predisposition Assessment (ATDPA)
- Educational Technology Predisposition Assessment (ETPA)
- Workplace Technology Predisposition Assessment (WTPA)
- Health Care Technology Predisposition Assessment (HCTPA)

Technology Device Predisposition Assessment (ATDPA) and the other measures in the suite of MPT instruments, supporting good validity and reliability (Scherer 2008).

While the MPT instruments were developed under the conceptual model of Matching Person and Technology, this multifaceted approach to delivering and assessing the impact of AT is also congruent with the ICF model (Scherer and Glueckauf 2005). The MPT takes a perspective of activities and participation measurement as well as a perspective measurement of environmental and personal factors. This is not surprising given Scherer's conscious effort to adhere to the terminology proposed by the ICF in the development of the MPTM and its corresponding instruments (Lenker and Paquet 2003).

The Quebec user evaluation of satisfaction with AT (QUEST 2.0)

The QUEST is a tool developed to assess the consumer's satisfaction with AT (Demers et al. 2002). Features of this assessment include: (i) its ability to test satisfaction across a wide range of AT devices; (ii) it's uses as both a clinical tool and a research measure, and (iii) its applicability to individuals ranging from later adolescence to the elderly. The instrument is rooted in the premise that satisfaction, as related to AT use, is based upon two underlying facets: devices and services.

The QUEST identified eight characteristics related to device satisfaction: comfort, weight, durability, adjustments, simplicity of use, dimensions, effectiveness, and safety. There are four components of AT service delivery: delivery, professional service, follow-up, and repairs/servicing (Demers et al. 2002). Consumers rate their experience with AT using a five-point Likert scale ranging from "not satisfied at all" to "very satisfied." It is self-administered via paper and pen or by interview for those who cannot complete independently (Demers et al. 2002). Scores can be calculated singly for the AT device, for AT services components, or as a total for the device and service components together. The psychometric properties of the instrument have been primarily tested by the instrument developers and have shown good validity and reliability (Demers et al. 2002). A strength of the QUEST is its generalizability toward a variety of AT interventions. However, it is focused solely on the outcome of the intervention and is therefore not designed to facilitate the AT delivery process.

The psychosocial impact of assistive devices scales (PIADS)

The PIADS is an instrument developed to measure three dimensions of the impact of AT: functional independence, well-being, and QoL (Day and Jutai 1996). It is a self-report questionnaire that consists of 26 items categorized within three subscales: competence, adaptability, and self-esteem. The 12 items representing competency are meant to reflect feelings of competency and efficacy by measuring the impact of AT on performance and productivity (Day and Jutai 1996). Six items reflect adaptability by capturing the technology user's willingness to take risks, try new things, or assume new roles because of the AT. The eight self-esteem items measure the impact of technology on the user's emotional well-being and self-confidence (Jutai and Day 2002). Each item is scored using a seven-point Likert scale ranging from −3 (maximum negative impact) to 0 (neutral or no impact) to +3 (maximum positive impact). A significant body of work exists measuring the psychometric properties of the PIADS, indicating good to excellent results (Jutai and Day 2002).

The PIADS has many strengths. It involves a comprehensive method of measuring the impact of AT with consideration of both personal and environmental factors that influence AT use. The tool also emphasizes activity capacity, performance, and participation, so aligns with the ICF framework (Jutai and Day 2002). Additionally, there may be predictive elements of this instrument, which, when completed a priori by the consumer, provide anticipation of the impact of a specific AT. This may provide insight into potential device use or discontinuance, thus potentially saving time and resources through prevention of an ineffective device.

Individually prioritized problem assessment (IPPA)

The IPPA is a client-centered, AT-specific instrument that was developed in response to a lack of appropriate existing measures in the field of health technology (Wessels et al. 2002). This interview-based assessment tool identifies prospective consumer problems in performing daily activities that might be reduced or eliminated because of AT intervention. Up to seven consumer goals may be identified, and an activity checklist is available to facilitate identification of problems (Wessels et al. 2002).

Once all of the problems are identified, the participant is asked to rate each problem according to the activity's level of importance (five-point Likert scale ranging from 1 "not important at all" to 5 "most important") and perceived difficulty in performing the activity (five-point Likert scale ranging from 1 "no difficulty at all" to 5 "too much difficulty to perform the activity at all"). The difficulty scores are weighted according to the importance scores and summed. That sum is divided by the number of problems identified and the result serves as the baseline score (Wessels et al. 2002).

With re-evaluation, several months after AT has been issued, the participant re-rates their difficulty in the activities/problems identified in the first assessment. The difference in the new score from the baseline score reflects the impact of the AT intervention. The psychometric properties of the IPPA were well established during its development (Persson 1997) and it has been used in several AT outcome studies; however, reliability, specifically inter-rater reliability, requires additional research (Wessels et al. 2002).

The IPPA is a practical tool in that it has a focus on the needs of the prospective AT consumer. The instrument aligns with the activity and participation component of the ICF as the user chooses meaningful activities that will facilitate their participation in expected life roles, while also assessing personal and environmental factors (Wessels et al. 2002).

SIVA cost analysis instrument (SCAI)

An important element in the evaluation of outcomes in AT is assessment of cost. Technology is continually advancing, with rising costs associated with providing technology to consumers. Healthcare practitioners are encouraged to consider the economic consequences of their decisions when recommending or prescribing AT (Andrich 2002). The SCAI is an instrument aimed to provide clinicians with a tool to calculate the costs associated with provision of AT services (Andrich 2002). This system, which is targeted at program outcomes rather than individual outcomes, consists of three steps: (i) describe the objectives of the AT program; (ii) estimate the sequencing and timing of all the interventions that form the program, and (iii) compile a cost calculation table for each AT intervention.

The SCAI was designed as an AT informative tool rather than contributing to AT decision-making. It has also been proposed as potentially useful for comparison of AT programs (Andrich 2002). In a response to the increasing demands for cost-effectiveness within healthcare and AT delivery, the SCAI is a feasible technique for implementation of a cost outcome analysis within individual AT programs.

Promising general outcome measures

Two existing instruments, the Canadian Occupational Performance Measure (COPM) and the Assessment of Life Habits (LIFE-H) show potential in outcomes measurement related to QoL, social participation, and performance of activities of daily living (ADLs).

The COPM

The COPM is an occupational therapy-based, client-centered tool developed as a clinical appraisal of occupational performance. The instrument is administered through a semi-structured interview consisting of five steps: (i) problem definition, (ii) problem weighing, (iii) problem scoring, (iv) reassessment, and (v) follow-up (Law et al. 1990).

Through an interview process, the clinician helps the participant to identify deficits in occupational performance areas and to establish goals for achievement. The participant is encouraged to think about problems in performance in the areas of self-care, productivity, and leisure to facilitate a comprehensive assessment of function. Once deficits are identified, the participant is asked to rate the importance of being able to perform the specified activity using a Likert scale of 1–10 (1 = *negative*; 10 = *positive*). This helps to prioritize goals. The participant is then asked to rate his or her current performance of the specified activities and satisfaction with that performance using the same Likert scale. The process is repeated after an intervention such as rehabilitation, or perhaps AT intervention.

The COPM's psychometric properties are well-developed (McColl et al. 2000) and it has been used to measure outcomes in a variety of populations (Bodiam 1999; Carpenter et al. 2001; Cup et al. 2003), including AT outcomes in adolescents with spinal cord injury (Mulcahey et al. 2004).

Strengths of the COPM include its focus on activities that are self-identified by the participant and its ability to measure the participant's internal judgment of changes in performance and satisfaction because of an intervention. The structure of the instrument offers great flexibility for measuring the impact of a wide variety of AT interventions. The participant could be guided to focus on occupational performance areas that could potentially change as the result of AT use.

The assessment of life habits (LIFE-H)

The goal of the LIFE-H is to document the quality of social participation in people with disabilities by capturing the way people complete ADLs and fulfill their social roles and expectations (Noreau et al. 2002). The instrument consists of a short form (69 items) that is used for screening and a long form (240 items) that is used for a more in-depth analysis of the various domains of social participation. The measurement scale reflects both the level of difficulty a person has while performing an activity or life habit and the type of assistance that is needed. These concepts are combined in one 10-point "accomplishment" scale (Noreau et al. 2002). The psychometric properties of the LIFE-H have been well established (Noreau et al. 2002, 2004). Like the COPM, the LIFE-H has been used with a variety of populations (Fauconnier et al. 2009; Noreau et al. 2002, 2004). The underlying concepts of the COPM and the LIFE-H are in congruence with the ICF model.

Research designs and methods

> Any research project should use strategies to ensure quality of the research and assure the researcher and consumers that the information is trustworthy, rigorous and authentic. The basic steps to any research project include: 1) develop a feasible, answerable research question; 2) complete a literature review to locate and analyze existing knowledge; 3) identify partners or mentors for research collaboration; 4) consultation with AT research stakeholders, including manufacturers of AT devices, consumers and AT service providers; 5) design a systematic study and research proposal with delineation on research participants, research design, procedures, assessments and instruments, data collection and analysis, and strategies/venues for dissemination.
>
> (Brandt et al. 2012a)

Of concern in AT outcomes research is: (i) creation of a team that provides interprofessional collaboration; (ii) clear definition of research purpose that addresses the following questions: Is the purpose an evaluation of an AT program intervention? Is the purpose to describe outcomes related to a device or service, product development, or development of a new instrument or assessment for AT? (iii) careful attention to feasibility issues; for example, does the team have the expertise to answer the question? Are the researchers able to generate an appropriate sample? Does the research team have the resources needed to complete the study? (Polit and Beck 2014).

Research methods for AT outcomes could be described in three major categories; quantitative, qualitative, and mixed methods (Brandt et al. 2012b). Additional methods include systematic literature review and methodological research to develop new products or assessments. Because research in AT outcomes is complex and should address many of the factors mentioned above, program evaluation methods are a relevant fit in designing outcome studies. Program evaluation research suggests mixed methods are most effective (Posavac and Carey 2003). This next section will explore each of these methods in detail as they relate to AT outcome research.

Experimental-type designs (quantitative)

Experimental-type designs (quantitative) use objective thinking and numeric data collection and statistical analysis methods to manipulate and control variables to test for the effectiveness of AT devices and services. Examples of quantitative methods and outcomes are presented in Table 5.3.

Table 5.3 Quantitative Designs and Outcomes.

Quantitative design	Examples
Descriptive research designs	Outcomes of pre and post AT numeric assessments, quality of life scales, caregiver assessments, activities of daily living (ADL) and instrumental activities of daily living (IADL) assessments, interviews, focus groups, and other methods to collect caregiver and end user opinions with no ability to imply cause and effect
Quasi-experimental research designs	Real-world applications; ethical concerns such as withholding treatment from a control group; counterbalanced designs, time series designs, single-subject research, cohort designs
Experimental research designs	Classic experimental design, Solomon four group designs
Meta-analysis	Statistical evaluation of multiple research studies

There are many practical decisions and concerns in choosing an experimental-type quantitative design for AT outcomes. Often it is difficult to obtain enough participants for a meaningful or powerful statistical analysis of data. The ethical considerations and practicality of using a control group are often a barrier to designing an experimental study. Longitudinal follow-up studies have the potential for addressing these concerns, especially with missing information or a high morbidity rate among participants in a study. Moreover, the AT research team may not have resources or expertise readily available for statistical analysis, appropriate selection of research design and procedures, or proficiency to implement complex designs. A careful review by the research team of these potential concerns prior to implementation of a study is essential.

Descriptive research

Descriptive quantitative research designs use statistical methods to describe participant characteristics and outcomes of AT prior to and after an intervention. They are limited in establishing cause and effect relationships, but are helpful in describing changes in performance, attitudes and opinions, and amount of use of the technology. Descriptive research is generally categorized as level-IV evidence. (Centre for Evidence-Based Medicine n.d.).

An example of a well-designed and rigorous descriptive study was completed by Demers et al. (2008). The authors completed a follow-up study of 139 participants for whom one or more mobility aids were recommended following hospitalization. Categories of AT use based on participant interviews were collected using Short Form 36 (SF 36) tool, a highly regarded measure of health-related QoL and identification of participant primary mobility aids. Comparisons between groups for seven different trajectories of use of mobility devices was made based on diagnosis, age, and SF 36 results in mental and physical functioning.

Moreover, this study described relationships among variables and use of mobility devices. For example, individuals in trajectory 5 group, who discontinued the recommended mobility device early after discharge, were found to have higher physical and mental functioning than the individuals in the other trajectories (Demers et al. 2008). Studies like this one can be repeated with various populations or used to generate patterns and relationships that can be further tested with experimental-type research.

Quasi-experimental research

Quasi-experimental research is denoted by a lack of a true control group or randomization, unlike true experimental design (Edmonds and Kennedy 2013). It is rated highly for ability to conduct experiments in real-world or naturalistic settings. It falls short of experimental research designs in internal validity. It is a type of research design with either inability to utilize a comparison or control group, or lack of randomization (Portney and Watkins 2015). Some basic quasi-experimental designs include: (i) cohort studies, in which equivalency among the groups cannot be guaranteed; (ii) time series designs that involve participants as their own controls and notes changes during the intervention implementation; (iii) counterbalance designs, in which participants receive multiple interventions and the timing of the treatment or control periods is randomized (Portney and Watkins 2015). Single-subject designs are classified as quasi-experimental research. This design is like group time series studies, with the timing of the control period used to compare outcomes measured during the intervention phase of the study. The participants act as their own controls (Creswell 2013; Ottenbacher 1986).

Watson et al. (2010) used a repeated-measures pretest–posttest quasi-experimental design to assess the effect of AT in a public school setting. This design was chosen to address a lower "n" and high levels of heterogeneity among the participants. The researchers utilized the Student Performance Profile assessment to establish the superior relative effectiveness of AT devices compared to other interventions in completion of individualized education plan (IEP) goals among 13 student participants (Watson et al. 2010).

Experimental research designs

The classic experimental design involves random selection of participants, random assignment of the participants to a control group or comparison group who receives standard intervention, and rigorous attempts to eliminate bias among the participants and researchers (Portney and Watkins 2015). Use of double-blind studies, in which the participant and the persons collecting data are unknown to each other, prevent the participants and the data collectors/evaluators from knowing who is receiving the experimental intervention and who is not. Additionally, this type of design aids in development of participant groups that are equivalent at the pretest phase of the study. This design is usually represented as shown below:

R	O	X	O
R	O		O

R = random assignment, O = an observation or measurement of the dependent variables, and X = the experimental treatment or intervention.

Two other basic experimental designs are the Solomon 4 group design:

R	O	X	O
R	O		O
R		X	O
R			O

and the posttest only control group design:

R	X	O
R		O

The latter two designs are more powerful for controlling the interaction between the pretesting procedures and the intervention. These experimental designs can be strengthened by replication of the "O" for observation of the long-term effects of the intervention (Campbell and Stanley 2010).

An example of a study utilizing an experimental research design was implemented by Tomita et al. (2007). The study involved 46 participants who received computers and X10 smart home technology with 67 individuals in a control group. The participants were characterized as home-based frail older adults who lived alone. The group receiving the intervention maintained physical and cognitive status, whereas the control group declined significantly in status. The strengths of this study included: (i) longitudinal follow-up over a two-year period; (ii) use of highly recognized and standardized assessments, Functional Independence Measure (FIM), Craig Handicap Assessment and Reporting Technique (CHART), and multiple measures including physical and cognitive function, ADL and instrumental activities of daily living (IADL) function, and living situation (Tomita et al. 2007). This study reported a statistically significant higher percentage of the participants in the intervention group that remained at home two years later.

Naturalistic design (qualitative)

Naturalistic designs (qualitative) are characterized by use of a subjective, reflexive approach with text, observational, or video data and analysis based on coding and thematic analysis (Creswell 2012; Patton 2015). The strength of qualitative research is the integration of the research question, the data, and the analysis of the data, all occurring simultaneously. Based on the perspective of the theoretical paradigm, there are a variety of qualitative research methods available (Corbin and Strauss 2014; Patton 2015). Qualitative research is useful in AT outcome studies for the attributes as presented in Table 5.4.

Methods used in qualitative research vary depending on the question being asked in the study, the study design, and the type of information needed by which informants address rigor, authenticity, and trustworthiness of the data being collected, analyzed, interpreted, and summarized. Some examples of methods used in qualitative research include interviews, focus groups, video or audiotaping of an event, review of documents, questionnaires, and observations (Creswell 2013; Patton 2015). Some researchers suggest that qualitative research is the best way of collecting PROs.

Qualitative research has traditionally been categorized into the following methods or designs: case study, ethnography, phenomenology, grounded theory, and biography (Corbin and Strauss 2014; Creswell 2012).

Table 5.4 Qualitative Research and AT Outcomes.

- Thicker and rich description of the person's experience with AT is possible
- Multiple viewpoints can be presented (e.g. consumer, caregiver, healthcare provider, researcher)
- Avoidance of ethical and practical AT outcomes issues that eliminate experimental-type designs as design choice
- Avoidance of longitudinal follow-up via experimental-type designs may be costly and prohibitive with large numbers of participants
- A high-quality study of fewer participants may provide better insight into the long-term effectiveness of AT devices and training
- Subjective data based on consumer's feelings and experiences are relevant to issues such as abandonment and quality of life

Case study: This method is used to improve understanding of a complex issue, person, or object through investigation of a single phenomenon in the unique context in which it occurs (Depoy and Gitlin 2016). Case studies emphasize detailed contextual analysis of a limited number of events or conditions and their relationships (Yin 2014).

A "case" can be any phenomenon, such as use of tablets among individuals with autism. The strength of case study methodology is the use of multiple data sources, so the phenomenon is explored from multiple view points and facets (Baxter and Jack 2008).

Ethnography: This is a qualitative design that represents the art and science of describing groups or cultures (Fetterman 2009). It is traditionally embraced in the field of anthropology, and its methods include immersion by personal experience, interviews, observations, and review of documents and artifacts (Genzuk n.d.). Ethnography describes cultural norms, perspectives, and characteristics and patterns specific to that culture (Polit and Beck 2014). Ethnographic research explores phenomena within cultural contexts, ideally conducted by researchers who are not part of the cultural group. It typically involves data collection in the field, taking an involved observational approach (Creswell 2012).

Phenomenology: Phenomenological methodology, based on the works of German philosopher Edmund Husserl, addresses research questions about meaning, in order to understand and describe how people experience their world (Richards and Morse 2012). The lived experience is critical to phenomenology, as well as the assumption that human existence is meaningful and of interest. Phenomenological inquiry is often targeted toward a rich understanding of the meaning of the lived experience. Methods used in phenomenology include interviews, participant observation, document review, and focus groups (Moustakas 1994).

Grounded theory: Grounded theory methods consist of systematic guidelines for collecting and analyzing data to form theoretical frameworks. These frameworks explain the collected data (Charmaz 2000). Grounded theory was developed by Barney Glaser and Anselm Strauss in 1967 as a challenge to the dominance of quantitative methods (Glaser and Strauss 1999). While quantitative methods stressed objectivity, replication of research, and testing of hypothesis, at this time qualitative research was impressionist, anecdotal, unsystematic, and biased.

Grounded theory answers process questions about changing experience over time, stages, or phases. It gives understanding to ways in which reality is socially constructed and develops a theory grounded in data (Richards and Morse 2012). Grounded theory is an appropriate methodology for researchers wanting to understand a process or situation from the participants themselves. While grounded theory has been shown to be one of the most commonly used qualitative methodologies in health research, there is disagreement about what is and what is not a grounded theory approach to research (Glaser 2002).

Differences in the grounded theory approach are also evident in terms of recommendations regarding the use of prior knowledge in studies. Examples of prior knowledge might include clinical training, beliefs, perspectives, and any background reading of the literature. Glaser (1992) asserted that researchers should avoid review of the literature in the area that is being studied as this could contaminate data analysis. In contrast to Glaser, Corbin and Strauss (2014) view pre-reading and reflection on prior knowledge as means to enhance theoretical knowledge and assist in generating the hypothesis for investigation during the data analysis. Charmaz (2014), like Corbin and Strauss (2014), noted that preconceived theoretical concepts can provide a starting point for looking at the data but should not be used to provide codes for analysis of the data.

Biography: A biographical study is an exhaustive account of a life experience that presents a comprehensive story utilizing documents, media, interviews, and other evidence available from past and present sources (Smith 1994). This design approach focus is on a narrative of a single life story experience (Roberts 2002).

An example of qualitative inquiry is a research study by Hemmingsson et al. (2009). The researched used qualitative methods to explore and understand student perspectives regarding the use of AT in mainstream schools. The strengths in this design included: (i) use of a variety of methods and participant-informants; (ii) longitudinal focus, and (iii) diversity of participants that displayed rich and thick description of the student perspectives. The authors identified the following themes from content analysis regarding adoption of AT in a school setting: (i) immediate ATD benefits for functioning; (ii) ATDs as a sign of deviance; (iii) ATDs seen as possessions, and (iv) ATDs as alien to the learning situation (Hemmingsson et al. 2009).

Mixed method design and program evaluation

Mixed methods is a design that involves both experimental-type (quantitative) and naturalistic (qualitative) procedures within a study. Mixed methods research is gaining popularity in the social and behavioral sciences (Bergman 2008). This increase in popularity may be attributed to the advantages of this type of research, such as it: (i) addresses research questions that other single methodologies cannot; (ii) provides better/stronger inferences; and (iii) provides an opportunity for presenting a greater diversity of views (Teddlie and Tashakkori 2010).

In addition, mixed methods research allows the researcher to use multiple methods possible to address the research question and therefore gain a better understanding of a research phenomenon and expand triangulation or confirmation of either a quantitative or a qualitative study alone (Creswell and Plano Clark 2010). Mixed methods research allows for a variety of approaches to conduct studies, for example, triangulated, embedded, explanatory, or exploratory design procedures (Creswell and Plano Clark 2010). Mixed method may be best suited for evaluating AT programs vs. outcomes related to specific technologies or services. Two additional examples of designs are: (i) concurrent design, a merger of the qualitative and quantitative studies in a parallel way; and (ii) sequential design, in which a stage of the one type of study (qualitative or quantitative) is completed with extended use of findings into the other type of study in a sequential approach (Creswell et al. 2008).

Program evaluation

Mixed method research design has potential for use in program evaluation and outcomes research. AT outcomes research is like program evaluation research for many reasons. For example: (i) many stakeholders are involved in the assessment, training, and implementation of AT; (ii) outcomes research relates to both quantitative and qualitative outcomes to thoroughly assess the impact of the interventions; (iii) program evaluation tends to include program development, with formative and summative components, which reflect the dynamic nature of AT provision (e.g. changes in funding sources and regulations, changes in the technology, training methods, intervention team structure and format, and environments or contexts); (iv) long-term AT outcomes may be better suited to mixed methods. Principles of program development and evaluation that could be applied to outcomes research in AT are provided in Table 5.5.

Goodman et al. (2002) utilized a program evaluation design to evaluate the effectiveness of a computer access training program for college students with disabilities. The multiple methods utilized in this study included Q sort, content analysis, pre- and posttesting of typing speed and accuracy, and quantitative assessment of adoption of the technology with a one-year follow-up. The authors applied a modification of the MPTM in this

Table 5.5 Principles of Program Development and Evaluation and AT Outcomes.

- Program evaluation requires input from multiple persons (stakeholders) at various stages of the process
- Program evaluation requires creation and assessment of program objectives
- Criteria for assessing program success are complex and not always agreed upon by all stakeholders
- A needs assessment is a critical component to the process
- Verification that services were provided as specified is an important component
- Outcome measures should assess the effectiveness of program objectives
- Information collected should help improve or maintain program quality
- Unplanned side effects should be considered
- Formative evaluations should be implemented to assess the process and the degree to which the program operates as would be expected
- Are program recipients actually benefiting from the program?
- Does receiving the service actually cause the change being measured?
- Can all stakeholders agree to what is a successful outcome and how it should be measured?
- Is there a cost–benefit analysis?
- Is this a short-term or long-term evaluation?
- Is there a timeline for regular monitoring of program effectiveness?
- Are the roles of the evaluators and potential biases clearly identified? (Posavac and Carey 2003).

study and utilized assessments from Scherer's (1991) model. The students who participated in this study reported that training was the most important factor that contributed to successful adoption of computer access technologies.

Methodological research, systematic literature reviews, and critical appraisals

Other methods related to AT outcomes include: methodological research; systematic literature reviews, and critical appraisals. These methods summarize and evaluate the quality of multiple research studies related to specific AT research questions, type of AT, or AT intervention. These methods enable critical review and evaluation of the strengths and limitations of various AT outcomes based on program evaluation and research findings.

Methodological research

Methodological research is the design, development, and evaluation of new assessments and instrument tools to measure outcomes. An example of a methodological study by Lenker et al. (2005) recommended constructs for measures used in AT outcomes research. Utilizing a systematic literature review approach, the authors identified seven outcome domains (usability, use, user satisfaction, functional level, QoL, role participation, and cost) that should be addressed by outcomes measures. Only a small percentage of the articles reviewed in this study reported outcomes for these domains and/or adequately described the psychometric properties of the measures actually used in these studies. Lenker et al. called for improvement and standardization of outcome measures in AT research.

Systematic literature review

Systematic reviews are a "scientific approach to collecting and synthesizing biomedical information to answer questions" (Nelson (2014), p. 1). Analysis of information in research studies through systematic review is used to support and develop evidence-based practice. Systematic literature review (SLR) components were delineated by Okoli and Schabram (2010) as an eight-step process that clearly differentiate it from a typical literature review. The eight steps include: (i) explain the purpose of the literature review; (ii) describe the protocol and training procedures; (iii) search for relevant literature; (iv) complete a practical screen of articles (using agreed-upon exclusion and inclusion criteria); (v) engage in a quality appraisal of articles; (vi) complete relevant data extraction; (vii) synthesize studies; (viii) compose the literature review (Okoli and Schabram 2010). Several examples of SLRs of AT outcomes research are summarized in Table 5.6.

Critical appraisal papers (CAP) are another form of evidence analysis that has gained popularity in many health professions, including medicine, occupational therapy, physical therapy, speech therapy, and other professions. These are short summary reports based on a focused clinical question and analysis of key interventions with application to practice. Table 5.7 addresses helpful resources for locating critical appraisal papers that report AT outcomes in Level 1 or 2 single studies, SLRs, or critical appraisals of evidence.

Evidence-based practice and levels of evidence

Sackett et al. (1996) created the evidence-based practice movement in medicine, which has been adopted by other health disciplines. Evidence-based practice (EBP) was defined as "the conscientious, explicit and judicious use of current best evidence in making decisions about the care of individual patients" (p. 71).

Moreover, third-party payers, consumers, and practitioners have established the need for increased accountability of service provision through EBP for health

Table 5.6 Systematic Literature Reviews of Outcomes in AT.

Authors	Outcomes	Methods	Results	Comments
Antilla et al. (2012)	Personal care and protection devices, personal mobility, adaptation of homes, communication, hearing aids, visual aids, other devices	Review of systematic literature reviews in AT – 2000–2010. Taxonomy of assistive technology device outcomes was utilized. 2210 citations reviewed – 44 SLR papers included in final review.	High-quality evidence reported in connection with home assessment, and hearing aids for limited populations (older adults at home and institutions, individuals with hearing loss). Moderate evidence found for benefits of absorbent insert pads for incontinence, hearing aids.	More well-designed outcomes studies looking at more frequently used AT were recommended.
Vincent and Routhier (2012)	Review of research designs in AT outcome studies	Reviewed 499 articles. Inclusion criteria: Published in English, associated to life habit domains of the Disability Creation Process (DCP), achieved in community setting. Exclusion criteria: non-commercial AT, non-specific AT, home modification technology, smart homes, and emergency call systems. Used DCP model to classify life habit domains (12 categories), and capabilities (10 categories).	19 studies met the inclusion criteria. Six of the studies were deemed experimental, four were quasi-experimental, and nine were non-experimental. 11 different types of AT were reported in the studies reviewed. Mobility was the life habit domain studied the most; motor activity was the most frequently studied capability.	Recommended designs that allow for measuring long-term effects, use of standardized tools that address life habits in the users' environments, and stronger research designs.
Sauer et al. (2010)	Employment for people with cognitive disabilities	Systematic literature review. Key terms: Primary: (i) cognitive disability, (ii) AT, and (iii) employment. Secondary: cognition, cognitive disabilities, developmental disabilities, mental retardation, impaired IQ, Down syndrome, autism, technology, devices, assistive technology devices (ATDs), jobs, sheltered workshops, supported employment, vocation and vocational training.	Positive outcomes were measured as a higher rate of accuracy and task completion, increased independence, and generalization of skills. A trend of moving from low- to high-tech visual and auditory cuing systems was discovered. Cuing systems are effective in teaching individuals with cognitive disabilities (CD) in both school and vocational settings. Only 36% of survey respondents indicated the use of an AT tool. The majority of respondents indicated that they did not use any accommodations and did not report their "mental limitations" to their employers.	74 000 articles received preliminary consideration, nine articles included after rigorous application of inclusion criteria. No level 1 evidence reported, most studies were level 2. 83% of articles studied accuracy, 63% of articles studied independence, and 38% studied generalization.

(Continued)

Table 5.6 (*Continued*)

Authors	Outcomes	Methods	Results	Comments
Souza et al. (2010)	Effects of mobility assistive technology (MAT) for individuals with multiple sclerosis.	Keywords: falls, mobility, multiple sclerosis (MS), cane, walker, wheelchair, assistive technology, and psychological problems. Peer reviewed journals related only to mobility problems in MS included. Quality of life, psychological aspects, new and emerging technologies, service delivery, and a variety of MAT were reviewed.	50 articles met the inclusion criteria. A limited number of articles with higher levels of evidence (LOEs) were found regarding the benefits of MAT use specifically for persons with MS. Most of the articles found were LOE IV ($n = 32$) and V ($n = 15$), followed by III ($n = 2$) and II ($n = 1$).	Future quantitative studies to provide higher levels of evidence were recommended. The article provided a clinical rationale for mobility devices and interventions-related outcomes.
Salminen et al. (2009)	Effectiveness of mobility device interventions in terms of activity and participation for individuals with mobility limitations.	20 key words utilized in search of articles without language restrictions. 1996–2008 date limitations. 1302 articles in preliminary review. Exclusion criteria: laboratory studies, studies with no primary focus on activity and participation. 9 articles selected that met full inclusion criteria.	One study was randomized controlled trial (RCT), four were controlled studies, and three were follow-up. Power wheelchairs, pushrim activated wheelchair, walkers, individually adjusted wheelchairs, and particular brands of walkers and wheelchairs were studied. Evidence was found that suggests mobility devices improve user's activity and participation, and increase mobility. Variables measuring user satisfaction, mobility, and quality of life were found to be statistically significant for improvement after intervention.	A list of measures was included (e.g. PIADS, QUEST) with descriptions of each and scaling information. A summary of strengths and weaknesses in reliability and validity was included. Several suggestions to improve the design of future studies were provided.
Henderson et al. (2008)	Impact on children with functional impairments, caregiver function. Many devices studied addressing computer access, communication, behavior changes, environment, and activity.	Systematic literature review. Inclusion criteria: Provision of an assistive device(s) (e.g. powered mobility as an alternative means of self-mobilization), clients under 19 years old, impact on social environment, primary research in refereed professional journals. Exclusion criteria: Assistive devices intended to enhance aspects of ordinary functioning (e.g. glasses, hearing aids, orthoses), modifications to homes and other physical environments, studies that focused solely on outcomes relating to the Body Structure and Function domain of the ICF. Cross-sectional studies and review articles.	Functional problems identified included accessing a computer ($n = 3$ studies), activity assistance ($n = 2$), behavior changes ($n = 3$), communication ($n = 30$), independent feeding ($n = 1$), living skills ($n = 1$), mobility ($n = 9$), modifying the environment ($n = 1$), nutrition ($n = 4$), and postural stability ($n = 2$). Study outcomes reported were mainly child-focused and could be classified as influencing activity, participation, and personal contextual factors, with only five studies primarily addressing caregiver-focused outcomes.	54 studies reviewed. Most were level 4 studies, with three studies classified as quasi-experimental or level 3 evidence.

Table 5.7 Databases and Resources that Provide Evidence for Effectiveness of AT.

Rehabilitation Measures Database	http://www.rehabmeasures.org/default.aspx
OT Seeker	http://otseeker.com
Evidence-Based Practice – American Occupational Therapy Association (AOTA)	https://www.aota.org/practice/researchers.aspx
Evidence-Based-Occupational Therapy – McMaster University	https://srs-mcmaster.ca/research/evidence-based-practice-research-group/
OT Search (AOTA database)	http://otsearch.aota.org
Centre for Evidence-Based Medicine – Oxford University	http://www.cebm.net
Cochrane Collaboration Library (for fee)	www.cochrane.org
Evidence-Based Practice and Research – American Physical Therapy Association (APTA)	http://www.apta.org/EvidenceResearch
OTDBASE (for fee)	http://www.otdbase.org
Campbell Collaboration	http://www.campbellcollaboration.org
Agency for Healthcare Research and Quality	www.ahrq.gov
What Works Clearinghouse – Educational Research[a]	http://ies.ed.gov/ncee/wwc
Center for Implementing Technology in Education[a]	http://www.air.org/project/center-implementing-technology-education-cited
National Center for Technology Innovation[a]	https://www.air.org/page/research-and-evaluation
Technical Assistance Center on Social Emotional Intervention for Young Children[a]	https://challengingbehavior.cbcs.usf.edu/about/index.html

[a] Resources cited in Peterson-Karlin and Parette (2007, p. 136).

professionals. There are EBP guidelines or position papers at the websites of most professional organizations, including the Rehabilitation Engineering and Assistive Technology Society of North America (RESNA) (http://www.resna.org/knowledge-center/position-papers-and-provision-guides).

Professionals and researchers working in the field of AT should be aware of the various levels of evidence used in SLRs or CAPs to judge the quality of research methods and outcomes reported in various studies (Brandt and Alwin 2012). In the development of a body of knowledge related to outcomes in AT practice, consideration of these levels of evidence, or evidence pyramids, should be consulted when designing a study, reading an outcomes paper, or evaluating existing evidence that is provided to support the value of an AT device, a program, or services.

There are many variations of the levels of evidence pyramids and some are more descriptive with more divisions within each level. Tomlin and Borgetto (2011) suggest qualitative studies should receive equal consideration in describing quality of research using levels of evidence pyramids. This model certainly fits well in AT outcomes research. Learning that occurs from in-depth interviews or observations of consumers of AT should be regarded with respect that is not necessarily given to articles of this type using traditional levels of evidence pyramids.

Summary

This chapter identifies categories of outcomes based on the ICF and other models of practice related to outcomes research in AT. Identifying and researching the outcomes reflecting all levels of the Human-Tech Ladder remain a challenge in the field yet are necessary to describe the full picture of AT-related outcomes. Factors to consider in designing high-quality outcome studies are discussed. Research methods and designs are summarized. Current evidence based on outcomes research on the effectiveness of AT in a variety of settings is reviewed. Resources such as suggested outcomes measures, individuals and groups with experience in outcomes research, journals, and organizations to support outcomes research are provided. Additionally, the Toolbox presents a guide design and implementation of AT outcomes research.

Along with the toolbox, the authors conclude this chapter with specific strategies to design and implement high-quality outcomes research in AT which include:

- a thorough review of previous literature;
- consultation with experts in the field;
- utilizing a model of practice or theory;
- inter-professional collaboration;
- consideration of all stakeholders in the study design and analysis of data;

- using measures that accurately, reliably, and effectively measure outcomes that are meaningful and based on improving QoL;
- choosing a design that most effectively answers the questions related to the study;
- improving skills needed to be a consumer of AT research such as thoughtful critique of existing research using levels of evidence pyramids or other tools to judge the quality of research outcomes and methods.

References

Andrich, R. (2002). The SCAI instrument: measuring costs of individual assistive technology programmes. *Technology and Disability* 14: 95–99.

Antilla, H., Samuelsson, K., Salminen, A.L., and Brandt, K. (2012). Quality of evidence of assistive technology interventions for people with disability: an overview of systematic reviews. *Technology and Disability* 24: 9–48.

Bailey, R.W. (1989). *Human Performance Engineering Using Human Factors/Ergonomics to Achieve Computer System Usability*, 2e. Englewood Cliffs, NJ: Prentice Hall.

Baxter, P. and Jack, S. (2008). Qualitative case study methodology: study design and implementation for novice researchers. *The Qualitative Report* 13: 544–559.

Bergman, M.M. (2008). The straw men of the qualitative-quantitative divide and their influences on mixed methods research. In: *Advances in Mixed Methods Research: Theories and Applications* (ed. M.M. Bergman), 11–20. London: Sage.

Bernd, T., Van Der Pijl, D., and De Witte, L.P. (2009). Existing models and instruments for the selection of assistive technology in rehabilitation practice. *Scandinavian Journal of Occupational Therapy* 16: 146–158.

Biering-Sorensen, F., Scheuringer, M., Baumberger, M. et al. (2006). Developing core sets for persons with spinal cord injuries based on the International Classification of Functioning, Disability and Health as a way to specify functioning. *Spinal Cord* 44: 541–546.

Bodiam, C. (1999). The use of the Canadian Occupational Performance Measure for the assessment of outcome on a neurorehabilitation unit. *The British Journal of Occupational Therapy* 62: 123–126.

Brandt, Å. and Alwin, J. (2012). Assistive technology outcomes research: contributions to evidence-based assistive technology practice. *Technology and Disability* 24 (1): 5–7. https://doi.org/10.3233/TAD-2012-0228.

Brandt, Å., Alwin, J., Vincent, C., and Routhier, F. (2012a). Designs in AT research: usefulness for therapists in clinical practice. *Technology and Disability* 24 (1): 49–58.

Brandt, Å., Alwin, J., Lenker, J.A. et al. (2012b). Classification of assistive technology services: implications for outcomes research. *Technology and Disability* 24 (1): 59–70.

Campbell, D.T. and Stanley, J.C. (2010). *Experimental and Quasi-Experimental Designs for Research*. Boston, MA: Houghton Mifflin.

Cardol, M., Brandsma, J.W., de Groot, I.J. et al. (1999). Handicap questionnaires: what do they assess? *Disability and Rehabilitation* 21 (3): 97–105.

Cardol, M., de Jong, B.A., van de Bos, G.A. et al. (2002). Beyond disability: perceived participation in people with a chronic disabling condition. *Clinical Rehabilitation* 16: 27–35.

Carpenter, L., Baker, G.A., and Tyldesley, B. (2001). The use of the Canadian Occupational Performance Measure as an outcome of a pain management program. *Canadian Journal of Occupational Therapy* 68: 16–22.

Centre for Evidence-Based Medicine (n.d.). OECBM 2011 levels of evidence system. Retrieved from https://www.cebm.net/wp-content/uploads/2014/06/CEBM-Levels-of-Evidence-2.1.pdf.

Charmaz, K. (2000). Grounded theory: objectivist and constructivist methods. In: *Handbook of Qualitative Research*, 2e (ed. N.K. Denzin and Y. Lincoln), 509–535. Thousand Oaks, CA: Sage.

Charmaz, K. (2014). *Constructing Grounded Theory: A Practical Guide Through Qualitative Analysis*. London: Sage.

Cieza, A., Stucki, G., Weigl, M. et al. (2004). ICF Core Sets for chronic widespread pain. *Journal of Rehabilitation Medicine* 44 (Suppl): 63–68.

Clayback, D., Hostak, R., Leahy, J.A. et al. (2015). Standards for assistive technology funding: what are the right criteria? *Assistive Technology Outcomes and Benefits* 9 (1): 38–53.

Cook, A.M. and Hussey, S.M. (2002). *Assistive Technologies: Principles and Practice*, 2e. St. Louis, MO: Mosby Elsevier.

Cook, A.M. and Polgar, J.M. (2008). *Assistive Technologies: Principles and Practice*, 3e. St. Louis, MO: Mosby Elsevier.

Cook, A.M. and Polgar, J.M. (2014). *Assistive Technologies: Principles and Practice*, 4e. St. Louis, MO: Mosby Elsevier.

Corbin, J. and Strauss, A. (2014). *Basics of Qualitative Research: Techniques and Procedures for Developing Grounded Theory*. Thousand Oaks, CA: Sage.

Creswell, J.W. (2012). *Qualitative Inquiry and Research Design: Choosing Among Five Traditions*. Newbury Park, CA: Sage.

Creswell, J.W. (2013). *Research Design: Qualitative, Quantitative, and Mixed Methods Approaches*, 4e. Thousand Oaks, CA: Sage.

Creswell, J.W. and Plano Clark, V.L. (2010). *Designing and Conducting Mixed Methods Research*. Thousand Oaks, California: Sage.

Creswell, J.W., Plano Clark, V.L., and Garrett, A.L. (2008). Methodological issues in conducting mixed methods research design. In: *Advances in Mixed Methods Research: Theories and Applications* (ed. M.M. Bergman), 66–84. London: Sage.

Cup, E.H.C., Scholte op Reimer, W., Thijssen, M.C.E., and van Kuyk-Minis, M.A.H. (2003). Reliability and validity of the Canadian Occupational Performance Measure in stroke patients. *Clinical Rehabilitation* 17 (4): 402–409.

Day, H. and Jutai, J. (1996). Measuring the psychosocial impact of assistive devices: the PIADS. *Canadian Journal of Rehabilitation* 9: 159–168.

Demers, L., Weiss-Lambrou, R., and Ska, B. (2002). The Quebec User Evaluation of Satisfaction with Assistive Technology (QUEST 2.0): an overview and recent progress. *Technology and Disability* 14: 101–105.

Demers, L., Fuhrer, M.J., Jutai, J.W. et al. (2008). Tracking mobility-related assistive technology in outcomes studies. *Assistive Technology* 20: 73–83.

Depoy, E. and Gitlin, L.N. (2016). *Introduction to Research: Understanding and Applying Multiple Strategies*. St. Louis, MO: Elsevier.

Duggan, C.H., Albright, K.J., and Lequerica, A. (2008). Using the ICF to code and analyse women's disability narratives. *Disability and Rehabilitation* 30 (12–13): 978–990.

Edmonds, W.A. and Kennedy, T.D. (2013). *An Applied Research Guide to Research Designs: Quantitative, Qualitative, and Mixed Methods*. Thousand Oaks, CA: Sage.

Fauconnier, J., Dickinson, H.O., Beckung, E. et al. (2009). Participation in life situations of 8–12 year old children with cerebral palsy: cross sectional European study. *BMJ: British Medical Journal* 338: b1458. https://doi.org/10.1136/bmj.b1458.

Fetterman, D.M. (2009). *Ethnography: Step-by Step*. Thousand Oaks, CA: Sage.

Fuhrer, M.J. (2001). Assistive technology outcomes research: challenges met and yet unmet. *American Journal of Physical Medicine and Rehabilitation* 80: 528–535.

Fuhrer, M.J., Jutai, J.W., Scherer, M.J., and Deruyter, F. (2003). A framework for the conceptual modelling of assistive technology device outcomes. *Disability and Rehabilitation* 25: 1243–1251.

Gelderblom, G.J. and de Witte, L.P. (2002). The assessment of assistive technology outcomes, effects and costs. *Technology and Disability* 14 (3): 91–94.

Genzuk, M. (n.d.). A synthesis of ethnographic research. Retrieved from http://www-bcf.usc.edu/~genzuk/Ethnographic_Research.html.

Gitlin, L. (1998). From hospital to home: individual variations in experience with assistive devices among older adults. In: *Designing and Using Assistive Technology* (ed. D.B. Gray, L.A. Quatrano and M.L. Lieberman), 117–135. Baltimore, MD: Paul H. Brookes.

Glaser, B. (1992). *Emergences vs Forcing: Basics of Grounded Theory Analysis*. Mill Valley, CA: Sociology Press.

Glaser, B.G. (2002). Constructivist grounded theory? *Forum: Qualitative Social Research* 3: 12. Retrieved from http://www.qualitative-research.net/index.php/fqs/article/view/825/1792.

Glaser, B.G. and Strauss, A.L. (1999). *The Discovery of Grounded Theory: Strategies for Qualitative Research*. Chicago, IL: Aldine.

Goodman, G., Tiene, D., and Luft, P. (2002). Adoption of assistive technology for computer access among college students with disabilities. *Disability and Rehabilitation* 24: 82–92.

Gray, D.B. and Hendershot, G.E. (2000). The ICIDH-2: developments for a new era of outcomes research. *Archives of Physical Medicine and Rehabilitation* 81 (Suppl 2): S10–S14.

Hemmingsson, H., Lidstrom, H., and Nygard, L. (2009). Use of assistive technology devices in mainstream schools: students' perspective. *American Journal of Occupational Therapy* 63 (4): 463–472.

Henderson, S., Skelton, H., and Rosenbaum, P. (2008). Assistive devices for children with functional impairments: impact on child and caregiver function. *Developmental Medicine & Child Neurology* 50: 89–98.

Higgins, J. and Green, S. (eds.). (2011). 17.1: What are patient-reported outcomes? *Cochrane Handbook for Systematic Reviews of Interventions. Version 5.1.0*. Retrieved from https://handbook-5-1.cochrane.org/chapter_17/17_1_what_are_patient_reported_outcomes.htm.

Jette, A.M., Haley, S.M., and Kooyoomijan, J.T. (2003). Are the ICF activity and participation dimensions distinct? *Journal of Rehabilitation Medicine* 35: 145–149.

Jutai, J. and Day, H. (2002). Psychosocial Impact of Assistive Devices Scale (PIADS). *Technology and Disability* 14: 107–111.

Jutai, J.W., Fuhrer, M.J., Demers, L. et al. (2004). A conceptual foundation for researching assisitve technology outcomes. Paper presented at the RESNA Annual Conference, Orlando, FL.

Jutai, J.W., Fuhrer, M.J., Demers, L. et al. (2005). Toward a taxonomy of assistive technology device outcomes. *American Journal of Physcial Medicine and Rehabilitation* 84: 294–302.

Law, M., Baptiste, S., McColl, M.A. et al. (1990). The Canadian Occupational Performance Measure: an outcome measure for occupational therapy. *Canadian Journal of Occupational Therapy* 57: 82–87.

Lenker, J.A. and Jutai, J.W. (1996). Assistive technology outcomes research and clinical practice: what role for ICF? Retrieved from https://static.aminer.org/pdf/PDF/000/288/762/the_study_of_assistive_technology_outcomes_in_the_united_states.pdf.

Lenker, J.A. and Paquet, V.L. (2003). A review of conceptual models for assistive technology outcomes research and practice. *Assistive Technology* 15: 1–15.

Lenker, J.A., Langton, T., Kniskern, J. et al. (2002). AT outcomes measurement. Assistive Technology Quick Reference Series. Retrieved from https://smartech.gatech.edu/bitstream/handle/1853/26270/ATOutcomes.pdf?sequence=1&isAllowed=y.

Lenker, J.A., Scherer, M.J., Fuhrer, M.J. et al. (2005). Psychometric and administrative properties of measures used in assistive technology device outcomes research. *Assistive Technology* 17: 7–22.

McColl, M.A., Paterson, M., Davies, D. et al. (2000). Validity and community utility of the Canadian Occupational Performance Measure. *Canadian Journal of Occupational Therapy* 67: 22–30.

Moustakas, C. (1994). *Phenomenological Research Methods*. London: Sage.

Mulcahey, M.J., Betz, R.R., Kozin, S.H. et al. (2004). Implantation of the Freehand System® during initial rehabilitation using minimally invasive techniques. *Spinal Cord* 42: 146–155.

Nelson, H.D. (2014). *Systematic Reviews to Answer Health Care Questions*. Philadelphia, PA: Lippincott Williams & Wilkins.

Noreau, L., Fougeyrollas, P., and Vincent, C. (2002). The LIFE-H: assessment of the quality of social participation. *Technology and Disability* 14: 113–118.

Noreau, L., Desrosiers, J., Robichaud, L. et al. (2004). Measuring social participation: reliability of the LIFE-H in older adults with disabilities. *Disability and Rehabilitation* 26 (6): 346–352.

Okoli, C. and Schabram, K. (2010). A guide to conducting a systematic literature review of information systems research. *Sprouts: Working Papers on Information Systems* 10 (26). Retrieved from https://pdfs.semanticscholar.org/31dc/753345d5230e421ea817dd7dcdd352e87ea2.pdf.

Ottenbacher, K.J. (1986). *Evaluating Clinical Change: Strategies for Occupational and Physical Therapists*. Baltimore: MD: Williams & Wilkins.

Patton, M.Q. (2015). *Qualitative Research & Evaluation Methods: Integrating Theory and Practice*, 4e. Thousand Oaks, CA: Sage.

Persson, J. (1997). An overview of the EATS project: effectiveness of assistive technology and services. In: *Advancement of Assistive Technology* (ed. G. Anogianakis, C. Buhler and M. Soede), 48–52. Amsterdam: IOS Press.

Peterson-Karlin, G.R. and Parette, H.P. (2007). Evidence-based practice and the consideration of assistive technology effectiveness and outcomes. *Assistive Technology Outcomes and Benefits* 4: 130–139.

Polit, D.F. and Beck, C.T. (2014). *Essentials of Nursing Research Methods, Appraisal and Utilisation*, 8e. Philadelphia, PA: Lippincott Williams & Wilkins.

Portney, L.G. and Watkins, M.P. (2015). *Foundations of Clinical Research: Applications to Practice*. Upper Saddle River, NJ: Pearson/Prentice Hall.

Posavac, E. and Carey, R. (2003). *Program Evaluation: Methods and Case Studies*. Upper Saddle River, NJ: Prentice Hall.

RESNA (2017). RESNA's guidelines and priorities for assistive technology and rehabilitation engineering research. Retrieved from https://www.resna.org/sites/default/files/legacy/RESNA%20research%20guidelines%20and%20priorities%20approved%2004142017.pdf.

Richards, L. and Morse, J. (2012). *Readme First for a User's Guide to Qualitative Methods*, 3e. Thousand Oaks, CA: Sage.

Roberts, B. (2002). *Biographical Research*. London: Open University Press.

Roelands, M., Van Oost, P., Depoorter, A., and Buysse, A. (2002). A social-cognitive model to predict the use of assistive devices for mobility and self-care in elderly people. *The Gerontologist* 42 (1): 39–50.

Rogers, E.M. (2003). *Diffusion of Innovations*, 5e. New York: Simon & Schuster.

Ruof, J., Cieza, A., Wolff, B. et al. (2004). ICF Core Sets for diabetes mellitus. *Journal of Rehabilitation Medicine* 44 (Suppl): 100–106.

Rust, K.L. and Smith, R.O. (2005). Assistive technology in the measurement of rehabilitation and health outcomes: a review and analysis of instruments. *American Journal of Physical Medicine and Rehabilitation* 84: 780–793.

Rust, K.L. and Smith, R.O. (2006). Perspectives of outcome data from assistive technology developers. *Assistive Technology Outcomes and Benefits* 3: 34–52.

Sackett, D., Rosenberg, W., Gray, J. et al. (1996). Evidence-based medicine: what it is and what it isn't. *British Medical Journal* 312, 88: 71. https://doi.org/10.1136/bmj.312.7023.71.

Salminen, A.L., Brandt, A., Samuelsson, K. et al. (2009). Mobility devices to promote activity and participation: a systematic review. *Journal of Rehabilitation Medicine* 41: 697–706.

Samsa, G.P. and Matchar, D.B. (2004). How strong is the relationship between functional status and quality of life among persons with stroke? *Journal of Rehabilitation Research and Development* 41 (3A): 279–282.

Sauer, A.L., Parks, A., and Heyn, P.C. (2010). Assistive technology effects on the employment outcomes for people with cognitive disabilities: a systematic review. *Disability and Rehabilitation: Assistive Technology* 5: 377–391.

Scherer, M.J. (1991). *The Scherer MPT Model: Matching People with Technologies*. Webster, NY: Scherer and Associates.

Scherer, M.J. (1998). *Matching Person and Technology*. Webster, NY: Institute for Matching Person and Technology.

Scherer, M.J. (2008). Matching Person and Technology assessment process. Matching Person and Technology. Retrieved from http://www.matchingpersonandtechnology.com.

Scherer, M.J. and Glueckauf, R. (2005). Assessing the benefits of assistive technologies for activities and participation. *Rehabilitation Psychology* 50 (2): 132–141.

Scherer, M.J., Jutai, J., Fuhrer, M. et al. (2007). A framework for modelling the selection of assistive technology devices (ATDs). *Disability and Rehabilitation* 2 (1): 1–8.

Schulz, R., Wahl, H.W., Matthews, J.T. et al. (2015). Advancing the aging and technology agenda in gerontology. *The Gerontologist* 55 (5): 724–734. https://doi.org/10.1093/geront/gnu071.

Smith, L.M. (1994). Biographical method. In: *Handbook of Qualitative Research* (ed. N.K. Denzin and Y.S. Lincoln), 286–305. Thousand Oaks CA: Sage.

Smith, R.O., Jansen, C., Seitz, J. and Longenecker Rust, K. (2006). The ICF in the context of assistive technology (AT) interventions and outcomes. *ATOMS Project Technical Report*. Retrieved from http://www.r2d2.uwm.edu/atoms/archive/icf.html.

Souza, A., Kelleher, A., Cooper, R. et al. (2010). Multiple sclerosis and mobility-related assistive technology: systematic review of literature. *Journal of Rehabilitation Research and Development* 47: 213–224.

Stucki, G. and Cieza, A. (2004). The International Classification of Functioning, Disability and Health (ICF) Core Sets for rheumatoid arthritis: a way to specify functioning. *Annals of the Rheumatic Diseases* 63 (Suppl 2): ii40–ii45.

Stucki, G., Ewart, T., and Cieza, A. (2003). Value and application of the ICF in rehabilitation medicine. *Disability and Rehabilitation* 25 (11–12): 628–634.

Stucki, G., Ustun, T.B., and Melvin, J. (2005). Applying the ICF for the acute hospital and early post-acute rehabilitation facilities. *Disability and Rehabilitation* 27 (7–8): 549–552.

Teddlie, C. and Tashakkori, A. (2010). Overview of contemporary issues in mixed methods research. In: *Handbook of Mixed Methods in Social and Behavioural Research*, 2e (ed. A. Tashakkori and C. Teddlie), 3–50. Thousand Oaks, CA: Sage.

Tomita, M.R., Mann, W.C., Stanton, K. et al. (2007). Use of currently available smart home technology by frail elders: process and outcomes. *Topics in Geriatric Rehabilitation* 23: 24–34.

Tomlin, G. and Borgetto, B. (2011). Research pyramid: a new evidence-based practice model for occupational therapy. *American Journal of Occupational Therapy* 65: 189–196. https://doi.org/10.5014/ajot.2011.000828.

Ustun, T.B., Chatterji, S., Bickenbach, J. et al. (2003). The International Classification of Functioning, Disability and Health: a new tool for understanding disability and health. *Disability and Rehabilitation* 25: 565–571.

Vincent, C. and Routhier, F. (2012). Designs in AT research: usefulness for therapists in clinical practice. *Technology and Disability* 24: 49–58.

Watson, A.H., Ito, M., Smith, R.O., and Andersen, L.T. (2010). Effect of assistive technology in a public school setting. *American Journal of Occupational Therapy* 64: 18–24.

Wessels, R., Persson, J., Lorentsen, O. et al. (2002). IPPA: individually prioritised problem assessment. *Technology and Disability* 14: 141–145.

World Health Organisation (2001). *International Classification of Functioning, Disability and Health*. Geneva, Switzerland: World Health Organization.

Yin, R.K. (2014). *Case Study Research: Design and Methods*. Thousand Oaks, CA: Sage.

Toolbox: Guide to design and implementation of outcomes research in AT

Resource	Citation	Comments/usefulness of resource
ATIA (Assistive Technology Industry Association	http://www.atia.org	The mission of ATIA is to serve as the collective voice of the assistive technology industry so that the best products and services are delivered to people with disabilities. They provide conferences, webinars, and resources to assist with AT outcomes research.
ATOB (*Assistive Technology Outcomes and Benefits Journal*)	https://www.atia.org/at-resources/atob	Journal devoted to outcomes research in AT co-sponsored by the Assistive Technology Industry Association and the Special Education Assistive Technology Center at Illinois State University.
ATOMS (Assistive Technology Outcomes Measurement System) Project	http://www.r2d2.uwm.edu/atoms	Assistive Technology Outcomes Measurement System website, University of Wisconsin, Milwaukee. Products link contains resources such as descriptions of models of practice in AT, databases, and outcomes bibliography with over 900 entries.
CATOR (Consortium for Assistive Technology Outcomes Research)	https://surgery.duke.edu/divisions/head-and-neck-surgery-and-communication-sciences/research/clinical-research/outcomes-measurement	Leaders in AT outcomes research (Lenker, Demers, DeRuyter, Fuhrer, Jutai) have collaborated to develop a program designed to advance the field.
CAT (Center for Assistive Technology, SUNY Buffalo	http://cat.buffalo.edu	This Center is producing outcomes research in AT including knowledge translation for technology transfer.
(CATEA) Center for Assistive Technology and Environmental Access	http://www.catea.gatech.edu	A multidisciplinary engineering and design research center dedicated to enhancing the health, activity, and participation of people with functional limitations through the application of assistive and universally designed technologies in real-world environments, products, and devices.
Closing the Gap	http://www.closingthegap.com/conference	Excellent conference with sessions devoted to outcomes research in assistive technology
CREATE (Center for Research and Expansion of Assistive Technology Excellence)	https://www.c4atx.com/	In 2001, Dunamis and the Dunamis Educational Foundation launched CREATE. Its purpose is to bring teachers, professionals, students, and parents together in a search for effective ways to apply assistive technology in the teaching/learning process.
CSUN, (California State University at Northridge) Conference	http://www.csun.edu/cod/conference	This university has supported an annual international conference on AT for 26 years. The conference is an ideal venue to share AT outcomes research and to see new and evolving assistive technology. The university is active in providing excellent certificates and degrees in AT.
Institute for Matching Person and Technology	http://matchingpersonandtechnology.com	Marcia Scherer's MPT Model, outcomes measures that are designed to apply her model, and many other materials helping address outcomes research are available at this site.
Intelligent Assistive Technology and Systems Lab (University of Toronto)	http://www.ot.utoronto.ca/iatsl/index.htm	A multidisciplinary group of researchers with backgrounds in engineering, computer science, occupational therapy, speech-language pathology, and gerontology. The goal of the center is to develop *zero-effort technologies* that are adaptive, flexible, and intelligent, to enable users to participate fully in their daily lives.
RESNA (The Rehabilitation Engineering and Assistive Technology Society of North America)	www.resna.org	This is the premier professional organization dedicated to promoting the health and well-being of people with disabilities through increasing access to technology solutions. They provide webinars, an annual conference, links to outcomes research resources, a listing of academic programs in AT, certification programs, and many other resources related to outcomes research in AT.
Trace Center, University of Wisconsin, Madison	http://trace.wisc.edu	Productive center devoted to dissemination of products, product development, computer access, and website design for accessibility. Many outcomes studies produced by faculty.
University of Pittsburgh- Center for Assistive Technology	http://www.upmc.com/Services/rehab/rehab-institute/services/cat/Pages/default.aspx	Centers devoted to product development and AT services with productive outcomes research.
University of Washington Project DO-IT	http://www.washington.edu/doit	Project DO-IT promotes the success of individuals with disabilities in postsecondary education and careers, using technology as an empowering tool. Includes the Center for Universal Design in Education. Faculty produce outcomes research.

6
Educational organizations

Kirk Behnke

Outline

Learning outcomes

After reading this chapter, you should be able to:

1. Describe legislation that provides technology and environmental interventions (TEI) to access the curriculum in K-12 educational settings.
2. List the technology and service provision mandates that are guaranteed by law to enable all students to access the K-12 curriculum.
3. Summarize a four-step process that can be used to incorporate a full range of low to high technology into the K-12 curriculum for students with disabilities.
4. Compare and contrast the concepts of Universal Design for Learning (UDL) assistive technology, instructional technology, and educational technology.

Assistive Technologies and Environmental Interventions in Healthcare: An Integrated Approach, First Edition.
Edited by Lynn Gitlow and Kathleen Flecky.

Companion website: www.wiley.com/go/gitlow/assitivetechnologies

Active learning prompts

Before you read this chapter:

1. Compare and contrast the Individuals with Disabilities Education Act (IDEA) and Section 504 of the Rehabilitation Act.
2. View this video http://www.youtube.com/watch?v=lNs88Ki1WSo and list some assumptions about assistive technology in schools.
3. Did you or anyone you know participate in special education in grade school? How do you feel about students who receive accommodations to participate in the classroom?

Key terms

Assistive technology device
Assistive technology service
Education for All Handicapped Children Act (EHA)
Free and appropriate public education (FAPE)
Individuals with Disabilities Education Act (IDEA)
Individualized education plan (IEP)
Technology-Related Assistance Act of 1988
Universal Design for Learning (UDL)

Introduction to educational organizations

According to Vicente's Human-Tech Ladder, organizational factors have an influence on technology. Organizational factors are described within the Human-Tech Ladder as systems related to management of persons and resources, communication among teams, and information sharing and organizational culture (Vicente 2006). This is certainly the case in educational organizations. The systems within the educational system are complex and consist of reward structures within the culture that can incentivize or de-incentivize technology (Vicente 2006). Organizational impact can vary from setting to setting as a supportive administration can incentivize and promote implementation of technology and environmental interventions (TEI) whereas a resistive administration can present de-incentives and barriers to its implementation.

Moreover, the political rung on the Human-Tech Ladder represents laws and regulations, budget allocations, and policies that impact technology (Vicente 2006). Regulations, policies, and legislation that shape implementation of TEI within educational institutions are essential to understand because laws and regulations dictate TEI service provision. Educational TEI service providers need a thorough understanding of the organizational and political factors within their school, district, and state settings as well as accessibility provisions in order to deliver effective TEI interventions. Please review Box 6.1 for an evidence-based practice application activity.

Evolution of access for children with disabilities: EHA 1975 – access to schools

The US Congress enacted the *Education for All Handicapped Children Act* (EHA) or Public Law (PL) 94-142 in 1975. The act required if public schools accepted federal funds they must have equal access to education for children with cognitive and/or physical disabilities (EHA 1975). Public schools were mandated to evaluate and create an educational plan for students with disabilities. The plan must include parent input and would emulate, as closely as possible, the educational experience of general education students (EHA 1975).

This act made it possible for parents of children with disabilities to dispute any plan-based decisions by the individualized education plan (IEP). This was not necessarily outlined in law before and therefore gave parents a major role in the educational planning process. If parents were to object to decisions made by the team, and once administrative efforts were exhausted, parents were then given opportunity to seek a judicial review of the administration's decision. Before the EHA was enacted, parents were able to take their disputes straight to the judiciary under the Rehabilitation Act of 1973. The previous mandatory dispute system of the EHA created a financial burden through the litigation pursuant to the Rehabilitation Act of 1973.

The EHA also states that students with disabilities should be placed in the least restrictive environment (LRE). LRE allows students with disabilities the maximum opportunity to learn, play, and socialize with general

Box 6.1 Here's the evidence

Prisner, C. (2003). Attitudes of elementary school principals toward the inclusion of students with disabilities. *Exceptional Children* 69(2): 135–145.

Key Words: inclusion, students with disabilities, principal's attitudes

Purpose: To identify the personal characteristics, training, and experience as well as attitudes of elementary school principals toward inclusion of students with disabilities and perceptions of appropriate placements.

Sample/Setting: 408 elementary school principals in a general education setting.

Method: Survey design.

Findings: Results indicated that 1 in 5 principals reported overall positive attitudes toward inclusion, whereas most were uncertain. Principals who reported more positive attitudes were more likely to place students with disabilities in the least restrictive environment. These principals also noted that their attitudes toward students with disabilities varied with the student's disability. Additionally, the principals indicated that their experiences with students with disabilities had an impact on their attitudes and student behavior and placement decisions were influenced by perceptions of the principal along with the individualized education plan (IEP).

Critical Thinking Questions:

1. Based on the findings of this study, what is significant about the perspectives of principals toward AT and students with disabilities?
2. What are the limitations of this study?
3. What implications does this study have for technology and environmental interventions (TEI) service providers who practice in educational settings?
4. What additional research questions would you investigate based on this study?

education students (EHA 1975). Before EHA, segregated and isolated schooling occurred when the nature or severity of the student's disability constrained education in a typical classroom environment. Children with these types of disabilities were viewed as not part of the mainstream of education. The law contains a due process clause that guarantees an impartial hearing to resolve conflicts between the parents of children with disabilities and the school system (EHA 1975).

This law was passed to meet four main goals:

1. To ensure that services are provided for those students designated with special education.
2. To oversee and ensure that school-based teaming made decisions on service provision to students with disabilities which are fair and appropriate.
3. To systematize data collection, monitoring, and management requirements for special education.
4. To offer funds which support states in the education of students with disabilities.

(EHA 1975; US Department of Education, Office for Civil Rights 2010)

IDEA 1990 – access to classrooms and related services

Please review Table 6.1 for relevant legislation related to educational organizations.

EHA was revised and renamed the *Individuals with Disabilities Education Act* (IDEA) in 1990 (PL 101-476). The amendments enacted in 1990 included two new special education categories of disability: autism and traumatic brain injury. The amendments also included services for older students with disabilities in the form of providing transition services. Last, but of course not least, was the introduction of assistive technology (AT) services (PL101-476). AT was not introduced in the IDEA – the definition and requirements were expanded to require AT, but PL 94-142 (1975) allowed for AT to be considered if needed for access to education in the IEP. The IEP is a written plan required by law to ensure that a young person with an identified disability from 3 to 21 years of age receiving special education has appropriate educational goals and services. (Please review Table 6.1 for relevant educational legislation).

AT devices and services were first defined in federal law in the *Technology-Related Assistance Act of 1988* (PL 100-407 1988). Often called the Tech Act for short, it was reauthorized in 1994 (PL103-218), 1998 (PL105-394), and 2004 (National Assistive Technology Act Programs 2017). IDEA of 1990 (PL 101-476) incorporated the AT definitions from the Tech Act with AT defined as an AT device or AT services.

AT devices are identified in the later version of IDEA as "Any item, piece of equipment or product system, whether acquired commercially off the shelf, modified, or customized, that is used to increase, maintain, or improve the functional capabilities of children with disabilities" (IDEA (PL 105-117) 1997). "Although the IDEA uses the term 'device', it is important to recognize that AT devices required by students with disabilities include hardware, software, as well as stand-alone devices per the federal definition above. Almost any tool can be considered to be an AT by this definition. Since the definition of an AT device is very broad, it can give IEP teams the flexibility that is needed to make decisions about appropriate AT devices for individual students" (Woods 2014, para. 4).

AT includes technologies that are generally considered instructional technology tools that can aid students with

Table 6.1 Relevant Educational Legislation.

1975	Education of the Handicapped Act (EHA)	Access to schools First legislation to address students with special needs attending their local public schools.
1990	Individuals with Disabilities Education Act (IDEA)	Access to classroom Legislation highlighted that students with special needs must not only have access to their local schools, but also to the grade level classroom. Included two new special education categories of autism and traumatic brain injury. Included AT devices *and* services.
1997	IDEA reauthorization	Access to general education curriculum Legislation mandated that students have access to the general education curriculum.
2004	IDEA reauthorization	Access to instructional materials Legislation mandated that local educational agencies (LEAs) provide core accessible instructional materials (AIM) for students who require them to access their curriculum.
2015	Every Student Succeeds Act (ESSA)	Implementation of Universal Design for Learning (UDL) in assessment and built-in accommodations

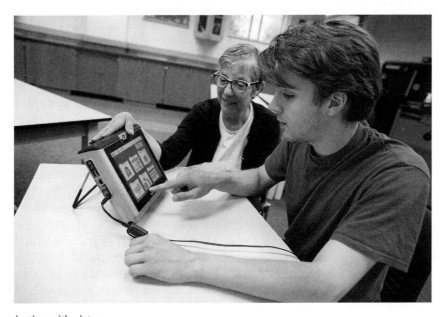

Figure 6.1 Communication with pictures.

accommodations or modifications to access educational goals and which are necessary and documented in the student's IEP. For example, a classroom tablet with a word processing program and word prediction can be considered AT for a student who demonstrates difficulty in writing and spelling if the IEP team has determined that it is educationally necessary in order to meet the educational goal.

AT devices can be on a continuum from no/low to mid to high tech. For example, a slant board is an AT device that may be used by a student who needs a specific angle to write – very much like the cover of an iPad. This will help a student with fine motor/physical disability to improve handwritten or typed communication by increasing the student's access angle (physical or visual).

Other devices are more high-tech tools, which tend to be more expensive and require more support. An example of a "high-technology" tool is an augmentative communication device (or software/app) in which a student types in messages on a communication display and these messages are read aloud via voice output (Woods 2014) Figure 6.1 displays a type of assistive communication device that uses pictures.

With the implementation of higher-tech devices, systems of support and services are crucial to support the success of the student using these tools. This leads to the second part of the AT definition, which defines *AT services* as any service that directly assists a child with a disability in the selection, acquisition, and use of an

AT device (Authority, 20 U.S.C. 1401(2), IDEA 2004). The term includes:

1. The evaluation of the needs of a child with a disability, including a functional evaluation of the child in the child's customary environment;
2. Purchasing, leasing, or otherwise providing for the acquisition of assistive technology devices by children with disabilities;
3. Selecting, designing, fitting, customizing, adapting, applying, retaining, repairing, or replacing assistive technology devices;
4. Coordinating and using other therapies, interventions, or services with assistive technology devices, such as those associated with existing education and rehabilitation plans and programs;
5. Training or technical assistance for a child with a disability or, if appropriate, that child's family; and
6. Training or technical assistance for professionals (including individuals or rehabilitation services), employers, or other individuals who provide services to employ, or are otherwise substantially involved in the major life functions of children with disabilities.

(Authority 20 U.S.C. 1401(2), IDEA, Section 300.6, 2004)

As stated in the IDEA definition, AT services are provided to assist in the selection, acquisition, and use of an AT device (IDEA 2004). An IEP team may tend to focus their energies on the device itself and discount AT services; however, as described previously in this chapter, AT services are critical to the student's successful use of the device. For some students, appropriate AT devices are identified through an evaluation, which the IDEA specifies must be conducted in the student's customary environment.

The phrase "customary environment," which is stated in the legislative history of the 1988 Tech Act, is intended to mean the various environments in which an individual engages in his or her major life activities. For example, for a school-age child, customary environments include the home and school environments (PL100-407 1988, p. 46). After a device has been selected to meet the student's needs, the next step or "service" is to provide the AT device for the student's use to access the educational curriculum. When a device or system of devices has been obtained and matched to individual tasks within the IEP, customization of the device(s) needs to be warranted for the best use from the student. All applicable individuals that work with the student, as well as the student herself/himself, should be trained in the use of the device(s). In addition, the device(s) should be made available for the student's use across instructional settings as needed and as designated within the IEP. This training includes IEP team members, family members (if the device is to be used in the home environment), and other team personnel such as paraprofessionals or relevant therapists.

IDEA (PL 105-117, 1997) entitled students with disabilities to an education which meets their individual needs in the least restrictive environment and at no cost to the student or parents. Special education can include more than academics: it also may include independent living skills and vocational training, therefore expanding services for children with disabilities in the educational environment (IDEA 1997).

IDEA (2004) also authorized related services, which "are required to assess a child with a disability to benefit from special education" (34 C.F.R. §300.34(a), IDEA 2004). Related services can include transportation or the services of health professionals such as audiologists, occupational therapists, physical therapists, psychologists, and speech therapists that can benefit students from special education.

IDEA 1997 – access to general education curriculum

With the reauthorization of IDEA in 1997 as the Individuals with Disabilities Education Act Amendments (IDEA 1997), school districts are now required under law to provide appropriate AT to students with disabilities when it supports their acquisition of a *free and appropriate public education* (FAPE). To support the inclusion and participation of students with disabilities in regular education classrooms, all IEPs developed for children identified as needing special education services must indicate that AT has been considered "to provide meaningful access to the general curriculum" (IDEA 1997). More specifically, IDEA indicates that AT devices and services must be made available to a child with a disability if required as a part of the child's special education plan, related service, or supplementary aids and services.

Since 1997, several clarifications from the Office of Special Education and Rehabilitative Services (OSERS) have been made regarding the use of AT by students with disabilities. One, which is important for families, is that school districts must provide AT at no cost to the family (Assistive Technology Training Online Project 2005). Interpretation of this law also means that school districts cannot ask families to provide AT through their private insurance.

Another example is that AT must be determined on a case-by-case basis as it is required if needed to ensure access to FAPE and access to the general curriculum.

Also, as may be the case for homework or out-of-school assignments, if the IEP team determines that AT is needed for home use to ensure FAPE, it must be provided. In addition, the student's IEP must reflect the nature of the AT and amount of supportive AT services required. This is a specific example where AT is not only a device but also a service.

IDEA 2004 – access to instructional materials

With the reauthorization of IDEA in 2004 as the Individuals with Disabilities Education Improvement Act (PL 108–446, 2004), Congress reaffirmed the strong emphasis in several areas originally made explicit in IDEA 1997. First, there is the expectation that the academic progress of *all* students will continue to increase and that progress will be measured through participation in statewide assessments so that the educational growth of all students is documented and schools are held accountable. As previously delineated in IDEA 1997, parents are to be actively involved in the development of the education programs of their children. Schools and families working together are to have high expectations for the educational achievement of every student and plan educational programs that lead to the achievement of those expectations.

Underscoring congressional intent that every student has the opportunity to make progress in the general education curriculum to the greatest extent possible, IDEA 2004 included a mandate that states provide accessible textbooks and core instructional materials to students with disabilities in a timely manner (Access to Instructional Materials 2006).

The Congressional intents are clear. All students are to have opportunities that enable them to achieve strong educational results; however, some students with disabilities require the support of AT devices and services for access to the curriculum, which includes access to instructional materials.

> Prior to the requirement that AT be considered during the development of the IEP for all students with disabilities, in many parts of the country, AT was either not considered at all for many students with disabilities, or the responsibility for AT decision-making was maintained by small district-level expert teams. Because Congress intends that all students have the AT devices and services that they require in order to benefit from their educational programs and participate in general curriculum, IDEA '97 shifted the responsibility for AT decision-making to the campus level, where it remains today, by including the requirement that each IEP team consider the student's need for AT as they develop the IEP. As mentioned above, the student and his or her parents/caregivers are part of the team along with education staff and other support staff depending on the child's needs. Each IEP Team has the responsibility to determine whether the student can work toward mastery of the goals and objectives set forth in his educational program, in the least restrictive environment without AT devices and services, or whether AT devices and services are required for the student to progress appropriately and benefit from a FAPE. In 2004, Congress also added requirements regarding accessible instructional materials.
>
> (Texas Assistive Technology Network (TATN) 2009a, Slide 7)

Although IDEA 2004 continues to make it clear that members of the IEP team must consider the student's need for AT, there is nothing in the law that prescribes *how* this is supposed to be done.

Reauthorization of IDEA

The definitions of an "assistive technology device" and "assistive technology services" remained unchanged until 2004, when, with the passage of the Individuals with Disabilities Education Improvement Act (PL 108-446), an exemption to the definition of an AT device was added to clarify a school system's responsibility to provide surgically implanted technology such as cochlear implants (IDEA 2004).

Section 602(1) of this Act clarifies that the definition of an AT device does not include a medical device that is surgically implanted or the replacement of such a device. Section 602(26) of the Act also stipulates that only medical services that are for diagnostic and evaluative purposes and required to assist a child with a disability to benefit from special education are considered a related service (IDEA 2004).

In addition, AT purchased by a school district belongs to the school district. The district is responsible for maintenance and repairs and insuring the device. A student does have the right to take a device home, if the equipment is needed at home or in the community so that a student may benefit fully from its use, as long as it is clear within the IEP. If a student moves or graduates from the public school system and equipment was purchased with a majority of school funds, the equipment stays within the school district (Millstone n.d.).

AT practitioners should become aware of the local and state policies or procedures to effectively support options for the transition of technology into the receiving environment. This could include joint funding by the school and vocational rehabilitation services, or even Medicaid or private insurance – dependent upon the end user and their financial situation. Check with your local, state, or regional procedures to support transitioning of tools and supports for users moving from the public school system.

Consideration of special factors

The IDEA lists five special factors that the IEP team must consider in the development, review, and revision of each child's IEP. Special consideration factors are as follows:

1. Behavior: Some children's behavior can impede their own learning or that of others. The use of positive behavioral interventions and supports (PBIS) along with other strategies and technologies can address the behavior and the manifestation of that behavior.
2. Limited English proficiency: A child with limited English proficiency and how they access their curriculum in either their native language, an adapted reading level, or iconic representation of key phrases.
3. Braille literacy: A child who is blind or visually impaired will need access to instruction in Braille, as well as reading Braille. All efforts should be supported to promote Braille literacy unless the IEP team determines after an extensive evaluation of the child's current level and potential for reading and writing skills that other appropriate reading and writing media should be in place for literacy.
4. Communication: The needs of the child who is deaf or hard of hearing can be complex. Consider the child's language and communication needs in the classroom and overall for opportunities for direct communications with peers and professional personnel. Augment the child's language and communication mode, academic level, and full range of needs, including opportunities for direct instruction in the child's language and communication mode.
5. Assistive technology: Of course, consideration of the child's needs for assistive technology devices and services to reach goals and objectives within the IEP. (IDEA 2004)

For many children, the first line of inquiry is whether the child's IEP can be implemented satisfactorily in the regular educational environment with the use of supplementary aids and services. Since AT devices or services can be provided as supplementary aids or services, a child's IEP team may need to consider whether a particular child requires a particular AT device or service, or whether school personnel require aid or support to enable a child with a disability to be educated satisfactorily in the regular education environment. For example, a supplemental aid/service can be providing large print or digital texts, which allow the student the opportunity to access classroom materials and participate in a classroom environment.

Section 300.320(a)(4) of IDEA (Office of Special Education and Rehabilitation Services, US Department of Education 2000) requires the IEP team to include a statement of the special education and related services and supplementary aids and services, based on peer-reviewed research to the extent practicable, to be provided to the child, or on behalf of the child. This would include any AT devices and services (determined by the IEP team) that the child needs in order for the child to receive a FAPE. Another topic that an IEP team may need to consider on a case-by-case basis is whether a child with a disability may need to use a school-purchased AT device in settings other than school, such as the child's home or other parts of the community, in order for the child to receive FAPE (IDEA 2004).

Consideration of AT in the IEP

As mandated by the IDEA as previously mentioned, IEP teams must document the student's need for AT devices and services within the IEP. AT may be addressed in one or more components of the IEP (IDEA 2004). The need for AT can be addressed in the IEP under the present levels of performance, as well as be a listing service of special education and related services, and in the annual goals, benchmarks, and objectives (IDEA 2004). AT may also be addressed in the supplementary aids and services section, in the modifications required for participation in statewide and district-wide assessments, and in the modifications and supports required for school personnel. AT must always be addressed in the consideration of special factors component of the IEP (IDEA 2004).

AT can be addressed and incorporated throughout the IEP. See Table 6.2 for relevant questions to address regarding educational AT.

SETT framework

In the AT application process, districts have used various models and structures from various parts of the country. Because each district follows their own state guidelines and setup processes specific to their needs, and because of the ever-changing nature of applying AT to fit student goals, specific evaluative AT process has not been established. One tool used to support teams and gather information to make sound AT decisions has been the SETT Framework (2005) established by Joy Zabala.

The SETT Framework is a framework that supports teams to gather, organize, and develop a plan to scaffold collaborative decisions about technology devices and

Table 6.2 Questions to Ask Regarding Educational AT.

Functional Individual Evaluation (FIE)	Is AT needed to increase, maintain, or improve the functional capabilities of a child with a disability? As part of the FIE, AT should be considered, explored, and clinicians should have a basic understanding as to how AT could be used to increase, maintain, or improve the functional capabilities of the student.
Present Levels of Academic and Functional Performance (PLAAFP)	Is AT specifically addressed? AT is frequently addressed in the present levels of performance component of the individualized education plan (IEP). This section provides a natural place to address AT needs as an integral part of the student's curriculum taking into account the student's strengths and weaknesses. When documenting AT in the present performance levels, the type of technology needed as well as the manner in which it will be used should be described.
Goals/benchmarks	Is AT listed as a condition to achieve the goal or benchmark? The use of AT is not the focus of the goal, rather the use of AT is needed to accomplish the educational or functional goal.
Accommodations	Is AT specified on the accommodations page? Within the IEP, the accommodations page is critical to help clarify how AT should be applied in various educational environments for consistency and effectiveness for the student.
State assessment	Is the use of AT needed as an accommodation to provide effective and equitable access to grade-level or course curriculum and assessment? If the technology is needed for the assessment, it should be provided throughout the year to support the learning of the content, not only for accessing the assessment.
Services	Are there any services needed to support AT implementation? Be sure to consider training, support, implementation within the educational environment, and other environments which may support the overall educational goal.
Deliberations	Is the use of AT clearly communicated and documented? The use of AT is like any other tool, it will need support, maintenance, training, and persons who will be responsible for these services. Remember to document persons responsible and due dates to meet implementation deadlines and accommodations.

services that foster the educational success of students with disabilities (Zabala n.d.). Zabala's work on the SETT Framework was originally developed to support AT selection and use in educational settings, and is the pinnacle of AT implementation plans. The SETT Framework has been used to guide decisions about a much broader range of educational services, and also, with minor adjustments, has been successfully used in non-educational environments and service plans (Zabala n.d.).

SETT is an acronym for Student, Environments, Tasks, and Tools. This framework looks at the student's needs first (S), in a specific environment (E), for a specific task (T). The framework is used to support the development and implementation of the tools (T) (Zabala n.d.).

Integration of a four-step process

Considering a student's need for AT is not a separate process, but should be embedded in the special education and IEP processes. AT consideration is embedded in the same way as any other special education service, related service, or supplementary aid/service. Although AT consideration occurs at all stages of the special education process, our focus will be on how the consideration is embedded into the IEP development process.

As an example, the Texas 4-Step Model (2009a) written by the Texas Assistive Technology Network (TATN) with leadership from Diana Carl and Joy Zabala, guides you through this process and mirrors the IEP development.

The consideration of whether or not a student needs AT is integrated into this process, and follows the same steps and takes place at the same time. When completed in the IEP sequence, the consideration of AT is a relatively brief, reasonably simple process during which IEP committee members determine if they have the information they need to make a decision or if more information is needed before a decision can be made. The Texas 4-Step Model shows the steps, which lead to responsive and responsible decision-making based on the student's needs, abilities, and educational program (TATN 2009a).

Step 1

Step 1 involves discussion of the student's present levels of academic and functional performance with the review of evaluation data. When the student's present levels of academic achievement and functional performance are discussed, it is important to note whether or not the student has been using AT as an accommodation or modification that has enabled them to reach the present level of performance in any area. Further, as the areas of need in the students' present levels of academic achievement and functional performance are discussed, it is critical to begin thinking about if and how technology might be included in the students' program to support increases in their educational performance (TATN 2009b).

In addition to direct recommendations about AT that some members of the evaluation team may offer, evaluation data can provide critical information that will be of significant use in making determinations about AT. For example, if during an evaluation for a suspected visual disability, data indicate that the student has difficulty seeing text of less than a certain size, it would be important to think about how AT can make all text accessible to the student. This example is one of the many ways that we think about a student's need for AT devices and services (TATN 2009b).

Step 2

As the goals and objectives are being developed in Step 2, IEP committee members must keep in mind that the goals and objectives need to be aimed toward what the student needs to be able to learn to do to participate in and benefit from the educational process, and not what the student is able to do at the time that the goals and objectives are being developed. As IDEA 2004 so firmly points out, high expectations, student progress, and student achievement are focal points of the special education process, and the goals and objectives in the IEP must reflect these expectations (TATN 2009b).

After the IEP committee determines what the student needs to learn and writes the goals and objectives, it is important to determine what specific tasks the student must be able to do to work toward mastery of those goals and objectives.

Step 3

In Step 3, IEP committee members think about what is happening in the classroom and other environments that enable students to make educational progress. In each educational environment, there are tasks that students need to be able to do in order to participate actively (TATN 2009a).

Note: You will also want to think about whether or not the core instructional materials used during these tasks are readily accessible (Braille, large print, digital, or audio) for this student or whether the student will need AT to access any accessible instructional materials (AIM).

As team members think about identified tasks, they determine if any of the tasks would be difficult or impossible for the student to work on at the appropriate level of independence.

Step 4

Finally, in Step 4, IEP committee members decide whether or not AT devices and services are required for the student to make progress in the educational program that has been developed. Team members come to one of three possible conclusions that will be discussed in depth shortly: (i) AT is not needed, (ii) AT is needed, or (iii) more information is needed (TATN 2009b). Decisions are documented in the IEP.

Discussion and decisions made in Step 4 follow logically from Steps 1, 2, and 3. The first three steps serve as the context and supporting data source for the decisions the IEP committee makes about the student's need for AT, just as they do for other supports and services (TATN 2009b).

Results of AT consideration

AT is not required

If, after completing the four steps of the consideration process, the IEP committee anticipates that the student will be able to make reasonable educational progress without AT devices and services, the team has a reasonable basis for determining that AT is not required at this time. This decision "at this time" does not mean that AT should not be reconsidered in the future (TATN 2009b).

When the decision is made that AT is not required, best practices require documentation of the basis of that determination. Documenting the process by which the decision was reached not only provides evidence of compliance with the legal requirement to consider a student's AT needs but allows all members of the IEP committee, including the student and parents, to understand how the decision was reached (TATN 2009b).

Many districts have included the documentation of AT consideration in their IEP forms. If it is not included in the forms in your district, a consistent place should be selected and used across the district. Wording should make it clear that AT has been thoughtfully considered by the IEP committee for each educational or functional goal of the student. Be sure to include evidence that supports the decision. The Quality Indicators for Assistive

Technology (QIAT) Leadership Team (2012) provides useful information on how to develop documentation in the IEP that clearly identifies AT consideration.

AT is required

In the following three scenarios, assistive technology (AT) is required:

- AT has been used to obtain present levels of academic achievement and functional performance and can adequately address the new goals and objectives.
- AT has been used to obtain present levels of academic achievement and functional performance, but different AT is needed to adequately address the new goals and objectives.
- AT has *not* been used previously but is needed to adequately address the new goals and objectives (TATN 2009b).

Within these three scenarios, AT is needed; however, in each circumstance review of data is essential to understand the existing technology and if it meets the needs of the student's new goals. The consensus of the IEP committee determines the goal and implements AT in order for the student to achieve that goal. IEP committee members are listed within the IEP for roles and responsibilities in order to support the technology in the environment for the student.

Also note, if technology is supported in the regular general curriculum (educational technology) for all students and it is the appropriate accommodation for a student with a disability, this technology should be written in the IEP to ensure that this educational technology is maintained and supported. In this instance, the educational technology is good for all students but it is now considered AT (required) for the student receiving special education.

More information is needed

The third possible result of the AT consideration process occurs when, after completing the four steps, members of the IEP committee are unsure about whether or not AT is required or are unsure about the nature of the AT that is required. The team will need more information before making a decision. When the committee reaches this conclusion, they make a request for assistance in gathering the additional information needed to make a decision, in a timely manner (TATN 2009b).

If more information is needed about the student and his functional needs in his educational environments, the team requests an AT evaluation and documents the evaluation in the IEP as an AT service to be provided to the student. Depending upon the needs of the student and the information that is needed, such an evaluation may be brief or may involve the participation of several people and/or trials with various types of AT (TATN 2009b).

If the committee knows what the student needs to be able to do and knows the characteristics of an effective system, but needs help to identify specific tools which have those characteristics, they will want to consult with others who have more experience with AT tools to get help determining which tools they want to try, or they may want to try out some tools before making a decision. When documenting that assistance is needed, document the type of assistance that is needed and include a time frame during which it is expected that a decision will be reached (TATN 2009b).

In regards to consideration of AT, it should be stressed that whatever decision is reached, the decision applies at this time. Consideration is an ongoing process that can be revisited at any point. At any time when the student is experiencing unpredicted difficulties in his educational progress or when changes in the student, the environments, and the tasks indicate that the student's needs are not being met with current tools, the IEP committee should reconvene to discuss AT options. These decisions will be revisited at least once a year, as the next IEP is being developed (TATN 2009b).

Other considerations

Universal design for learning

As technology develops and becomes more apparent in our society, the use of non-traditional types of AT has evolved with universal accommodations. Such features include the use of smartphones with voice output navigation tools for persons with visual impairments; amplification and volume controls on mobile devices; speech recognition tools for input and processing of data and text. These are only a few of the many types of readily available technology features embedded within commercial technology devices. As we move toward more educational and/or mobile technology devices, the author wishes (and optimistically hopes) that these devices bring more accessible opportunities to a variety of persons with specialized needs.

Typically, US society has "accommodated" persons with disabilities after-the-fact; meaning that persons with disabilities were thought about *after* the design or program was put into place and then accommodations were made for those in the "margin" (Sanford 2012). Back in the 1980s, with the help of the American's with Disabilities Act (ADA) and its subsequent amendments, a concept called "universal design" was offered. This architectural concept took the idea of designing buildings or structures with accessibility in mind, therefore creating a seamless accessibility, rather than retrofitting (Institute for Human Centered Design n.d.). The idea caught on very quickly with architects, not only because it was a law, but also because to build accessibility within the design phase was less expensive than retrofitting structures for accessibility and gave a unique design perspective.

The idea of universal design was applied to learning and students who were marginalized in the classroom, such as gifted/talented, English as a second language, and, of course, students with learning needs such as special education. *universal design for learning* (UDL) was coined by the Center for Applied Special Technology (CAST), which was founded in 1984. CAST has earned international recognition for its innovative contributions to educational products, classroom practices, and policies (National Center on Universal Design for Learning at CAST 2015).

The concept of UDL is a framework and set of principles for building curricular design to give all students equal opportunities to learn. UDL provides a framework to create instructional goals, methods, materials, and assessments that support student mastering of content. It is a flexible approach to curriculum delivery and student learning which can be customized to address individual educational needs (Rose et al. 2014).

The three fundamental principles of UDL are based on brain-based research to address the three brain networks for learning: recognition networks (the "what" of learning), the strategic networks (the "how" of learning), and the affective networks (the "why" of learning) (Rose et al. 2014). Each UDL principle aligns with the networks for learning, which are (i) provide multiple means of representation (e.g. present materials/lessons in a variety of formats to reach individual learning or accessibility preferences – videos, lectures, books, magazines, websites, workbooks, articles, etc.), (ii) provide multiple means of action and expression (e.g. provide choices in assignments or tasks to support individualized action/expression), and (iii) provide multiple means of engagement (e.g. variety of materials or lessons which support the provision of and maintaining student engagement of the materials). Under each principle are guidelines and checkpoints to help curriculum developers provide flexible approaches and strategies to reach to all student learning needs (Rose et al. 2014).

For more specific information on UDL, go to the National Center on UDL at www.udlcenter.org.

UDL will become more prevalent as good teaching models surface to address the dynamic changing face of today's public school classrooms where diversity of children's cultures, learning needs, and socioeconomic, ethnic, and other issues are now being addressed to help learners' identify their own learning needs, and hopefully address a more flexible learning environment to foster mastering of learning. UDL also takes into consideration no-tech, mid-tech, and high-tech applications to facilitate digital-native learning needs (Rose et al. 2014).

AT, Ed Tech, and instructional technology

Through UDL, digital natives using readily accessible technologies in the educational setting, and the use of instructional technologies throughout schools, the blending of these and assistive technologies has become evident. Many educational professionals are excited to see the expanded use of technology in the schools for all students. The technology, if readily accessible, can give many students more opportunities for learning and showing what they know through a variety of tools. On the other hand, if the technology is mandated for use by all students and it is not fully accessible for students with special needs, then the technology can actually be yet another literal bump in the road (National Center on Accessible Educational Materials [AEM] 2006).

For example, the use of an interactive whiteboard (IWB), a large interactive display that connects to a computer and a projector and displays the computer's desktop onto the board's surface, can serve as a great way to include technology in lesson plans and provide the three principles of UDL.

Users, such as teachers and students, control the computer using a pen, finger, stylus, remote pad, or other device, which may be good for those with learning disabilities where physical manipulation of ideas or concepts can make learning much more visual and concrete. However, students with visual impairments may not be able to see the concepts on an IWB, making the concepts inaccessible to them. Great care must be taken as we approach the next generation of technology for classroom use tools, and with regard to how educators address flexible options within the curriculum as well as flexible tools in order to access, manipulate, and assess learning for all students (National Center on Accessible Educational Materials [AEM] 2006).

Students with 504 plans, english language learners (ELL), or struggling students

For those students who may not be eligible for special education services, or for parents who decide not to have their children enrolled in special education, there is another option for schools to provide a FAPE. Section 504 of the Rehabilitation Act of 1973, PL 93-112, 87 (Section 504 of the Rehabilitation Act of 1973, 34 C.F.R. Part 104 2015) protects the rights of individuals with disabilities in programs and activities that receive federal financial assistance. Section 504 also provides that: "No otherwise qualified individual with a disability in the United States … shall, solely by reason of her or his disability, be excluded from the participation in, be denied the benefits of, or be subjected to discrimination under any program or activity receiving Federal financial assistance …" (US Department of Education, Office for Civil Rights 2010).

This regulation requires a school district to provide FAPE to each qualified student with a disability who is in the school district's jurisdiction, regardless of the nature or severity of the student's disability. This means that a student may not necessarily qualify for special education services via an IEP but may need basic accommodations in order to support their learning. Once the student is entitled to FAPE through Section 504, an educational plan must be developed and appropriate services, and/or technology, can be implemented in order to meet the student's educational or functional goals through that designated accommodation or 504 plan.

There are several reasons Section 504 and the ADA have become more prominent in public schools, but the primary reason is that Section 504 and the ADA use a different definition of *disability* and a different approach to eligibility than does the IDEA, resulting in many children who are not eligible under IDEA being protected by Section 504 and the ADA (Wright and Wright 2008).

Regardless of the specific reason for the increase in attention to Section 504 and the ADA, more and more parents are beginning to request services, technologies,

Box 6.2 Case study

Aiden has been identified with the diagnosis of developmental dyslexia and speech-language impairment. This impacts his ability to decode written words and express himself as he would like to. He is a 12-year-old boy who was referred by the teacher for an AT evaluation and specifically for the purpose of acquiring recommendations for equipment or software to support his written communication skills.

Aiden is in the seventh grade and his attitude toward learning and reading is good, but he is frustrated by not being able to comprehend written words and is unable to independently communicate his frustrations. Aiden has had ongoing evaluations regarding his academic challenges, including but not restricted to psychological and speech/language evaluations. He lives at home with his parents and siblings. He plays soccer and enjoys snowboarding. Aiden's outlook on school and attending class is good and he seems to enjoy learning, especially with the help of his para-educator. He states that he does not have problems taking notes as he receives handout notes and he uses a highlighter to mark key points. He also states that he has no difficulty with remembering homework or managing his time.

During the assessment process, Aiden was interviewed to determine his educational needs per his IEP team request. He was given a demonstration of and was asked to complete some tasks using the following AT devices in order to address his needs of taking notes during class:

1. Pulse Lifescribe Pen, (a "pen" type of recording device to help support notetaking);
2. Intel Reader (a portable scanning device to help capture printed notes and store and read them digitally);
3. SOLO™ software (a suite of technology interventions to support reading, writing, word completion, and drafting).

During the interview, Aiden was able to stay on tasks for one hour, listened attentively, and followed instructions given to him verbally. However, Aiden had difficulty with note taking, organizing his work, and managing his time. This was also noted in the referral from the teacher. Aiden lacked insight into his learning difficulties. This is very typical of students with learning disabilities. It will be important for him to be able to articulate his learning difficulties and advocate for what he needs as he looks toward transitioning beyond school.

He gravitated toward the SOLO software, which was similar to a tool he has used in the past. The suggestion made for the assessment was to trial SOLO for a while, along with providing a laptop and training not only him but for also for his para-educator and teacher so that they would understand how the software works and how to support him in becoming more efficient in his notetaking and in future written work as well. It was also determined that a membership to http://Bookshare.org would be beneficial so that his textbooks and other possible materials could be made available to him electronically and could be read with the software to support reading comprehension. With the various features of SOLO, Aiden would be given tools to help him become more effective and successful in his classroom and homework assignments.

As part of IDEA and the AT definitions, the IEP supported Aiden by first addressing his present levels of performance, then identifying which areas of need should be addressed and recommending an AT evaluation to address these needs and what tools, if any, could support Aiden in successfully fulfilling his educational goals. The AT devices were provided to Aiden in a variety of environments, based on his needs to accomplish his educational goals for that task. IDEA dictates that Aiden should receive those AT devices and services in order to meet his goals in his IEP.

and protections under these two acts. As a result, schools must learn the legal requirements of these acts and specific actions and services that are required.

The kinds of 504, and even special education, accommodations that schools can provide will vary and may not be consistent even in the same school. These accommodations will be made based on school resources, needs of students, etc. as we discussed earlier in the SETT Framework. The 504 evaluation team, like the special education team, decides which accommodations will best support a particular student in her own environment and specific task. For example, a student who has a reading disability of dyslexia and only needs access to screen reading tools in order to learn from the assigned curriculum qualifies for 504 simply because he cannot access the textbook visually alone. This provides services to the student in the learning environment to meet the needs of his 504 plan.

Summary

To summarize, the material in this chapter has provided an overview of the organizational influences that impact TEI intervention in educational settings. Best practice guidelines are presented to help practitioners work within the varying organizational settings environments they may encounter. The following case study (Box 6.2) illustrates the application of the chapter's content.

References

Access to instructional materials (2006). 34 CFR 300.172. Retrieved from https://www.law.cornell.edu/cfr/text/34/300.172.

Assistive Technology Training Online Project (2005). Retrieved from: https://www.humancentereddesign.org/inclusive-design/history.

Education for All Handicapped Children Act of 1975 (1975). Pub. L. No. 94-142, 20 U.S.C., § 1401, Part H, §677.

Individuals with Disabilities Education Improvement Act of 2004 (2004). Pub. L. No. 108-446, 20 U.S.C. § 1400 *et seq.*

Individuals with Disabilities Educational Act Amendments of 1990 (1997). Pub. L. No. 105-117, 111 Stat. 37.

Institute for Human Centered Design (n.d.). Inclusive design. Retrieved from https://www.humancentereddesign.org/inclusive-design/history.

Musgrove, M. (n.d.). Who pays for assistive technology? Parents or schools? Retrieved from https://www.understood.org/en/school-learning/assistive-technology/assistive-technologies-basics/who-pays-for-assistive-technology-parents-or-schools.

National Center on Accessible Educational Materials [AEM] (2006). Need for AEM. Retrieved from: http://aem.cast.org/aem-center/about-aem-center.html#.WRCuj9y1vcs.

National Center on Universal Design for Learning at CAST (2015). About Universal Design for Learning. Retrieved from http://www.cast.org/our-work/about-udl.html#.Vc0KoCxViko.

National Assistive Technology Act Programs (2017). The Assistive Technology Act: and the Basics of the 2004 Law. [PowerPoint slides]. Retrieved from https://www.at3center.net/repository/atactinformation.

Office of Special Education and Rehabilitation Services, US Department of Education (2000). A guide to the individualized education program. Retrieved from https://www2.ed.gov/parents/needs/speced/iepguide/iepguide.pdf.

Rehabilitation Act of 1973 (1973). 29 U.S.C., §504.

Rose, D.H., Gravel, J.W., and Gordon, D. (2014). Universal design for learning. In: *SAGE Handbook of Special Education*, 2e (ed. L. Florian), 475–491. London: Sage.

Sanford, J. (2012). *Universal Design as a Rehabilitation Strategy: Design for the Ages*. New York: Springer.

Section 504 of the Rehabilitation Act of 1973 (2015). 34 C.F.R. Part 104. Retrieved from http://www.ecfr.gov/cgi-bin/text-idx?tpl=/ecfrbrowse/Title34/34cfr104_main_02.tpl.

Technology-Related Assistance Act (1988). PL 100-407.

Texas Assistive Technology Network (2009a). The Texas 4-Step Model: Considering assistive technology in the IEP Process. [PowerPoint slides]. Retrieved from https://www.texasat.net/Assets/consid-notes-color-rev-121008(1).pdf.

Texas Assistive Technology Network (2009b). Training Modules Home. Retrieved from https://www.texasat.net/training-modules/training-modules-home.

The QIAT Leadership Team (2012). Quality indicators for assistive technology. Retrieved from http://www.qiat.org/indicators.html.

US Department of Education, Office for Civil Rights (2010). Free appropriate public education for students with disabilities: requirements under Section 504 of the Rehabilitation Act of 1973. Washington, DC: Author. Retrieved from http://www2.ed.gov/about/offices/list/ocr/docs/edlite-FAPE504.html.

Vicente, K. (2006). *The Human Factor: Revolutionizing the Way We Live with Technology*. New York: Routledge, Taylor & Francis Group.

Woods, R. (2014). Definition of assistive technology. Retrieved from http://www.gpat.org/georgia-project-for-assistive-technology/pages/assistive-technology-definition.aspx.

Wright, P. and Wright, P. (2008). Key differences between Section 504, the ADA, and the IDEA. Retrieved from http://www.wrightslaw.com/info/sec504.summ.rights.htm.

Zabala, J. (2005). Using the SETT Framework to level the learning field for students with disabilities. Retrieved from http://www.joyzabala.com/uploads/Zabala_SETT_Leveling_the_Learning_Field.pdf.

Zabala, J. (n.d.). SETT Framework. Retrieved from www.joyzabala.com.

7

Technology, employment, and disability: Creating a technology accessible vocational environment: Legal and organizational considerations

Wendy Strobel Gower and LaWanda Cook

Outline

Learning outcomes

After reading this chapter, you should be able to:

1. Explore the critical nature of an accessible technology environment within an organization.
2. Understand the benefits of accessible technology and providing reasonable accommodation in the workplace.
3. Understand the impact of the Americans with Disabilities Act in ensuring an accessible workplace for employees with disabilities.

Active learning prompts

Before you read this chapter:

1. Explore the Ease of Access Center in the Windows operating system.
2. Explore the accessibility features of the MAC operating system.
3. What do you think are the biggest barriers to employment for people with disabilities?
4. Develop an elevator speech that you might use to approach an employer about the benefits of accessible technology in the workplace.

Assistive Technologies and Environmental Interventions in Healthcare: An Integrated Approach, First Edition.
Edited by Lynn Gitlow and Kathleen Flecky.

Companion website: www.wiley.com/go/gitlow/assitivetechnologies

Key terms

Universal design (UD)
Accessible electronic and information technology
Assistive technology (AT)
Americans with Disabilities Act (ADA)
Reasonable accommodation (RA)

Introduction

People with disabilities make up at least 10% of the US working-age population (Erickson et al. 2015), but only 5.5% of the workforce (US Census 2015). Those that are employed are often reluctant to identify themselves due to fear of a negative reaction from their managers and coworkers (von Schrader et al. 2014). Disparities are significant for people with disabilities in terms of both access and experiences in the workplace, and many employers have not been successful in making change within their organizations.

For many people with disabilities, accessible technology is a necessary element to securing access to the workplace. A recent study conducted by the Society for Human Resource Management (SHRM) (2016) found that two-thirds of organizations are leveraging mobile recruiting through career websites, online job postings, and online application processes. Social media is becoming an increasingly popular recruitment tool, with 84% of companies using social media for recruitment purposes and an additional 9% exploring its use (SHRM 2016). As illustrated by this data, companies are increasingly commonly use eRecruting tools to bring job seekers into their organizations. According to the Partnership on Employment and Accessible Technology (PEAT) (2015), employers are using online tools to find, attract, assess, interview, and hire new personnel. A survey conducted by this organization found that design features of these systems, because of a lack of accessibility, tend to screen out many people with disabilities.

These design features included complex navigation, timeout restrictions, poor screen contrast, poorly written instructions, form fields that lack labels, and many other common website accessibility mistakes (Partnership on Employment and Accessible Technology 2015).

Technology is common at every stage of the employment life cycle and therefore it can continue to pose barriers even after employment has been successfully secured. PEAT (n.d.) defines six stages of the employment life cycle and lists examples of the accessible technology considerations at each stage. These stages along, with technology considerations, are:

1. Recruiting (e.g. corporate websites, pre-employment screening tools, digital interview technology)
2. Hiring and on-boarding (e.g. corporate intranets, job training, online benefits administration forms)
3. Work immersion and productivity (e.g. technology infrastructure, travel booking systems, office equipment)
4. Career advancement (e.g. learning management systems, training modules, performance review systems)
5. Retention (e.g. online employee assistance program (EAP) systems and locations, employee resource groups (i.e. internal communication channels (slack channels) or training opportunities)
6. Post-employment and retirement (e.g. online benefits administration tools) (PEAT n.d.)

Failure to consider accessible technology at each of these stages of employment can make it difficult to ensure the full participation of people with disabilities in the workplace. Today, nearly every kind of work requires the use of technology. Both skilled and unskilled positions frequently require employees to use some type of technology (Purcell and Rainie 2014).

Waiters and waitresses enter orders into a computerized system, janitorial staff clock in and out using a computerized process, and office employees spend the majority of their time in front of a computer. However, not everyone is able to access that technology in the same way. Disability plays a role in the way that people access technology, as does aging and experience with technology. Every organization must consider these individual differences when planning its technology infrastructure. This is an example of the impact of the organization rung on the Human-Tech Ladder (Vicente 2006).

Creating an ideal technology organization

Accessible technology can play a critical role in the accommodation and inclusion of individuals with disabilities in the workplace (Parks and Sedov 2016). Employers must plan to create an accessible technology environment in the workplace. In order to do so, it is necessary to assess the current level of accessibility in existing technology. This can be done by working directly with the technology vendor or conducting user testing to ensure access is possible using common access tools. When purchasing enterprise level software, it is necessary to understand if it has on-ramps for assistive and accessible technologies (US Department of Justice 2015; Voluntary Product Accessibility Template® [VPAT®] 2017). Identification of which access technologies are supported by the enterprise level solutions your organization uses can ease the burden of the organization as they seek to understand what reasonable accommodations to offer to employees. If you know your systems work with Job Access with Speech (JAWS) (screen reading software) and MAGic® (screen magnification software), those are the tools that are offered as access solutions for employees with disabilities who need them. As we will discuss later in this chapter, it is the employer who decides which accommodations to implement, as long as those tools are effective for the employee. If an employee is accustomed to another solution, you may have to offer training to ensure that accommodation's effectiveness. A well-thought-out approach to an accessible technology infrastructure will help to ensure that the organization saves money and time by providing a technology that easily adapts to individual needs.

In order to ensure the success of a technology environment within an organization, all pieces of the technology environment must work together. Consider the diagram in (Figure 7.1).

As illustrated by Figure 7.1, there are three components to ensuring access to technology in the workplace: (i) a universally designed environment and technology, (ii) accessible information technology, and (iii) assistive technology that provides on-ramps to the company's technologies platforms when needed. A universally designed environment and technology is the first critical component in ensuring access for the majority of the people who will interface with it. Universal design (UD) is the term introduced by architect Ron Mace to describe the concept of designing an environment and the products within it to be usable to the greatest extent possible by everyone, regardless of their age or disability (Center for Universal Design 2008). Simply put, UD means accessible to most. Figure 7.2 demonstrates an example of UD through the use of an adjustable work desk.

The Center for Universal Design (1997) outlines several principles for UD that are critical to its implementation. These principles include:

1. Equitable use: The design is useful and marketable to people with diverse abilities.
2. Flexibility in use: The design accommodates a wide range of individual preferences and abilities.
3. Simple and intuitive use: Use of the design is easy to understand, regardless of the user's experience, knowledge, language skills, or current concentration level.

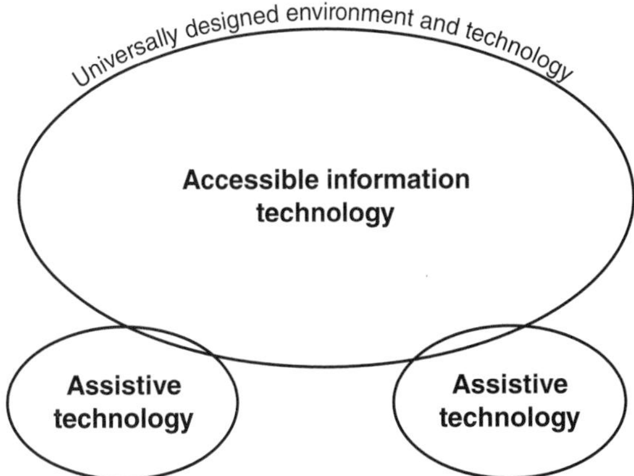

Figure 7.1 Ideal organizational technology environment. Source: Cornell University (2012).

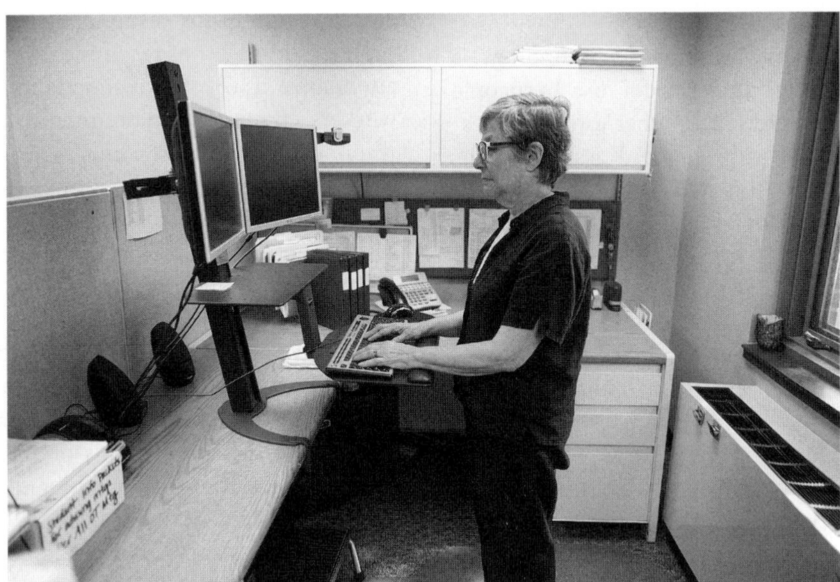

Figure 7.2 Individual working at an adjustable work station.

4. Perceptible information: The design communicates necessary information effectively to the user, regardless of ambient conditions or the user's sensory abilities.
5. Tolerance for error: The design minimizes hazards and the adverse consequences of accidental or unintended actions.
6. Low physical effort: The design can be used efficiently and comfortably and with minimum fatigue.
7. Size and space for approach and use: Appropriate size and space is provided for approach, reach, manipulation, and use, regardless of user's body size, posture, or mobility.

Although the concept of UD comes from the field of architecture, it can be applied in other contexts, including devices, processes, and workplace elements (Loy 2007). The concept of UD encourages organizations to recognize that "normal" is difficult to define and that a well-designed environment will allow for individual variation in the way that a person engages with an environment. Nicholas et al. (2011) reported that Walgreens incorporated the principles of UD in designing its distribution center in Anderson, South Carolina, where 40% of the 700 employees have disabilities. The company's universally designed distribution center includes automated guided vehicles that can be easily used by all employees, adjustable workstations, and an easier-to-use computer interface that features a simple touch screen available on a graphic user base. Reportedly, these changes have simplified operations at the distribution center making it easier for all employees to learn essential components of the center's operation; it has also made it easier to assign workers to different jobs within the center, since everyone has a better understanding of how the tasks within each job contribute to the others and to the overall operation (Nicholas et al. 2011).

Accessible electronic and information technology is technology that has been designed for use by people with a wide range of abilities. It is either directly accessible or it is compatible with standard assistive technology (University of Washington 2012). Mainstream operating systems that many of us use every day ensure access to the majority of their users through integrated accessibility features. Windows offers an Ease of Access Center that is accessible through the computer's control panel. A setup wizard walks the user through how to maximize the accessibility features for optimal use. The Ease of Access Center offers a screen magnifier, an on-screen keyboard, a narrator, and high contrast. For example, the user can optimize the visual display by increasing the contrast on the screen, can turn on a magnifier to increase the size of the content on a screen, and can change the display effects on the computer so it is easier to use. The user can also turn on a narration feature to read the text displayed on the screen or to access audio description in videos that have that feature. Users who are blind, people with cognitive disabilities, or individuals who operate the computer without a mouse can make optimum use of use of the computer system given these features. The Windows operating system (OS) Ease of Access Center also allows users to optimize the system for use with assistive technology.

Apple products also offer built-in accessibility features. Facetime can be used to enhance communication for people who are deaf or hard of hearing, VoiceOver is a screen reader that can be used on Macs and in web-based applications, and Switch Control is available for Mac Devices in the MacOS to ensure access for people with physical disabilities.

There are many benefits to accessible electronic and information technology. A recent study commissioned by Microsoft found that over 80% of organizations in Europe agree that a "robust accessibility strategy" contributes to a more diverse workplace, improves workplace productivity, reduces recruitments costs, and ensures compliance with federal mandates. These robust accessibility strategies can also expand the talent pool of people who can easily apply for and attain positions within the organization. An accessible technology infrastructure also assists with retaining employees who have acquired a disability (Parks and Sedov 2016). These findings are supported by the Job Accommodation Network (JAN), which has done a yearly study on the benefits of costs and benefits of job accommodations since 2004. This study found several direct and indirect benefits of accommodation in the workplace from survey respondents. Direct benefits included retaining valuable employees (90% of respondents), increased employee productivity (73% of respondents), increased employee attendance (56% of respondents), and savings on workers' compensation or other insurance costs (38% of respondents). Indirect benefits to survey respondents included improved interactions with coworkers (64% of respondents), increased company morale (63% of respondents), increased company productivity (56% of respondents), and improved interaction with customers (45% of respondents) (Loy 2016).

Assistive technology (AT) is the third critical component of an ideal technology environment. When a person has unique access needs, AT environments allow the addition of specialized tools or AT to better meet the person's needs. Assistive technologies are personal devices that can be used to help someone with a disability to complete specific tasks. The Assistive Technology Act defines an AT device as "any item, piece of equipment, or product system, whether acquired commercially, modified, or customized, that is used to increase, maintain, or improve functional capabilities of individuals with disabilities (Assistive Technology Act 2004)." Using this definition, AT includes products that are specifically designed for people with disabilities as well as any other products that someone with a disability might find useful in overcoming the functional limitations associated with their disability. For instance, an electronic letter opener is a piece of general office equipment that could be used by someone with a disability to open letters when they do not have the hand strength to open them manually. In this case, the electronic letter opener, a convenience for office workers, is a type of AT for the worker with limited hand strength.

Assistive devices can be added to a well-designed technology environment to meet the needs of one individual. Examples include things like a screen magnification program such as MAGic that can magnify images on a personal computer from 1 to 60 times its normal size or a screen reader such as JAWS that can allow someone who is blind to effectively use web pages and screen content (Figure 7.3). While the accessible electronic and information technology described above offers these features, assistive technologies like JAWS and MAGic allow customization of these features well beyond those that are built in to these existing operating systems.

A well-designed technology environment will ensure that the AT that an individual needs will be compatible with the technology infrastructure of the company. As mentioned in previous chapters, technology interventions must be considered in the context or environments where they will be used. The case study in Box 7.1 illustrates the consequences of failing to design an ideal technology environment.

While this case presents a complex solution, not all technology and environmental interventions (TEIs) are complex. Sometimes, the simplest solution is the easiest to implement and use, and it is often the most effective. In the case study in Box 7.2 a business evaluated its options for accommodating an employee with a learning disability and identified the simplest, most cost-effective solution.

As previously mentioned, making technology-related accommodations in the workplace requires that the entire technology environment be taken into consideration. Additionally, the employer must balance the needs of the business with the needs of the individual. In the case study in Box 7.3 a business had to assert its customers' right to privacy in determining what accommodation would be reasonable for a receptionist with a disability.

Box 7.1 Case study 1

A data entry clerk in a small office was unable to use a keyboard due to a disability and required the use of speech-to-text technology to maintain the organization's database. The company was using a Microsoft Access database specially designed for its use by a consultant. When this technology was designed, the consultant did not design it to be compatible with assistive technology. In order to accommodate the employee, the company had to pay the consultant to build a bridge between the database and the assistive technology in order for the person to complete data entry tasks.

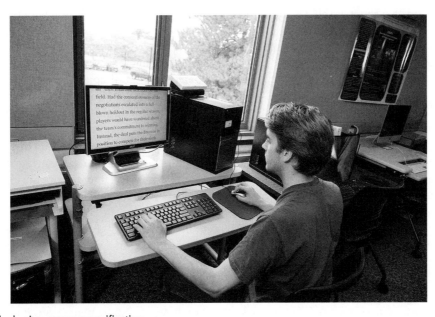

Figure 7.3 Individual using screen magnification.

Box 7.2 Case study 2

An employer wanted all new project ideas presented in writing prior to discussion with the work team. An employee with a learning disability was not accustomed to working on a computer and found it difficult to master commonly available screen reading technology. The employer found an online service known as iDictate (www.idictate.com) that would allow the employee to present his ideas to a transcriptionist over the phone at a cost of about one cent per word. The transcriptionist would then email the final document to the employee to share with his supervisor.

Box 7.3 Case study 3

A woman who did not have the use of her hands as a result of a brain stem injury worked as a receptionist in a small office. As part of her regular job duties, she had to take telephone messages. She proposed to her employer that she use the conversation record feature available on the phone so that she could record conversations and transfer the messages after each call using speech-to-text software. Her employer stated that this request was not reasonable as recording clients' conversations violated customers' right to privacy. An alternative solution was proposed that allowed the receptionist to use a tape recorder to record phone messages. She asked the caller to say and spell their name and she would repeat the information into the tape recorder. She could play back this information at a later time and send an email message to the appropriate colleague with the contents of the message. This solution was effective for the person with a disability and allowed the business to maintain the privacy rights of its customers.

As discussed later in this chapter, the TEIs provided to the employees in the examples above are a form of what is referred to by the Americans with Disabilities Act (ADA) as "reasonable accommodation."

The Americans with Disabilities Act (ADA)

No discussion about technology in the workplace would be complete without mention of the ADA. The ADA is a civil rights law passed in the United States that prohibits discrimination against people with disabilities in all areas of public life, including employment, in participating in state and local government programs and services, and in accessing privately owned businesses. While the ADA is United States legislation, it has been used as a foundation for international disability legislation (Prince 2010; Szymanski 2009). Please refer to Chapter 4 for references to international disability laws. The ADA provides the legal basis for employers to make what is referred to as reasonable accommodation, which in many cases may include some type of technology. Before continuing discussion of technology, however, a brief overview of this important legislation is warranted. According to the ADA National Network (2015), the purpose of the law is to ensure that people with disabilities have the same rights and opportunities as everyone else. The ADA has five titles, each covering a different aspect of community life. Title I is designed to help people with disabilities access the same employment opportunities and benefits available to people without disabilities. Title II prohibits discrimination on the basis of disability by public entities, which are programs and services offered by state and local governments. Title III prevents places of public accommodation (privately owned businesses that offer services to the public) from discriminating against people with disabilities. Title IV mandated the telephone relay service that allows people who are deaf and hard of hearing to gain access to the telephone. Title V contains miscellaneous provisions that deal with relationships with other laws, state immunity from financial damages, protections against retaliation and coercion, and attorney's fees (ADA National Network 2015).

Title I of the ADA protects qualified individuals with disabilities from discrimination as they apply for a job, when they are working, and as they take advantage of the benefits and privileges of employment. According to the US Equal Employment Opportunity Commission (US EEOC) (2017), a qualified individual with a disability is a person who "meets the legitimate skill, experience, education, or other requirements of an employment position that he seeks or holds, and who can perform the essential functions of the job with or without reasonable accommodations." Further, the ADA requires that employers provide reasonable workplace accommodations to employees who meet the legal definition of "person with a disability" to maintain or enhance their job performance (Gold et al. 2012). The ADA defines a person with a disability as an individual with a physical or mental impairment that substantially limits one or more major life activities; a record of such an impairment; or being regarded as having such an impairment (Regulations to Implement the Equal Employment Provisions of the Americans with Disabilities Act, as amended 2011). Reasonable accommodations provided to individuals with disabilities include changes that make the job application process accessible to candidates with disabilities, changes in the work setting or the way that the job is typically done, and changes that enable an employee with a disability to enjoy equal benefits and privileges of employment (US EEOC 1999).

The process of providing reasonable accommodation is intended to be interactive (US EEOC 2002), thus it is rarely straightforward for the employee or the employer. In fact, between 2005 and 2010, 28.2% of the charges filed by employees with disabilities against their employers allege failure to respond appropriately to requests for reasonable accommodation (von Schrader 2011). Unfortunately, in the nearly 25 years since the ADA was initially passed, case law had so limited who fits this definition that very few people could actually take advantage of the protections offered by the law. The majority of cases that were brought to the courts stopped at proving whether or not someone had a disability, and the issue of whether or not discrimination occurred was never addressed. In order to restore the original intent of the law, to prevent discrimination against people with disabilities, the ADA Amendments Act (ADAAA) was passed in 2008 and went into effect in January of 2009 (US EEOC 2017).

The ADAAA retained the original definition of disability provided by the ADA, but urged the courts to view disability broadly and maintain the focus of legal proceedings around the ADA on whether or not discrimination occurred. The ADAAA was specifically crafted to reverse the courts' prior misinterpretations of the original intent of the ADA (US EEOC 2002). In Sutton v United Airlines (1999), and two other cases decided on the same day (often referred to as the Sutton Trilogy), the Court ruled that in determining whether a plaintiff has a substantial limitation the courts should consider the person's condition in its corrected state. In other words, if a person's diabetes was controlled by insulin, the individual would not have a disability that would qualify for protection under the law. Similarly, an individual who, due to an amputation, had a prosthetic limb would not be considered to have a disability, under this interpretation of the law. Additionally, in Toyota v Williams (2002), the court found that in order for an individual to have a qualifying disability, the physical or mental impairment must prevent or severely restrict a major life activity, leaving a very narrow definition of disability.

Congress instructed the EEOC, the agency charged with enforcing the employment provisions of the ADA, to revise its ADA regulations to reflect the ADAAA's interpretation of disability. On March 25, 2011, the EEOC published the new regulations incorporating the ADAAA's changes, which took effect on May 24, 2011. The Title I regulations released by the EEOC provide practical and consistent standards to follow by providing rules of the full intent of the law. The regulations state that:

> The primary purpose of the ADAAA is to make it easier for people with disabilities to obtain protection under the ADA. Consistent with the Amendments Act's purpose of reinstating a broad scope of protection under the ADA, the definition of "disability" in this part shall be construed broadly in favor of expansive coverage to the maximum extent permitted by the terms of the ADA. The primary object of attention in cases brought under the ADA should be whether covered entities have complied with their obligations and whether discrimination has occurred, not whether the individual meets the definition of disability. The question of whether an individual meets the definition of disability under this part should not demand extensive analysis.
>
> (Regulations to Implement the Equal Employment Provisions of the ADA 2011, p. 4)

In addition, the regulations for Title I of the ADA state that mitigating measures should not be considered when determining whether or not someone has a disability. For example, if a person has diabetes that would qualify as a disability under the law, he or she is considered under the law to have a disability whether or not the diabetes is controlled with insulin.

Further, if an individual has a relapsing or remitting condition that, when active, meets the definition of disability under the ADA, the person is protected under the law, even when not currently experiencing significant limitations of the condition. For instance, if a person has multiple sclerosis (MS) with episodic exacerbations, the individual still qualifies for coverage under the ADA, even when she or he is not significantly limited by the condition. This is because when the condition is active, the person experiences significant difficulty with one or more major life activities.

These important distinctions in the definition of disability expand the number of people with disabilities eligible for the protections of the law. These legal protections include the right to request and receive reasonable accommodations. Further, with the ADAAA, the EEOC clarified "physical or mental impairment" to include any physiological disorder or condition, cosmetic disfigurement, or anatomical loss affecting one or more body systems, such as neurological, musculoskeletal, special sense organs, respiratory (including speech organs), cardiovascular, reproductive, digestive, genitourinary, immune, circulatory, and endocrine impairments. The ADAAA further clarifies that any mental or psychological disorder, such as intellectual disability (formerly termed mental retardation), organic brain syndrome, emotional or mental illness, and specific learning disabilities, are also covered under the law [Section 1630.2(h)]. The EEOC went so far as to provide a list of conditions that should be easily found to qualify as disabilities under the ADAAA, such as cancer, diabetes, and HIV (Regulations to Implement the Equal Employment Provisions of the ADA 2011; US EEOC 2017). However, it is important to remember that not every condition will meet the definition of disability provided by the ADAAA. The EEOC notes that many factors are taken into consideration when assessing how a condition impacts major life activities, including consideration of the difficulty, effort, or time required to perform a major life activity; pain experienced when performing a major life activity; the length of time a major life activity can be performed; and/or the way an impairment affects the operation of a major bodily function (Regulations to Implement the Equal Employment Provisions of the ADA 2011; US EEOC 2017).

The ADA and reasonable accommodation

The ADA and the ADAAA require that employers provide reasonable accommodation to qualified individuals with disabilities who apply for jobs or are employees in their organization unless doing so would result in an undue hardship (US EEOC 2002). The EEOC (2002) defines an accommodation as "any change in the work environment or in the way things are customarily done that enables an individual with a disability to enjoy equal employment opportunities" (para. 5). They define three categories of reasonable accommodation:

1. Modifications or adjustments to a job application process that would allow someone to be considered for a position.
2. Modifications or adjustments to the work environment or the way that work is customarily held or performed that would allow someone to perform the essential functions of the job.
3. Modifications or adjustments that enable the employee with a disability to enjoy equal benefits and privileges of employment that employees without disabilities enjoy.

Accommodations are for an individual's employment needs. Therefore, employers are not responsible for purchasing technology for an employee's or applicant's personal use, such as a wheelchair, hearing aid, or eyeglasses (US EEOC 2002).

Not all accommodations provided under the ADA will be technology related. The EEOC defines a number of options, including job restructuring, modified work schedules, changes in policies, and reassignment to a vacant position, as well as acquiring or modifying equipment, as some of the ways to potentially accommodate individuals with disabilities. Employers do not have to eliminate essential functions of the job as a reasonable accommodation, nor do they have to lower production standards that are required of all employees (US EEOC 2002). In one study, employers reported a variety of accommodation solutions. These solutions included changes in work schedules (22.9%), purchasing technology (12.7%), modification to the work site (5.3%), reassignment (9.8%), educating coworkers (4.1%), providing a service such as a sign language interpreter or reader (2.9%), or changing a workplace policy (2.5%) (Hartnett et al. 2011). Accommodations provided under the ADA are to assist employees with disabilities in performing essential job functions. Employers are often concerned that providing accommodations to employees with disabilities will be viewed as favoritism or special treatment. All employees should be advised that accommodations are provided in accordance with the law and are available to any employee who qualifies for them.

The accommodation process

The ADA states that reasonable accommodation requests do not have to be in writing or contain any specific legal language. This can create confusion for some managers and supervisors, as they may not recognize an employee's statement or request as a request for an accommodation. Employers are encouraged to err on the side of caution and ask the employee for clarification or bring in human resources to ensure that the appropriate protocol is followed (JAN 2011). Organizations should begin the interactive reasonable accommodation discussion process if an employee states that because of a medical condition or disability they are unable to or are having difficulty performing some aspect of their job. It is also important to note that third parties can initiate reasonable accommodation requests on behalf of an individual. For example, if a doctor sends a note to the workplace stating that the individual cannot use his hands to type, this would initiate a request for a reasonable accommodation on the individual's behalf. The EEOC (2002) also states that family members or friends of the employee with a disability can initiate a reasonable accommodation request. An employer may require documentation of a disability to verify the need for a reasonable accommodation in situations where the employee's disability or need for an accommodation is not immediately obvious. Keep in mind that medical documentation should be limited to the impact of the disability on the job. Employers are not entitled to the employee's entire medical history as a result of a reasonable accommodation request (US EEOC 2002).

Employers are advised to respond to reasonable accommodation requests expeditiously (US EEOC 2002), meaning they should begin the interactive process shortly after the request is received. It is best for the employer to keep the employee informed about the status of the request so that the employee or applicant with a disability is aware of the progress being made and is aware of any delays that might arise. Both the employer and the employee should maintain documentation of involvement in the interactive process (JAN 2011). If it is necessary for the individual to file an EEOC charge for failure to accommodate, the court generally finds the party who failed to respond in the interactive process at fault.

An employee can request a reasonable accommodation at any point in the employment process, even if she or he did not disclose the disability at the time of hire. It is very important that the individual request an accommodation as soon as they recognize that they are having difficulty with some aspect of their job. An employee should not wait until they have performance problems to request a reasonable accommodation. Even if the employee meets the definition of a person with a disability under the ADA, they are responsible for their work performance and subject to any consequences of poor performance for work completed prior to disability disclosure (US EEOC 2011).

As stated previously, any form of disclosure of disability and request for an accommodation should trigger the employer to begin an informal accommodation discussion. During this conversation, the employer may ask for documentation of disability, ask what job tasks are impacted by the disability, and ask about the type of accommodation that the employee or applicant is seeking. While the employee does not have to name a specific accommodation, they should have information about how their disability is impacting their work (US EEOC 2002). In one study, it was found that employers actually wanted employees to present "compelling arguments" about which specific job functions must be modified or accommodated (Gold et al. 2012). The employee is usually the best source of information as to what solution will be most effective for them but they may need assistance in thinking through how the functional limitation of the disability relates to the essential job functions. Service providers, including but not limited to certified rehabilitation counselors, occupational therapy practitioners, AT practitioners, and psychologists, can play a key role in providing support to people with disabilities even before the reasonable accommodation is requested (Bishop and Johnson 2017). Decisions about what technology solution will be put into place are based on the functional limitation associated with the disability as well as the skills or optimal areas of function, the essential functions of the job, and the setting in which the work is performed.

There are many resources available that can help employers to determine what type of accommodations might work for the person. The Job Accommodation Network (https://askjan.org) and the ADA National Network (https://adata.org) are excellent sources of information on potential technology aids for a variety of disabilities. It is important to provide the simplest solution that will meet the person's needs. The goal is not to have the technology replace the person's skills, but to enhance their skills so that they can perform the essential functions of the job effectively and efficiently. Simple solutions are usually easier to learn to use, easier to support, present fewer chances of problems with compatibility with the organization's technology infrastructure, and are more cost-effective. When exploring AT options, the employer should consider the availability of a vendor who can support the technology and provide service and training when necessary. If an employer chooses to use a solution that does not have this support, they should consider who in their organization can provide technology-related support to the employee. This helps to ensure that the final accommodation provided to the employee is as seamless as possible. If an organization is unsure of what technology solution would be most effective for the employee, it is possible to try many devices and software solutions before purchasing them. For example, many software solutions provide trial versions that may be downloaded at no cost.

While employers have reported that most workplace accommodations cost under $500 and that the majority of accommodations cost nothing to implement (Loy 2016), cost is still a concern for some employers. There are tax credits for employers who make certain kinds of accommodations. For example, the Disabled Access Tax Credit (Title 26, IRS Code, Section 44) is available to eligible businesses that provide adaptive equipment or modification of equipment, as well as other types of accommodations (Adaptive Environments Center 1992).

According to the ADA, the employer makes the final decision about what accommodation will be put into place. However, that accommodation must be effective. For example, if a legal secretary requires voice-input software in order to perform the essential functions of her job, the employer would have to provide a solution that could understand the vocabulary associated with that position. While standard voice-input software is available for relatively low cost, it does not contain the vocabulary to be effective in the job tasks associated with being a legal secretary. The employer would have to provide a higher-cost solution, such as Dragon NaturallySpeaking Legal, that contained the appropriate legal vocabulary. In order to ensure that an accommodation is effective, the employer should make sure that any training that the employee needs to use the technology solution is provided to the team that works with the employee. This can include both the employee and their immediate supervisor. Any coworkers or departments that will be supporting the technology (i.e. IT department) should be provided with training on the technology as well.

Once an accommodation is put into place, it is important to monitor the solution to ensure that it is effective for the employee. There are many reasons why an accommodation may not be effective: the employee's disability changes, the technology infrastructure of the workplace changes, or the job itself changes as new duties are assigned (JAN 2011). The employer should plan to check with the employee on a regular basis to ensure that the accommodation continues to be effective for the employee, especially if they notice that production levels are not being maintained or the person is continuing to have difficulty completing the essential job function for which they received the accommodation. Ongoing communication between the employee and the manager should be encouraged.

One final consideration when discussing accommodations is the notion of stigma. The Human-Tech Ladder reminds us that the psychological impact of technology must be considered when matching a person with technology (Vicente 2006). Although TEI can be tremendously helpful, not all people with disabilities are eager to use these kinds of resources at work.

Research has demonstrated several factors, including social pressures and perceived stigma, unattractive product design, and concern on the part of family members that an individual's reliance on TEI may hinder the learning of important skills such as telling time, can influence one's decision to use job accommodations (Parette and Scherer 2004; Resnik et al. 2009). However, when ordinary items are used as TEI or when the technologies are the same as those used by people without disabilities, job accommodations need not be stigmatizing

Box 7.4 Here's the evidence

Anand, P., and Sevak, P. (2017). The role of workplace accommodations in the employment of people with disabilities. *IZA Journal of Labor Policy* 6(1): 1–20.

Key Words: vocational rehabilitation, employment, workplace accommodations, disability

Purpose: The purpose of this article was to analyze a recent survey of disability employment to identify: (i) employment barriers faced by people with disabilities, (ii) availability of workplace accommodations, and (iii) worker characteristics. By understanding the characteristics of workers who report barriers to employment that could be overcome by accommodations as well as understanding those who do not receive them, the authors hope that vocational rehabilitation agencies can increasingly identify workplace barriers and accommodations for those who can benefit from them.

Sample/Setting: Data from the Survey of Disability and Employment (August 15, 2014–December 15, 2014) from Mississippi, New Jersey, and Ohio were analyzed. This survey contains information on the employment history and workplace and social supports for people who applied for vocational rehabilitation services during the dates mentioned above.

Method: Data analysis consisted of using descriptive statistics and regression analysis and involved three main components. First, the authors looked at workplace barriers identified by non-working respondents to see if they could be addressed by workplace accommodations. Next, a regression analysis was conducted to examine the relationship between obtaining workplace accommodations and employment status. The final analysis investigated the characteristics of people with disabilities who receive and do not receive accommodations.

Findings: The most common reported barrier to work was a person's condition, which prevents them from working. Other barriers reported included inability to find a job, being discouraged from previous attempts at working, employers who will not give the respondent a chance, and lack of skills. Inaccessible workplaces were mentioned by about one third of the non-working respondents. Also mentioned was lack of transportation. At least one third of the non-working group stated they would be more likely to be employed if workplace accommodations were provided. Those with higher levels of education were more likely to be employed. Workplace accommodations positively correlated with current employment included flexible work schedules, receiving help with transportation, and having a personal care attendant or assistant. Those with less education, poor health, or physical disability were less likely to receive workplace accommodations, and perceived workplace accessibility as a barrier to employment.

Critical Thinking Questions:

1. After reading this research article, what do you understand to be the limitations of this research? Are there any limitations not stated?
2. What other findings did you take away from this article?
3. What implications does this article have for practice?

and can serve to enhance social interaction and inclusion in the workplace (Robitaille 2010). For example, a worker with attention deficit disorder who benefits from the accommodation of being able to wear headphones at work is not going to stand out as different from his colleagues if others also use headsets while performing job-related tasks. Likewise, the calendars and alarm features on smartphones enable people with and without disabilities to keep track of obligations. The common use of such items can create a way for employees with and without disabilities to relate to each other simply as people, without the stigma that can be associated with AT devices which single out the user as different. Please review Box 7.4 for research of workplace accommodations using technology.

Summary

The ADAAA has realigned the spirit of the ADA with the letter of the law and refocused prevention of discrimination of people with disabilities in the workplace.

Unfortunately, the law alone cannot serve as sufficient motivation to create environments that are inclusive to people with disabilities. Accessible technology can help to create work opportunities and to enhance the lives of individuals with and without disabilities in the workplace. Service providers play an important role in educating employers about the importance of accessible technology in the workplace. Service providers can also be a source of information for employers about the importance of developing proactive strategies and policies for ensuring effective workplace practices for employees with disabilities. Without inclusive policies and practices in place, it can be very difficult for a person with a disability to receive the support necessary from their employer to be successful in the workplace. It is critical that service providers form partnerships with champions of disability in the business community to ensure that work environments are inclusive and encourage the success of all job seekers and employees. Additionally, service providers must also provide support to the individual with a disability around issues such as disclosure of disability and what accommodations might help them to be successful on the job. Service providers play a critical role as both educators and advocates in increasing the employment rates of people with disabilities.

References

ADA National Network (2015). An overview of the Americans with Disabilities Act. Retrieved from https://adata.org/factsheet/ADA-overview.

Adaptive Environments Center (2007). Fact sheet 4: tax incentives for providing business accessibility. Retrieved from https://www.ada.gov/archive/taxpack.pdf.

Assistive Technology Act of 2004 (2004). 29 U.S.C. 3002.

Bishop, M.and Johnson, E. (2017). Workplace accommodation. Retrieved from https://www.aesnet.org/clinical_resources/practice_tools/employment_resources/workplace_accomodation.

Center for Universal Design (1997). *The Principles of Universal Design*, Version 2.0. Raleigh, NC: North Carolina State University.

Center for Universal Design (2008). About universal design. Retrieved from https://www.ncsu.edu/ncsu/design/cud/about_ud/about_ud.htm.

Cornell University (2012). Accessible technology in the workplace. Retrieved from https://www.northeastada.org/talking-to-managers/9.

Erickson, W., Lee, C., and von Schrader, S. (2015). *Disability Status Report: United States*. Ithaca, NY: Cornell University Yang-Tan Institute (YTI).

Gold, P.B., Oire, S.N., Fabian, E.S., and Wewiorski, N.J. (2012). Negotiating reasonable workplace accommodations: perspectives of employers, employees with disabilities, and rehabilitation service providers. *Journal of Vocational Rehabilitation* 37 (1): 25–37. https://doi.org/10.3233/JVR-2012-0597.

Hartnett, H.P., Stuart, H., Thurman, H. et al. (2011). Employers' perceptions of the benefits of workplace accommodations: reasons to hire, retain and promote people with disabilities. *Journal of Vocational Rehabilitation* 34: 17–23. https://doi.org/10.3233/JVR-2010-0530.

Job Accommodation Network (JAN) (2011). Effective accommodation practices series: the interactive process. Retrieved from https://askjan.org/publications/Topic-Downloads.cfm?pubid=962701.

Loy, B. (2007). Universal design and assistive technology as workplace accommodations: an exploratory white paper on implementation and outcomes. Retrieved from https://askjan.org/publications/Topic-Downloads.cfm?pubid=63941.

Loy, B. (2016). Workplace accommodations: low cost, high impact. Retrieved from https://askjan.org/publications/Topic-Downloads.cfm?pubid=962628&action=download&pubtype=pdf.

Nicholas, R., Kauder, R., Krepcio, K., and Baker, D. (2011). *Ready and Able: Addressing Labor Market Needs and Building Productive Careers for People with Disabilities through Collaborative Approaches*. New Brunswick, NJ: National Technical Assistance and Research Center to Promote Leadership for Increasing Employment and Economic Independence of Adults with Disabilities.

Parette, P. and Scherer, M. (2004). Assistive technology and stigma. *Education and Training in Developmental Disabilities* 39 (3): 217–226.

Parks, S. and Sedov, V. (2016). Accessing the value of accessible technologies for organizations: a Total Economic Impact™ study. Retrieved from https://blogs.microsoft.com/uploads/prod/sites/73/2018/10/5bc08e8059d68-5bc08e8059d6bMicrosoft-TEI-Accessibility-Study_Edited_FINAL-v2.pdf.pdf.

Partnership on Employment and Accessible Technology (PEAT) (2015). Is HR tech hurting your bottom line? A Report on PEAT's 2015 erecruiting research findings. Retrieved from http://www.peatworks.org/talentworks/resources/survey-report.

Partnership on Employment and Accessible Technology (PEAT) (n.d.). Accessible technology and the employment lifecycle. Retrieved from http://www.peatworks.org/talentworks/resources/employment-lifecycle.

Prince, M. (2010). What about a disability rights act for Canada? Practices and lessons from America, Australia, and the United Kingdom. *Canadian Public Policy. Analyse de Politiques* 36: 199–214.

Purcell, K. and Rainie. L. (2014). Technology's impact on workers. Pew Research Center. Retrieved from http://www.pewInternet.org/2014/12/30/technologys-impact-on-workers.

Regulations to Implement the Equal Employment Provisions of the Americans with Disabilities Act, as Amended (2011). 29 C.F.R. 1630.

Resnik, L., Allen, S., Isenstadt, D. et al. (2009). Perspectives on the use of mobility aids in a diverse population of seniors: implications for intervention. *Disability and Health Journal* 2 (2): 77–85.

Robitaille, S. (2010). *The Illustrated Guide to Assistive Technology and Devices: Tools and Gadgets for Living Independently*. New York: Demos Medical Publishing.

von Schrader, S. (2011). *Calculations from EEOC Integrated Mission System*. Ithaca, NY: Cornell University, RRTC on Employer Practices Related to Employment Outcomes Among Individuals with Disabilities.

von Schrader, S., Malzer, V., and Bruyère, S. (2014). Perspectives on disability disclosure: the importance of employer practices and workplace climate. *Employee Responsibilities and Rights Journal* 26 (4): 237–255.

Society for Human Resource Management (SHRM) (2016). SHRM survey findings: using social media for talent acquisition – recruitment and screening. Retrieved from https://www.shrm.org/hr-today/trends-and-forecasting/research-and-surveys/Documents/SHRM-Social-Media-Recruiting-Screening-2015.pdf.

Sutton v United Airlines (1999). 527 U.S. 471.

Szymanski, C. (2009). The globalization of disability rights law – from the Americans with Disabilities Act to the UN Convention on the Rights of Persons with Disabilities. *Baltic Journal of Law & Politics* 2 (1): 18. http://dx.doi.org.ezproxy.ithaca.edu:2048/10.2478/v10076-009-0002-z.

Toyota Motor Mfg., KY, Inc. v Williams (2002). 534 U.S. 184.

US Census (2015). Table S1811, selected economic characteristics for the civilian noninstitutionalized population by disability status. 2011–2015 American community survey 5-year estimates [Data file]. Washington, DC.

US Department of Justice (2015). Software accessibility checklist. Retrieved from https://www.justice.gov/crt/software-accessibility-checklist.

US EEOC (1999). The Americans with Disabilities Act: a primer for small business. Retrieved from https://www.eeoc.gov/eeoc/publications/adahandbook.cfm.

US EEOC (2002). Enforcement guidance: reasonable accommodation and undue hardship under the Americans with Disabilities Act. Retrieved from http://www.eeoc.gov/policy/docs/accommodation.html.

US EEOC (2011). The Americans with Disabilities Act: applying performance and conduct standards to employees with disabilities. Retrieved from https://www.eeoc.gov/facts/performance-conduct.html.

US EEOC (2017). Questions and answers on the final rule implementing the ADA Amendments Act of 2008. Retrieved from https://www.eeoc.gov/laws/regulations/ada_qa_final_rule.cfm.

University of Washington (2012). What is accessible electronic and information technology? Retrieved from https://www.washington.edu/doit/what-accessible-electronic-and-information-technology?1110=.

Vicente, K. (2006). *The Human Factor: Revolutionizing the Way People Live with Technology*. New York: Routledge, Taylor & Francis Group.

Voluntary Product Accessibility Template® (VPAT®) (2017). Wikipedia entry on VPAT. Retrieved from https://en.wikipedia.org/wiki/Voluntary_Product_Accessibility_Template.

8

Technology and environmental interventions for the home environment

BevVan Phillips

Outline

Assistive Technologies and Environmental Interventions in Healthcare: An Integrated Approach, First Edition.
Edited by Lynn Gitlow and Kathleen Flecky.

Companion website: www.wiley.com/go/gitlow/assitivetechnologies

Learning outcomes

After reading this chapter, you should be able to:

1. Identify key factors that influence successful technology and environmental intervention (TEI).
2. Explain how design concepts of accessibility, universal design, adaptability, visitability, and home design impact decision-making for TEI in a client's home.
3. Describe the role of the client as part of a home modification assessment and intervention planning team.
4. Explain how funding, codes, and guidelines for home modifications affect technology and environmental modifications in a client's home or residence.
5. Describe the various qualifications and perspectives of professionals who assess, design, implement, and evaluate home modifications.
6. Identify structural aspects of the private home and assistive technology factors that guide TEI.
7. Identify aspects of the Human-Tech Ladder relevant to TEI in home environments.

Active learning prompts

Before you read this chapter:

1. If you went home today using a wheelchair for mobility, list the areas of your home in which you would have difficulty gaining access.
2. If you were living with a person diagnosed with Alzheimer's disease, sixth stage, identify the areas within your home that might pose safety risk(s).
3. Search for and review information about the US Accessibility Standards for public places. These standards apply to residences or homes if they are incorporated into local building codes and they form a starting point for design of a person's residential access. One online source of information is www.ada.gov.
4. Search for the definitions of the following terms: accessibility, adaptability, visitability, and universal design.
5. List potential professionals in your region that you would contact to provide home modifications or assistive technology. Provide a brief statement regarding what this professional's role would be as part of a TEI team and how they would be paid for services.

Key terms

Accessibility
Adaptability
Building code
Funding
Monetary value
Structure
Team director
TEI team
Universal design
Visitability
Zoning

Technology and environmental intervention for the home environment

In this chapter, various factors that influence successful technology and environmental interventions (TEI) in home settings and the role of persons involved in the TEI process will be investigated. The basic structural and technology concepts needed to assess, design, implement, and evaluate home modifications will be presented. This chapter will give the reader an opportunity to envision how human factors, structural design, and technology interplay within home environments. Additionally, the reader will gain knowledge on how to assess the ability to work as part of an interprofessional team in order to match TEI for a client's unique lifestyle.

Modification of home environments to best fit the capacities, abilities, and interests of clients with or without disabilities is partially a result of the ongoing evolution of the home building industry. Residential home designs have evolved in ways that make everyday living safer and more convenient. Consider how relatively easy it is to use and care for a modern toilet than to do so for the previously common toilets outside the home, referred to as outhouses. Although outhouses are still used in the United States and other countries today, those of us who have never lived with one may not realize they needed to be maintained or even moved to handle accumulations of waste. This home environmental modification – the modern toilet – was made possible by technology innovation and municipal infrastructure for managing supply and waste water.

The need for and appearance of these innovations can be viewed as creative responses to physical and psychological factors identified in the Human-Tech Ladder (Vicente 2006). The ability to accomplish innovation is possible when teams or organizations share creative designs and building materials and when policies are generated to implement home modifications (Vicente 2006). Enhancement in residential home design is only possible due to improvement in technology, an increased body of knowledge about the relationship of structure to safety and consumer comfort and demand. Moreover, organizational and political factors such as creation of building codes evolve to meet public safety concerns. Consider how much more uniform and safer stairs are constructed in homes built under current codes compared to stairs constructed 100 years ago with stair tread depth and rise height unregulated! The building industry has also been changed by legislation related to persons with disabilities. For example, the 1988 amendments to the Fair Housing Act delineated design modifications applicable to multifamily dwellings, which involved features to improve physical accessibility (Fair Housing Accessibility FIRST n.d.). Moreover, aspects of the American with Disabilities Act Guidelines (2010) are incorporated into building codes applicable to private residences (International Code Council 2012). Vicente's (2006) Human-Tech Ladder reminds us how the political and organizational factors, such as building codes and federal legislation, are instrumental in influencing how technology in turn impacts the individual and society.

This chapter will first consider the key factors that influence successful TEI, followed by an examination of how the design concepts of accessibility, universal design, adaptability, visitability, and home design impact TEI decisions in a client's home setting. Next, the role of the client as part of the TEI team will be illustrated in order to appreciate the client as a creative force and decision-maker in home modification planning and implementation. Key information related to funding, building, and planning codes and guidelines will be presented with an opportunity for readers to relate this information to TEI. The role of the client, TEI professionals on the team, and other professionals will be examined in the process and successful completion of home modification. Finally, structural aspects of the private home setting and factors related to assistive technology (AT) will be highlighted as they pertain to TEI, and a summary synopsis will be presented of how the Human-Tech Ladder is relevant to home environments.

Key factors that influence successful TEI

Many of the factors considered by health professionals in order to create the best match of TEI to client needs can be relevant within the home environment, but there are also factors unique to this environment. This author has identified five key factors that must be considered to match technology and structural modifications in the home environment in order to achieve the best possible home solutions for a client or family. These five factors complement each other and support one another for optimal functioning. A visual is presented in Figure 8.1 with labels for each as one of the five lines in a simple cross-section of a home. This figure can be used when working with clients on the potential complexity of a successful TEI, as it is easy to understand if the home setting is incomplete, that is, if all five factors in the visual have not been accounted for.

The five factors are: (i) person and family; (ii) funding, codes, and laws; (iii) professionals in the home modification process; (iv) physical structure of the home; (v) characteristics of the technology used or that will be used by the client in the home. The design process involving successful TEI is not a simple or black and white process. There is no clear answer that works in every home modification situation, nor is it a purely subjective process of interpretation of client desires or goals. A successful intervention using the five factors can be envisioned as similar to any therapeutic

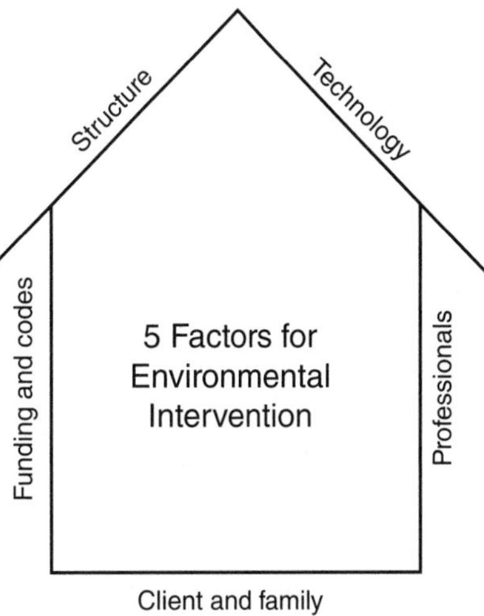

Figure 8.1 Five factors for successful home modification: five sides of a home.

intervention. It is a dynamic process of evaluation and interpretation (DeJonge and Cordiner 2011) of client goals and abilities with intervention based on an understanding of the intervention tools, residential structure and technology, and the relationships, roles, and responsibilities of each member of the team. Moreover, while it depends on the assessment tools that one chooses, more often than not assessment of the TEI outcome may not be a formal process; rather, it is generally the client's assessment in terms of satisfaction.

Issues that may impede successful TEI using the five factors are: (i) information needed from multiple professional agencies with different viewpoints on TEI; (ii) funding and rules varying from one home modification situation to another; (iii) no clear TEI team director or leader coordinating the TEI process from start to finish. As emphasized in Vicente's Human-Tech Ladder, the importance of the team cannot be overlooked in this area. Without a designated TEI team and team leader or director, there may be challenges on agreement of goals, communication, lack of involvement, unclear roles, and responsibilities, and a successful outcome is at risk.

Successful TEI in home settings requires shared knowledge from disparate fields. Additionally, knowledge related to human factors similar to those discussed in the Vicente Human-Tech Ladder (2006), such as physiology and psychology, as well as an understanding of disease and illness processes and rehabilitation, are essential. Also, knowledge of residential construction, home design, and building codes and laws, as well as of technology commonly used in the home and the TEI process, is required. TEI team members need to have an understanding of and training in team skills, especially recognition of the roles of other professionals and their expertise on the team, as well as cooperation, conflict resolution, consensus, and coordination (See Chapter 9 for further information on best practices related to teams). Finally, the client who will live with the TEI outcomes wants something that matches their perception of what their home should look like and that fits with the level of change they are prepared to make at the time of intervention.

Design concepts

Several different design concepts, or combinations of concepts, can be used in the TEI home modification process, although the overall goal remains to change the structure and technology within the environment to make the home meet the living needs of the client and family. It may be necessary to determine if the client's goals are to increase access, decrease access, or guide access. Limiting or guiding physical access may be optimal when modifying homes for people with dementia or brain injuries. It is possible to work toward increasing and decreasing access for the same client. Consider how you would problem-solve making bathing an easier process for a person who can walk who demonstrates symptoms of Alzheimer's disease and arthritis. You might design modifications to guide them away from potentially unsafe areas of the home, such as stairs to the basement, while also thinking of modifications to guide them toward the bathroom. You might be planning modifications to increase their safe access to the tub or shower that would also make caregiving easier for those providing bathing services.

Accessible design

Accessible design is the "design of a space that allows a person with a disability to make the greatest possible use of a space. It targets a specific client with a disability" (Wade and Rancourt 2002). Generally speaking, the goal of accessible design is to compensate for a deficit in performance (Sanford 2012). What creates confusion is that in private residences, the word "accessible" can mean several different things. It can denote that the dwelling meets minimum requirements for what an agency or funding source defines as accessible housing or it may mean that an intervention is matched to a client's unique needs or abilities. Mandatory requirements vary by program and generally apply to commercial, federal, or third-party-funded projects. Some funding sources have specific definitions of accessibility which must be met whether or not they are needed or desired by the client. When persons with disabilities are provided choices that match their unique needs, those modifications may not work well for others.

If an accessible design is not as useable for others in the home and is not integral to the environment, it may not be considered desirable by those who don't need it. For example, a low counter height used in preparation of a meal by a client who is short-statured may be unuseable for others. Grab bars positioned for a client who uses only the left upper extremity may not be positioned for usability for others with different physical abilities.

Home modification designers and their clients need to be aware that accessibility features may have a negative impact on the *monetary value* of the home. The value of the home on the real estate market is influenced by the perceptions of potential buyers. If features are not considered desirable, they could reduce a potential buyer's interest in a home and therefore reduce perceived value and number of potential buyers. Extended time on the market and fewer potential buyers may diminish a seller's room for negotiation. For example, a ramp or

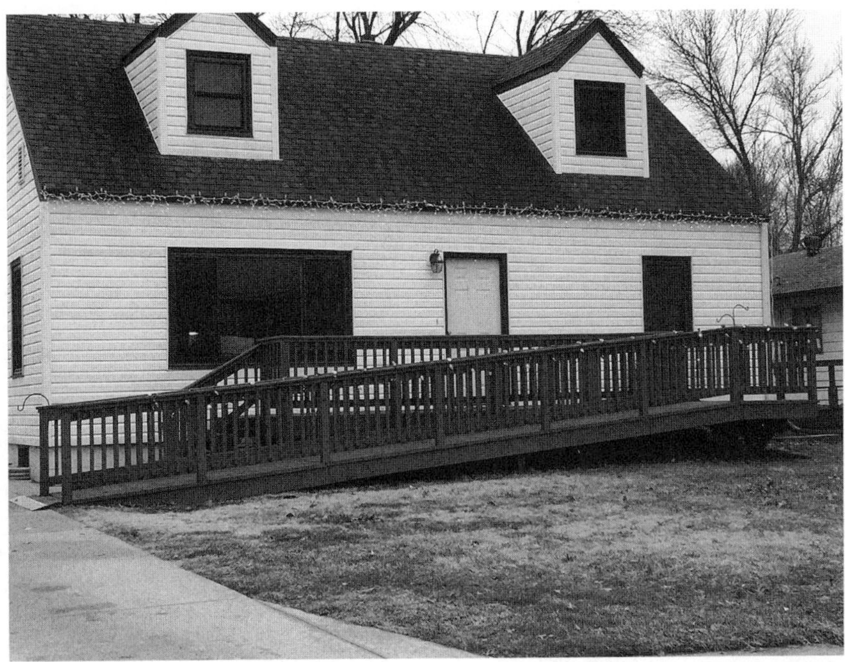

Figure 8.2 House with a ramp.

vertical platform lift is of no use to the majority of potential future buyers, so it will not typically enhance the home's monetary value. The example in Figure 8.2 shows an example of a ramp.

Modification of existing homes that eliminate bedrooms to provide space for larger bathrooms or hallways may negatively affect municipally assessed monetary value. When it is not possible to create a functional solution that is useful for other people or one that blends in with the existing structure, consider trying to make the access feature one that is easily removed if needed for resale of the home. Conversely, there are fewer homes on the market with access features than without them, so there are fewer potential selections for a buyer looking for one. This may create high perceived value for a home with accessible features that meets that buyer's requirements for location and price. It is important to educate clients about options and the consequences of those options. There is nothing wrong with a client making a choice to implement an accessible feature that meets a unique need yet may not be desirable to others. The client does need to have the information of options and consequences of options to make an informed choice.

Universal design

Universal design is 'the design of products and environments to be usable by all people, to the greatest extent possible, without the need for adaptation or specialized design" (Center for Universal Design 2008) and will typically be attractive to, and therefore more valuable to, a wide range of individuals. Universal design is not a specific set of requirements, but a collection of seven principles with guidelines and key elements of these principles. These principles are defined below and are illustrated in Figures 8.3–8.9, with other examples offered on the following website: http://www.ncsu.edu/ncsu/design/cud/pubs_p/docs/poster.pdf.

1. Equitable use: the design is useful and marketable to people with diverse abilities.
2. Flexibility in use: the design accommodates a wide range of individual preferences and abilities.
3. Simple and intuitive use: use of design is easy to understand regardless of the user's experience, knowledge, language skills, or education level.
4. Perceptible information: the design communicates necessary information effectively to the user, regardless of ambient conditions or the user's sensory abilities.
5. Tolerance for error: the design minimizes hazards and the adverse consequences of accidental or unintended actions.
6. Low physical effort: the design can be used efficiently and comfortably and with minimum fatigue.
7. Size and space for approach and use: appropriate size and space is provided for approach, reach, manipulation, and use regardless of user's body size, posture, or mobility (Center for Universal Design 2008).

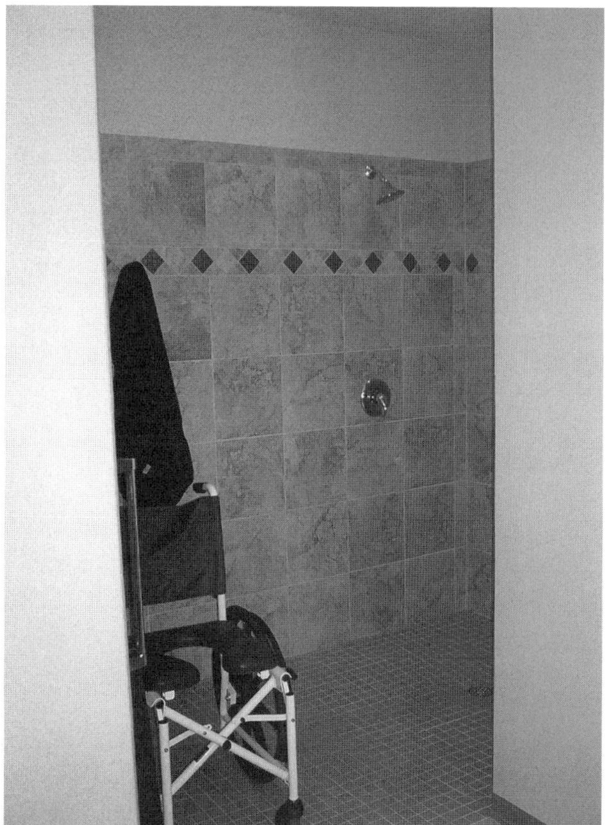

Figure 8.3 0 threshold shower.

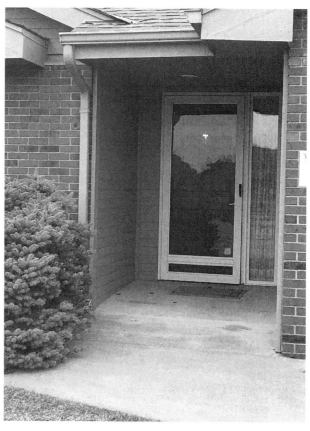

Figure 8.5 0 step entry without steps.

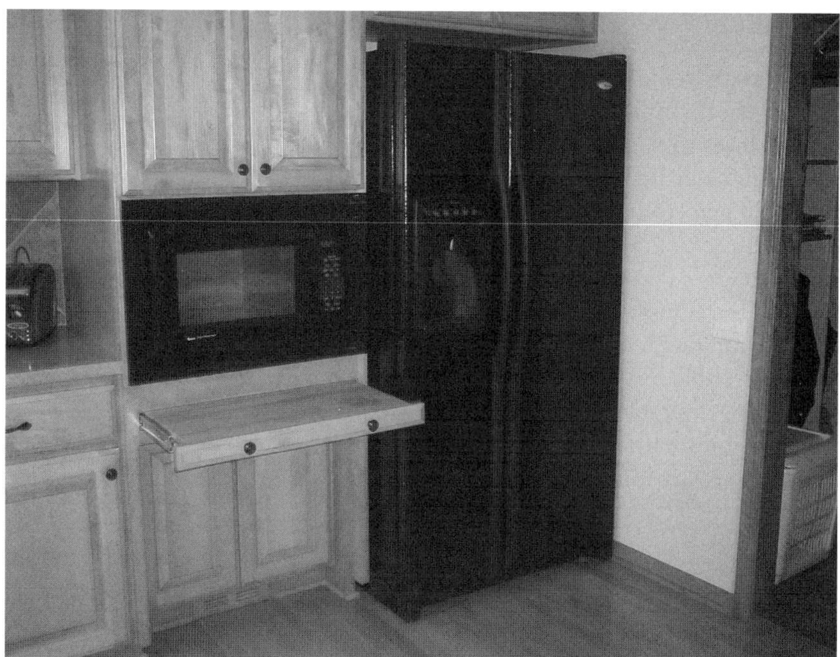

Figure 8.4 Counter height microwave.

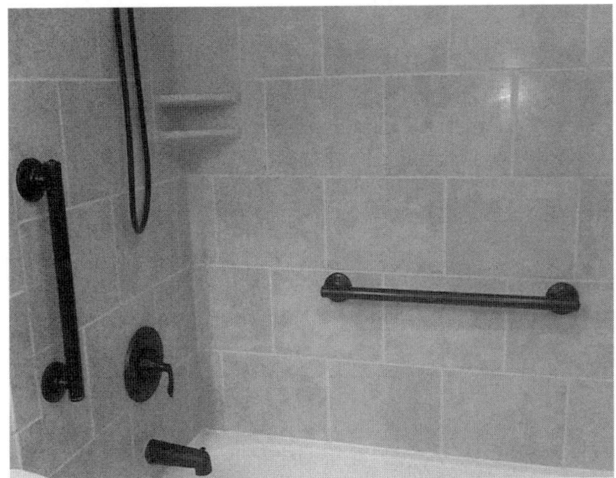

Figure 8.6 Bathroom grab bars in contrasting color.

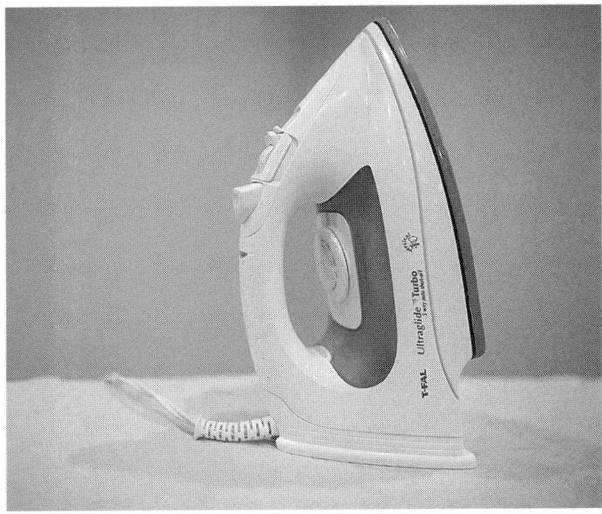

Figure 8.7 Iron with auto-shut off feature.

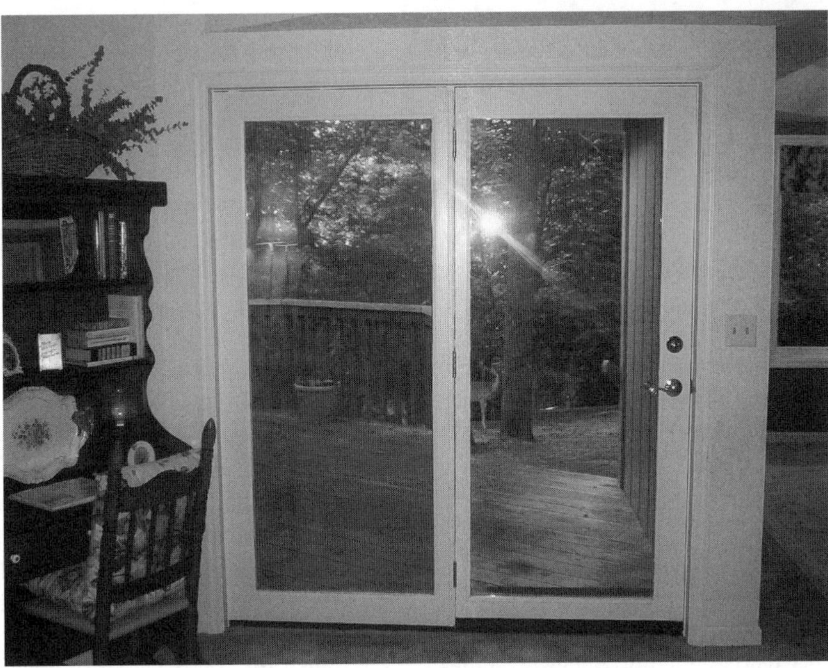

Figure 8.8 Patio door with lever handle.

Adaptable design

Adaptable design is a concept of addressing changing needs over time. It may not provide for a high level of accessibility, but it allows for a space to be easily changed as needed (Wade and Rancourt 2002). Specific definitions for the term have been developed by agencies with regulatory control such as the Department of Housing and Urban Development (HUD) and incorporated into standard definitions of the American National Standards Institute (ANSI) and Uniform Federal Accessibility Standards. The concept of addressing changing needs over time is congruent with the social movement of Aging in Place and works well for individuals with progressive diseases (Steinfeld and Maisel 2012). It also is suitable for clients who are not ready emotionally or financially to commit to a large accessibility remodeling project.

An adaptable design is one in which elements can be added to or removed relatively easily, as opposed to other types of modifications or structures which may need to be added or removed at great effort or expense (Center for Universal Design 2006). The concept of

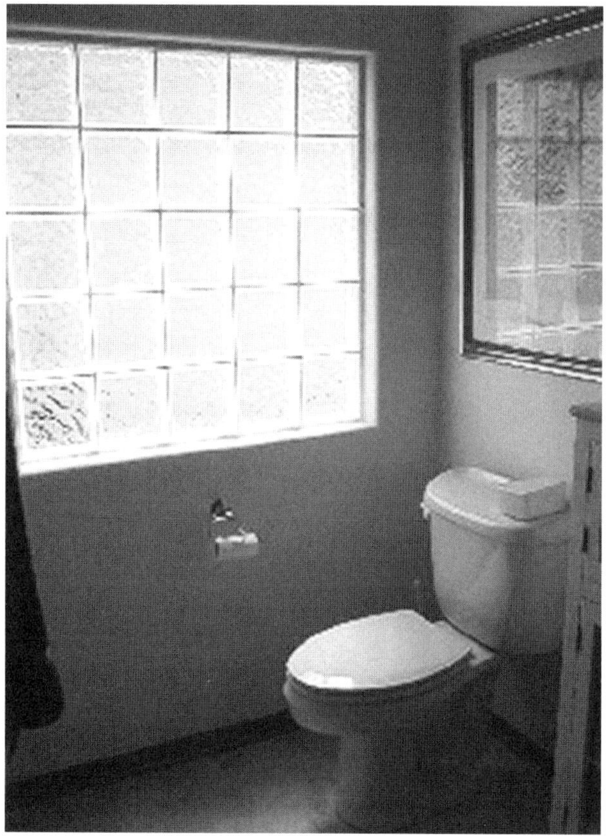

Figure 8.9 Roomy access to toilet.

adaptation may also be used to provide initial accessibility which can later be changed if there is no longer a need for such modification. This is beneficial when a client recovers from an illness or injury or develops skills over time and no longer requires compensation through environmental modification.

Adaptable design can also be employed when a client anticipates the need to restore a dwelling to its original design in the near future, for example, when a client enters hospice, or for those who frequently change dwellings.

Consider the case study in Box 8.1.

Visitability

Visitability describes the movement to change housing policy so that local legislation would apply to all new homes constructed, not just homes impacted by funding from federal or state sources, Concrete Change (Guzman et al. 2017). The goal of this change is to strive for all new homes to be accessible to visit for persons with mobility concerns. Learn more about Concrete Change and visitability at the organizations' website: www.concretechange.org.

There are numerous resources available at this website, including a train the trainer webinar on the principles of visitability. Based on this organization, 57 local and state visitability laws were passed between 1991 and 2008. According to visitability standards, three minimum accessible housing features should be required:

1. At least one zero-step entrance approached by an accessible route on a firm surface no steeper than 1 in. rise for every 12 in. of length, from a driveway or public sidewalk.
2. Wide passage doors.
3. At least a half bath or powder room on the main floor.

Disability rights groups have advocated for visitability to be recognized as a legislative issue, which then influences policy and funding. The following example from a press release illustrates how the top rung of the Vicente's Human-Tech Ladder, legislation and policy, influence funding and thus TEI. Please review Box 8.2. Are there examples of press releases, news articles, or blogs like this in your state or local community?

Forgiving home design

Many people who experience impairment in cognition or judgment can live at home if the home is designed to support their abilities in a safe home setting. It may involve reducing access to areas in which a person may injure themselves or become frustrated with challenges, as well as using environmental modifications to minimize distraction, provide simpler choices, or guide safe behaviors. Forgiving designs for persons living with brain injuries, dementias, or developmental disabilities or mental health issues can make the difference between living with limited choices or in an unsafe home and living well at home. "There are three main characteristics of a forgiving home design: 1) the potential for accidents are recognized and minimized; 2) the potential for failure and upsets are recognized and minimized; 3) injury and trauma are minimized when accidents occur" (Warner 2000, p. 358).

Strategies that contribute to a forgiving home are "creating clear and open pathways, removing furniture that is easy to trip over, providing soft and stable furniture that can be relied on in a fall or will not cause bruises or cuts" (Warner 2000, p. 358). Using the environment itself to simplify decision-making is also beneficial, such as a night light to direct one's path to the bathroom or to disguise or add a barrier to stair access poised as a safety hazard. Figure 8.13 provides an example of a forgiving home strategy.

Warner (2000) noted the creation of zones within the home as another strategy for supportive and forgiving environments for persons experiencing

Box 8.1 Case study

As noted above, both accessible and adaptable design can be beneficial to enhance a client's ability to access and live in home environments. This case, which illustrates applying accessible, adaptable, and universal design strategies, is about an 84-year-old man who weighed 285 pounds and was 6 ft 1 in. tall. He had lived alone in his home settings, but his son, your client, reported that he needs increasing assistance with household management and self-care. His son related that his father, Bill, suffered from pneumonia and was subsequently hospitalized for months. As Bill recovered he was moved to a rehabilitation setting where he regained the ability to walk short distances of up to 10 ft alone with the use of a walker.

His family's plan was to move Bill to live with his daughter in her home, where he would receive home care. The healthcare professional in charge of home access and modifications reviewed Bill's medical history. This included pain in the hips and knees due to osteoarthritis and a history of two reported falls with minor injuries when he was living alone. The professional also noted there seemed to be a reduction in daily mobility due to deconditioning after his recent hospitalization. After discussion with Bill and his family about potential changes he might experience in his abilities and the challenges of living independently alone in the future, he and his daughter decided that Bill would move into her home and she would provide care as needed for Bill, even if his abilities declined again.

Bill's daughter's home was a small two-bedroom residence with narrow doorways throughout the house. Doors to the bathroom and Bill's bedroom required 90° turns off of a 34 in. hallway. The opening from the living room to the kitchen/dining room was 28 in. Bill reported that he would be discharged from the rehabilitation setting with a standard width walker and a wheelchair with a 20 in. seat width. There was room to add a 36-in.-wide door in the bathroom and a 32-in. door for his bedroom, but Bill would not be able to maneuver his wide wheelchair through the door from the living room and from the narrow hallway into either bedroom or bathroom. The bathroom was 5 ft wide with 31 in. between the toilet and the bathroom wall. What strategies would be used for Bill to live in his daughter's home?

Access to the home was achieved with use of a shallow wooden ramp with handrails, built over the existing steps. Four doors were modified to provide access to the bedroom and bathroom. A 3-ft doorway was created to the bedroom through the living room wall, and the existing bathroom and bedroom doors were widened to 36 in. and 32 in., respectively. Bill moved from the living room to his bedroom using the 3-ft door and from the bedroom directly to the bathroom. His daughter planned to remove the door and repair the living room wall when it was no longer needed (accessible design). The area between the living room and kitchen was widened from a doorway to a 5-ft-wide arch, thus making it possible for Bill to access the kitchen and dining room table and increasing his mobility around the table. This strategy opened the rooms for Bill and made the house seem larger to his daughter, the homeowner (universal design).

A Superpole fits between the toilet and the floor to increase the set height. Bill found it easier now to sit and rise from the toilet without the space between the toilet and wall being reduced, as would occur with use of a toilet with an elongated bowl. Additionally, this assistive device would not require special cleaning compared to a typical riser that sits on the top of the toilet bowl. Moreover, a Superpole with Superbar, as shown in Figure 8.10, provided a grab bar at the toilet and to assist Bill with transfers on the tub bench.

His daughter planned to remove the SuperPole at some point in the future but keep the grab bars for her own use (adaptive design). She eventually also opted to remove the tub and replaced it with a roll-in shower, but in the interim, Bill used the tub transfer bench as he already owned it and was familiar with its use. Within a year, his daughter added a rolling shower chair and hired a caregiver to assist Bill with bathing (adaptive design). Examples of home modification changes are illustrated in Figure 8.11 and Figure 8.12.

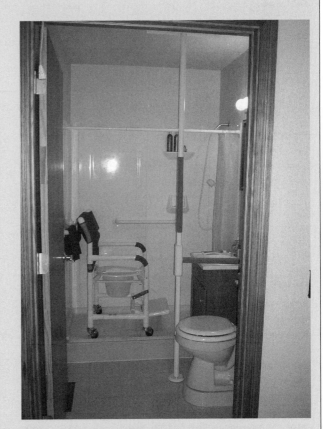

Figure 8.10 Superpole with Superbar. Source: Picture taken by author.

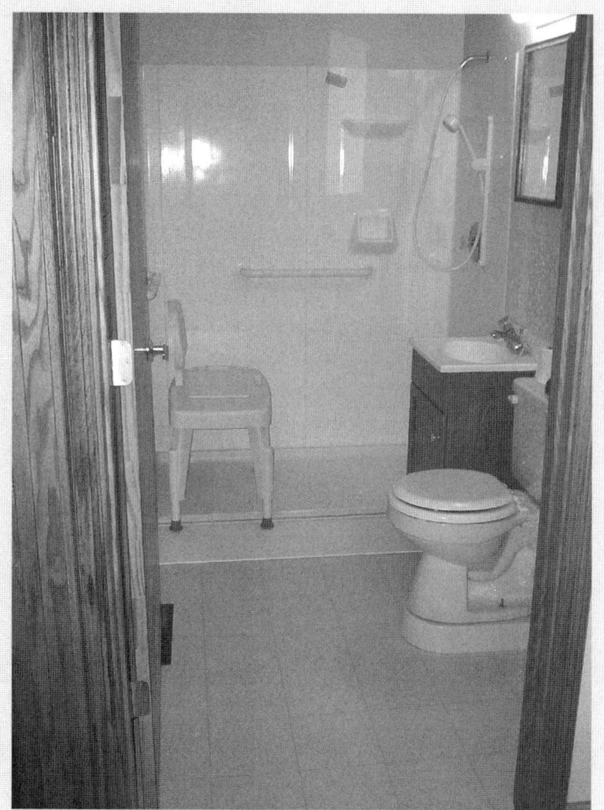

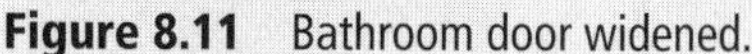

Figure 8.11 Bathroom door widened.

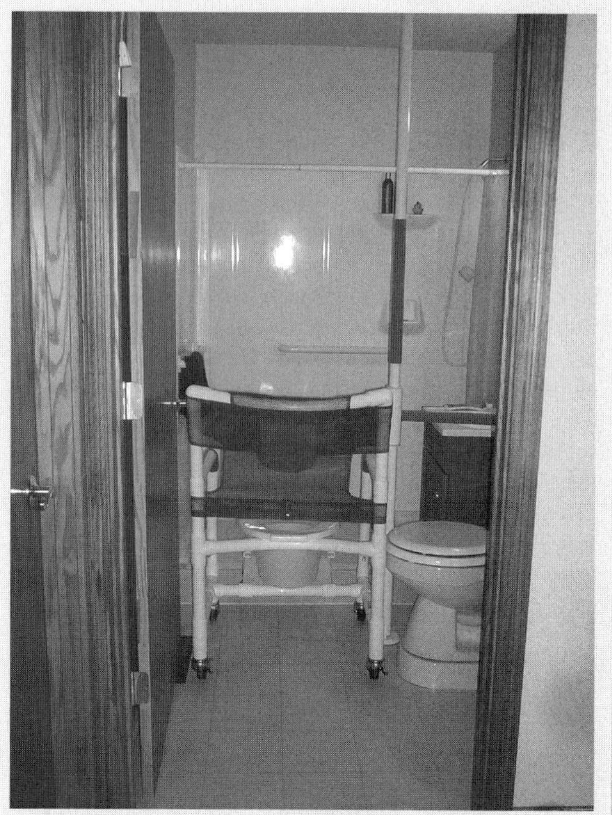

Figure 8.12 Wide rolling bath chair.

Box 8.2 Visitability press release

Disability Community Pushes Visitability Tax Credit through New York Legislature

June 25, 2015 – After years of advocacy from members of the Disability Community, the Senate and Assembly have both passed a visitability tax credit this year. The Center for Disability Rights applauds passage of the legislation (SB.2967A/AB.1276), which was introduced in by Senator DeFrancisco and Assembly Member Lavine, and which creates a tax credit of up to $2,750 for purchasing a home that is universally visitable or for modifying a home in order to make it universally visitable. Universal visitability modifications require, among other things, at least one wheelchair-accessible entrance at ground level, at least one accessible bathroom on the same floor as the entrance, and doors and doorways with a minimum 32″ clearance. For modifications of an existing residence, the tax credit will be 50% of the cost of modifications, to a maximum of $2,750. Members of New York State ADAPT and the Center for Disability Rights have traveled from Rochester to Albany many times in support of this bill, which was proposed by disability advocates at the New York Association on Independent Living. The bill passed due to the work of the Disability Community, particularly those members who put in hours of advocacy on the phone, driving back and forth to Albany, and meeting with legislators again and again over the years. "I'm excited about what this means for community integration," said Jensen Caraballo, a wheelchair user and member of New York State ADAPT who will benefit from this law. "The bill means that more homes will be places where people with disabilities are included, not excluded. It means visiting family and friends in their homes instead of them having to visit my home. Disabled people will be able to take for granted a lot of things that non-disabled people already take for granted." A lack of visitable housing in New York excludes people with disabilities from the social life of our communities. "Without universal visitability, people with disabilities are excluded from events like a summer barbecue, a holiday party at the boss's house, or a meet-the-candidate event for a local politician," said Adam Prizio, Manager of Government Affairs at the Center for Disability Rights. "This tax credit gives all New Yorkers – not just people with disabilities – a real financial incentive to make their homes visitable." The bill passed the Senate on June 18, 2015, and the Assembly last night. It will be sent to Governor Cuomo for signing. The bill was strongly supported by the Disability Community in New York, which has advocated for its passage for many years. (Center for Disability Rights 2015)

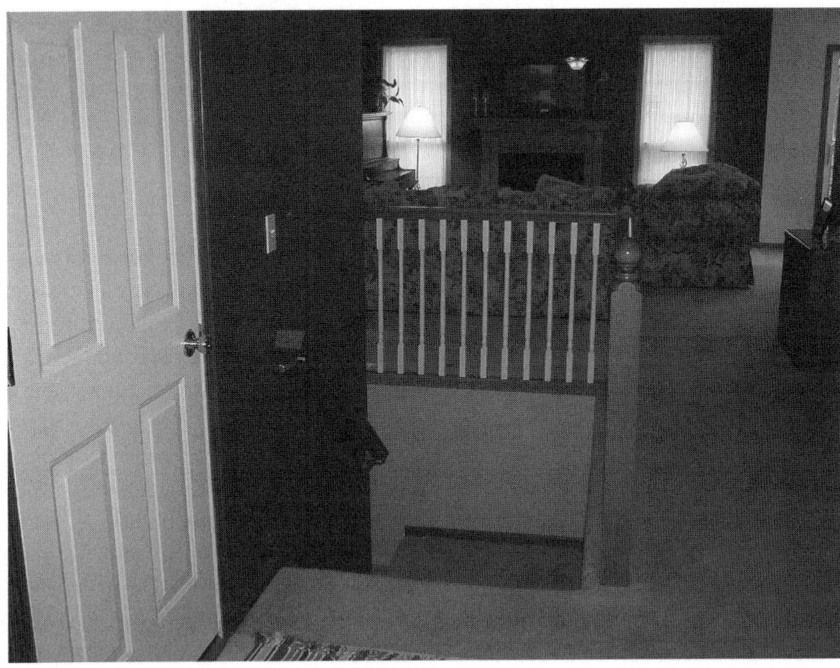

Figure 8.13 Gate at top of stairs.

dementia and their families. These zones consist of: (i) danger zones: areas that are unsafe, kept off limits, or used to store valuables or breakable or unsafe items – these can be created using locks, alarms, or wandering notification devices; (ii) respite zones: areas for caregiver sanctuary and uninterrupted rest; (iii) safe zones: as much of the home that is possible to make safe and available for independent movement and occupation (Warner 2000).

In sum, the various design concepts presented above – accessibility, universal design, adaptability, visitability, and forgiving home design – can be beneficial for home environment TEI.

The role of the client

The client is the key individual in the process in TEI, whether the person knows it or not, or is prepared for it or not. The client and family members are the ones who will remain in the home environment and use the space long after other members of the team are gone. They are typically the ones who are paying for home modifications and much of the technology and equipment. They are certainly the ones impacted by the intervention and its monetary value. Their goals, abilities, and challenges form the starting point for TEI goal setting, planning, implementation, and evaluation. Of all those on the TEI team, they are the ones whose lives are changed for better or worse by the TEI process and product.

The client or a designated family member should function as the team leader or director of the TEI team, not only due to their central role, but because they may be the only persons involved in the TEI process from start to finish. Consider a person whose home modification process begins in a hospital setting. The client is working with professionals who focus on the client's healthcare needs, and initiation of the home modification process is part of the client's discharge plan. Typically, these professionals are not the ones involved with the team technology and environmental home intervention and it is highly unlikely that they will be working with the client after the intervention or evaluating the success of the intervention. If there are technology and structural changes as part of the TEI, there is likely to be a variety of professionals as part of the TEI team (Ainsworth and DeJonge 2011).

The client may not be willing or able to assume a leadership role as team director for a variety of reasons. If one is physically or mentally unable to assume this role, generally a family member is invited, such as a family caregiver. Occasionally, a client or family member is uncomfortable or unable to assume the director decision-making role, or they are intimidated by the professionals on the team. If the client or family leader is not guided and supported in the TEI process as an educated decision-maker, even if they are reluctant to assume the role, the chances of a successful TEI and home modification process and product are diminished. It is unlikely that other team members will fully understand the client's preferences, goals, and perspective about their abilities, challenges, and what their home should look like on completion. A poor modification may seem to be successful for other members of the team, but it may make the client feel disabled, disfigured, disenfranchised, or different (Tanner 2011a).

Clients who are willing to participate as directors also need accurate information to make informed decisions. Often clients do not have the knowledge and skills to determine relevant technology, environmental modifications, cost, maintenance, funding sources, or how to work with technology specialists or building professionals. Since there is no one specific TEI home modification profession, many clients do not realize they will need to research options to make good TEI decisions. Clients and caregivers may struggle to gain some control in healthcare decisions and find that home modifications and the TEI process may be one area in which they can exert control.

The strategies to facilitate a successful home modification result in which the client has an important and educated role as director of the TEI process will vary, but consider the scenarios and suggestions noted in Box 8.3.

Reflect upon similar scenarios you may have had with a client. Consider how these suggestions might be incorporated into an intervention plan.

Finally, to end this chapter section, reflect on the scenarios presented and your own experiences with clients to thoughtfully address the reflective questions in Box 8.4 on the client role in TEI in the home environment.

Funding, codes, and guidelines

Funding must be addressed even before professionals engage in the TEI process and aspects of home modification, structure, environmental, and technology issues are addressed. Without a means to pay for home environmental modifications, it is not likely that a change will be made. Third-party funding sources have stipulations about what clients they serve, the manner in which their money can be utilized, and what may be considered for funding. Building codes and zoning regulations provide rules for what can be done to structurally alter a home and what portions can be modified. *Zoning* is defined as land use or type of dwelling or building allowed in a given area (US Department of Housing and Urban Development [HUD] 2008). It includes setbacks (distance a structure must be back from the edge of the lot), width of side yard, and the percentage of the lot that the dwelling can occupy (Proctor 2000). If zoning will not permit additions to a home, or placement of permanent accessible features in a yard, a client may need to engage in a civil process to obtain a variance in zoning or to modify their plan. As the author has discussed in the previous section on accessibility, building codes may define accessibility if the guideline has been incorporated into international building codes (International Code Council 2012) or local codes or ordinances, or if the dwelling is federally funded (HUD 2008).

Some professionals and clients do not understand the scope of the American with Disabilities Guidelines or Fair Housing Laws for residential dwellings (Ainsworth et al. 2011). There is a great deal of misunderstanding about responsibility for payment for home modifications under these legislative measures. Federal laws that prohibit discrimination against persons with disabilities prohibit a landlord from refusing to allow a person to make reasonable accommodations at the renter's own expense (Fair Housing Accessibility FIRST n.d.). The landlord can expect that modifications that substantially change their property will be restored at the renter's expense. Communication and collaboration with a landlord are fundamental prior to any design or planning. Modifications in some federally funded housing might be paid for at the housing provider's expense, if there is no administrative or financial hardship to the housing provider.

Clients need assistance to understand what potential funding sources are available and what will be provided by funding and why it will be provided. Clients who begin the TEI home modification process at a healthcare medical setting may assume home modifications and technology will be provided by the same system that provided medical care funding, especially if they perceive home modification needs to be due to a medical issue. Typically, this is not the case, as the medical care funding is not designed to provide assurance of living at home (Sanford 2012). Some AT is provided by medically based or vocationally based funding. Medicaid Community Waiver programs are designed to support persons at home instead of in an institutional setting (Eldercare Locator n.d.). Please refer to Box 8.5 for questions to consider for funding issues.

Funding that does provide for home modifications may have prohibitions regarding cost of items outside its scope or have parameters that must be adhered to as part of the TEI home modification plan. An example of this type of funding is the *Specially Adapted Housing Grant for US Veterans* (US Department of Veterans Affairs n.d.). Long-term care insurance and Worker's Compensation and other types of insurance or litigation settlements may provide home modification sources.

When exploring funding options, it is important to fully understand rules associated with funding (Tanner 2011b). Table 8.1 has examples of funding resources for home modification to explore.

Box 8.3 Scenarios and suggestions for home modification

Scenario	Suggestions
Scenario: clients defer to you or other professionals for decisions related to their home.	• Be clear that there is a wide range of options by giving two extremes, such as taking a door off its hinges or widening a door, which will incur framing, wall repairs, floor, and floor covering repair, electrical repairs, and the of cost of a new door. Help the clients understand they must be involved to express preferences and establish a realistic budget. Make sure the clients understand that they are the ones to make sure the TEI plan is carried out successfully. They do not have to know what to do, but should be able to articulate what they want to accomplish in order to lead the TEI process. They also need to understand how home modifications impact function. For example, a subcontractor may increase the size of a sink, instead of following the size specified by the other members of the TEI team. The primary contractor may have been told, but plan details may not have been communicated to subcontractors. If the clients are asked by the subcontractor if they would like a larger sink, they need to have the right information to make an informed and educated decision as to the impact of a larger sink. • Build on client responses based on their ability to take in and process new information, to collaborate on plan details. • Be willing to work as a temporary team leader in the TEI process as needed when the clients have related to you that they do not have the time or energy to lead. Be obvious that you expect them to delegate. Report to them with progress using the language you would use to report to a team leader
Clients are willing to direct the TEI home modification process, but you perceive their decisions as uneducated or irrational.	• Try to avoid the situation by being clear with your language. Do not ask clients for solutions; ask them for their goals or what they would like to do in their home space. Remember that clients may not understand the difference between stating a goal and identifying solutions for the goal. Discuss goals clearly before you discuss solutions with clients in order to hear their perspectives and preferences first before collaborating with them on options for solutions. There is less risk that they will think you are disagreeing with them or limiting their control. It may avoid a situation in which clients feel they need to defend a decision that may have been made without all the pertinent information. Be cautious about labeling decisions as irrational. It may only mean you do not understand or agree with your clients' vision or perspectives. Ask them to describe their plan step by step, record it, and, without judgment, ask about details or steps that may help you better understand their perspective or any errors in logic. Once you can articulate their perspective, you can consider whether additional information is needed by the clients or work to incorporate aspects of the clients' plan. • It may be easier for clients to understand options if they are given examples about other clients who had good or bad TEI experiences or results. Providing real-life examples, without identifying information to honor confidentiality, may enhance the clients' ability to understand aspects of technology and home modifications and how they impact function.
Clients have a different perspective on their ability to function or expectation for recovery than their health professionals or other TEI members, or their expectation regarding the extent of recovery or potential change in function is not known.	• Provide clear statements of recovery, based on evidence-based resources within your scope of practice that are relevant to the client's abilities to understand. • Provide suggestions for temporary modifications as well as more permanent solutions that match the client's ability to process and understand a realistic outcome based on current best evidence of their recovery. Work with solutions that can be modified to accommodate changes in the client's function, whether they progress or decline. For example, if a client plans to replace their tub with a walk-in shower, but there is a significant possibility of use of a rolling shower chair in the future, suggest a shower unit that is a roll-in shower, but have a faux threshold caulked in place. Review Figure 8.10 for an example of a roll-in shower unit.

Box 8.4 Active learning questions on the client role

Situation	Question
Think about a situation you may have experienced in which a client's goal or plan differed from those of the healthcare professionals.	• How do you think the client felt in knowing that there were differences? • How did the differences between the client and the professionals come to be resolved? • Could any of the strategies in the scenario-suggestion section of this chapter be helpful in this case? Which ones?
Reflect on a situation in which you were challenged with disagreement or resistance in communicating with a client.	• How did you feel? • How do you think the client felt? • Would you benefit from learning how different clients perceive their role and communicate it? • How would you modify your communication style in working with clients to honor their central role?

Box 8.5 Active learning questions on funding

Funding issue	Question
Review information you learned about funding sources in Chapter 4.	• Which of these funding sources might apply to technology and environmental modifications in the home? • What funding sources beyond those presented in Chapter 4 will be applicable?
Reflect on the TEI process and home modifications in a traditional hospital setting.	• How much assistance could a healthcare professional in a traditional hospital setting provide on funding information? • What if your client or their caregiver is not able to search for funding? What would you do?

Table 8.1 Funding Resources for Home Modification.

Resource	Contact information
Home modification and repair funds from Title III of the Older Americans Act	These funds are distributed by your local area agency on aging (AAA). To contact your local AAA, call the Eldercare Locator (1-800-677-1116) or visit the Eldercare Locator website at www.eldercare.gov.
Rebuilding Together, Inc. (Income-based)	http://rebuildingtogether.org
How can I pay for home modifications?	https://eldercare.acl.gov/Public/Resources/Factsheets/Home_Modifications.aspx
The National Directory of Home Modification and Repair Resources	http://gero.usc.edu/nrcshhm/directory
Home Access Program	http://www.homeaccessprogram.org/index.html
Handi-Ramp Foundation	https://www.handiramp.com/
How to pay for it?	http://www.infinitec.org/funding-tips-in-general
Mortgage and home loan help guide for the disabled	https://www.mortgageloan.com/disabilities

Moreover, in using funding sources, the team should not assume that the client will only request the options that the funding sources provide. For example, a basic floor-based lift with a hydraulic mechanism may be the system provided by a medical third-party payer, such as Medicare or private medical insurance. However, the client may opt for a ceiling-based lift that requires less floor space or one that the client can operate independently. The space saving convenience and independent use are not fundable justifications for many medical payment systems, but it may be important enough to the client to pay privately for features that match their goals and preferences (DeJonge et al. 2011; Tanner 2011a).

TEI home modifications are often self-funded, for many persons simply like to do it, as with other home remodeling projects. One way of viewing this is to compare the remodeling needed to update a bathroom to make it useable for growing children, to the remodeling to modify a bathroom for a person using a new wheelchair. Both projects are aimed to benefit the homeowner and make a space more functional and pleasing. Moreover, the potential for an accessible home to reduce the likelihood of injury, reduce caregiving costs, and improve quality of life are important for the self-funder, but not a primary concern for medically based, educationally based, or vocationally based funding sources (DeJonge et al. 2011).

It is important to discuss with the self-funder client the consequences of home modifications and indirect or long-term costs. For example, a straight short wooden ramp with a rise of less than 18 ft will initially cost less than a vertical platform lift but will generally require more physical effort to navigate. If a client has a progressive disease or is at an age at which physical strength for themselves or caregivers is expected to decrease, the initial investment in the lift will cost less than beginning with a ramp and adding a lift later, and will avoid having to curtail activities due to the physical effort of using the ramp.

Moreover, any intervention or piece of AT equipment that does not function in the manner that the client needs or is not long-lasting is useless for the client regardless of how inexpensive it may be. For example, the purchase of a bath bench at a yard sale or pharmacy instead of a tub transfer bench is not useful if the client cannot safely step over the side of the tub. Finally, a consequence of TEI home and environmental modifications may be the long-term consideration of whether the modification enhances or detracts from the monetary value of the home. Taxes are paid on residential assessments based on square footage, features, and condition (Internal Revenue Service 2014). When potential buyers apply for a mortgage, sale price is not only based on comparison of similar homes, but on the desirability of the home to the buyers themselves.

Qualifications and perspectives of home modification professionals

The qualifications, perspectives, and communication among the various professionals involved in the TEI process impact the result for the client. The opportunity for the participants to develop unity of focus and a true team approach is limited, as noted in Chapter 9 on teams. Unless one home modification professional works with a client from the beginning to the end of the home environmental modification process, the opportunity for miscommunication, error, and a less than desirable result is high. The various professions and trades involved have different skill sets and perceptions and work with different funding sources, so they may be focused on different aspects of the project. They may be involved in one stage of the TEI process and not be in communication with, or even be aware of, professionals involved in other stages of the intervention. Once again, this is a good reason to have an educated client as the team director, especially in settings where the home modification process commences when a person is under medical care. It is also a reason to seek out and work with professionals who are willing to listen to the client and work as part of an informal or formal intervention team.

It is important to understand the role and scope of each professional and the role of each in the different phases of the home modification process. If a medical professional encounters an issue outside their scope of practice, they need to refer to and rely on other professionals with relevant expertise. If not self-employed, professionals need to be cognizant of your facility or organization's rules about referrals and recommendations. Some prohibit referrals outside of the organization; others have lists of approved vendors and referral sources. Communicate with your client about referrals, as the client may perceive you have a business relationship with them. Keep in mind that professionals who are not in healthcare may not be familiar with the Health and Insurance Portability and Accountability Act (HIPAA), although they may have their own professional standards related to client confidentiality (US Department of Health and Human Services 2013). It is important to communicate as a team regarding how client information will be shared and with whom.

Professionals in the building industry, such as architects and interior designers, require specific education and training with requisite national and state regulation, certification, and licensing. Others, such as general contractors, may not require specific educational standards and their licensure requirements can vary from state to state (HUD 2008). It is prudent to contact the licensing agency in your city or state to determine which types of building professionals must be licensed in your area. Where a license is required or not, a builder or contractor must have knowledge of applicable building codes and building structures and systems; they must also have liability insurance and the ability to organize and manage projects (National Association of Home Builders n.d.-a). Because a contractor will typically be responsible for code compliance and errors in construction, they tend to be more comfortable with previously used and familiar structural techniques and structural products. Please refer to Box 8.6 for questions related to working with a home modification professional.

Many clients do not realize the breadth of knowledge needed for building and design and may assume that any contractor can produce safe and effective structural work. Clients may engage family members or unlicensed, unqualified persons to build unsafe or structurally unsound products to save money. It is important to communicate with clients that replacing a structure, limiting access due to an unsafe structure, or removing a structure due to a building code violation is an unnecessary cost.

Box 8.6 Active learning questions and home modification professionals

Home modification issue	Questions
Policies and referral	• Why would an organization or facility have a policy regarding making referrals to other medical or building professionals? • How would you go about finding out what the policy is?
Educational and licensing	• Create a chart listing the educational and licensure requirements of the following professionals in your area, as well as strategies for locating/evaluating skills for that professional. o Architect o Contractor o Building trade specialist such as an electrician or plumber o Interior designer o Technology supplier and/or durable medical equipment (DME) / home medical equipment (HME) provider o Funding professional o Medical professional • How might each of the professionals be reimbursed? • What role or responsibility would each professional assume on a TEI home modification intervention?

There are several ways to locate professionals for building and technology needs. For example, clients can request recommendations from others who have home modifications.

With personal referrals, you can request information about how well the professional worked with the client on goals, communication style, and areas of expertise and skill set.

Additionally, consumer protection agencies such as the Better Business Bureau can help the client determine general information about the professional, their organization, length of business practice, and complaint history (Better Business Bureau n.d.). Investigation of professional designations related to disability or aging or specific practice areas can be very helpful. For example, the National Association of Home Builders collaborated with Home Innovation Research Labs, National Association of Home Builders 50+ Housing Council, and the American Association for Retired People to develop the Certified Aging in Place Specialist (CAPS) certification (National Association of Home Builders n.d.-b).

The National Directory of Home Modifications and Repair Resources has pertinent national or local directories of professionals, agencies, and organizations with expertise in home modifications (National Directory of Home Modifications and Repair Resources n.d.). There may be local associations, councils, and networking groups for various professionals with expertise in home modifications. Some are chapters of national associations, such as the National Aging in Place Council (NAIPC), others are unique to the area. Area agencies on aging, state assistive technology programs, or a local center for independent living may be able to provide information about home modification resources.

Home medical equipment or durable medical equipment suppliers and technology specialists are involved in the TEI home modification process when provision and evaluation of equipment, assistive technology, and education are needed for its use (Homemods.org 2019). The Rehabilitation Engineering and Assistive Technology Association of North America (RESNA) offers certification in two areas that provide pertinent expertise and skills for the TEI home modification process (RESNA 2014). For example, if one looks at the exam outline for one of the RESNA certifications, the assistive technology professional (ATP), the outline delineates that the test contains content on assessing and providing intervention in environmental intervention (RESNA 2014). Another example of a specialty certification in home modification is one available for occupational therapy practitioners

(American Occupational Therapy Association n.d.). A final one that I mention in this chapter is the Certified Environmental Access Consultant (CEAC). Accessible Home Improvements of America offers this certification (Accessible Construction Inc. n.d.).

The method of funding and professional payment for home environmental modification will often influence what services a professional provides and their level of involvement in different stages of the TEI home modification (The Council for Disability Rights n.d.). Clients need an awareness of how various professionals are paid for services, for example, medical professionals may be paid whether a home modification is implemented or not, other professionals are paid on commission, while some are paid only if the product or service is delivered (Sanford 2012; Tanner 2011a). Refer to Chapter 4 on funding for a review of funding and payment. The client may pay for services of a professional for consultation but have access to many money-saving options, since the professional receives payment regardless of the cost of options. Services may be paid for by a third party, such as insurance, which then defines the scope of the service.

The stage of the TEI process a professional engages in impacts communication and eventual outcome. For example, a healthcare professional working with a client may or may not be able to complete an on-site visit. Without this visit, a lack of general information about client factors, AT, and environmental modifications may mean that other professionals are left to make a great deal of assumptions and interpretation. When on-site visits are part of a client's healthcare services, discharge is typically timed to allow the client maximum rehabilitation time but may not provide adequate time for other professionals to design, plan, and implement home modification changes if significant structure changes are needed.

Structural aspects and technology factors

The existing home structure has a great impact on the best options for home modification. A colleague who has been a home remodeler for over 20 years related to this author that anything can be made accessible if the homeowner and clients do not care about the cost or what the product looks like. However, most homeowners and clients do care, so the underlying structure and style of the house affects what is economically, functionally, and aesthetically a good match for TEI home and environmental modifications. Unless you are the TEI team member professional responsible for code compliance and implementation of structural interventions, it is not essential to understand every detail, but everyone should have a basic understanding of the structure and style implications to support effective communication among the team. For example, the amount and size of plumbing waste pipe sloped for good drainage is not need-to-know information for the team, but everyone should be aware that the waste pipes need to be sloped so all are running toward the soil stack in the home. General knowledge of plumbing systems will enable an understanding of why a professional would suggest that moving a wall of plumbing or a toilet perpendicular to underlying joists would be more expensive than a plan to modify fixtures while working off the same wall or within the same joist cavity.

This section will present introductory concepts regarding typical residential home structures for the professionals on a TEI home modification team to make relevant suggestions to clients and building professionals that best fit client abilities, preferences, and needs. If further information and study is desired, resources about structural design and modification are provided at the end of this chapter. Please refer to Box 8.7 for questions related to structure and technology.

In addition to housing structure, building codes in force at the time of construction will impact design, planning, and implementation of structural changes. Typically, if an area of the home is no longer code

Box 8.7 Active learning related to structure and technology

Structure and technology issue	Questions
Identification of home structures	• Locate a residence near where you live with an unfinished basement and attic. • Search and identify supply and waste plumbing, heating and air ductwork, and joists.
Home structure cost	• In what situations might a client want to spend more money initially on a project with modifications that involve moving walls, plumbing, or heating, ventilation, and air conditioning (HVAC)? • When might a person want to use equipment solutions over structural changes? • In contrast, when might a person want to use structural changes over equipment solutions?

compliant, it will need to be brought up to current codes during the remodeling process, depending on the amount of work planned and rules requiring permits in that location (American National Standards Institute 2012; International Code Council 2012). The consequences of codes may be that the code compliant process becomes larger than the home modification process itself. For example, homes built prior to a mechanical ventilation bathroom requirement may use an operable window as ventilation. However, current International Residential Code (International Code Council 2012) requires that, at a minimum, a bathroom fan pulling 50 cubic feet per minute (cfm) with exhaust to out of doors be installed when any structural work is done in the bathroom (International Code Council 2012). Once again, reliance on a competent building professional is essential to identify these issues and bring this information to the team.

Structure: Plumbing systems

It is important for professionals on the TEI home modifications team to understand basic elements of plumbing that impact modifications of areas of the home with a water supply or waste disposal. There are two basic subsystems in residential plumbing systems: water supply and drain/waste/vent systems (DWV). Figure 8.14 illustrates an example of a DWV behind the walls and between the floors.

The water supply system must have adequate pressure to deliver water flow at the desired temperature to each of the water fixtures in the house even when more than one fixture is used (International Code Council 2012). The DWV system is responsible for moving waste water and solids within the water out of the house into a septic or municipal waste system and relies on gravity and atmospheric pressure to perform (International Code Council 2018; Wormer 1998). This is the reason that pipe diameters and maximum or minimum pipe slopes are so important, with this information extensively conveyed in building codes (Ripka 2011). Traps are covered sections of pipes with standing water located at the fixtures to block sewer gases from entering the home. They perform with vent lines to link back up with the soil stack for venting through the roof. Venting provides discharge for sewer gases and equalized atmospheric pressure with the DWV system to allow liquids and solids to flow down the pipes (International Association of Plumbing and Mechanical Officials 2015; Wormer 1998).

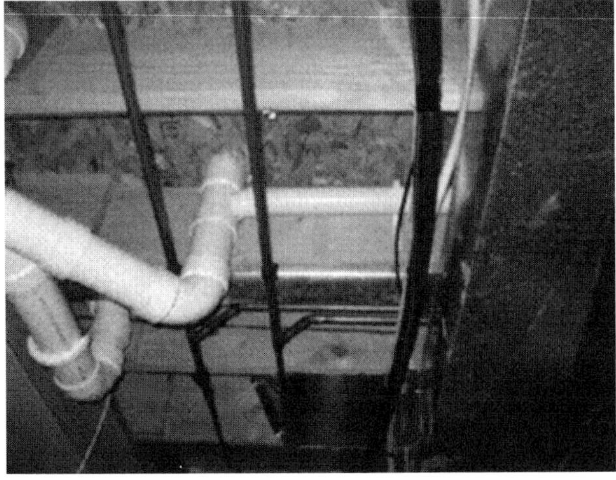

Figure 8.14 Water supply drain/waste/vent (DWV) system.

Structure: Electrical systems

There are three issues related to electricity that impact electrical selections in the home modification process: capacity, moving switches, and code requirements for location and clearance (National Fire Protection Association 2013). Improperly controlled electricity can be dangerous and thus, professional electricians and the electrical industry is highly regulated (Thiele 2019). New electrical work and existing electrical systems impacted by home modifications require permits and inspection for safety. Moreover, electrical supply for the average residence has increased over the years from systems with plug fuses to 240-volt systems with circuit breakers (Rockis et al. 2010). The fuse system continues to be safe, and found in many homes, but is inadequate for most current households with a multitude of electrical devices. Even a 100 A 240-volt system may not be adequate for additional circuitry (Thiele 2019). At any rate, expanding capacity is the expertise of a licensed electrician and can be costly (Mullin and Simmons 2015). Newer electrical fixtures often require a dedicated circuit, so TEI home modification professionals need to read the specifications of suggested products carefully. For example, a professional on the team may want to recommend a light and heat to provide additional quick location heating for a client who chills easily, but this suggestion requires a dedicated circuit (Brown et al. 2005).

Common home modification recommendations call for moving switches or adding outlets for assistive equipment such as power-operated beds, chargers for wheelchairs, powering lights and small appliances, and fixtures for environmental control units. The addition of outlets to provide this needed electrical power is safer than overloading a circuit with extension cords, especially in an older home. Additionally, moving a switch to provide room for a widened door or to position a switch to within a client's reach can be a simple or complicated process (Mullin and Simmons 2015). The scope of these tasks depends on the direction of wiring to and from the device, any hidden structures between the current and desired location, and whether adequate slack or extra wiring is available. Any challenges related to these three issues may require extra time and cost due to electrician time and cost and additional building inspection time and cost (Brown et al. 2005). There are numerous residential codes that regulate switch and outlet placement (International Code Council 2018; National Fire Protection Association 2013). Caution is important when placing switches and outlets in wet areas, such as bathrooms, and a ground-fault circuit interrupter (GFCI) must be used to protect outlets in these areas.

Finally, professionals on the TEI home environment modification team need to consider outside the house as part of the living space. When designing and planning for decks, landings, and ramps, the location of the electrical service to the house must be identified for safety purposes (Rockis et al. 2010). Electrical wiring may be above ground running from a pole into and out of the house. There must be at least 10 ft of space between a walking surface and the lowest point of the wiring for electrical service (International Code Council 2018). This distance reduces the likelihood that a person standing on the surface will accidentally contact the wire with a ladder or other tool.

Structure: Heating, ventilation, and air conditioning systems

Home modification teams need to have a basic understanding of heating and cooling systems to relate to the specialized professionals that address this complex system. The issues that impact modifications typically relate to adding capacity when additions to the home are recommended and an awareness of the ductwork that may need to be moved with significant structural changes (Plumbing-Heating-Cooling Contractors National Association 2005). If the heating and cooling system is forced air, ductwork will distribute this air.

Figure 8.15 is an example of heating and air conditioning ductwork. The large rectangular ducts in the figure are for main line runs; the smaller circular ducts are individual feeds to specific registers. Typically, there are also cold air returns to return air to the furnace. The size of the system and the number and location of registers and cold air returns all impact the system efficiency. These systems are regulated by building codes (International Code Council 2018).

When suggesting home modification recommendations, professional team members will want to know the location of registers and returns and the pathway of the ductwork. Be aware that the need to move registers or ductwork due to movement of plumbing or structures such as doors, walls, or fixtures may require additional cost and time (International Association of Plumbing and Mechanical Officials 2015).

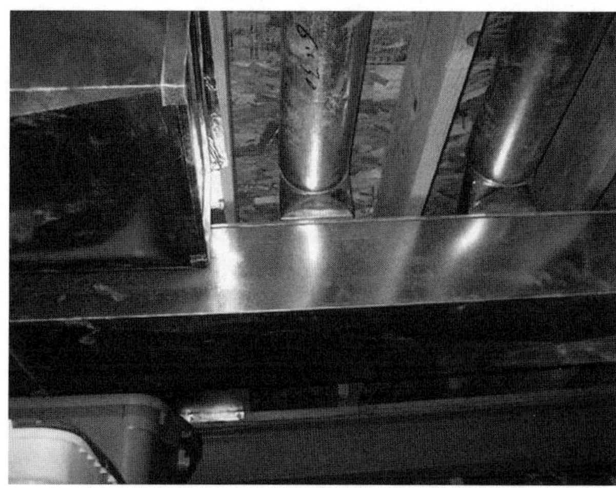

Figure 8.15 Heating and air conditioning ductwork.

Structure: Floor joists, wall framing, and roof systems

A relevant visual for those new to home and environmental modifications is to think of floor joists, wall framing, and roof systems as like the skeletal system of the body. It is easy to imagine how all other systems of the house are hung from, supported by, and attached to them. While it is necessary to rely on the building professionals on your TEI team to identify and develop strategies and techniques for the structure of the home, as noted throughout this chapter, other team members, such as the client, home designer, and AT specialists need a general understanding of these systems to make informed decisions. Lack of awareness and communication can create costlier and time-consuming as well as ineffective modifications.

Joists

Joists are horizontal framing pieces typically spaced 16 in. or 24 in. apart as measured from the center of one joist to the next, or "on center" (OC). They function to take the load of the floor or the roof (Feirer et al. 1997). The type and direction of floor joists impact home modification if you need to move plumbing or HVAC ductwork (Ripka 2011). An example of a structured I-beam joist is presented in Figure 8.16.

Structured I-beam or I-joists are engineered for efficient use of wood and produce joists that are lighter

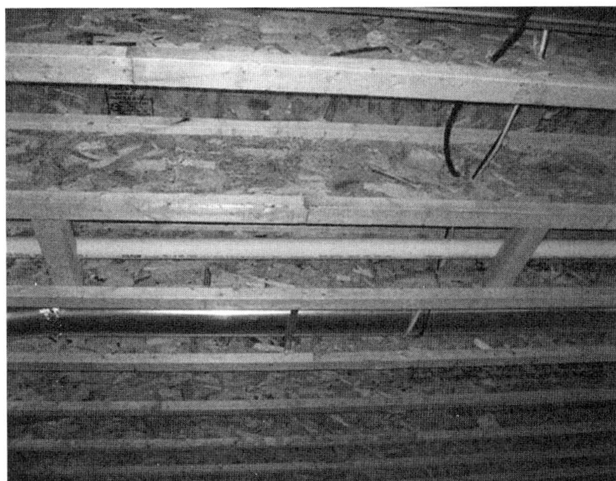

Figure 8.16 Structured I-beam joist.

but have a higher load-bearing capacity than solid lumber sawn joists. The top and bottom part of the I-joists are called chords, which are united by a center piece called the web, which should never be cut (Feirer et al. 1997). The type of joist in a home will impact what types of AT, such as ceiling-based lifts, can be suspended from the joists or how a contractor would recess a shower pan into an existing floor. The services of structural professionals such as architects and structural engineers may be needed to determine what modifications to joists can be made without jeopardizing the structural integrity of the home.

Studs

Studs are vertical pieces used in framing within walls. Understanding the purpose of studs in the home and the various methods for attaching grab bars enables the TEI home modification team members to work collaboratively with contractors in placement of grab bars and other AT equipment. Commonly, studs are 16 in. or 24 in. OC, though this may be adjusted to accommodate doors, windows, and other walls (Koel 2013). Studs will usually be 2×4 in. or 2×6 in. and serve to bear the weight of the roof structures down to the floor joists (Feirer et al. 1997). The size, height, and spacing of studs are regulated by building codes (International Code Council 2018). Studs tend to be oriented so the narrow side faces the interior or exterior of the room and not wide enough to have all three holes in a three-hole assistive device commercial-type grab bar over the stud (Miller and Miller 2009). A health professional and an AT specialist will tend to focus on grab bar placement best suited for client balance and mobility. However, a contractor or structural specialist will aim for how well the bar can be attached to the structure of the house. It is important to communicate the focus of each professional's expertise to achieve the best fit for the client.

Roof systems

There is a variety of technology employed for roof structures, dimensions, and spans or lengths of horizontal sections. All three of these features are dependent on the type of construction, attributes, and dimensions of material used and all are regulated by building codes (IRC 2009). The type of roof structure will impact a home modification when the team is planning to remove or move walls as well as hang assistive equipment from a ceiling, such as a ceiling-based lift. With ceiling joists, an interior wall can assist in support of the load of the ceiling and the roof along with exterior walls (Huth 2012). When the roof trusses span the entire width of the house, only the exterior walls can carry the roof and ceiling loads. It is important for TEI home modification team members to be aware that load-bearing walls can be modified, but the building professional needs to have the knowledge and skills to employ techniques that do not compromise the roof and ceiling stability. Often, replacing or redirecting support will make modification of the load-bearing wall cost more than modification of the non-load-bearing or partition wall (Miller and Miller 2009).

In sum, structural changes may have more impact, either positive or negative, on the monetary value of a client's home than AT equipment, which typically can be removed. While health professionals and AT specialists' input can enhance the design of the space and support a client's ability to use the environment in a myriad of ways, an understanding and appreciation of structural features will enhance collaboration with the client and other team members to problem-solve and provide solutions that can be realistically accomplished within a budget and aligned with client abilities and preferences (Ainsworth and DeJonge 2011).

The human-tech ladder and technology relevant to TEI in the home

Technology and client factors as well as organizational and political factors are essential to consider when designing, planning, implementing, and evaluating home environmental modifications (Vicente 2006). With the trend toward increasing efficiency and ease of living at home, technology and client factors, such as need for convenience and universal design, are becoming more strongly aligned. For example, consider touch-free faucets as an innovation in home design. A client who has difficulty operating knobs or levers can use this faucet independently to turn water on or off. Moreover, the faucet is also convenient and features universal design for any person to turn the water on or off if one's hands are full or dirty. The professionals on a TEI home modification team need to be aware of and utilize innovative household technologies as well as assistive technologies for use in the home to provide a range of client factors, such as physical and psychological, as well as options in terms of solutions (Vicente 2006).

Clients need opportunities to engage with technology and learn why professionals on the TEI team recommend different options, what the technological properties of options are, and what impact the options have on how clients engage with their home environment (Ainsworth and DeJonge 2011; Center for Assistive Technology Act Data Assistance 2018).

Additionally, clients' comfort levels and experiences with using technology influence how readily technology will be accepted and used in the home. They may need assistance in fully understanding how to evaluate technology, such as identification of skills required to use a device, or how the assistive equipment will need to be maintained, or how long the technology will last, and what impact technology will have on the aesthetics and value of their home. Assessments that may be applicable for home modification are addressed in Table 8.2.

Healthcare and AT professionals may need to provide information on and analysis of how the technology interplays with clients' abilities, such as strength, balance, vision, and cognition, in performing an important activity of daily living. Clients may not be familiar with newly acquired AT such as a scooter or be able to anticipate the potential for barriers in their home. Through education and communication as part of the AT process, clients may feel more confident to evaluate technology options themselves and make informed technology decisions (Ainsworth and DeJonge 2011).

An entry-level health professional without experience in AT on a regular basis may provide service delivery for technology such as built-up handles on tools and utensils or bathroom equipment such as bedside commodes or benches as part of their daily practice experiences with clients. Additional expertise and training to educate clients on more complex technology and services is often required (RESNA 2014). For example, a recommendation for lever door handles and a magnetized door stop is an AT service that may require less expertise and training for the health professional or team member than the service process of evaluation and specifications of recommendation for a wheelchair control system.

In many chapters of this text, options for AT ranging from low tech to high tech are presented. Many of these options can be utilized in a variety of settings, such as the home. Whether the technology is focused on enhancement of mobility, seating, communication, hearing, vision, transportation, or leisure activities, the TEI team will want to consider together if and how the structure and properties of the home support their use by the client in desired and meaningful ways. The home is one of the most valued settings for clients to enjoy life and engage in valued activities (Tanner 2011b).

Table 8.2 Assessment Tools for Home Modifications.

Assessment tool	Elements included in assessment
Home safety self-assessment tool (HSSAT) http://sphhp.buffalo.edu/rehabilitation-science/research-and-facilities/funded-research/aging/home-safety-self-assessment-tool.html	An assessment consisting of sections on self-assessment of home safety, home modification providers along with local service providers
The AARP HomeFit Guide http://www.aarp.org/livable-communities/info-2014/aarp-home-fit-guide-aging-in-place.html	An assessment and educational features which can be helpful for making a home accessible
Cornell Gerontological Environmental Modification (GEM) http://0104.nccdn.net/1_5/3d5/1bd/166/VNAABP_Gerontological-Environment-Modifications--Environmental-Assessment.pdf	A tool to identify problems and solutions for home environments
Comprehensive Home Evaluation Report https://www.youtube.com/watch?v=cY1tvACR7PI	The CHER® (Comprehensive Home Evaluation Report) is an innovative web- based tool that provides a unique way to produce a home modification evaluation or assessment report.
Comprehensive assessment and solution process for aging residents https://www.ehls.com/wp-content/uploads/2015/07/CASPAROverview.pdf	A free assessment tool for home modification.

As noted by Vicente (2006), technology is continually evolving. Home technology is no different. Consider the improved safety of newer irons on the market that can turn off after a period of disuse. These devices present a significant safety feature that likely prevents burns and household fires. On the other hand, the complexity of some home technology items may create a hindrance to use, or as Vicente (2006) noted, "technology running amok" (p. 27).

The author of this chapter met a woman who changed stoves three times after moving into a new home from one she had lived in for many years. This woman found digital controls complex and, frankly, irritating, so she reduced her cooking activities to those accomplished through use of a toaster oven and microwave. She finally found a used stove with what she called "old-fashioned" controls. This is an example of what Vicente (2006) would call not paying attention to psychological factors impacting technology: instead of trying to change this woman's human nature responses, the technology can be modified to take advantage of natural tendencies of home nature.

With numerous options for technology, it is now possible to use the Internet to research with the client and the TEI home environment modification team hundreds of technology products for the home. With the access to these products comes the need to be educated and informed consumers of technology. Keeping up to date on technology and equipment, what potentially will work in the home setting, what knowledge and skills are required for use, as well as cost, maintenance, and longevity, can be an overwhelming task. Box 8.8 is an example of a worksheet to guide the TEI team in technology decisions.

Box 8.8 Technology worksheet

Assistive technology information for product and design recommendations
Activities of daily living (ADL) category
Product name
What product does/how it works
Is it for independent/dependent use or both?
Abilities required to use it
Abilities it can compensate for
Maintenance required and durability
General cost and potential funding sources
Where can it be obtained?
Other notes

Summary

One's home influences the ability to live safely and fulfill desired and needed roles and activities. Vicente's model of the Human-Tech Ladder (Vicente 2006) lends itself well to understanding the complexity of the process of applying TEI in the home environment. Human factors, such as physical, psychological, organizational, and political, interact and impact successful home modifications (Vicente 2006). Technology choices and environmental intervention provide an opportunity for a best fit for a client in their home, if the TEI team process is collaborative, knowledgeable, skillful, and systematic in design, planning, decision-making, implementation, and evaluation of home modifications. The client is the key team director, regardless of complexity of funding, design, structures, team professionals, and final product. Please refer to Box 8.9 and consider questions related to AT issues.

Professionals assisting clients with TEI in their homes need to learn to identify roles and collaborate with other professionals and be open to learning more about how design concepts, funding, codes, laws, structure, and technology interplay in successful home modifications.

Box 8.9 Active learning questions related to AT

AT issue	Questions
Experience with assistive technology	• Complete the Technology Worksheet in Box 8.8 in relation to a familiar example of AT you have used with clients. In contrast, complete the worksheet with a form of AT with which you are unfamiliar. Is your thinking process different for each example? How so? • Where could you get additional information to accurately match an example of unfamiliar technology for a client?
Client potential for AT	• Compare two homes in terms of fixtures such as refrigerators or washers displaying different features. Using the Technology Worksheet in Box 8.8, describe examples of compensations related to these technology features that you could suggest for a client's physical, mental, or sociocultural limitations or barriers.

References

Accessible Construction Inc. (n.d.). Certified Environmental Access Consultant (CEAC) Accessible Design & Consulting Inc.. Retrieved from https://www.accessibleconstruction.com/ceac/.

Ainsworth, E. and DeJonge, D. (2011). The home modification process. In: *An Occupational Therapist Guide to Home Modification Practice* (ed. E. Ainsworth and D. DeJonge), 87–111. Thorofare, NJ: Slack.

Ainsworth, E., DeJonge, D., and Sanford, J. (2011). Legislation, regulations, codes, and standards influencing home modification practice. In: *An Occupational Therapist Guide to Home Modification Practice* (ed. E. Ainsworth and D. DeJonge), 49–65. Thorofare, NJ: Slack.

American National Standards Institute (2012). Homepage. Retrieved from http://www.ansi.org/default.aspx.

American Occupational Therapy Association (n.d.). Specialty certification in environmental modification. Retrieved from http://www.aota.org/Education-Careers/Advance-Career/Board-Specialty-Certifications/EnvironmentalModification.aspx.

Americans with Disabilities Act of 1990 (1990). Pub. L. 101-336, 42 U.S.C. § 12101.

Better Business Bureau (n.d.). Homepage. Retrieved from www.bbb.org.

Brown, M., Rawtani, J., and Patil, D. (2005). *Troubleshooting of Electrical Equipment and Control Circuits*. Philadelphia, PA: Elsevier.

Center for Assistive Technology Act Data Assistance (2018). AT Act data brief series. Issue 10. Retrieved from https://catada.info/assets/files/AT_Report_FY17_FinalAccessible.pdf.

Center for Disability Rights (2015). Disability community pushes visitability tax credit through New York legislature. Retrieved from http://cdrnys.org/blog/press-releases/disability-community-pushes-visitability-tax-credit-through-new-york-legislature/.

Center for Universal Design (2006). Definitions: accessible, adaptable, and universal design. Fact sheet 6. Retrieved from http://www.ncsu.edu/ncsu/design/cud/pubs_p/docs/Fact%20Sheet%206.pdf.

Center for Universal Design (2008). About UD. Retrieved from https://projects.ncsu.edu/design/cud/about_ud/about_ud.htm.

DeJonge, D. and Cordiner, R. (2011). Evaluating clients' home modification needs and priorities. In: *An Occupational Therapists Guide to Home Modification Practice* (ed. E. Ainsworth and D. DeJonge), 113–138. Thorofare, NJ: Slack.

DeJonge, D., Jones, A., Phillips, R., and Pynoos, J. (2011). Approaches to service delivery. In: *An Occupational therapist's Guide to Home Modification Practice* (ed. E. Ainsworth and D. DeJonge), 17–31. Thorofare, NJ: Slack.

Eldercare Locator (n.d.). Home improvement assistance. Retrieved from https://eldercare.acl.gov/Public/Resources/Factsheets/Home_Modifications.aspx.

Fair Housing Accessibility FIRST (n.d.). Fair Housing Accessibility FIRST: requirements. Retrieved from http://www.fairhousingfirst.org/fairhousing/requirements.html.

Feirer, J.L., Hutchings, G.R., and Feirer, M. (1997). *Carpentry and Building Construction*. New York: McGraw-Hill.

Guzman, S., Viveiros, J. and Salomon, E. (2017). Insight on the issues: expanding implementation of universal design and visitability features in the housing stock. Retrieved from https://www.aarp.org/content/dam/aarp/ppi/2017/06/expanding-implementation-of-universal-design-and-visitability-features-in-the-housing-stock.pdf.

Homemods.org (2019). National directory. Retrieved from http://www.homemods.org/FAQ/index.shtml.

Huth, M.W. (2012). *Residential Construction Academy: Basic Principles for Construction*, 3e. Clifton Park, NY: Delmar Cengage Learning.

Internal Revenue Service (2014). Publication 530 Tax information for homeowners. Retrieved from http://www.irs.gov/publications/p530/ar02.html.

International Association of Plumbing and Mechanical Officials (2015). *2015 Uniform Plumbing Code*. Ontario, CA: Author.

International Code Council (2012). 2012 International residential code for one and two family dwellings. Retrieved from https://basc.pnnl.gov/resources/2012-irc-international-residential-code-one-and-two-family-dwellings.

International Code Council (2018). International plumbing code. Retrieved from https://codes.iccsafe.org/content/document/751?site_type=public.

Koel, L. (2013). *Carpentry*, 6e. Orland Park, IL: American Technical Publishers.

Miller, M. and Miller, R. (2009). *Carpentry & Construction*, 5e. New York, NY: McGraw-Hill.

Mullin, R.C. and Simmons, P. (2015). *Electrical Wiring Residential*, 18e. Stamford, CT: Cengage Learning.

National Association of Home Builders (n.d.-a). Homepage. Retrieved from www.nahb.org.

National Association of Home Builders (n.d.-b). Certified Aging-in-Place Specialists (CAPS) Retrieved from http://www.nahb.org/en/learn/designations/certified-aging-in-place-specialist.aspx.

National Directory of Home Modifications and Repair Resources (n.d.). Homepage. Retrieved from http://www.homemods.org/directory.

National Fire Protection Association (2013). *National Electrical Code*. Quincy, MA: Author.

Plumbing-Heating-Cooling Contractors National Association (2005). *National Standard Plumbing Code Illustrated*. Falls Church, VA: Author.

Proctor, T. (2000). *Building Trades Printreading-Part 2*, 3e. Homewood, IL: American Technical Publishers.

Rehabilitation Engineering and Assistive Technology Association of North America (2014). ATP exam outline. Retrieved from http://www.resna.org/get-certified/atp/exam-outline/atp-exam-outline.

Ripka, L.V. (2011). *Plumbing Design and Installation*, 4e. Orland Park, IL: American Technical Publishers.

Rockis, G.J., Rockis, S.M., and Proctor, T.E. (2010). *Residential Wiring*, 3e. Orland Park, IL: American Technical Publishers.

Sanford, J. (2012). *Design for the Ages: Universal Design as a Rehabilitation Strategy*. Philadelphia, PA: Springer.

Steinfeld, E. and Maisel, J. (2012). *Universal Design: Creating Inclusive Environments*. Hoboken, NJ: Wiley.

Tanner, B. (2011a). The home environment. In: *An Occupational Therapist Guide to Home Modification Practice* (ed. E. Ainsworth and D. DeJonge), 3–16. Thorofare, NJ: Slack.

Tanner, B. (2011b). History and future of home modification services. In: *An Occupational Therapist Guide to Home Modification Practice* (ed. E. Ainsworth and D. DeJonge), 67–83. Thorofare, NJ: Slack.

The Council for Disability Rights (n.d.). Home modification – funding sources. Retrieved from http://www.disabilityrights.org/mod3.htm.

Thiele, T. (2019). How electrical service panels have evolved. Retrieved from: https://www.thespruce.com/service-panels-changed-in-the-1900s-1152732.

US Department of Health and Human Services (2013). Summary of the HIPPA Privacy Rule. Retrieved from https://www.hhs.gov/hipaa/for-professionals/privacy/laws-regulations/index.html.

US Department of Housing and Urban Development (2008). *The Fair Housing Act Design Manual: A Manual to Assist Builders in Meeting the Accessibility Requirements of the Fair Housing Act*. Washington, DC: Author.

US Department of Veterans Affairs (n.d.). VA home loans. Retrieved from www.benefits.va.gov/homeloans/adaptedhousing.asp.

Vicente, K. (2006). *The Human Factor: Revolutionizing the Way People Live with Technology*. New York: Routledge, Taylor & Francis Group.

Wade, C. and Rancourt, H. (2002). *NABH Student Builder Home Modifications Remodeling for Today and Tomorrow*. Upper Marlboro, MD: NABH Research Center.

Warner, M. (2000). *The Complete Guide to Alzheimer's: Proofing Your Home*. West Lafayette, IA: Purdue University Press.

Wormer, A. (1998). *The Builder's Book of Bathrooms*. Newtown, CT: Tauton Press.

9

Working and communicating in face-to-face teams

M. Gayl Bowser

Outline

Assistive Technologies and Environmental Interventions in Healthcare: An Integrated Approach, First Edition.
Edited by Lynn Gitlow and Kathleen Flecky.

Companion website: www.wiley.com/go/gitlow/assitivetechnologies

Learning outcomes

After reading this chapter, you should be able to:

1. Describe the difference between a team and a working group.
2. Identify three research-supported benefits of working in teams.
3. List a range of definitions of teams and discuss the implications of using various definitions in your AT/TEI practice.
4. Describe the differences between multidisciplinary, interdisciplinary, and collaborative teams.
5. Define and describe an assistive technology team decision-making process.
6. Recognize and address common types of team dysfunction.

Active learning prompts

Before you read this chapter:

1. Think of one of the teams you work with either professionally or in your private life.
   In your opinion, how well does this team function? Is it empowered to make a decision or does your team allow one or two individuals to make the decisions? How does the team's system of functioning affect the success of its work?
2. When you have participated as a member of a team that worked well, how did that team function? What do you believe made the team's work effective?
3. When you have participated on teams that support people with disabilities, how has the individual with a disability been included? How has that person's family been included on the team?
4. In your own words, define the term team. What do you feel your role should be on a team that addresses assistive technology/environmental intervention needs of a person with a disability?
5. Describe the role that you believe assistive technology/environmental intervention teams should play in helping individuals with disability to use technology?

Key terms

Human-Tech Ladder
Teams
Effective teamwork
TEI
Team functioning

Introduction

In Chapter 1, the Human-Tech Ladder was presented. The *Human-Tech Ladder* is a five-level visual model to conceptualize human factors, such as physical, psychological, team, organizational, and political human factors, that interact with technology as seen in Figure 9.1. The quotation from Vicente below illuminates the importance of the team human factor in engagement with technology.

> The physical and psychological levels [of the Human-Tech Ladder] do a relatively good job of describing an individual person, but people don't usually work in isolation.
>
> Many jobs require us to function in a team consisting of two or more people who need to communicate with each other and coordinate their respective actions to achieve individual and common goals … For instance, if teams are to function efficiently, explicit goals and priorities should be identified and communicated among the members so that they can all paddle in the same direction and thereby achieve a synergistic effect as opposed to having each member go off in a different and conflicting direction and consequently dilute the team's effectiveness (Vicente 2006, p. 56).

From over 20 years of research in healthcare fields, we know that better patient care and lower levels of patient mortality are evident when health professionals work together in multidisciplinary teams (Borrill et al. 2000; West 2002; West et al. 2006). Similar research in the fields of education, business, and human services also demonstrates the value of teamwork to accomplish tasks, make changes, and create innovation and improve the quality of services (Clark 1994; Johnson et al. 1983; Kagan 1991; West 2002).

In this chapter, the *Team* rung on the Human-Tech Ladder proposed by (Vicente 2006, p. 61) will be addressed in application to teamwork in assistive and environmental intervention technology. Recall from previous chapters that *TEI* is the shortcut term for technology and

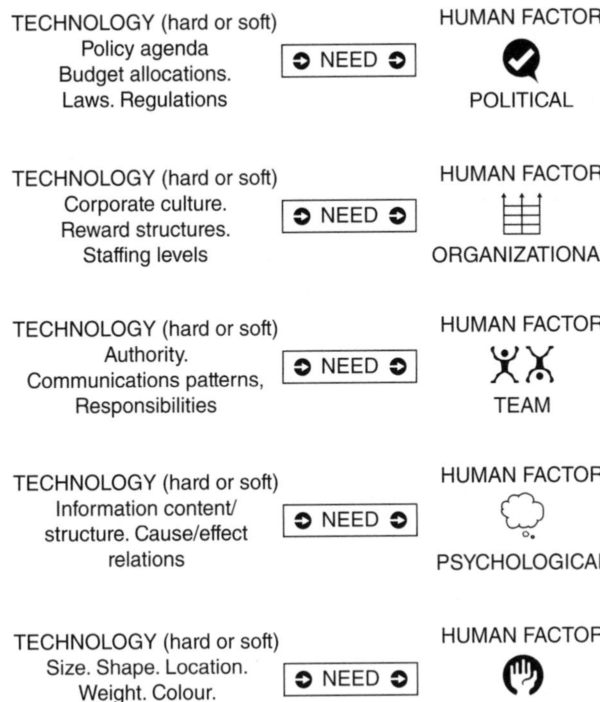

Figure 9.1 Human-tech ladder. Source: Reproduced with permission of Taylor & Francis.

environmental intervention. This term represents the interrelated connection between technology and environmental factors in the assistive technology (AT) process.

Basic information about teamwork will be examined in relationship to how teams differ from other kinds of groups along with the benefits and drawbacks of working in teams. What is known about AT teams and how they function will be examined along with suggestions for strategies to address teamwork barriers when they arise. Finally, new and creative ways will be explored in terms of teamwork strategies that maximize efficient use of time, resources, and the expertise of team members who provide support for individuals who use AT.

What is a team?

A *team* is a group of people who work together toward a common goal. Many groups are called teams, but for a real team to exist, there must be a compelling team purpose that is distinctive and specific to the group that requires its members to roll up their sleeves and accomplish something beyond individual products (Katzenback and Smith 1993). A team is not simply appointed. To develop as a team, individuals must work together to build an effective working relationship that uses each person's knowledge, skills, and interests and complements the individual's strengths with the strengths of other team members. At least part of a team's time together must be devoted to developing and maintaining the team's identity as well as completing the tasks that the team was created to accomplish. See Table 9.1 for specific differences between a working group and a team.

When teamwork is effective, a group of individuals with diverse training and knowledge come together to contribute ideas, information, and direction based upon their unique perspective.

Effective teamwork is also dependent upon individual team members' ability to share their knowledge and opinions and collaborate to make appropriate decisions that can be successfully implemented.

Table 9.1 Comparison of Characteristics of Teams and Groups.

Working group	Team
• A strong, focused leader is appointed.	• Leadership is shared among members.
• The general organizational mission is the group's purpose, with short-term projects and assignments.	• There are specific, well-defined goals that are unique to the team and members value the goals.
• Effectiveness is measured indirectly by the group's influence on others.	• Effectiveness is measured directly by assessing team accomplishments.
• Individual accomplishments are recognized and rewarded.	• Team efforts are celebrated as well as individuals' contributions to the team.
• Different individuals may join the group for specific tasks or projects.	• Membership is ongoing; change requires re-establishment of norms, roles, identity.
• Members bring their own information, may or may not contribute, and are not concerned with the group as a whole.	• Team members work at maintenance tasks to ensure that the team can work effectively.
• Meetings are efficiently run and last for short periods of time.	• Meetings have open-ended discussion and include active problem-solving.
• In meetings, members discuss, decide, and delegate.	• In meetings members discuss, decide, and do real work together.
• Decisions may or may not be made by consensus. Leader may seek input, but decide by authority rule.	• Decisions are made by consensus.

Source: Adapted from Johnson and Johnson (2006).

Why work in teams?

Michael West, in *Effective Teamwork: Practical Lessons from Organizational Research* West (2012), identified seven evidence-based reasons why a team approach is effective and frequently used in medical, educational, and business environments. He makes the following key points and supports them with research about team functioning:

- Teams are a very good way to enact organizational plans.
- Teams enable organizations to speedily develop and deliver products and services.
- Teams can integrate with other teams and link in ways individuals cannot.
- Teams enable organizations to learn more effectively.
- Team-based organizations focus on improvement and promote change.
- Organizations that are team-based can be managed more effectively.
- Teams can undertake system-wide change (West, 2012, pp. 17–19).

When applied to an individual's use of AT and the provision of AT/TEI services to support that use, these seven points help to explain why best practice guidance, legal mandates, and procedural guidelines about AT and TEI include an emphasis on team involvement, as noted in the next section.

Teams are a good way to enact AT plans

Teams are an effective way to create and implement comprehensive plans that are needed when an individual begins to use AT. Initially these team plans focus on an individual's need for AT and the trial of a variety of high-tech and low-tech AT tools to determine which work well to help the individual overcome barriers to performance in the context of the person's everyday routines and environments.

Most individuals who use AT use it in many activities and many environments. Because of the need for consistency between these environments, additional plans are made for training and regular use of the AT once it has been chosen. A team-based structure allows for greater fidelity of plan implementation. Successful implementation of AT/TEI typically requires many people to collaborate.

Acquisition of the AT, training for those who will implement its use daily, monitoring its effectiveness, and troubleshooting and repair are all part of AT implementation and may be most effectively accomplished by a combination of individuals whose knowledge and skills complement and support each other. If these individuals have formed a team, then they already know how to work together to build on each other's skills. Review Box 9.1 for a case scenario of teamwork with Michael. See the supplemental chapter material on the companion website for an AT Implementation Plan that can be used to guide your teamwork.

> **Box 9.1** Teamwork with Michael
>
> The team that supports Michael in his group home includes several staff members with whom he has bonded, his mother and older sister, and a friend that he met in high school. When Michael began to use his new tablet device for communication, his team met to identify ways that they might support him in learning to communicate in this new way. The daytime manager of the group home agreed to learn the operation of the tablet and be available for troubleshooting when other people, including Michael, couldn't make it work the way they wanted it to. As the team brainstormed places in Michael's day when he might practice using the device for communication, they agreed that one option was for Michael to go to the local coffee shop to order his favorite caramel macchiato latte drinks. Several staff members agreed to go with him every morning at first to help him learn the steps of ordering with a communication device. But eventually, Michael said, he wanted to do it himself.

Teams can develop and deliver services quickly

When team members each take part of the responsibility for the team's work goal and function interdependently, teams can work faster and more effectively. In a team-based AT model, there is less need for a hierarchy of expert involvement that slows decision-making. Each member of the team is empowered to take action. If one individual working with a client who needs AT takes full responsibility for AT assessment, decision-making, or integration, the processes are much slower and may result in a reduced focus on use in everyday environments.

For example, if multiple team members collect environmental data about the vocabulary needs of an individual who will use augmentative communication, that data can then be combined to ensure faster and more comprehensive assembly of the needed vocabulary. Time is saved if people working in teams can perform activities formerly performed by individuals.

Teamwork helps distribute the workload in a way that is both effective and efficient. An effective team can divide tasks and collaborate, making everyone's job easier. For instance, if a device for trial needs to be rented and

Box 9.2 Teamwork with George

Before his stroke, George was in contact with hundreds of friends around the country who shared his interest in Civil War memorabilia. After his stroke, George had a very hard time typing on his computer keyboard and felt a real loss because he was unable to keep in contact with his network of friends. He and his support team met to try to figure out how he could reconnect. One team member mentioned that George might be able to use speech recognition on his cellular phone to send texts and emails. Another team member knew about a speech recognition program that is a little more accurate that could be used on George's computer. Everyone agreed that speech recognition would be worth trying, but George wanted a more immediate solution. His occupational therapist (OT) agreed to contact a local AT loan program and borrow a large-key keyboard for George to try. The team felt that he might be able to type using the larger keys with high contrast letters, but wanted to try this option before George purchased a similar device. George's son, Daniel, agreed to be the go-to person for his technology use and coordinate the team's efforts to help George get back to the business of connecting with his friends.

Box 9.3 Teamwork with Maria

Maria got her first powered wheelchair when she was seven, but at the age of 12 she had outgrown it and no more modifications were possible. When she visited the hospital wheelchair clinic to be fitted for a new and improved chair, the physical therapist (PT) asked if Maria was using any AT at school. Maria's family knew that the school was looking at providing her some adapted equipment for computer access. The private speech and language clinician with whom she worked also wanted to provide her with an augmentative communication device to help her repair communication breakdowns when her speech was hard to understand.

After some consultation and planning, it was decided that the school team, and, in particular, the PT on that team, would coordinate all of these efforts. The school team planned weekly meetings to coordinate all the equipment efforts and both the hospital PT and the private speech-language pathologist attended some of the team meetings using two-way video conferencing. When this was not possible, they both provided email updates that were sent the day before the regularly scheduled meetings.

programmed for an individual, one team member may be assigned to contact with vendors, while another is skilled at programming the device and observes the settings where it will be used. They are more efficient working together than either would be working alone. Please review Box 9.2 for examples of teamwork with the client, George.

Teams can integrate with other teams

A variety of teams may be asked to contribute to decisions related to AT selection, adaptation, or use. These might include a medical assessment team, a team that develops an individualized service plan, the service delivery team, and a specialized AT team that may provide initial assessment information and recommendations. Another example would be a team that is involved in making home modification recommendations. One individual may receive services from all teams in separate settings.

Team members need to be able to work together to accomplish specific tasks and goals but also to work across team boundaries to ensure good communication and a common direction. Yet, in a study of school-based AT teams across the United States, team-building issues were identified by AT team members as one of the greatest challenges to providing successful services (DeCoste et al. 2005).

To ensure that information is shared effectively and used in real-world environments, it is important that individuals with disabilities and their advocates are included on teams that consider AT/TEI. When there is at least one team member who can report on the activities of other teams and the impact that these activities will have on an individual's AT use, AT can be better integrated with the work of medical, vocational, and other types of rehabilitation teams to ensure a comprehensive approach to services. An example of this type of team reporting is presented in the case in Box 9.3.

Teams enable groups to learn more effectively and retain learning

Effective provision of AT services requires each individual involved in selection, acquisition, and use of the technology to develop his or her individual knowledge base, and also to work cooperatively with others. No one individual knows everything that is needed to help clients use AT/TEI or to provide related services that are meaningful and useful across the full range of daily environments. Each team member brings a specific set of skills and knowledge to the team and shares that expertise with other team members.

Because of this shared knowledge set, teams are able to learn more effectively, be more creative, and maintain team function over time. Additionally, when one team member leaves, the knowledge base of the team is not lost. The case presented in Box 9.4 demonstrates how each team member's unique skill set worked to coordinate a successful TEI outcome for Frankie.

Box 9.4 Teamwork with Frankie

Frankie used a single switch on her wheelchair to run both her communication device and her computer. She used row/column scanning for both devices and was able to communicate using full sentences and also to do her office data entry work with the same switch. She pressed the switch by moving her knee upward to a spot where the switch was mounted under her wheelchair tray.

When Frankie's PT began to notice that she was developing additional tightness in her hip, the team wondered if her frequent switch use was having an impact. Frankie's care assistant agreed to work with her to try to identify a new placement for the switch and they found that Frankie had good control of her right elbow and could move it backward to activate a switch placed just behind her elbow. Once Frankie had some practice with the new switch site, she was able to use both her knee and her elbow for her work and communication. The care assistant and the PT developed a schedule to ensure that the switch was not placed in the same place for too many days in a row so that Frankie's muscles would have a chance to recover from frequent use. She also began a daily series of exercises provided by her OT to ensure that her shoulders and elbow would remain flexible despite extended switch use at the elbow. The team agreed to review Frankie's range of motion in the affected joints as well as her work performance every two months.

Teams promote change

Team members with different points of view provide multiple ways to look at a problem. Each member is likely to have different ideas about how to solve an identified problem. Each group member's knowledge can be combined to bring new ideas and concepts to the AT process. Innovation is promoted when a team-based approach is used (Sacramento et al. 2006). See the case of Tomeo in Box 9.5 for an example of how this works.

Teams can manage AT recommendations and activities effectively

Effective planning and problem-solving require multiple perspectives so that potential problems can be avoided if possible, or handled quickly if not avoidable. Discussion during the planning stage can often illuminate potential problems that, if not attended to, would diminish the effective use of AT.

A case coordinator, a disability advocate, or a self-advocate can more easily keep track of the activities of several teams and collect and apply the recommendations of all the individuals who make up those teams. Teamwork reduces the number of individual recommendations that must be addressed and helps to combine and synthesize them into a more holistic focus on the needs of the person who will use the AT. The case in Box 9.6 illustrates this concept.

Box 9.5 Teamwork with Tomeo

While Tomeo didn't want to call attention to his hearing impairment, he really could not understand much of what was going on in his college classes. He and his counselor from the college's office of disability services called a meeting with Tomeo, his instructors, and their AT support specialist to see what could be done. Since Tomeo did not understand American Sign Language (ASL), a sign language interpreter was not really an option. Tomeo's hearing aids were not sufficient for him to catch all of the conversations in class. Tomeo shared with the team that the hardest activities for him were classes where there was very large group instruction with auditorium seating and classes where there was a lot of small group work that created a lot of noise. One instructor asked whether lectures in the auditorium classroom might be amplified for all the students since there were others who had difficulty hearing the lectures. Tomeo's microbiology instructor agreed that Tomeo and his work group could use a small office space off the main microbiology lab to do their project work so that there was less noise and distraction. With these two innovative modifications, Tomeo was able to understand what was being said around him and was more successful in completing his coursework.

Box 9.6 Teamwork with Helga's Daughter

When Helga's daughter announced that she wanted a destination wedding on the beach in Maui, everyone was puzzled about how Helga would be able to attend. Her multiple sclerosis (MS) had advanced to a place where she required the use of a powered wheelchair for independent mobility, and everyone agreed that there was no way that the chair would work on a sandy beach. Helga wanted to give her daughter the exact wedding she wanted and was unwilling to say that there had to be a change in venue to accommodate her mobility needs. An emergency meeting of Helga's team was called. Helga's husband said he would just carry her to the beach. Someone else suggested a stretcher arrangement with a seat back that could be carried by the ushers. One team member was aware of special wheelchairs that were designed to be driven on sand. Another team member suggested a golf cart with sand tires such as those used on links golf courses. After discussion and brainstorming, Helga's team was able to quickly identify several solutions that would enable her to attend her daughter's perfect wedding.

AT teams can undertake system-wide change

An essential element of team functioning is one of self-evaluation of the work of the team. There are a variety of

Box 9.7 Teamwork with Rehabilitation Staff

The staff at Smithville Hospital and Rehabilitation center was aware that many of the AT recommendations they made were not implemented. They were frustrated that they worked hard in the AT clinic to identify the best technology solutions for their patients but that work seemed to go to waste. They decided to initiate a review of the AT services they provided, to examine the kinds of recommendations they were making and the ones that were most likely to be followed, and to interview patients who were both successful and unsuccessful with AT use. The data review showed that many of the reports they wrote were written in medical jargon that their patients did not really understand and that patients who did understand the recommendations often felt that the technology was too complicated for them to use. As a result of this investigation, they adopted a new approach to AT recommendations that they described as "The simplest tool to overcome the barrier." They also developed an ongoing data collection and follow-up system to determine whether the changes they made had the desired effects for patients.

AT self-assessments that can be used by AT teams who provide services to multiple individuals (Bowser and Reed 2012; QIAT 2012; QIAT-PS 2012). When self-assessments are completed and plans for improvement of AT services are developed, a team approach to systems change is generally more effective than individual effort (West 2012). See the case in Box 9.7 for an example of how this self-assessment process worked in the setting.

Elements of effective teamwork

No matter what the team structure, each team functions differently. Some teams may be very efficient while the work of others may stagnate. One team may typically stay focused on the task at hand, while another strays easily to related or even unrelated tasks. The reasons for differences in performance among various teams may include the differing nature of their tasks, sets of instructions, time constraints, and funding for services, and differences in personalities and interaction styles of team members.

In order to grow from a working group into an ongoing and effective team, attention must be paid to several aspects of the team. One well-established conceptualization of team building that seems to fit well with a focus on AT is that of Adair (1986). In this model, each group or team is unique but they all share three common needs: (i) to achieve the task or tasks which they are supposed to accomplish, (ii) to build the team, and (iii) to develop the skills of individual team members. Figure 9.2 demonstrates the ways in which these

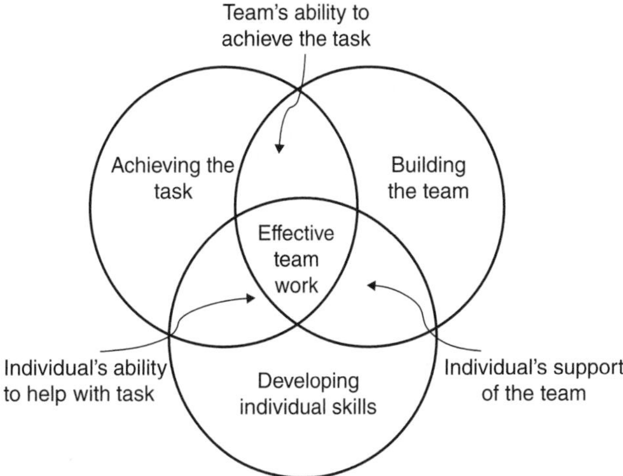

Figure 9.2 Three aspects of team functioning.

three aspects of team function overlap in six areas of team function.

Team leaders and collaborative teams that examine their own structures and functioning can have a significant impact on team function when they attend to the circle overlap areas in Figure 9.2.

Individual's ability to help with the task

In the overlap area between developing individual skills and achieving the team's task, teams may sometimes focus on helping team members to develop new skills to accomplish the team's goals. In this area, professional development may be required to increase individual team members' abilities. For an AT team, this may include training in device operation but could also focus on data collection, technology integration into activities of daily living, or even report writing for AT funding.

Individual's support of the team

When team members seem to be "outsiders," the overlap between the development of individual skills and teamwork skills comes into focus. Team members may need support in learning new collaboration or team membership skills. In addition, the team may need to learn to support a member who has trouble with teamwork. Individual support and mentoring is often required in this situation.

Team's ability to achieve the task

The third overlap in Figure 9.2 is between building the team and achieving the task. It is in this area that team management and coordination are most needed. An effective team finds a balance between team-building activities that bring members closer together and task-focused activities that may require individual actions and an emphasis on goals. In order to build the team's ability to achieve the task, members may need to identify new resources. These may include time, money, additional sources of expertise, or additional supports for the team itself.

When a team establishes a balance between each aspect of team functioning, teamwork is effective, productive, and satisfying to team members. A well-defined team structure is at the center of all aspects of team function.

Structures of AT teams

AT teams are found in hospitals and clinics, in local schools and school districts, in rehabilitation programs, and in a variety of other settings. They are funded by government agencies, insurance, rehabilitation services, and privately. Despite the variety of funding streams, geographical location, expertise, and philosophy, AT/TEI teams all come together to work toward the common goal of providing high-quality services for individuals with disabilities.

AT teams vary widely in makeup, function, and goals (DeCoste et al. 2005). In some settings, the group referred to as an AT team may be a group of professionals who primarily focus on the AT needs of a wide variety of individuals. They may receive specific AT referrals, complete AT assessments, and make recommendations to those with primary responsibility for the implementation of the program. In other cases, the group that provides direct services to the individual with a disability may also directly address that individual's AT needs as part of the team's goals. No matter what the team structure, a primary function of the team is to determine what information is available and what other information might be needed to make an AT recommendation, and to identify sources of expertise about that information.

Contributions of individual team members

While few teams will have all the members listed below, each team member who helps to address the AT needs of a person with a disability contributes unique information to the conversation. When additional expertise is needed, teams may invite new members with the needed skills to participate.

- *Client and, when appropriate, family members:* Clients and their families are the overall experts about their own lives. When clients and their families do not participate and support the selection and acquisition of AT there is clear evidence that the technology is more likely to be underused or abandoned, even if appropriate and useful technology has been selected (Scherer and Glueckauf 2005).
- *Occupational therapist:* "Occupational therapy (OT) is a health and rehabilitation profession that strives to maximize individuals' independence in the daily occupations they pursue. OT teaches clients skills for daily living and provides specialized assistance, enabling them to lead independent, productive and satisfying lives" (American Occupational Therapy Association [AOTA] 1997). In the area of AT, OTs are essential in recommending the location or position of devices and determining the most likely means of access. OTs have skills in planning accommodations, designing customized equipment, guiding client instruction, and recommending AT accommodations such as adapted computer access or cognitive supports. Additionally, occupational therapists are able to evaluate and provide interventions for environmental adaptations.
- *Physical therapist:* The American Physical Therapy Association identifies complex rehabilitation technology (CRT) as a subset of AT. CRT includes but is not limited to individually configured manual wheelchair systems, power wheelchair systems, adaptive seating systems, alternative positioning systems, and other mobility devices. PTs contribute to an AT team by performing client evaluations and environmental reviews, developing plans of care, helping to identify goals for the use of AT, customizing the technology, and providing training and follow-up. PTs also work with clients to "address and prevent body structure and functional limitations to maintain or increase their activity and participation in society …" (American Physical Therapy Association, 1997, p. 1).
- *Rehabilitation counselor:* A rehabilitation counselor is a generalist who works with a person – usually a disabled adult. They work with clients to develop a plan to access whatever rehabilitation services are needed. The main goal of rehabilitation counselors is empowerment to maximize functioning and return clients to work and/or greater independence (Infinitec 2013). Rehabilitation counselors may refer clients to AT services in order to help them maximize their independence. When rehabilitation counselors are members of a team that considers AT, they can help to coordinate AT services and ensure follow-up for the team's recommendations.
- *Rehabilitation engineer (RE):* Rehabilitation engineers work in many areas relative to AT. Some are involved in research and work on developing devices, or developing standards for a particular category of devices. Others work in private industry in the development of

products for the consumer. Many REs are involved in direct service delivery. They may work with an individual client's team to determine needs and employ or even create new AT to meet those needs. (Rehabilitation Engineering Society of America n.d.).

- *Social worker:* Social workers are skilled at finding resources for people. They research the kinds of help people need and they make plans to provide that help. They might find a career training program, a mentor, or a disability expert when the AT team determines that is needed (Bureau of Labor Statistics 2010). Social workers who participate on an AT team might find funding resources, medical providers, classes, or support groups to help clients learn about how to use their AT.
- *Speech-language pathologist (SLP):* SLPs are trained to work with individuals of all ages who experience difficulties in communicating (American Speech Language Hearing Association, ASHA n.d.). SLPs cover areas such as augmentative and alternative communication, environmental control, and aids to daily living. They may provide direct and/or consultative assessment and treatment services using one or more types of technology. As a member of an AT team, their skills are also critical in the selection of vocabulary and designing content and layout of communication systems. SLPs can provide training and suggest ways to maximize a client's speech, language, and communication opportunities throughout the day.
- *Teachers:* For clients enrolled in elementary school, general education and special education teachers contribute expertise in cognitive development, play/social development, behavior management, pre-vocational and vocational skill development, academic instruction, and the demands of educational environments. Educators can help teams identify opportunities for use of AT in daily schedules, implement, supervise, and train students to use devices, and integrate the use of AT into everyday routines and activities. For some students, specific expertise will also be needed from teachers of students with visual impairments (TVIs) and teachers of students with hearing impairments (THIs) (Bowser and Reed 2012)
- *Technology consultant:* AT consultants are generally professionals from other disciplines who have spent extra time and effort to learn the use and operation of a variety of AT devices. Technology consultants can be instrumental in determining specific technologies a client needs from a wide array of brands and options. As team members, they provide expertise about wide range of AT devices, including vendor contact information, operation, and functional use.
- *Vendor:* Vendors are often the most knowledgeable source of information about the technologies that they distribute. They can contribute to team knowledge by providing information that helps the team understand the particular features of devices or durable medical equipment such as wheelchairs and speech-generating devices (SGDs). They may also assist in assessments. When teams work with vendors, it is important to remember that they are often experts in their own products but may not know about the full range of AT options available to the client.

Team operation

Professionals and consumers of AT/TEI services identify the characteristics of the teams that they work with and understand how the team's models of operation affect the way team members work together and the services provided.

There are three primary ways that AT teams may operate. Teams may be multidisciplinary, interdisciplinary, or collaborative.

Multidisciplinary teams

Multidisciplinary teams have historically been based on a medical model of intervention (Bodine and Melonis 2005). Multidisciplinary teams consist of professionals from several disciplines, including AT, who work independently of each other (Fewell 1983). While they may share the same space and even work side by side, they function separately and interact minimally (Clark 1994). Recommendations regarding AT services are based on team member area of expertise. Professionals on multidisciplinary teams function as independent specialists who provide parallel services but have built-in formal mechanisms for communication. For example, each team member might conduct an independent assessment of an individual's AT needs, but then meet for a formal case conference to share their findings and plans (American Occupational Therapy Association, AOTA 1997).

Interdisciplinary teams

The interdisciplinary team model of AT services is a model in which team members make a strong commitment to frequent collaborative communication. Team members collaborate to design an AT intervention strategy that combines the most important objectives of each discipline and maximizes the potential for a positive outcome. Interdisciplinary teams use the many unique viewpoints of team members to produce integrated plans for clients (AOTA 1997, p. 85) Most often, each professional is responsible for his or her own area of expertise and the part of the AT plan related to that area. Unlike multidisciplinary teams, these teams encourage team members to share their information and discuss individual results (Fewell 1983).

Collaborative teams

In a collaborative AT team model, it is assumed that no one person or profession has an adequate knowledge base or sufficient expertise to complete all the functions associated with providing AT services. Professionals and family members as well as individuals with disabilities and those who advocate for them, all communicate and collaborate with one another to make meaningful decisions and to provide appropriate and effective services. All team members are involved in planning and monitoring AT goals and procedures, although each team member's responsibility for the implementation of the plans may vary. Team members can be considered as sharing joint ownership and responsibility for intervention objectives (ASHA n.d.; Wilcox et al. 1991).

The collaborative AT team model (also known as a transdisciplinary model) is an outgrowth of dissatisfaction with the multidisciplinary model, which can be fragmented among different specialty areas, deficit-based, and remediation-oriented. In this model, teams form a more unified approach to working together, often crossing boundaries of expertise and information sharing (Sarason and Lorentz 1998).

> Individuals, including parents, siblings and community members who are familiar with the student, exchange knowledge, information and skills and then the intervention plan is carried out. During the decision-making process, the collective sharing and wisdom of the group allows for the creating of many alternatives for education services. The goals of the services relate to the whole student rather than discipline-specific goals.
>
> (Bodine and Melonis 2005, pp. 212–213)

There is no evidence that one model of teamwork for an AT team is better than another. The model of AT service delivery that will work best depends upon the goal of the team, available personnel and financial resources, population density, geography, and the availability of assistance from other resources and services. However, when using the International Classification of Functioning, Disability and Health (ICF) (WHO 2001) as a basis for AT decisions, the team charged with implementation of the final plans will need to be able to share information and resources and make rapid decisions about strategic use of AT. In this case, a collaborative team model is likely to yield the most effective implementation.

How do collaborative AT teams function?

In addition to nurturing team function, valuing each team member, and being willing to take the time to learn to work together, teams need to develop a set of operating procedures that ensure that they can, indeed, work as a team. Setting norms for schedules, communication, facilitation, record keeping etc. must be done at the outset of the team's work (Johnson and Johnson 1983).

One of the most critical components of AT teamwork is a clearly defined decision-making process that teams use as they work together to make AT decisions, as illustrated in the team working together in Figure 9.3.

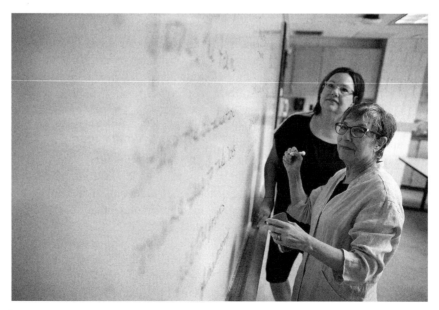

Figure 9.3 Team collaboration.

Team decision-making for AT can be divided into two parts: (i) gathering information, and (ii) analyzing that information to make a decision or recommendation.

Information gathering starts with the individual and the specific functional capabilities that may be increased, maintained, or improved through the use of AT. Information can be gathered from chart and file reviews, histories, formal or informal testing, or interviews with the individual or those familiar with the individual and observations. In order to assemble the entire range of information that is needed, teams must be familiar with the environments in which the person who uses AT typically spends time. If team members are not familiar with all of the environments, environmental observations are completed as part of information gathering with an eye to the supports that are already in place for the tasks/activities (Zabala 2005).

Once information and data are gathered, teams analyze the information and make a decision about what AT is most likely to be useful. Making effective decisions about the recommendation for purchase and use of AT requires the collaborative efforts of several individuals. The team that makes decisions about AT should include the individual for whom the AT is being considered and their advocates. They should be equal, participating members of the AT team, not brought in after the decision has been made (Cook and Polger 2007).

Using an effective decision-making process requires team members to employ a variety of skills that are separate from the technical skills they may have needed during data gathering. These include communication skills and group process skills. Communication skills include but are not limited to active listening, negotiation, providing non-threatening feedback, and accepting criticism without becoming defensive (Dettmer et al. 2003). Group process skills include a variety of group tasks that become important when working as part of a team, one of the most important being the effective use of an agreed-upon group decision-making process.

The value of using a clearly defined decision-making process in team decision-making has for many years been identified within the fields of rehabilitation, education (Gordon 1977; Schmuck and Runkel 1994), and early intervention (Prentice and Spencer 1985). Although awareness of the importance of using a decision-making process has been evident in the literature for more than 30 years, many team members are still not receiving training in this important area. The key elements or steps of an effective decision-making process include:

1. problem identification – the identification and definition of a specific problem;
2. solution generation – the suggestion of possible solutions;
3. solution selection – the evaluation of suggestions and choosing of a solution, to create an action plan;
4. implementation – the carrying out of the plan; and
5. follow-up – meeting again to evaluate the solution.

(Bowser and Reed 2012, p. 23)

Step 1: Problem identification

During the problem identification step, it is important for the team to address not only the characteristics of the individual, but also those of the environments in which the individual functions, and the tasks that need to be done. Many times when technology is abandoned, it is because only the physical, psychological, and social characteristics of the individual are addressed, with little attention paid to the settings in which the device will be used or the specific tasks that the individual really needs to address (Cook and Polger 2007). In education and many other settings, the SETT (Student, Environments, Tasks, and Tools) Framework (Zabala 2005) is used. The SETT Framework suggests that teamwork about technology needs should focus on the personal characteristics and interests of a student (or individual who needs AT), the environment, including physical characteristics of the setting as well as environmental demands and physical arrangements, and the tasks and specific activities that the individual needs to be able to do in each environment. This focus is helpful in clearly identifying and defining the problem in order to guide the team in identifying appropriate technology tools and other solutions. Other models such as the Assistive Technology Service Method (ATSM) (Elsaesser 2011) and the Matching Person and Technology (MPT) model (Scherer 2004) take similar approaches to the definition of characteristics of a quality AT assessment.

Step 2: Solution generation

When generating solutions, teams use brainstorming rules to create a climate of trust. This means that all suggestions are recorded in a way that is visible to all, no comments are allowed, and no judgments are passed. The goal is to generate as many ideas as possible.

Step 3: Solution selection

As alternatives are discussed and evaluated, it may become apparent that some items are very similar or that others make an excellent sequence of steps. New suggestions may be added at any time. During solution selection, the team discusses the value and relationship of the many suggestions. It is often helpful to categorize suggestions into "Things we can do tomorrow," "Things we can do in a month," and "Things we may want to consider later." The Action Plan is then created to include a timeline and the persons responsible for each of the solutions or steps that were selected.

Step 4: Implementation

During implementation, teams arrange to follow the plan they made during solution selection. For that to happen, everyone on the team needs to be aware of the plan and his or her role in it (Prentice and Spencer 1985). Implementation is the step of the decision-making process that informs teams about the quality of their solution.

Step 5: Follow-up

At a predetermined interval after the assessment and implementation, follow-up or monitoring must take place. If monitoring does not take place according to the original plan, a variety of problems can arise and go unaddressed as each team member focuses on their own assignment, but does not have the opportunity to get the "big picture" that comes from a team discussion. Plans should be adjusted or changed based on the data that are collected.

When all members of the team follow an AT process, they "paddle in the same direction" with a synergistic effect, rather than going off in different and conflicting directions and consequently diluting team effectiveness (Vicente 2006, p. 56). When little attention is paid to process, individual styles of thinking and communicating can result in team conflict and confusion.

When team issues arise

There are two primary types of issues influencing effective team functioning: structural issues and relational issues. Structural issues are those issues surrounding the organization of the team and expectations for functioning within the organizational model. The team's primary goal and purpose and resource management combine to create structure for a team (Bodine and Melonis 2005, p. 219). Common structural issues found in teams can include:

- models of service delivery that restrict the functioning of the team;
- lack of team goals and purpose;
- lack of self-evaluation systems to provide teams with effectiveness information;
- inadequate team membership or composition;
- team referrals and how that process is organized;
- service organization and delivery that does not match the individual's needs or environments;
- ineffective resource management;
- lack of information and training;
- unavailable equipment.

(Beukelman and Mirenda 1998, p. 126; DeCoste et al. 2005).

Relational issues in teams encompass the interactions among team members. They impact how the team functions and the quality and quantity of teamwork. The relational performance of a team includes the dynamic, multilevel nature of teamwork (Bodine and Melonis 2005, p. 219).

Common relational issues in teams include:

- frequent violation of the implicit and/or explicit social norms of communication established by the group;
- frequent disagreements and internal conflicts;
- lack of a safe environment for team members to express their feelings and opinions;
- unequal or dysfunctional interactions among members;
- poor or inactive administrative support;
- inability to give and receive criticism, resolve conflicts, and view the world from others' perspectives;
- processes that cause some members to feel devalued or marginalized;
- hierarchical structures of team functioning;
- group-think – convergence on a particular interpretation just to achieve team harmony;
- tendency of team members to agree with opinions expressed by those who are hierarchically senior to them in the group;
- loss of effort – people may work less hard in teams than if they alone were responsible for task outcomes;
- production blocking – lack of focused teamwork in favor of team member interaction;
- freeloading, perpetual lateness, or work avoidance by members;
- lack of positive interdependence (all for one, one for all)

(Beukelman and Mirenda 1998, pp. 126–127; Vicente 2006, pp. 34–54, West 2012, pp. 21–23; Zaccaro et al. 2009).

West (2012) suggests the following strategy to avoid both structural and relational team issues: The basic conditions for effective teamwork include having a real team whose membership is clear, which is of the right size, relatively stable in membership, and working on a task that requires teamwork. The team must have an overall purpose that adds value and which is translated into clear challenging team objectives. And the team needs the right people as team members with the required skills in the right roles. They must be enablers not derailers – people who support effective teamwork through their behaviors, not people who sabotage, undermine, or obstruct teams functioning (p. 4).

Summary

Often on an AT/TEI team, there are people with medical, rehabilitation, technological, and educational or vocational backgrounds. They all have valuable experience that can be brought to the team's work. Together with the individual who needs AT/TEI and advocates for that individual, they contribute a broad range of relevant experience to the team's deliberations. It is important that all team members are involved in team processes, so that this wide experience is available as a resource. Creativity and innovation are promoted through the cross-fertilization of ideas when a team approach is used (West 2002).

Equally important is the fact that involving everyone from the beginning is vital in order to gain commitment and reduce resistance (Heller et al. 1998). When some team members are not included in the process of problem identification, information gathering, brainstorming, solution selection, implementation, and follow-up, they are less likely to adopt or support the plan for AT use and may even create resistance (Bowser and Reed 2012).

Staff who work in teams report higher levels of involvement and commitment, and studies also show that they have lower stress levels than those who do not work in teams (Richter et al. 2011). Many team members argue that it is just more fun to work in teams.

Despite the benefits of working in teams, there are many factors that limit the use of teamwork as a strategy for providing AT services. Time, distance, the nature of funding sources, and the need to involve people from multiple agencies, all come together to restrict professionals' abilities to meet and work as teams. One solution to this growing problem may be the increased use of electronic resources and distance communication strategies to facilitate teamwork activities. In many environments, the answer may be increased use of virtual teamwork in AT services. With readily available technology and some creative thinking on the part of the team, all essential team members can be included in the AT teamwork regardless of distance and time limitations. In the following chapter, the essential elements of virtual teamwork and ideas for its application to AT services will be presented as a follow-up to this chapter. Please review Box 9.8 for an example of how a team collaborates using best evidence for a client.

Box 9.8 Here's the evidence

Gupta, R., Davis, E., and Horton, C. (2013). Interval examination: building primary care teams in an urban academic teaching clinic. *Journal of General Internal Medicine* 28(11): 1517–1521. doi: https://doi.org/10.1007/s11606-013-2598-7.

Key Words: team-based care, primary care redesign, patient-centered medical home, medical student and residency education

Purpose: Investigated how to develop team-based care in a hospital clinic.

Sample/Setting: Team workers at San Francisco General Hospital's General Medicine Clinic. Bottom Line: Team care increased access, continuity, and quality of care in this setting.

Critical Thinking Questions:

1. After reading this research article, what do you understand to be the limitations of this research? Are there any limitations not stated?
2. What implications does this article have for practice?

References

Adair, J. (1986). *Effective Team Building*. Aldershot: Gower.

American Occupational Therapy Association (AOTA) (1997). *Occupational Therapy Services for Children and Youth Under the Individuals with Disabilities Act*. Bethesda, MD: AOTA.

American Physical Therapy Association (APTA) National Governance Board (2012). Provision of assistive technology. Retrieved from http://www.apta.org/uploadedFiles/APTAorg/About_Us/Policies/Health_Social_Environment/ProvisionAssistiveTechnology.pdf#search=%22assistive%20technology%22.

American Speech-Language-Hearing Association (ASHA) (1997). Position statement: multiskilled personnel. *Journal of Speech-Language-Hearing Association* 39 (2): 13.

Bodine, C. and Melonis, M. (2005). Teaming and assistive technology in educational settings. In: *Handbook of Special Education Technology: Research and Practice* (ed. D. Edyburn, K. Higgins and R. Boone), 209–227. Whitefish Bay, WI: Knowledge by Design.

Beukelman, D.R. and Mirenda, P. (1998). *Augmentative and Alernative Communications: Management of Severe comMunication Disorders in Children and Adults*, 2e. Baltimore, MD: Paul H. Brookes.

Borrill, C., West, M., Shapiro, D., and Rees, A. (2000). Team working and effectiveness in the NHS. *British Journal of Health Care Management* 6: 364–371.

Bowser, G. and Reed, P. (2012). Education tech points profile of assistive technology services. In: *Education Tech Points: A Framework for Assistive Technology*, 3e. Retrieved from www.educationtechpoints.org.

Bureau of Labor Statistics (BLS) (2010). Social workers. Retrieved from https://www.bls.gov/ooh/community-and-social-service/social-workers.htm.

Clark, P.G. (1994). Social, professional and educational values on the interdisciplinary team: implications for gerontological and geriatric education. *Education Gerontology* 20: 35–51.

Cook, A. and Polger, J.M. (2007). *Cook and Hussey's Assistive Technologies: Principles and Practice*, 3e. St. Louis, MO: Mosby Elsevier.

DeCoste, D.C., Reed, P., and Kaplan, M.W. (2005). *Assistive Technology Teams: Many Ways to Do It Well.* Roseburg, OR: National Assistive Technology in Education Network.

Dettmer, P.L., Thurston, P., and Dyck, N. (1993). *Consultation, Collaboration, and Teamwork for Students with Special Needs.* Boston, MA: Allyn & Bacon.

Elsaesser, L. (2011). Assistive Technology Service Method. National Disability Authority, Centre for Excellence in Universal Design, Assistive Technology and Knowledge Translation seminar, Dublin, Ireland.

Fewell, R.R. (1983). The team approach to infant education. In: *Educating Handicapped Infants: Issues in Development and Intervention* (ed. S.G. Garwood and R.R. Fewell), 299–322. Rockville, MD: Aspen.

Gordon, T. (1977). *Leader Effectiveness Training - LET: The No-Lose Way to Release the Production Potential in People.* Toronto: Bantam.

Heller, F., Pusic, E., Strauss, G., and Wilpert, B. (1998). *Organizational Participation: Myth and Reality.* New York: Oxford University Press.

Infinitec (2013). Rehabilitation counselor. Retrieved from www.infinite.org/careers-in-at.

Johnson, D. and Johnson, F. (2006). *Joining Together: Group Theory and Group Skills*, 9e. Boston, MA: Allyn & Bacon.

Johnson, D., Johnson, F., and Maruyama, G. (1983). Interdependence and interpersonal attraction among heterogeneous and homogeneous individuals: a theoretical reformation and meta-analysis of the research. *Review of Educational Research* 53 (1): 5–54.

Kagan, S.L. (1991). *United We Stand: Collaboration for the Child Care and Early Intervention Services.* New York: Teachers College Press.

Katzenback, J. and Smith, D. (1993). *The Wisdom of Teams.* Cambridge, MA: Harvard Business School Press.

Prentice, R. and Spencer, P. (1985). *Decision-Making for Early Services: A Team Approach.* Elk Grove Village, IL: American Academy of Pediatrics.

QIAT (2012). Quality indicators for assistive technology services. Retrieved from www.qiat.org.

QIAT-PS (2012). Quality indicators for AT in post-secondary education. Retrieved from http://www.qiat-ps.org.

Rehabilitation Engineering Society of America (RESNA) (n.d.). ATP general info. Retrieved from https://www.resna.org/atp-general-info.

Richter, A.W., Dawson, J.F., and West, M.A. (2011). The effectiveness of teams in organizations: a meta-analysis. *The International Journal of Human Resource Management* 22: 2749–2769.

Sacramento, C.A., Chang, S.M.W., and West, M.A. (2006). Team innovation through collaboration. In: *Innovation Through Collaboration* (ed. M.M. Beyerlein, S.T. Beyerlein and F.A. Kennedy), 81–112. St. Louis, MO: Elsevier.

Sarason, S.B. and Lorentz, E.M. (1998). *Crossing Boundaries.* San Francisco: Jossey-Bass.

Scherer, M. (2004). *Matching Person and Technology Process and Accompanying Assessment Instruments* (Rev. ed.). Webster, NY: Institute for Matching Person & Technology.

Scherer, M. and Glueckauf, R. (2005). Assessing the benefits of assistive technologies on activities and participation. *Rehabilitation Psychology* 50 (2): 1–10.

Schmuck, R. and Runkel, P. (1994). *The Handbook of Organization Development in Schools.* Palo Alto, CA: Mayfield.

Vicente, K. (2006). *The Human Factor: Revolutionizing the Way People Live with Technology.* New York: Routledge, Taylor & Francis Group.

West, M.A. (2002). Reflexivity revolution and innovation in work teams. In: *Product Development Teams: Advances in Interdisciplinary Studies of Work Teams* (ed. M. Beyerlein), 1–30. Greenwich, CT: JAI Press.

West, M.A. (2012). *Effective Teamwork: Practical Lessons from Organizational Research.* Chichester: Wiley.

West, M.A., Markiewicz, L., and Dawson, J.F. (2006). *Aston Team Performance Inventory: Management Set.* London: ASE.

Wilcox, M.J., Kouri, T.A., and Caswell, S.B. (1991). Early language intervention: a comparison of classroom and individual treatment. *American Journal of Speech-Language Pathology* 1: 49–61.

World Health Organization (2001). *International Classification of Functioning, Disability and Health.* Geneva, Switzerland: World Health Organization.

Zabala, J. (2005). Ready, SETT, go: getting started with the SETT framework. *Closing the Gap* 6: 1–3. Retrieved from www.joyzabala.com.

Zaccaro, S.J., Heinen, B., and Shuffler, M. (2009). Team leadership and team effectiveness. In: *The Organizational Frontiers Series. Team Effectiveness in Complex Organizations: Cross-Disciplinary Perspectives and Approaches* (ed. E. Salas, G.F. Goodwin and C.S. Burke), 83–111. New York: Routledge.

Additional resources

Institute of Medicine (2014). *Establishing Transdisciplinary Professionalism for Improving Health Outcomes: Workshop Summary.* Washington, DC: The National Academies Press.

Mitchell, P., Wynia, M., Golden, R. et al. (2012). Core principles & values of effective team-based health care. Discussion paper, Institute of Medicine, Washington, DC.

World Health Organization (2007). Team building. Retrieved from http://www.who.int/cancer/modules/Team%20building.pdf.

10

Working and communicating in virtual teams

M. Gayl Bowser

Outline

Learning outcomes

After reading this chapter, you should be able to:

1. Define virtual team and virtual teamwork.
2. List at least three aspects of virtual work that affect how individual teams work together.
3. Name types of technology used by virtual teams.
4. Describe advantages and disadvantages of virtual teamwork for individuals, teams and organizations.
5. Describe four ways in which assistive technology teams can enhance their function by working in a virtual environment.
6. Apply research-based operating characteristics of effective virtual teams, including effective communication and leadership strategies.

Assistive Technologies and Environmental Interventions in Healthcare: An Integrated Approach, First Edition.
Edited by Lynn Gitlow and Kathleen Flecky.

Companion website: www.wiley.com/go/gitlow/assitivetechnologies

Active learning prompts

Before you read this chapter:

1. Think of one of the teams you work with either professionally or in your private life.
   a. How frequently does your team use computer-mediated communication strategies? What percentage of time does your team meet face-to-face?
2. What is your experience of working in a virtual team? What do you like about it? What are the disadvantages that you see?
3. How have you used virtual teamwork strategies in your professional work? Have you ever participated on a team focused on the needs of an individual with a disability that used computer-mediated strategies for communication and teamwork? What is your perception of how these strategies worked for the person served by the team?
4. Which aspects of assistive technology selection, acquisition, and use might best be done through face-to-face teamwork? Which might lend themselves to a virtual team environment?

Key terms

Virtual teams

Virtual teamwork

Introduction

Virtual teams are defined as two or more persons who work together on a mutual goal or work assignment, interact from different locations, and therefore communicate and cooperate by means of information and communication technology (Bell and Kozlowski 2002; Hertel et al. 2005). The following is a description of the activities that one virtual team leader engaged in on a selected day.

A day in the life of a virtual team member

1. I completed a phone interview with a new consultant who might be joining the team.
2. I did follow-up by email with the consultant to confirm agreed-upon next steps.
3. I used the Doodle easy scheduling tool to identify a day and time (http://doodle.com) for the next team meeting.
4. I reviewed the client's current rehabilitation plan and suggested changes using the *Track Changes* function in the team's word processing software.
5. I posted the suggested changes in the plan to a Dropbox cloud sharing folder (www.dropbox.com) for team review.
6. I sent an email to all team members (including the new consultant) about the revised plan's location in the cloud and announced the schedule for the meeting.
7. I hosted a video conference meeting with the team for planning a trial period of assistive technology (AT) use.
8. I did online research about the variety of AT devices that are available and might meet the client's needs.
9. I used a university online publications database to locate research for evidence about the efficacy of using this type of device for clients with this disability.
10. I wrote a request to the rehabilitation agency for funds to rent the device the team has identified and submitted the request electronically by attaching it to an email.
11. I completed a virtual home visit with the family of this individual. Three other team members used the same video conferencing tool to participate in the home visit.
12. After the conference, I sent a tweet (www.twitter.com) to two team members. I invited them to meet me for coffee after work so that we could catch up on news of our families and friends.

Working and communicating in virtual teams

The use of document sharing sites, web-based meeting tools, email, video conferencing, and social media sites is changing the nature of the way AT teams work. It is now possible to create a team that includes people from multiple remote locations who can share ideas, jointly create documents and explore options for people with disabilities. Some virtual teams may even work without ever coming together in person. Currently, most teams work virtually to some degree. Many teams use computer mediated communication for most of their work and others–especially those whose members are located in different countries or at great geographic distances – may never meet in a face-to-face environment. In the previous chapter, the characteristics of effective teams and effective teamwork were discussed. While these characteristics apply equally as well to virtual teams, there is evidence that virtual teams have unique ways of operating and functioning.

Many researchers have attempted to define the term *virtual teamwork* by identifying the various dimensions of the team's functioning. Dimensions identified have included synchronous communication, face-to-face meetings, proportion of members who work in the same location, degree of physical distance, and percentage of use of computer-mediated communication tools (Cohen and Gibson 2003; Kirkman and Mathieu 2005; Martins et al. 2004). For each of these dimensions, a continuum of virtual teamwork exists that can impact the functioning and effectiveness of the team. Figure 10.1 illustrates the range of ways that virtual teams can be structured.

Chudoba et al. (2005), identified six additional factors that affect the way virtual teams interact once the basic work structure has been established. They include geography, time zone, culture, work practices, organization, and technology. If all team members live in the same city, virtual team meetings can be alternated with face-to-face contacts. But if all team members live in different countries, time zones, national holidays, and daily work schedules will all affect how often and for how long the team can meet, and such teams may meet less frequently or collaborate in different ways between team meetings.

No matter what the team structure, team membership is ongoing; effectiveness is measured; and there are specific team goals that are valued by the members. In all effective teams, members discuss, decide upon, and do real work together. However, despite their commonalities with face-to-face teams, successful virtual teams present some unique challenges. Technology applications, communication strategies, and team leadership must all be addressed differently when a team works in a virtual environment.

When working in a virtual environment to provide AT services for an individual, the team may include people from multiple service settings, multiple agencies, and even multiple geographic locations. It is not uncommon for a team to include family members, the school, and medical service providers in the individual's hometown, experts in a particular AT area from a nearby clinical setting, and specialists who may be located in distant geographic locations. When location, costs of travel, and time constraints affect the ability of these team members to work together, virtual teamwork strategies may provide a solution.

Project ECHO® (Extension for Community Healthcare Outcomes) (http://echo.unm.edu/) is an example of a virtual medical teamwork project. It is funded by the Robert Wood Johnson Foundation, the New Mexico Legislature, the University of New Mexico, and the New Mexico Department of Public Health. Project ECHO helps physicians and other medical providers such as community health nurses and physician's assistants to "safely and effectively treat chronic, common, and complex diseases in rural and underserved areas, and to monitor outcomes of their treatment" (Arora n.d.). Research about Project ECHO has demonstrated that it "can improve access to primary and specialty care for patients with complex needs while also reducing the cost of care by utilizing a multidisciplinary team- based approach" (Arora n.d.). Project ECHO offers virtual clinics in topics such as Dementia Care Diabetes and Cardiovascular Care, Hepatitis C Community Clinic, HIV/AIDS, and Rheumatology. The use of video conferencing technology allows local medical providers to talk with experts in healthcare about their patients without leaving their offices. The project has

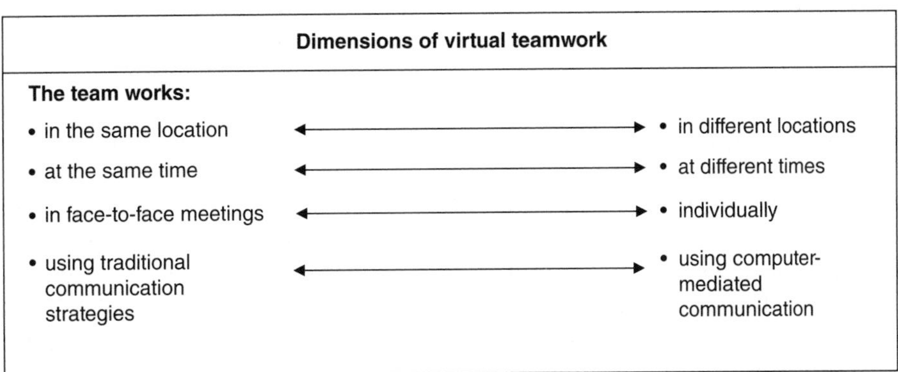

Figure 10.1 Dimensions of virtual teamwork.

demonstrated that the virtual clinic model supports best-practice care and reduces disparities and variation in care for underserved populations. Project ECHO does not see patients. Its Tele-ECHO clinics connect primary care partners (PCPs) to specialists who help co-manage rural and underserved patients with common chronic conditions.

Benefits and drawbacks of virtual teamwork

Virtual teams offer additional benefits for the individual, the team, and the organization that sponsors the team (Hertel et al. 2005). Numerous authors have examined the advantages and drawbacks to working in a virtual environment (DeRosa 2008; DeRosa and Lepsinger 2010; Hertel et al. 2005; West 2012).

Advantages to virtual teamwork

- *For the individual*, virtual teamwork offers flexibility and autonomy. Not only are schedules for working independently flexible, but the work environment can be flexible too. In the example of virtual teamwork activities provided at the beginning of this chapter, several of the non-confidential actions of the virtual team member were completed in a coffee shop where the team leader used a computer with access to the Internet.

  Virtual teamwork allows the individual to create a personal balance between work and non- work life. Parents of young children can work during nap time or after children go to bed.

  Consultants can provide services to clients in other locations by taking a break from the vacation they take with their family to attend a virtual meeting.

  For everyone who participates on a virtual team, there is less travel time and less expense involved in attending meetings. Treatment models such as Project ECHO are designed to meet the needs of clients in very remote locations. With needed supports, people with disabilities are more easily included on the team because they do not have to travel long distances to meet with their service providers.
- *For the team as a whole,* virtual teamwork also has benefits. Virtual teamwork generally implies more flexibility in scheduling and meeting arrangements. Perhaps the greatest benefit for the team of virtual teamwork is the flexibility of including new team members. In a virtual team, members can be selected because of their skills rather than because of their geographic location. This means that there is a larger pool of skilled people to choose from. Teams have the potential for increased diversity, and the integration of the person with a disability on an AT team is frequently easier because of the virtual work style.

  Because it is possible to meet with all team members without travel time or expenses, virtual teams are more often able to include all team members in team discussions and decisions. When an AT team makes a decision about use of an AT device, it is possible for the people who will be responsible for daily supports and services to discuss their concerns and needs with experts who make recommendations. As a result, virtual team strategies can increase buy-in for implementing consultant recommendations and increase consultants' understanding of the important factors in the individual's environment.
- *For the organization,* virtual teamwork allows teams to increase their speed of response to issues that arise. If team members do not have to be in the same location to respond, as a team, to a problem that arises, it is possible to solve problems more quickly. Site or home visits are less often needed, which reduces the cost of travel and office expenses (Hertel et al. 2005).

Overall participation on successful virtual teams can mean empowerment for team members, the teams, and the agencies that sponsor them. However, there are also disadvantages to working in a virtual team environment. Note Figure 10.2 for a visual example of team collaboration.

Drawbacks of virtual teamwork

- *For the individual,* virtual teamwork can offer more flexibility, but virtual teamwork strategies that allow teams to meet at any time may result in increased invasion of non- work time by the virtual team (Hertel et al. 2005).

  Research has shown that if team members can see just a quick glance of the actions of their colleagues, they will be able to coordinate their respective tasks (Kiesler and Cummings 2002). This is not possible in a virtual team, which adds one more factor to the difficulty of team collaboration.

  Virtual team members may experience feelings of isolation when face-to-face meetings are not a part of the team's work plans. Decreased interpersonal contact with other team members can result in reduced informal conversations and reduced opportunities to build friendships. Because members are often at a distance in their daily lives, virtual team members have more limited communication options. This factor increases the potential for misunderstandings and conflict between team members (Hertel et al. 2005).

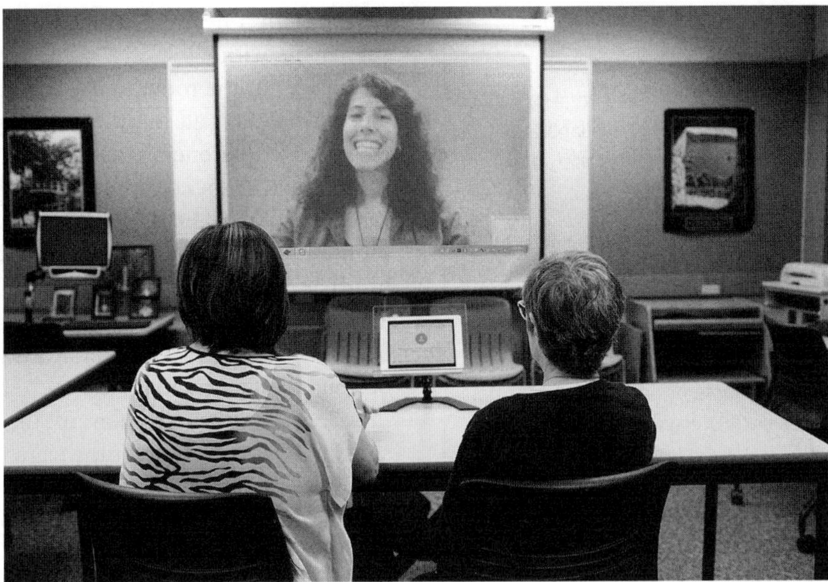

Figure 10.2 Virtual team collaboration.

- *For the team as a whole,* communication problems may be exaggerated. Computer-mediated communication strategies often result in a loss of non-verbal cues to meaning, and communication problems may be exaggerated. It is more difficult to establish shared meaning without non-verbal cues so building consensus among team members as to the course of action to be taken may be more difficult (Nunamaker et al. 2009).

  There is a potential for teams to be less productive because of the complicated nature of the communication technology. When too much meeting time is spent in providing technical assistance and troubleshooting, teams lose valuable time for teamwork. While teams have the potential to assemble and respond to difficulties more quickly, if strategies are not developed to prevent it from happening, both synchronous and asynchronous communication technologies can delay the response and work of the team (Hertel et al. 2005).

  Because they do not know each other as well, because they do not have as many non-verbal cues to respond to, and because the work of the team may not be equally visible to all team members, there is a potential for reduced team-member ownership of the goals and reduced productivity (Dempster 2005).
- *For the organization,* reduced costs of travel and office space may be offset by increased need for more sophisticated technology. Hardware, software, and team-member training may be needed in order to ensure effective teamwork (Nunamaker et al. 2009).

  Virtual teams that work in human service environments have the potential to breach confidentiality unintentionally. Insecure networks, emails forwarded to people who are not on the team, and information sharing sites without proper encryption can result in violations of privacy rules for the individual with a disability (Brebner n.d.).

  Supervision and team leadership for virtual teams are more difficult. Virtual team leaders may never meet some of the team members they supervise. This can result in a variety of interpersonal issues that must be addressed directly with the team member (Dempster 2005).

In his discussion of effective teamwork, Vicente (2006) stated, "Key factors such as communication, authority, responsibility and priority setting must all be taken care of, otherwise the team members won't be able to coordinate their respective actions" (p. 155). The need to address these key factors for teams in virtual work environments is even greater than for teams that work face-to-face. Review the research evidence for teamwork in Box 10.1.

Considerations for using virtual team strategies in client-focused teams

Virtual team strategies can be used in many ways. Virtual teams can write grants, create new software, make plans for programmatic changes, or investigate the uses of new technologies.

When teams use virtual meeting and working strategies in order to address the needs of specific clients, the client's knowledge of the technology, the accessibility of the virtual teamwork technology, and confidentiality must be carefully addressed.

Box 10.1 Here's the evidence

Catagnus, R.M., and Hantula, D.A. (2011). The virtual Individual Education Plan (IEP) team: Using online collaboration to develop a behavior intervention plan. *International Journal of e-Collaboration (IJeC)* 7(1):30–46.doi:10.4018/jec.2011010103.

Key Words: behavior intervention plan, e-collaboration, online platform, virtual collaboration, virtual IEP team

Purpose: Explore use of an online venue for a virtual team to develop a student behavioral intervention plan.

Sample/Setting: Convenience sample of professional educators working in a private school for children with disabilities.

Bottom Line: Virtual team collaboration offers an efficient model for professional educators.

Critical Thinking Questions:

1. Having read this research article, what do you understand to be the limitations of this research? Are there any limitations not stated?
2. What implications does this article have for practice?

Client's familiarity with technology

Client, family, and advocates' participation on an AT team helps to ensure effective use of AT and reduce the likelihood of technology abandonment (Scherer 2004). If clients and their supporters are to be effective participants in virtual teamwork activities, the team must ensure that they have access to the technology needed for virtual activities and that they understand its use.

When clients are expected to use technology independently in projects like the Virtual Home Visiting Project (Fiechtl et al. 2011), an essential component of the team's activities must be training and, when needed, the provision of technology and resources used by other team members. One way to ensure optimal client participation is to arrange for the client and at least one technology-savvy team member to be in the same location and use the technology together when virtual teamwork activities occur. Without the needed support, technology may become an additional barrier to client participation.

Accessibility

When a client or other virtual team member with a disability participates in virtual teamwork, special care must be taken to make sure that the technologies used are accessible and compliant with legal mandates such as the Americans with Disabilities Act (ADA) and Section 504 of the Rehabilitation Act (Section 504) (ADA 1990; Rehabilitation Act 1973). For example, working in a virtual team, using conference calls would pose no barriers for a person with a visual impairment; however, a person with a hearing impairment would be unable to participate without special accommodations such as an interpreter in the room or the use of a relay operator to write what is said in the meeting. Virtual meeting or video conferencing tools such as *Adobe Connect* (http://www.adobe.com/products/adobeconnect.html) and Blackboard Collaborate (https://www.blackboard.com/online-collaborative-learning/blackboard-collaborate.html) each have different accessibility features. Some allow users to use their AT devices in the meeting while others do not. If a client or team member needs this option, the team should ensure that the conferencing product allows connection of the specific device or software that is needed for the team member.

Confidentiality

When the work of a team focuses on individual clients, special care must be taken to ensure the confidentiality of client information. A number of professional organizations such as the Ethics Committee for Dieticians (Ashley 2002), the National Association of Social Workers and the Association of Social Work Boards (2005), and the National Association of School Psychologists (Harvey and Carlson 2003) have begun to develop standards of practice for virtual client consultations and treatment. Brebner (n.d.) hypothesizes that in cases where medical treatment is provided by a physician through digital means (i.e. telemedicine):

> … obligations, appropriately, are placed on both the distance provider and the local site. The service must be provided in a private setting with a digital line. The consumer must be educated about the nature and purpose of the equipment, any potential breaches of confidentiality inherent in the technologies deployed and questioned regarding the level of satisfaction with the service.

The professional ethics of each team member do not change because the team is a virtual one. Each profession has its own rules, standards, and guidance regarding confidentiality, and these apply to services provided through the use of technology as well as in face-to-face settings.

Virtual AT teams

To the degree that they are used by an AT team, virtual teamwork strategies can allow people who live and work at a distance from each other to come together to focus on an individual's AT goals. Most teams focused on selection, acquisition, and use of AT devices meet in a face-to-face setting on occasion, and use virtual meeting strategies to augment the team's work toward achieving goals. However, it may be possible that some team members attend all meetings virtually in order to augment the information, skills, and plans of the face-to-face team.

When teams work in a virtual environment, they may include only regular team members, or they may include outside members, such as a consultants, personal care assistants, or specialists. Virtual teamwork can help AT teams to include new people in the work of the team without extensive travel or costs. Teams concerned with providing and supporting the use of AT for individuals with disabilities may be able to identify and include expert consultants through the use of video conferencing, voice conference calls, or even commonly used social media options such as Skype or ooVoo. This strategy can allow a clinical provider such as an occupational therapist (OT) or a speech-language pathologist who is an augmentative and alternative communication (AAC) specialist to participate and provide guidance during a meeting that takes place in the individual's home, school, or local rehabilitation center.

One other common use of computer-mediated strategies by AT teams is for training. If team members need training in order to operate an AT device, there are multiple virtual options available. Vendor websites often offer step-by-step training videos for their products and there are many university- and government-sponsored websites which provide similar training options. Several subscription services exist which provide online training options for a large variety of software and hardware applications. A list of online tutorials about the use of AT devices is provided in the training resources section at the end of this chapter.

Clients, family members, and caregivers can also participate virtually in team consultations and planning about AT. Commonly available social media such as Skype or Google Video Chat can be used to allow their participation as well as helping other team members to complete virtual home visits and view other client environments. In the Virtual Home Visits Project, completed by Utah State University, investigators found the following advantages to the use of virtual home visits in an early intervention program.

- Decrease cost: *interventionists travel less, save salary/ benefits, mileage reimbursement*
- Prevent missed visits: *weather, illness*
- Increase compliance with IDEA timelines: *service delivery, 45-day IFSP, 90-day transition*
- Increase service opportunities: *children and families in rural/frontier areas*
- Enhance parent skills: *promote parent use of developmental strategies*
- Facilitate team participation in meetings: *scheduling, distance* (Fiechtl et al. 2011)

Especially after AT has been selected and integration of the technology into everyday routines and activities is the goal, use of virtual home visits can help AT teams to work together, problem-solve, and plan for increased integration of AT. Successful virtual home visits require new skills for the AT service provider. In addition to understanding and operating the technology used by the team, the Virtual Home Visits Project also found that project's service providers needed additional training in the use of coaching strategies (Fiechtl et al. 2011). Please review the Toolbox at the end of this chapter for resources for training in a virtual environment.

Steps for creating a virtual team

Virtual teamwork has long been used as a strategy in business. Pape (1997) describes the strategy used by the Verifone company to develop and manage virtual teams in a multinational work environment. The company's process includes the following steps:

1. Define a purpose
2. Recruit members
3. Determine duration
4. Select technology tools.

Clearly defined steps and guidelines like those used by Verifone can help AT teams to use virtual strategies to enhance their work. In the following discussion, these steps have been listed and discussed in terms of their application to AT processes.

1. Define a purpose for the virtual AT team
   It is important for the team to identify precisely what defines success in its work. Will all AT selection, acquisition, and use activities be addressed by the virtual team, or will face-to-face meetings be used for some of the work? AT teams that plan to work virtually should ensure that all startup issues have been addressed and recorded. The team leader may need to remind people frequently of their responsibilities to the team and the scope of the virtual teamwork.
2. Recruit members to the virtual team
   The size of a virtual AT team will depend on the needs of the individual and the expertise of the existing team members. Most virtual teams should have between three and seven members to work most effectively (Pape 1997). A team with too many members can make it difficult for each individual to contribute meaningfully. However, education and

rehabilitation agencies and others who provide AT services may need to be included to ensure adequate services as well as funding for the devices. As the team membership is defined, it may be necessary to identify a core AT team as well as individuals who will be included in team communications but may not be heavily involved in the day-to-day work of the team.

Once the team has been defined and identified, team-building activities and team training can be an essential component of building an effective team. Team members may not be together often during their work, and, because of distances between their physical work sites, may not have the opportunity to have impromptu conversations. It is essential that they have opportunities to get to know each other in more structured ways to ensure effective team function.

3. Define the ways the team will function
   Verifone uses the term *duration* to describe not only the timelines for the team's work but also how the team will function, who will lead, and individual team-member responsibilities. An AT team should describe team duration before work toward goals is begun.

   Teams should also describe what they feel they will be able to do in a virtual work environment and other activities that may need to be completed face-to-face.

For example, when one team began to look for AT that would help their client to remember his daily schedule, they felt that they could examine a wide range of devices without a face-to-face meeting. Once the team settled on three device choices, some team members took the client shopping to try them. The team came together in a teleconference to discuss the outcome of his trial use of each device, select one option, and identify a funding source. All applications for funding and purchase activities were completed without a face-to-face meeting. When the device had been acquired, members of the AT team provided five face-to-face training sessions for the client, his family, and his caregivers. Following initial training, videoconference home visits were held every other week to help him use the device in everyday routines and activities.

Leadership and virtual team function

Team leadership becomes even more important when team members are unlikely to see or interact with each other in person. It's important for a virtual team to have an assigned leader who is responsible to help the team set performance expectations and model virtual team behaviors. A virtual team leader can enhance the work of the team with frequent check-ins that help members keep track of work progress and goals.

Effective virtual team leaders communicate with team members on a predictable schedule between team activities (Hambley et al. 2007). One role of virtual team leaders is to help members understand their roles within the structure of the team. AT team members frequently come from several different agencies or organizations. In a virtual work environment, AT team members may feel isolated and become disengaged without frequent support and communication.

Communication challenges are more pronounced in virtual AT teams. Effective virtual teams find ways to overcome these challenges with frequent check-ins, confirmations of communications received, and interpersonal communications outside of the formal team meetings. Trust is a top factor for virtual team success but trust builds when team members follow through on commitments and hold one another accountable for results (DeRosa 2008; DeRosa et al. 2004).

To ensure that team functions and operations are implemented in an AT team, training is needed. Training in the use of the communication technology is only one aspect of team training in virtual teams. Training in the human factors of virtual teamwork is essential.

> In any complex technological system, the system design isn't complete unless or until the training program is specified.
>
> (Vicente 2006 p. 162)

4. Select technology tools for the team and train people how to use them

A common error among virtual teams is selection of technology for computer-mediated communication before the purpose, membership, and function of the team is defined. Teams should wait to select communication technology modes until a complete picture of the team has been described. Choosing electronic communication strategies after teams are established ensures that the technologies used will best fit the needs of all team members and functions.

The choice of technology should be based on the team's goals and on the ways and amount that a team plans to function in a virtual environment (National Research Council 2015; Watkins 2013).

There are synchronous meeting tools such as Adobe Connect, Elluminate, GoTo Meeting and Webex that allow users to hear each other and see the work being created on a computer screen. Virtual meeting tools are particularly useful for meetings where a document like an AT Implementation Plan is being developed. Video chat options such as Skype, Google Chat, and FaceTime, allow team members to see each other during discussion but do not allow everyone to see a document or video of a client. Video chat tools are particularly good for smaller meetings that are used for progress reports or team check-in because they can provide information about the everyday environment(s) where the AT is to be used. Asynchronous group productivity tools such as Google Docs can be used to create drafts and edit documents between meetings when members are not all able to meet at the same time (National Research Council 2015).

When groups consider choices of technologies that can offer help to build an online team, it is generally true that the simplest tool that will support planned team activities is the best one (Watkins 2013). Tools which are difficult to understand or use because they have more options than the team needs, have the potential to interfere with teamwork and make virtual team activities more difficult.

Regardless of the tools that are chosen for the team's activities, the context of the work is more important than the tool. Virtual teams should spend some initial time reviewing and selecting technology applications that will facilitate the work that they are doing. Once the tools are chosen, virtual teams need access to tech support so that they do not lose valuable teamwork time with technical difficulties. In many successful virtual teams, a new team role may emerge. One or more individuals who are experienced with the technology may be assigned as the tech-support person on the team to teach others how to manage the technology in non-meeting time.

What makes virtual teams successful?

> The basic conditions for effective teamwork include having a real team whose membership is clear, which is of the right size, relatively stable in membership and working on a task that requires teamwork. The team must have an overall purpose that adds value and which is translated into clear challenging team objectives. And the team needs the right people as team members with the required skills in the right roles. They must be enablers not derailers – people who support effective team working through their behaviors, not people who sabotage, undermine or obstruct teams functioning.
>
> (West 2012, p. 4)

DeRosa and Lepsinger (2010) identified nine practices for optimal virtual team performance.

1. Team members demonstrate a high level of initiative.
2. Team members are willing to assume leadership responsibility.
3. Teams have a shared process for decision-making and problem-solving.
4. Team members are clear about how their work contributes to the success of the organization.
5. Team members provide timely feedback to one another.
6. Team members trust one another to get things done.
7. Team members are willing to put in extra effort to get things done.
8. Team members work together effectively.
9. Team members help one another achieve team goals.

These practices, combined with expertise in AT and a commitment to address the independence and functional capabilities of individuals with disabilities, can enable AT teams to use computer-mediated communication and virtual teamwork strategies to enhance their work.

> Yes, there are many questions that remain to be investigated; but if we concentrate on the human factor and make it central to the technological world in which we now live, that world could be a completely different place – safer, healthier, more productive and sustainable and more humane.
>
> (Vicente 2006, p. 5)

Summary

As we have seen in Chapters 9 and 10, teams are critical to the successful use of technology and environmental intervention (TEI). Bringing together a variety of people, including clients, professionals, and caregivers,

Box 10.2 Case study

Instructions: Using the information from the chapter and the Toolbox, describe how this team scenario might use virtual methods to work on its goals.

The staff at Smithville Hospital and Rehabilitation center was aware that many of the AT recommendations they made were not implemented. They were frustrated that they worked hard in the AT clinic to identify the best technology solutions for their patients but that work seemed to go to waste. They decided to initiate a review of the AT services they provided, to examine the kinds of recommendations they were making and the ones that were most likely to be followed, and to interview patients who were both successful and unsuccessful with AT use. The data review showed that many of the reports they wrote were written in medical jargon that their patients did not really understand and that patients who did understand the recommendations often felt that the technology was too complicated for them to use. As a result of this investigation, they adopted a new approach to AT recommendations that they described as "The simplest tool to overcome the barrier." They also developed an ongoing data collection and follow-up system to determine whether the changes they made had the desired effects for patient.

to solve human problems turns out to create solutions that are greater than the sum of the parts (Vicente 2006). This being said, teams face many challenges, which need to be worked out in order for their work to be effective (Demris 2006). The previous chapter, on face-to-face teams, provides guidelines and strategies that can help all TEI teams function effectively. In this chapter, we see that the use of technology has transformed and expanded the traditional notion of team to one that utilizes various forms of communications technology to cast a wider net in order to meet clients' TEI needs. While virtual teams have additional challenges, this chapter demonstrates the potential they have to meet the needs of clients who formerly may not have had access to resources now available through these virtual teams. Although more research is needed to address the challenges presented by virtual teaming (Demris 2006), the opportunities presented by these teams continue to flourish and grow. Please review Box 10.2 for a case to apply your understanding of information in this chapter.

References

Americans with Disabilities Act of 1990 (1990). Pub. L. No. 101-336, 104 Stat. 328.

Arora, S. (n.d.). Project ECHO. University of New Mexico. Retrieved from http://echo.unm.edu/FAQ.html.

Ashley, R.C. (2002). Telemedicine: Legal, ethical, and liability considerations. *Journal of the American Dietetic Association* 102: 267–269.

Bell, B.S. and Kozlowski, S.W.J. (2002). A typology of virtual teams: Implications for effective leadership. *Group and Organization Management* 27: 14–49.

Brebner, E. (n.d.). Confidentiality, and legal components of telemedicine. University of Aberdeen. Retrieved from http://www.vannas.se/Sve/Filarkiv/V%C3%A5rd-%20och%20omsorgsn%C3%A4mnden/Confident.pdf.

Chudoba, K.A., Wynn, E., Lu, M., and Watson-Manheim, M.B. (2005). How virtual are we? Measuring virtuality and understanding its impact in a global organization. *Information Systems Journal* 15: 279–306.

Cohen, S.G. and Gibson, C.B. (2003). In the beginning: introduction and framework. In: *Virtual Teams that Work: Creating Conditions for Virtual Team Effectiveness* (ed. C.B. Gibson and S.G. Cohen), 1–13. San Francisco: Jossey-Bass.

Dempster, M. (2005). Team building key for virtual workplace. *Business Edge Magazine* 5 (27): Retrieved from http://www.businessedge.ca/.

Demris, G. (2006). The diffusions of virtual communities in health care: concepts and challenges. *Patient Education and Counseling* 63: 178–188.

DeRosa, D. (2008). Collaborating from a distance: success factors for top performing virtual teams. Onpoint Consulting. [white paper].

DeRosa, D. and Lepsinger, R. (2010). Leading from a distance: five best practices for virtual team leaders. Retrieved from http://info.onpointconsultingllc.com/docs/Leading_from_a_Distance_Five_Best_Practices_Release.pdf.

DeRosa, D., Hantula, D., and D'Arcy, J. (2004). Trust and leadership in virtual teamwork: a media naturalness perspective. *Human Resource Management* 43: 219–232.

Fiechtl, B., Rule, S. and Olsen, S. (2011). Virtual home visits: participant responses and outcomes. Paper presented at the American Council on Rural Special Education Annual Conference, Albuquerque, NM (March 24–26).

Hambley, L.A., O'Neill, T.A., and Kline, T.J.B. (2007). Virtual team leadership: the effects of leadership style and communication medium on team interaction styles and outcomes. *Organizational Behavior and Human Decision Processes* 103 (1): 1–20.

Harvey, V.S. and Carlson, J.F. (2003). Ethical and professional issues with computer-related technology. *School Psychology Review* 32 (1): 92–107.

Hertel, G., Geister, S., and Konradt, U. (2005). Managing virtual teams: a review of current empirical research. *Human Resource Management Review* 15: 69–95.

Kiesler, S. and Cummings, J.N. (2002). What do we know about proximity and distance in work groups? A legacy of research. In: *Distributed Work* (ed. P. Hinds and S. Keisler), 57–82. Cambridge, MA: MIT Press.

Kirkman, B.L. and Mathieu, J.E. (2005). The dimensions and antecedents of team virtuality. *Journal of Management* 31: 700–718.

Martins, L.L., Gilson, L.L., and Maynard, M.T. (2004). Virtual teams: what do we know and where do we go from here? *Journal of Management* 30: 805–835.

National Association of Social Workers (NASW) & The Association of Social Work Boards (ASWB) (2005). *NASW and ASWB Standards for Technology and Social Work Practice*. Washington, DC: NASW Press.

National Research Council (2015). *Enhancing the Effectiveness of Team Science* (ed. N.J. Cooke and M.L. Hilton) Committee on the Science of Team Science Board on Behavioral, Cognitive, and Sensory Sciences, Division of Behavioral and Social Sciences and Education. Washington, DC: The National Academies Press Retrieved from https://www.nap.edu/read/19007/chapter/1.

Nunamaker, J.F., Reinig, B.A., and Briggs, R.O. (2009). Principles for effective virtual teamwork. *Communications of the ACM* 52 (4): 113–117.

Pape, W. (1997). Group insurance. *Inc.* (15 June). Retrieved from http://www.inc.com/magazine/19970615/1409.html.

Rehabilitation Act of 1973 (1973). Pub. L. No. 93-112, 87 Stat. 394.

Scherer, M. (2004). *Matching Persons with Technology Processes and Accompanying Assessment Instruments (Rev. ed.)*. Webster, NY: Institute for Matching Person & Technology.

Vicente, K. (2006). *The Human Factor: Revolutionizing the Way People Live with Technology*. New York: Routledge, Taylor & Francis Group.

Watkins, M. (2013). Making virtual teams work: ten basic principles. *Harvard Business Review* (27 June). Retrieved from https://hbr.org/2013/06/making-virtual-teams-work-ten#.

West, M.A. (2012). *Effective Teamwork: Practical Lessons from Organizational Research*. Oxford: Blackwell.

Toolbox: Resources for Training in a Virtual Environment

Sources of Online Videos and Tutorials about AT

Compiled by Gayl Bowser, Independent Consultant

AbililtyNet Fact Sheets and Skill Sheets – www.abilitynet.org.uk/expert-resources/factsheets AbilityNet is a UK pan-disability charity which is committed to creating a world where information and communication technologies (ICT) is not a barrier to people but rather enables them to live their lives to achieve their full potential whether at home, through education, or in work. Videos include:

- Choosing your preferred colors in Windows
- Choosing your preferred colors in your browser
- Choosing your preferred text style in Windows
- Choosing your preferred text style in your browser
- Making the text insertion point and text select cursor more visible in word processors

AEM Product Tutorials – http://aem.cast.org/about/quick-start-educators.html#.XKZNBcR7k2w

Assistive Technology in Arizona – http://www.atarizona.com/
AT Arizona staff training program videos and documents for general disability, blind or visually impaired clients, deaf or hard of hearing clients, ergonomics and physical considerations, learning disabilities, cognitive challenges, augmentative and alternative communication and computer skills for professionals.

Atomic Learning – https://www.atomiclearning.com/accessible-instruction
Atomic Learning offers a subscription service for technology training. However each video tutorial series offers a few free sample tutorials and demonstrations. Atomic Learning's Assistive Technology Collection includes short show-and-tell video tutorials with voice narration.

Boardmaker 6.0 Tutorials – https://screencast-o-matic.com/channels/cXnQlzVbB
Video Board Maker 6.0 + tutorials created by Aaron E. Marsters

Bookshare – http://www.bookshare.org/_/help/training/upcoming Webinars

Bookshare offers a variety of online training opportunities including complimentary webinars and video training modules to help clients use text-to-speech software applications
California School Library Association – http://discoveringat.csla.net
This tutorial is offered by the California School Library Association and TransAccess, a community-based organization that provides persons with disabilities access to computer adaptive technology and career transition services so that they can achieve their desired education and employment and improve their quality of life. Modules include Assistive Technology Hardware Solutions and Assistive Technology Software Solutions

Freedom Machines – www.freedommachines.com
Freedom Machines presents histories of people ages 8–93, whose talents and independence are enhanced by access to enabling technologies. The site posts video clips of real people using assistive technology.

Georgia Project for Assistive Technology (GPAT) – www.gpat.org
The GPAT, a unit of the Georgia Department of Education, supports local school systems in their efforts to provide AT devices and services to students with disabilities. The devices section of the website offers multiple tools lists, tip sheets, and links to vendor sites.

High Incidence Assistive Technology (HIAT) – http://www.montgomeryschoolsmd.org/departments/hiat/tech_quick_guides
The High Incidence Assistive Technology Program of Montgomery County Public Schools in Maryland is an extensive collection of Technology Quick Guides and Video Tutorials at its resource website. The guides are available to all site visitors and are appropriate for adults as well as students in school.

Iris Center – https://iris.peabody.vanderbilt.edu
The IRIS Center for Training Enhancements offers free online interactive resources that translate research about the education of students with disabilities into practice. The materials cover a wide variety of evidence-based topics, including behavior, response to intervention (RTI), learning strategies, and progress monitoring. The AT module offers an overview of AT and explores ways to expand students' access to it in the classroom.

Kurzweil Education Systems – https://www.kurzweiledu.com/experience-kurzweil/video-library/video-library.html
The website offers a video Gallery of people using Kurzweil software. This site also links to other Kurzweil success stories.

Landmark College – https://intranet.landmark.edu/tls/OnlineTraining.cfm
Online Tutorials, handouts, tip sheets, and screencasts.

Microsoft Accessibility Products – https://www.microsoft.com/en-us/accessibility

Adobe Acrobat Pro	Inspiration
Choosing AT	Kurzweil 3000
Classroom	Microsoft Office 2010
Instruction Click,	Moodle
Speak Computer	PowerPoint
Basics	WebNotes
Dragon NaturallySpeaking	WordTalk
File Management	
GroupWise	

These step-by-step tutorials introduce the user to some of the most commonly used accessibility features in Microsoft products. The instructions show you how to use the mouse or keyboard to navigate, select options, and change settings. The information is presented in a side-by-side format so that you can see at a glance how to use the mouse, the keyboard, or a combination of both.

Pennsylvania Assistive Technology Network – http://pattanat.framewelder.com
The training videos included on the site were developed to increase the skills of individualized education plan (IEP) and other team members in the following areas: assessing AT needs; selecting and adapting AT for the student; implementing and integrating AT devices and services; and increasing independence for students with disabilities. These videos address specific AT topics from the above areas for the purpose of providing guidance to teams as they work with clients with disabilities.

Premier Assistive Technology – http://www.premierathome.com/support/Videos.php
Premier Assistive Technology offers a series of training videos to show you how to use the company's products. Each video is designed to be from 5 to 10 minutes in length. The videos can be played from the website.

NATRI Video Tutorials – http://natri.uky.edu/assoc_projects/viewer/index.html
Visit the Assistive Technology Viewer from the NATRI (National Assistive Technology Research Institute) to see short videos for Input Devices, Communication, Mobility, and Vision Aids, Switches, Alternative Keyboards, Workplace Technology, and Software.

SET-BC – www.setbc.org
The SET-BC website offers tip sheets and videos about AT. Videos on this site are organized by topic.

Tobii ATI Training Resources – https://www.tobiidynavox.com/en-US/support-training/webinars/
This vendor's video tutorials, quick-start guides, and manuals help clients use their products.

Washington Assistive Technology Act Program – http://worksource.uwctds.washington.edu/videos.htm
Video Tutorials about ReadPlease, WordQ, WYNN, ZoomText, JAWS, and Kurzweil. Learning Videos about Seating and Positioning, Pointing Devices, Keyboards, and Accessibility Options.

11

Technology and environmental intervention: Psychosocial considerations

Michèle Verdonck

Outline

Assistive Technologies and Environmental Interventions in Healthcare: An Integrated Approach, First Edition.
Edited by Lynn Gitlow and Kathleen Flecky.

Companion website: www.wiley.com/go/gitlow/assitivetechnologies

Learning outcomes

After reading this chapter, you should be able to:

1. Discuss the value of applying a client-centered approach to technology and environmental interventions (TEI) through seeking to understand the lived experience.
2. Describe psychosocial challenges involved in TEI use.
3. Explain the phenomena of continued TEI use despite challenges encountered.
4. Compare the experience of "hassles" with the experience of "engagement" in TEI use.
5. Describe how TEI users evaluate the personal fit of TEI.
6. Discuss the varied meanings attributed to TEI use in the lived experience.
7. List five take-home messages applicable to your experience as a TEI user or as a service provider.

Active learning prompts

Before you read this chapter:

1. Think about what it would be like to use a smartphone for the first time with no previous experience. Answer the following questions:
   - Do you know how to use it?
   - Do you want to use it?
   - Is it easy or difficult?
   - Does it make sense?
   - Is it fun?
   - Do you like using it?
   - How does learning to use it make you feel?
   - How would you like it to work?
2. After reviewing the following case scenario, answer the questions that follow.
   Dylan has a 15-year-old automatic car, affectionately called "the Rust-bucket." The Rust-bucket is not a great looking car but is very comfortable to drive in traffic. Long journeys, however, are tedious as the Rust-bucket has a low top speed. Dylan decides to replace the car with a new sporty convertible. The new car, a manual (stick shift), looks great and was sold to Dylan as "an easy car to drive." Dylan loves the look of the new car and he feels great sitting in the driver's seat.
   During his first week driving the car he stalls several times a day while adjusting to the new demand of using a clutch, a far cry from "easy to drive." He also discovers that driving in traffic in a manual car is far more demanding than driving his old automatic. On the other hand, he is enjoying the onlookers who cast appreciative looks when he is sitting in traffic with the top down. He has also begun to travel further afield on the weekends on longer trips.
   - Discuss how Dylan feels about the new car.
   - What do you think the long-term outcome of this new car will be?
   - Relate this story to a person replacing their old TEI with new TEI.
   - Can you identify some themes which may be universal to all users of TEI?
3. After reviewing the following case scenario, answer the questions that follow.
   Susan has mastered control of her previously unused in-car satellite navigation system in rush-hour traffic to find another way home. She had previously considered the technology to be "not for me."
   - How might she feel after this experience?
   - How might she feel about that device now?
4. Consider the following statements and answer the questions that follow.
   If we ask users what they think about their TEI or about the possibility of using TEI, their responses will range from "it is amazing" and "I wouldn't be without it," to "I hate using it," "that wouldn't suit me," "it is not reliable," and "I wish it was more normal looking."
   - Why might users respond in this way?
   - What psychological or social factors impact TEI use?
5. Watch the TED video: Sue Austin deep sea diving … in a wheelchair: http://www.ted.com/talks/sue_austin_deep_sea_diving_in_a_wheelchair.html
   - What assumptions do you have about what it is like to use a wheelchair?
   - What does having a wheelchair mean to Sue?
   - What new associations can you attribute to wheelchair use having watched this video? (prompts: stigma, enjoyment, freedom)

Key terms

Abandonment
Autonomy
Becoming
Being
Belonging
Doing
Engagement
Environmental control system (ECS)/ Environmental control units ECU/ electronic aids to daily living (EADL)
Incorporation
Lived experience
Non-use
Phenomenology
Psychosocial considerations
Technology and environmental interventions (TEI)
Wheelchairs

Technology and environmental intervention: Psychosocial considerations

We are all technology users. The technology we use is diverse, ranging from smartphones to wrist watches for some people or bent spoons to powered wheelchairs for others. As users of technology we are all able to relate to the psychosocial factors involved with technology and environmental intervention (TEI). This chapter will draw on your own experiences as a technology consumer as well as your understanding of the use of technology from other consumers. Some effort has been made previously to delineate between different types of technology and patterns related to the use of specific types of devices. However, this chapter is written with the assumption that psychosocial factors involved with TEI use can span across all device types and all environmental interventions. Some use will be made of specific examples but in each case the reader is urged to apply the same concepts to other devices or interventions and evaluate the fit themselves.

Psychosocial considerations and the human-tech ladder

Vicente's (2006) Human-Tech Ladder as presented in Chapter 1 has five rungs, the second of which is the psychological rung (see Figure 11.1).

This rung refers to how technology fits/relates to/suits/meets users' psychological status. This chapter focuses on this rung in attending to the individual psychosocial experiences of TEI. *Psychosocial considerations* presented here are the personal factors influencing a person in his or her immediate environment. Psychosocial factors are closely related to sociocultural aspects and may be considered to be part of the same construct; however, for ease of learning, this chapter focuses on the person/consumer/user of TEI and their personal perspective. Chapter 12 details social and cultural aspects focused on the person's wider context and complements this chapter's perspective on the individual aspect.

In addition to the Human-Tech Ladder model, other assistive technology models incorporate psychosocial elements. Their associated assessment tools and outcome measurements can be useful for both research and service provision in considering psychosocial aspects. Refer to Tables 11.1 and 11.2 and additional chapters in this text that address specific assessment tools and outcome measures for more information on these tools.

The focus of this chapter is the psychological rung explored as the personal lived experiences of using TEI supported by evidence provided by qualitative studies of TEI use. Psychosocial considerations are explored in

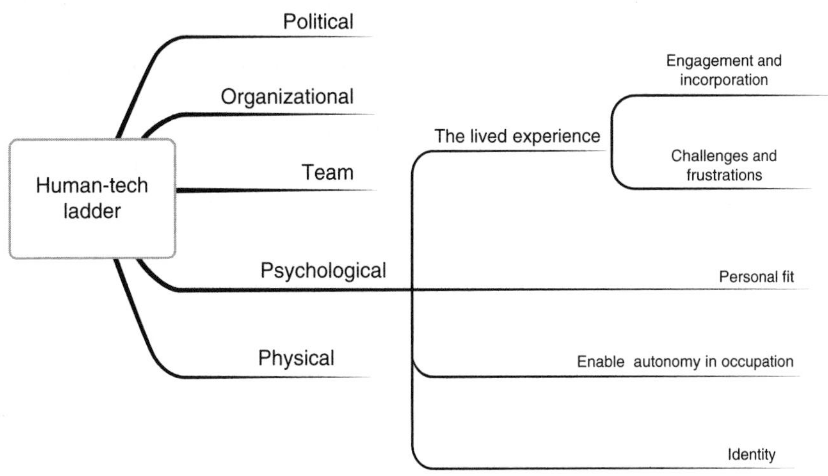

Figure 11.1 Psychosocial considerations and the Human-Tech Ladder. Source: Reproduced with permission of Taylor & Francis.

Table 11.1 Psychosocial Elements Included in Some Technology Models.

Model	Psychosocial elements included in the model
Human Activity Assistive Technology, HAAT model (Cook and Polgar 2015)	Human-tech interface (part of assistive technology domain) Social context Cultural context
International Classification of Functioning, Disability and Health (ICF) (World Health Organization 2001)	Participation Environmental factors – social cultural context Personal factors
Matching Person and Technology Model (Scherer 2005).	• Environmental factors (milieu) • Individual characteristics Motivation, personality, expectations, sense of control, sense of status associated with device use, self-esteem • AT device characteristics Aesthetics, usability
Canadian Model of Occupational Performance (Law et al. 1996)	• Person Affect, spirituality • Environment Social, cultural
Rogers' Perceived Attributes Theory (Lenker and Paquet 2003)	"Relative advantage" (benefit from use) "Compatibility" (social-cultural fit) "Complexity" (ease of use) "Trialability" (opportunity for pre-use trial) "Observability" (how visible the device is) "Re-invention" (modification, possible adaptability of device) "Change agents" (facilitators of device acquisition)
Assistive devices utilization in activities of everyday life (Krantz 2012)	• Person's expectations and experiences o Assistive device – Usable – Useworthy o Activity o Doable o Do-worthy o Relationship of expectation and intention with experience and outcome

Table 11.2 Assessment Tools and Outcome Measures.

Tool/outcome measure	Psychosocial elements included in assessment
Assistive Technology Device Predisposition Assessment (ATD PA) (Scherer et al. 2005)	Temperament and personality factors Psychosocial arena – environment
Québec Users Evaluation of Satisfaction with Assistive Technology (QUEST) (Demers et al. 2002)	Personal satisfaction with milieu, person, and technology
Psychosocial Impact of Assistive Devices Scale (PIADS) (Jutai and Day 2002)	Competence, Efficiency, quality of life, independence Adaptability Well-being, ability in new situations, willingness to take chances Self-esteem Happiness, embarrassment, sense of control, self-confidence self-esteem

four sections below: the lived experience of TEI; personal fit of TEI, TEI to enable and disable occupation, and TEI and identity.

The lived experience of TEI

There is an increased interest in understanding "the *lived experience*," as evidenced by outcome measurement research that acknowledges that this user-centered perspective is an essential component to understanding assistive technology outcomes (Lenker et al. 2013). Exploring lived experience requires an alternative to direct questioning or measurement. This is why phenomenological inquiry can be so informative. *Phenomenology* is a philosophy based on the exploration of the human experience as it is perceived by an individual (Creswell 1998). Similarly, a client-centered approach seeks to understand the user's perspective, which includes understanding what it is like to experience TEI. Thus, phenomenology is a potentially useful philosophical approach for client-centered study of TEI use.

Exploring the lived experience involves consideration of the interaction of several personal factors, including personality, self-esteem, identity, temperament, peer support, and attitudes. This means that there is no simple answer but rather several interrelated factors to consider for each individual and all of his or her TEI. With a focus on users' experiences rather than a device-specific investigation, the shared phenomenon of using any TEI is presented. Evidence is provided by users of several TEI types with the assumption that the psychosocial experience can be similar irrespective of the device.

Consider your answers to Learning Prompt 1. We are all technology users able to provide different and unique answers. Answers to Learning Prompt 1 will span both positive and negative experiences, and may be grouped into difficulties and successes. Adopting a phenomenological perspective seeks to gain some understanding of what it is like to use TEI. TEI use can be described as a transactional experience of balancing the hassle or effort of TEI use with the engagement and successful integration of TEI into everyday activities (Verdonck et al. 2014). The "using" TEI is also likely to be an ambivalent experience for some (see Box 11.1). Similarly, a metasynthesis of qualitative studies exploring the meaning of wheelchairs and scooters also found that the experience was dynamic and complex (Ripat et al. 2018).

Engagement and incorporation

Use of technology can be satisfying and allow *engagement* in occupation through *incorporation* into daily life. TEI are intended to provide positive effects, and it follows that experienced TEI users report personal improvements or improved capacity through use.

> I would say your technology is your lifeline … it opens up a world of opportunities
>
> (Shinohara and Wobbrock 2011, p. 708)

> TEI just makes my life better
>
> (Lenker et al. 2013, p. 377)

> I love my water leveller, I really like that because it means that I can function competently … it makes me feel real good.
>
> (Lupton and Seymour 2000, p. 1856)

For some, TEI can be incorporated into daily life to the extent that it becomes considered integral and "part of me" (Palmer and Seale 2007) or "as an extension of the

Box 11.1 Here's the evidence

Dahler, A., Rasmussen, D., and Andersen, P. (2016). Meanings and experiences of assistive technologies in everyday lives of older citizens: a meta-interpretive review. *Disability and Rehabilitation: Assistive Technology* 11(8): 619–629.

Key Words: ambivalence, autonomy, independence, elders, assistive technology, systematic review

Purpose: The purpose of this study was to synthesize the findings from qualitative studies investigation of the experiences and meanings of assistive technology from the perspectives of elders. In this case, the technologies were those that help and support elders in their homes or institutional settings, as opposed to technologies that are used as treatment interventions, such as telemedicine.

Sample: Sixteen articles were included.

Method: A systematic search was undertaken using a variety of search indexes with the goal of covering research from different theoretical and professional perspectives. The review was limited to articles published in English, Danish, Swedish, and Norwegian languages between 1/1/2004 and 08/01/2015. Search terms included technology, assistive technology (AT), assistive device, ambient assisted living, welfare technology, health technology, congregate housing, and medical technology. These terms were combined with patient perspective, user perspective, independent living, everyday life, activities of daily living, and lived experience.

Findings: A range of themes emerged from the literature that were described under three main headings. The first theme deals with expectations, views, and experiences that elders have prior to using AT themselves. The theme reveals that while elders have a hard time keeping up with new developments in technology, they see the potential it has to be helpful. Additionally, they are worried about admitting they need AT as it signals that they are aging. Lack of knowledge about AT and privacy concerns present barriers to AT use. The second theme revolves around the acquisition process. Acquisition and acceptance are found to be stressful. Trust in the experts you deal with and feeling that they are giving you the right information is a helpful prerequisite for AT use, as is self-confidence. Training that is tailored to the elder client is critical. The physical environment can be a barrier to AT use. A variety of reasons are presented that impact acceptance or resistance to AT use. Theme three revealed different aspects of elders use of AT and included: variation, ambivalence, participation, power (in terms of capital), independence, becoming a burden, safety, autonomy, and privacy. Overall findings reveal that while elders have positive attitudes toward technology, acceptance is influenced by various factors.

Critical Thinking Questions:

1. What are the limitations of this study?
2. If you designed a study to examine the perceptions of AT users, what would you want to know? How would you design the study?
3. After reading this article, what additional research do you believe is needed in addition to that already discussed in the study?

body" (Blach Rossen et al. 2012). A phenomenological study of Danish elders who use assistive technology indicated that assistive devices that are "well incorporated" were considered positively (Häggblom-Kronlöf and Sonn 1999).

Mobility technology was considered by users, caregivers, and service providers to have a positive effect on emotional health, including reduced depression, decreased anxiety, and improved mood (Hammel et al. 2013). Similarly, Lenker et al. (2013) found that TEI users reported improved subjective well-being, including improved self-esteem, personal fulfillment, and improved quality of life related to TEI use.

Moreover, it is not uncommon to observe people enjoying the use of their technology, whether it be mainstream technology or assistive technology. Refer back to Learning Prompt 4. Sue Austin demonstrates her enjoyment as a TEI user. TEI can enable "just having fun" (Hammel et al. 2013) through participation in enjoyable activities such as watching television, listening to music, conversation, or playing games (Verdonck et al. 2018). The actual use of an assistive device can also be inherently enjoyable, as described by James, a 28-year-old student:

> It's great to have something (ECS/EADL) that you can just go into and just mess around with it … it was just playing around. It was like a new toy. And it is like a new toy to someone. It's a good toy.
>
> (Verdonck et al. 2014, p. 74)

James also described staying up all night, enabled to watch an entire box set of a television series using a new *environmental control system* (ECS), a feat not previously possible. Such a description suggests the achievement of a state of flow which occurs when an activity is all-encompassing and one becomes fully engaged in doing that activity (Csikszentmihalyi 1990).

Technology can be used in an unstructured, spontaneous way that is enjoyable.

> Just to mess around with it and usually you'd have an hour anyway to find something … just like mess about, turn up the volume, turn down the volume.
>
> (Verdonck et al. 2014, p. 74)

This vague enjoyable experience of using technology is in direct contrast with the scientific norm of measuring tangible productivity using technology but certainly promotes an inclusive approach to enabling people with disabilities to enjoy the same types of pleasurable experiences as their non-disabled peers.

Consider Learning Prompt 3. There is achievement in skill acquisition and mastering control of a device. Overcoming the challenges of TEI use and working out how to use a device can itself be an enjoyable experience with an element of achievement (Häggblom-Kronlöf and Sonn 1999; Myburg et al. 2017). Refer back to Learning Prompt 1. Mastering control of a smartphone can be enjoyable when one can proficiently use it to email, phone, surf the web, and possibly even edit photographs or map your latest walking trail.

Enjoyment may stem from the unexpected nature of successful use and benefits. A retired school teacher with little previous computer experience did not think that she would be able to use a tablet computer after suffering a cervical spinal cord injury. Six months after she was discharged from rehabilitation, she reported how she now loved her tablet and was able to play games, read books, and send emails (F. Maye, personal communication, June 9, 2013).

Furthermore, use of TEI can also be humorous. The unexpected ability offered by technology can allow the user to surprise others. Users may find it humorous to experience a new ability, such as being able to hide from a caregiver when first in a powered wheelchair, to make an unexpected trip to the pub or change the TV channel during a partner's favorite show (Verdonck et al. 2014). This can enable social participation in unexpected ways which many able-bodied people take for granted.

Psychosocial frustrations and challenges

Review Learning Prompt 1 again. When using technology for the first time, it is seldom without frustration or challenge. If one chose to not use the smartphone as described, this could be classed as *abandonment* or *non-use*. The latter is the preferred term in this chapter as it reflects choice over failure. Non-use of assistive technology is a dominant focus of the literature (Pape et al. 2002; Phillips and Zhao 1993; Ravneberg 2012). Instead of focusing on non-use, phenomenological inquiry rather seeks to understand what it is like to use TEI, which may inform our understanding of non-use.

Using technologies can involve a steep learning curve because one needs to work hard to become a proficient user. Erikson et al. (2004) described four stages of TEI use specifically focusing on ECS: (i) plunging in; (ii) landing and feeling comfortable; (iii) incorporating into daily activities; and (iv) taking off in the future. If users are given TEI without supporting the learning process and anticipating some challenges, it seems unlikely that they will reach "incorporation" and "taking off." Learning how to use technology can be difficult and can result in anxiety and stress (Davenport et al. 2012). In addition, some users may fear that expressing difficulty with TEI may perpetuate others' misperceptions of the users' individual incompetence (Martin et al. 2011).

People who live with a disability rely on routine and habits, with some having become accustomed to dependency (Verdonck et al. 2014). The introduction of TEI requires adjustment to habits and routines, and despite appreciating the possible benefits a TEI may provide, for some the change to routine may not be worth the benefit. It follows that both the introduction of assistive technology for computer use and the introduction of TEI have been recommended to start early in rehabilitation to allow their use to become routine for the user and easier to integrate into daily life (Folan et al. 2013; Verdonck et al. 2014).

While not widely reported in the academic literature, successful TEI users may experience frustration. This frustration is easily understood when referring back to Learning Prompt 2. Despite upgrading to a fancy car, it is likely that the driver will be frustrated by the need to use a clutch and physically change gears in heavy traffic. This new car may require significant effort. On the other hand, the older car may be frustrating because it is much slower, making a weekend trip tedious.

In a study of experienced ECS users' attitudes toward their technology, Palmer and Seale (2007) reported that some users described ECS as "extremely limiting," that they "could be better," and they had "good points and bad points." It is interesting to note that these users also described their technology as "indispensable," illustrating a shared perception of both positive and negative aspects.

The use of TEI requires making several adjustments to routines of everyday life, adaptations, and renegotiations (Ravneberg 2012). Häggblom-Kronlöf and Sonn (1999) described modification as a positive process of overcoming the hassles of using the AT or as pragmatic adaptation. Successful use of technology involves regular effort in terms of maintaining the technology to suit ones changing needs and contexts. This requires self-tailoring, involving trial and error and ongoing adjustment, as described by users of mobility technology (Hammel et al. 2013). Frustrations with the technical aspects involved in using devices can limit long-term adoption.

Psychosocial frustration and challenges with the system

In addition to frustration with the learning process, users also express frustration with "the system." This refers to the organizational and political rungs of the Vicente Human-Tech Ladder model (Vicente 2006). Users have to constantly work to ensure that they have the TEIs that meet their needs, which involves self-advocacy and seeking equitable funding (Hammel et al. 2013). Focus group findings describe how users found the TEI acquisition process a "headache," which "required energy" involving "lengthy periods of hassle and frustration" (Lenker et al. 2013). There may be differences of perception of need between users and organizations, providers and clinicians.

> I think I mentioned it once to the OT. ... and it was the whole fobbing off thing. ... you can't blame her for thinking about it as, "there are other people who need more essential things than you need a TV control." But in my eyes (sniggers), ... I think that was every bit as essential as an airbed for somebody else. Maybe that's being selfish but ... they think the money can go towards something. Something better but, better in my eyes is one of those (an ECS). (James).
>
> (Verdonck et al. 2014, p. 73)

A young Irish lady, Emily, who had participated in a tedious ECS assessment, expressed her frustration with not acquiring the essential technology, "It's just a kick in the teeth" (Verdonck et al. 2014, p. 73). She had anticipated having several devices to enable her both to access a computer and to control her home environment following her assistive technology assessment. In reality, no technology was supplied, so she described how she began to adjust her own perception of what she needed by finding ways to cope without TEI. She used care assistants to pre-program her television and ensured her family was scheduled to be available at other times. Her family built a small extension to their family home to accommodate Emily and her partner when accessible accommodation was not forthcoming.

For Emily and others who do not have access to TEI, their frustration with the lack of supply may contribute to non-use at a later stage and can change their perceptions of need. Moreover, Gramstad et al. (2013) explored Norwegian elders who were waiting to received ordered TEI and discovered that, instead of having articulated their TEI requirements, the elders had endured difficulties associated with living without TEI by adjusting their daily activities and expectations to overcome or ignore their possible TEI needs. Some of these users were unaware of their need (Gramstad et al. 2013).

Personal fit of TEI

Every TEI user evaluates their individual need and use of TEI and the value they place on it based on their psychosocial perspective. Krantz (2012) describes two elements affecting the individual's thoughts about using assistive technology and the activities performed when using those devices. The first is expectations of the user, which encompass the pre-use thoughts, perceptions, and attitudes about the TEI. The second is experience derived post-use.

Expectations are based on knowledge of TEI. Knowledge is based on personal experience as well as on the opinions of others. Users and potential users actively seek advice from peers, with relevant experience, through support networks both physical and virtual (Hammel et al. 2013). In addition, trials by the user are essential for providing opportunities to form realistic expectations of the TEI (Folan et al. 2013; Verdonck et al. 2014).

Users ask themselves, "is it usable, and is it worth using?" (Krantz 2012). Answering the question "Is it usable?" on a personal level involves evaluating the persons own capacity to use the TEI. Do they think they have the required skills and knowledge? Are they comfortable using the TEI? Their evaluation may be based on previous experience of either successful or unsuccessful use of the same or similar technology. Answering the question "Is it usable?" on a practical level relates to functions and features. Users are concerned about device reliability, size, and appearance (Blach Rossen et al. 2012). In addition, users want TEI to be easy to install or set up and simple to use (Davenport et al. 2012). Functionality and features are not specifically psychosocial domains and relate more to the individual devices and technologies which are addressed in other chapters of this textbook. However, users do have individual perceptions of device features and functions which cannot be ignored, and service providers need to be aware of these contributing factors to the psychosocial impact of TEI (Verdonck et al. 2009). Aesthetic considerations are reasons for non-use and need to be considered a psychosocial consideration of TEI (Phillips and Zhao 1993; Ravneberg 2012; Shinohara and Wobbrock 2011).

> I like things attractive. Whatever adaptive equipment, I want it to look nice. You know, you got everybody with their iPods and their iPads and their Blackberries, you know, and they're whipped out, they're small … and they're nice looking … And, as a blind person, yeah, maybe I don't see it, but other people see it, and I want it to be, you know, just as glamorous as the next guy.
>
> (Shinohara and Wobbrock 2011, p. 709)

It is easy to understand the preference to have the best-looking TEI. There is an obvious preference for mainstream devices over traditional unattractive assistive technologies. As technologies become even more integrated into everyday life, designers of TEI need to consider aesthetics as a priority over function (Shinohara and Wobbrock 2011).

Usability

Without previous realistic experience of TEI, a user is unable to accurately evaluate if a TEI is useable. It follows that some TEI users are surprised by TEI due to their inaccurate pre-use perceptions. They can be surprised if TEI are easy to use, if they are simple, if TEI suit them as a user despite previous perceptions that the TEI would "not suit me" (Verdonck et al. 2014). Surprise when it does work and does suit the user may facilitate continued TEI use and incorporation into everyday life. For example, refer to Learning Prompt 1 for an example of a technology that you may have been surprised to incorporate into your everyday life.

Users may also consider the cost of the effort to use a TEI compared with the benefits, described by new ECS users who, "seemed to ask themselves is the hassle worth it?" (Verdonck et al. 2014, p. 75). For experienced speech-driven-ECS users, enduring the "struggle" with reliability of their devices was favored over the alternative of relying solely on switch access (Judge et al. 2009).

For some, TEI may not be worth using because it may only offer some but not full function, and some but not full access (Phillips and Zhao 1993). In addition, specialized assistive technology still lags behind most mainstream technology, making it unsatisfactory in comparison (Copley and Ziviani 2004; Shinohara and Wobbrock 2011). Users want devices to be compatible, durable, suitable for customization, and ideally "available any place" (Lenker et al. 2013).

Asking someone what they think about a single item or device is also problematic as they may not be able to consider one device in isolation. "Participants found it hard to evaluate the outcomes of a single piece of technology since they did not conceptualise use in this way" (Hammel et al. 2013, p. 303). For example, power wheelchair users did not consider their wheelchairs to be the only important aid in everyday life (Blach Rossen et al. 2012). With increasing "connectivity" between devices, this is pertinent. User evaluation involves several items across various settings in a transactional balance, making the task of understanding the experience more complex.

The experience of technology for people with disabilities has been described as a love/hate relationship (Lupton and Seymour 2000). TEI can be both enabling and disabling. In a retrospective longitudinal Danish study, meanings attributed to TEI where found to be ambivalent. TEI use was considered normal and as well as a sign of old age: pleasant and also unpleasant, safe but unsafe, usable and inappropriate, essential and cumbersome, aiding respect and making one feel afraid, causing indifference and also embarrassment (Häggblom-Kronlöf and Sonn 2007). It follows that a meta-interpretive review of assistive technology experiences for older adults also showed conflicting meanings (Dahler et al. 2016). Similarly, in a metasynthesis the meaning ascribed to wheelchairs and scooters was described as a "dynamic duality" encompassing both enabling and disabling experiences (Ripat et al. 2018).

TEI to enable autonomy in occupation

Autonomy is cited by several qualitative studies as a benefit to TEI use (Blach Rossen et al. 2012; Davenport et al. 2012; Folan et al. 2013; Häggblom-Kronlöf and Sonn 1999; Hammel et al. 2013; Iacono et al. 2013; Lenker et al. 2013; Verdonck et al. 2011). *Autonomy* is considered to include organizing one's own social roles, affairs, and relationships (participation) as well as feeling comfortable with the way of living (self-determination) (van de Ven et al. 2008). Relevant literature includes several supportive quotations about autonomy facilitated through the use of TEI:

> I am in charge.
>
> (Hammel et al. 2013)

> (It) allows me to be master of my own domain.
>
> (Lenker et al. 2013, p. 377)

> (You can) do what you want to do, where you want, with whom you want.
>
> (Hammel et al. 2013, p. 303)

> Gives you the choice to choose what you want to do.
>
> (Verdonck et al. 2011 p. 275)

> (I can) go where I want to and function as I want.
>
> (Hammel et al. 2013, p. 297)

> (I) can do what I want, when I want it.
>
> (Ripat and Strock 2004, p. 69; Ripat and Woodgate 2011)

> Control over personal space and activity.
>
> (Rigby et al. 2000)

The use of TEI may provide the ability to express one's own choices (Hooper et al. 2018). Ironically, the choice afforded to one through the use of TEI must be balanced by reports that some have no choice in using TEI as they have "no alternative" (Häggblom-Kronlöf and Sonn 1999). The user may be "forced to accept" the TEI. For some the extent of their impairment dictates their need for assistive technology and thus an enforced "value." For example, a person who has had their legs amputated requires a wheelchair or prosthetic limbs, and even if they dislike the wheelchair or prosthetic limbs they will be reliant on them and have a value forced on them through necessity.

Facilitation of autonomous physical tasks is an inherent function of TEI. This outcome is the easiest aspect to measure. For example: how far can someone walk with crutches versus without them. Users find it easy to express the tangible physical benefits of using TEI, such as improved mobility, access to computers, and being able to dress or eat without being dependent on others. Hemmingsson et al. (2009) provide the example of a school boy who is an indoor crutch user but outdoors he is faster than his class mates when playing catch because he uses a wheelchair. TEI can also enable productivity in terms of work: "being able to find a job," to "keep a job," or even "just getting your foot in the door" (Hammel et al. 2013, p. 298).

TEI does not, however, negate disability. It cannot fully replace lost function. TEI may only allow "taking back a little of what they had lost," which may have significant meaning and value for a person (Verdonck et al. 2018). Some other people may not consider TEI to be "amazing" and may be annoyed at others' positive attitudes to their TEI. It may be considered patronizing that others refer to their TEI as "amazing" when to them it may only provide limited assistance. The reliance on technology or environmental accommodation may itself be considered disabling (Korotchenko and Clarke 2014; Verdonck 2012).

Being

Use of TEI can enable "being" as well as "doing." As humans, "we take time to reflect, be introspective or meditative, (re)discover the self, savour the moment, appreciate nature, art or music in a contemplative manner and to enjoy being with special people" (Hammell 2004).

Being is not a measurable quantity and is highly individualized (Wilcock 1999). It relates to the ability to spend time alone (refer to Learning Prompt 5). Sue Austin describes the freedom she experiences in her powered wheelchair. The freedom to be alone has been expressed by other powered mobility users (Boss and Finlayson 2006) and by ECS users (Myburg et al. 2017; Verdonck et al. 2011). Time alone is important because it facilitates privacy for people whose daily lives may be characterized by time spent predominantly with caregivers and family members.

Using TEI may allow one to feel less needy. Life with a disability has been described as involving a state of being continually indebted. Galvin and Donnell (2002) describe reliance on others as living with "perpetual obligation" that requires "irrevocable gratitude" which involves constant apologizing and thanking of others. In contrast, if TEI enables autonomy, users may be able to spend time with significant others on an equal footing (Hammel et al. 2013). This may allow a change in relationships between user and carers or family members, with interactions based on more than physical need alone (Davenport et al. 2012; Iacono et al. 2013; Verdonck et al. 2011):

> I can make phone calls which is great because it means I can be on my own in the house, and I mean, that is a complete change of life experience, instead of having people worrying – oh Jane is on her own if the house goes on fire. I can now be on my own and it just makes such a huge difference.
>
> (Verdonck et al. 2011 p. 275)

Sense of security

TEI may facilitate feeling safe and secure when alone. TEI users feel secure if they know that they can call for help if needed using an alarm system or physically leave a dangerous situation in a power chair in an adapted environment. The physical support or external safety offered by TEI is complemented by the psychological support of internal security (Häggblom-Kronlöf and Sonn 1999; Myburg et al. 2017). When users have reliable TEI, they can feel safer alone and have "peace of mind" (Hooper et al. 2018). They may feel more self-confident, less vulnerable, and less anxious (Hammel et al. 2013). Service providers, teams, and organizations may focus on the physical safety of avoiding ill health. In contrast, the psychological element of the feelings associated with TEI use is far more important to the individual and likely to impact on continued use or non-use.

Social participation

In addition to physical participation, TEI can also enable social participation. Improved physical mobility offered through wheelchair use in an accessible modified environment allows community mobility and social integration (Lenker et al. 2013). The use of a powered wheelchair was described by users as a tool to enable one to "meet other people" and to participate in sport and club activities (Blach Rossen et al. 2012; Fomiatti et al. 2014). Social *belonging* can also be a virtual experience. Stroke survivors described how "connected" they became through computer use (Dorey et al. 2007). A person with cerebral palsy describes her computer as providing,

> an opportunity to meet other people and it's an opportunity I wouldn't have without it (computer) because my disability makes it awkward to meet people and the bulletin board is another avenue to meet people.
>
> (Lupton and Seymour 2000, p. 1857)

Computers can facilitate the formation of virtual communities of people with similar life situations. Virtual interaction can also allow a level playing field as the person's disability can be hidden and they can function as an equal.

TEI and identity

TEI use can influence identity, and how each individual incorporates their TEI into their identity is personal (Krantz 2012). How does the TEI relate to who we are? TEI can be perceived as a sign of deviance. TEI can label a person as disabled and impose a stigma on device use (Hemmingsson et al. 2009; Parette and Scherer 2004).

> Yes, it was really a shock. Many red lamps were installed. It looked like flashers on the car. Just that it is red lamps, small triangles around the house. When somebody was at the doorbell or when the phone rang, it shone red all over the house. It is very nice, but it is like – look at me, I have a hearing problem! (Hanna laughed).
>
> (Ravneberg 2012, p. 266)

TEI may also label a person as vulnerable and possibly a target for wrongdoers, (Hemmingsson et al. 2009; Shinohara and Wobbrock 2011). Whether a user perceives TEI as stigmatizing is influenced by society and cultural context (as discussed in Chapter 15). Beliefs, attitudes, values, and traditions may lead to personal reluctance or embarrassment.

> It's no fun and people stare and make a long detour round you and you come to town … you feel a bit vulnerable.
>
> (Häggblom-Kronlöf and Sonn 1999, p. 165)

It is common for wheelchair users to postpone the use of a powered wheelchair to avoid the associated personal identification issues (Blach Rossen et al. 2012). Accepting TEI may also be considered to be "giving up" and accepting one's loss of function (Gramstad et al. 2013). The need for TEI can also be considered a sign of failure, that one is unable to engage in previous occupations without the assistance of TEI, and can provoke a feeling of inadequacy within the user. TEI may be considered a foreign object outside of an individual's personal identity, and may be considered an unwanted burden (Hemmingsson et al. 2009).

Conversely, the label provided through the use of TEI may be viewed as a positive. It may act as a signal to others to accommodate the users' disability, such as moving out of the way of a white cane. Danish elders described how using a device can signal your need for assistance and help others treat you with respect (Häggblom-Kronlöf and Sonn 1999). TEI can allow you to be "just like everyone else" if it is discreet or hidden or virtual (Shinohara and Wobbrock 2011).

TEI may also provide a new ability or competence:

> I think [proficiency in computer use] has a social significance in the way you deal with other people and I think that rubs off. If other people see that you are competently doing and confident in what you're doing, then I think they treat you differently.
>
> (Lupton and Seymour 2000) p. 1857)

Similarly, people with tetraplegia incorporated computers into their lives to return to previous roles or to engage in new roles. For this group, computers were instrumental to their rehabilitation (Folan et al. 2013).

Take-home messages: What does this all mean for you and the TEI user?

This chapter has discussed three questions: What is it like to use TEI? What do users think of TEI? What does using TEI mean? The response for each of these questions is influenced by a wide range of individual psychosocial factors. In exploring these questions, the reader will have gained some insight into possible psychosocial factors to consider in connection with TEI use. The principle take-home messages from this exploration of the lived experience of TEI are discussed below.

TEI use involves effort, challenges, and frustrations

Users require support to overcome the challenges involved with TEI use in order to allow incorporation into daily lives and activities. The interplay of hassle and engagement is a dynamic process where overcoming some hassle can result in improved engagement. Engagement may, in turn, result in some hassle possibly threatening the ongoing engagement. Anticipating the hassle may prepare the user and allow for the formulation of realistic expectations. Service providers may tend to focus on the positive benefits of TEI use, but preparing users for the difficulties prior to experiencing the benefits is advised. The user cannot be a passive recipient of TEI and needs to be engaged in its use and incorporation into their daily life. Introducing TEI into a treatment plan as early as possible can help with its successful incorporation into a user's routine.

TEI use can be fun

It is possible that some users may enjoy the actual process of **becoming** accustomed to using TEI and mastering technology to best suit individual needs. This involves constant adjustment and a dynamic engagement with the hassle. When supporting TEI use it may be helpful to focus on the possible enjoyment of the learning process in a bid to cope with the expected and unexpected frustrations.

TEI user expectations and choices based on real-life experience

It is best that people not be given TEI without first experiencing the use of TEI. Each person has different psychosocial factors which influence their experience of technology. Incorporation of TEI is best facilitated through matching one's experience with one's expectations. Having accurate expectations requires access to realistic information about devices and their functions or actual trial thereof. Users need to be supported through the decision process of considering if TEI is worth using and if it is useable.

Non-use of TEI is an acceptable and expected outcome

A primary concern with TEI provision is abandonment or non-use, which is well documented in the literature (Copley and Ziviani 2004; Johnston and Evans 2005; Phillips and Zhao 1993; Scherer 2005; Wessels et al. 2003). For some the benefits of TEI use may not be worth the hassle involved. The choice to not use TEI should not be based on an opinion but should instead be a decision made following realistic opportunities to use TEI. It follows that successful use may be an unexpected outcome of this experience, or alternatively that TEI might not meet the users' expectations and be considered not worth using.

Aesthetics influences use and non-use and associated social participation

The appearance of devices is integral to their acceptance and is related to possible stigmatization. If devices are discreet they are easier to incorporate into life. Effort needs to be made to provide and to design devices that meet mainstream norms and are socially acceptable. TEI can enable the user to engage in social and community activities. They may, however, also stigmatize or label a person, which can then be perceived by the user as further disabling.

Meanings and experiences of TEI can be contradictory

People's experience of and the meaning attributed to TEI is unlikely to be polarized. If given the opportunity, it is possible that users will attribute both positive and negative meaning to TEI. This means that when using clinical evaluation tools it is important to explore their personal perspective in more detail to understand the nuanced experience, which may contribute to non-use or difficulty in incorporation.

TEI enables "being" as well as "doing"

Identified benefits of TEI may be neither tangible nor measurable. TEI may contribute to the ability to simply "be," to experience true privacy, to enjoy one's own company, and to be alone. TEI use may provide psychological comfort, allowing a person to feel safe and confident. The psychological benefit of being able to do things using TEI must also be considered. TEI that is incorporated into daily life can improve a user's autonomy.

Summary

The psychosocial factors involved in TEI use are complex and varied. Adopting a phenomenological approach can be beneficial in understanding TEI use from an individual user's perspective. This involves asking what using TEI is like, what users think of TEI, and what TEI use means. Using TEI involves challenges and hassle. Users experience frustrations with the use of TEI and with the political and organization aspect of TEI provision. Learning to use TEI requires support in overcoming hassles and facilitating engagement with TEI to incorporate it into daily occupations. Incorporation of TEI can be enjoyable and even humorous. Users consider personal fit by asking themselves if the TEI is useable and if is it worth using. Their answers can be contradictory, with both positive and negative answers. TEI has many meanings to users. Primarily, TEI enables users to "do" activities. In addition, it allows them to "be" alone or engage in non-purposeful but meaningful activities. Social participation and belonging are also facilitated by TEI use. TEI can cause stigmatization or provide a useful label, both of which influence identity. TEI may enhance autonomy and be considered an enabler for some, while for others it may be a disabler and reduce autonomy. The choice to use or not to use TEI involves a complex process influenced by several psychosocial aspects and both use and non-use should be considered reasonable outcomes of a TEI intervention if the personal lived experience is understood.

References

Blach Rossen, C., Sorensen, B., Wurtz Jochumsen, B., and Wind, G. (2012). Everyday life for users of electric wheelchairs – a qualitative interview study. *Disability and Rehabilitation. Assistive Technology* 7 (5): 399–407. https://doi.org/10.3109/17483107.2012.665976.

Boss, T.M. and Finlayson, M. (2006). Responses to the acquisition and use of power mobility by individuals who have multiple sclerosis and their families. *The American Journal of Occupational Therapy* 60 (3): 348–358.

Copley, J. and Ziviani, J. (2004). Barriers to the use of assistive technology for children with multiple disabilities. *Occupational Therapy International* 11 (4): 229–243.

Cook, A.M. and Polgar, J.M. (2015). *Assistive Technologies: Principles and Practice*, 4e. St. Louis, MO: Mosby, Elsevier.

Creswell, J.W. (1998). *Qualitative Inquiry and Research Design: Choosing Among Five Traditions*. Thousand Oaks, CA: Sage.

Csikszentmihalyi, M. (1990). *Flow*. New York: Harper & Row.

Dahler, A.M., Rasmussen, D.M., and Andersen, P.T. (2016). Meanings and experiences of assistive technologies in everyday lives of older citizens: a meta-interpretive review. *Disability and Rehabilitation: Assistive Technology* 11 (8): 619–629. https://doi.org/10.3109/17483107.2016.1151950.

Davenport, R.D., Mann, W., and Lutz, B. (2012). How older adults make decisions regarding smart technology: an ethnographic approach. *Assistive Technology* 24 (3): 168–181. https://doi.org/10.1080/10400435.2012.659792.

van de Ven, L., Post, M., de Witte, L., and van den Heuvel, W. (2008). Strategies for autonomy used by people with cervical spinal cord injury: a qualitative study. *Disability and Rehabilitation* 30 (4): 249–260.

Demers, L., Weiss-Lambrous, R., and Ska, B. (2002). The Quebec users evaluation of satisfaction with assistive technology (QUEST 2.0): an overview of recent progress. *Technology and Disability* 14: 101–105.

Dorey, B., Reid, D., and Chiu, T. (2007). Stroke survivors' experiences of computer use at home. *Technology and Disability* 19 (4): 179–188.

Erikson, A., Karlsson, G., Soderstrom, M., and Tham, K. (2004). A training apartment with electronic aids to daily living: lived experiences of persons with brain damage. *American Journal of Occupational Therapy* 58 (3): 261–271.

Folan, A., Barclay, L., Cooper, C., and Robinson, M. (2013). Exploring the experience of clients with tetraplegia utilizing assistive technology for computer access. *Disability and Rehabilitation: Assistive Technology* 10 (1): 46–52. https://doi.org/10.3109/17483107.2013.836686.

Fomiatti, R., Moir, L., Richmond, J., and Millsteed, J. (2014). The experience of being a motorised mobility scooter user. *Disability and Rehabilitation: Assistive Technology* 9 (3): 183–187. https://doi.org/10.3109/17483107.2013.814171.

Galvin, J.C. and Donnell, C.M. (2002). Educating the consumer and caretaker on assistive technology. In: *Assistive Technology: Matching Device and Consumer for Successful Rehabilition* (ed. M.J. Scherer), 153–167. Washington: American Psychological Association.

Gramstad, A., Storli, S.L., and Hamran, T. (2013). "Do I need it? Do I really need it?" Elderly people's experiences of unmet assistive technology device needs. *Disability and Rehabilitation: Assistive*

Technology 8 (4): 287–293. https://doi.org/10.3109/17483107.2012.699993.

Häggblom-Kronlöf, G.H. and Sonn, U. (1999). Elderly women's way of relating to assistive devices. *Technology and Disability* 10 (3): 161–168.

Häggblom-Kronlöf, G.H. and Sonn, U. (2007). Use of assistive devices – a reality full of contradictions in elderly persons' everyday life. *Disability and Rehabilitation: Assistive Technology* 2 (6): 335–345. https://doi.org/10.1080/17483100701701672.

Hammel, J., Southall, K., Jutai, J. et al. (2013). Evaluating use and outcomes of mobility technology: a multiple stakeholder analysis. *Disability and Rehabilitation: Assistive Technology* 8 (4): 294–304. https://doi.org/10.3109/17483107.2012.735745.

Hammell, K.W. (2004). Dimensions of meaning in the occupations of daily life. *Canadian Journal of Occupational Therapy* 71 (5): 296–305.

Hemmingsson, H., Lidström, H., and Nygård, L. (2009). Use of assistive technology devices in mainstream schools: students' perspective. *The American Journal of Occupational Therapy* 63 (4): 463–472.

Hooper, B., Verdonck, M., Amsters, D. et al. (2018). Smart-device environmental control systems: experiences of people with cervical spinal cord injuries. *Disability and Rehabilitation: Assistive Technology* 13 (8): 724–730. https://doi.org/10.1080/17483107.2017.1369591.

Iacono, T., Lyon, K., Johnson, H., and West, D. (2013). Experiences of adults with complex communication needs receiving and using low tech AAC: an Australian context. *Disability and Rehabilitation: Assistive Technology* 8 (5): 392–401. https://doi.org/10.3109/17483107.2013.769122.

Johnston, S.S. and Evans, J. (2005). Considering response efficiency as a strategy to prevent assistive technology abandonment. *Journal of Special Education Technology* 20 (3): 45–50.

Judge, S., Robertson, Z., Hawley, M., and Enderby, P. (2009). Speech-driven environmental control systems – a qualitative analysis of users' perceptions. *Disability and Rehabilitation: Assistive Technology* 4 (3): 151–157.

Jutai, J. and Day, H. (2002). Psychosocial Impact of Assistive Devices Scale (PIADS). *Technology and Disability* 14 (3): 107–111.

Korotchenko, A. and Clarke, L.H. (2014). Power mobility and the built environment: the experiences of older Canadians. *Disability & Society* 29: 431–443. https://doi.org/10.1080/09687599.2013.816626.

Krantz, O. (2012). Assistive devices utilisation in activities of everyday life – a proposed framework of understanding a user perspective. *Disability and Rehabilitation: Assistive Technology* 7 (3): 189–198. https://doi.org/10.3109/17483107.2011.618212.

Law, M., Cooper, B., Strong, S. et al. (1996). The person-environment-occupation model: a transactive approach to occupational performance. *Canadian Journal of Occupational Therapy* 63 (1): 9–23.

Lenker, J.A., Harris, F., Taugher, M., and Smith, R.O. (2013). Consumer perspectives on assistive technology outcomes. *Disability and Rehabilitation: Assistive Technology* 8 (5): 373–380. https://doi.org/10.3109/17483107.2012.749429.

Lenker, J. and Paquet, V. (2003). A review of conceptual models for assistive technology outcomes: research and practice. *Assistive Technology* 15 (1): 1–15.

Lupton, D. and Seymour, W. (2000). Technology, selfhood and physical disability. *Social Science & Medicine* 50 (12): 1851–1862. https://doi.org/10.1016/S0277-9536(99)00422-0.

Martin, J.K., Martin, L.G., Stumbo, N.J., and Morrill, J.H. (2011). The impact of consumer involvement on satisfaction with and use of assistive technology. *Disability and Rehabilitation. Assistive Technology* 6 (3): 225–242. https://doi.org/10.3109/17483107.2010.522685.

Myburg, M., Allan, E., Nalder, E. et al. (2017). Environmental control systems – the experiences of people with spinal cord injury and the implications for prescribers. *Disability and Rehabilitation: Assistive Technology* 12 (2): 128–136. https://doi.org/10.3109/17483107.2015.1099748.

Palmer, P. and Seale, J. (2007). Exploring the attitudes to environmental control systems of people with physical disabilities: a grounded theory approach. *Technology and Disability* 19 (1): 17–27.

Pape, T.L.-B., Kim, J., and Weiner, B. (2002). The shaping of individual meanings assigned to assistive technology: a review of personal factors. *Disability and Rehabilitation* 24 (1): 5–20.

Parette, P. and Scherer, M. (2004). Assistive technology use and stigma. *Education and Training in Developmental Disabilities* 39 (3): 217–226.

Phillips, B. and Zhao, H. (1993). Predictors of assistive technology abandonment. *Assistive Technology* 5 (1): 36–45.

Ravneberg, B. (2012). Usability and abandonment of assistive technology. *Journal of Assistive Technologies* 6 (4): 259–269. https://doi.org/10.1108/17549451211285753.

Rigby, P., Renzoni, A. M., Ryan, S. et al. (2000). Exploring the impact of electronic aids for daily living upon persons with neuromuscular conditions. Paper presented at the Tri-Joint Congress 2000, Toronto, Ontario, Canada, May 24–27.

Ripat, J. and Strock, A. (2004). Users' perceptions of the impact of electronic aids to daily living throughout the acquisition process. *Assistive Technology* 16 (1): 63–72.

Ripat, J. and Woodgate, R. (2011). The intersection of culture, disability and assistive technology. *Disability and Rehabilitation: Assistive Technology* 6 (2): 87–96. https://doi.org/10.3109/17483107.2010.507859.

Ripat, J., Verdonck, M., and Carter, R.J. (2018). The meaning ascribed to wheeled mobility devices by individuals who use wheelchairs and scooters: a metasynthesis. *Disability and Rehabilitation: Assistive Technology* 13 (3): 253–262. https://doi.org/10.1080/17483107.2017.1306594.

Scherer, M.J. (2005). *Living in the State of Stuck: How Assistive Technology Impacts the Lives of People with Disabilities*, 4e. Brookline, MA: Brookline Books.

Scherer, M.J., Sax, C., Vanbiervliet, A. et al. (2005). Predictors of assistive technology use: the importance of personal and psychosocial factors. *Disability and Rehabilitation* 27 (21): 1321–1331. https://doi.org/10.1080/09638280500164800.

Shinohara, K. and Wobbrock, J.O. (2011). In the shadow of misperception: assistive technology use and social interactions. In *Proceedings of the SIGCHI Conference on Human Factors in Computing Systems*, Vancouver, Canada (May 7–12). New York: ACM.

Verdonck, M. (2012). The meaning of environmental control systems (ECS) for people with spinal cord injury: an occupational therapist explores an intervention. PhD dissertation. University College Cork. Retrieved from http://hdl.handle.net/10468/582.

Verdonck, M., Chard, G., and Nolan, M. (2011). Electronic aids to daily living: be able to do what you want. *Disability and Rehabilitation: Assistive Technology* 6 (3): 268–281. https://doi.org/10.3109/17483107.2010.525291.

Verdonck, M., Steggles, E. and Chard, G. (2009). Experiences and desires of people with tetraplegia living with and without electronic aids to daily living: an Irish focus group study. Retrieved from https://www.resna.org/sites/default/files/legacy/conference/proceedings/2009/JEA/Verdonck.html.

Verdonck, M., Steggles, E., Nolan, M., and Chard, G. (2014). Experiences of using an environmental control system (ECS) for persons with high cervical spinal cord injury: the interplay between hassle and engagement. *Disability and Rehabilitation: Assistive Technology* 9 (1): 70–78. https://doi.org/10.3109/17483107.2013.823572.

Verdonck, M., Nolan, M., and Chard, G. (2018). Taking back a little of what you have lost: the meaning of using an environmental control system (ECS) for people with high cervical spinal cord injury. *Disability and Rehabilitation: Assistive Technology* 13 (8): 785–790. https://doi.org/10.1080/17483107.2017.1378392.

Vicente, K. (2006). *The Human Factor: Revolutionizing the Way We Live with Technology*. New York: Routledge, Taylor & Francis Group.

Wessels, R., Dijcks, B., Soede, M. et al. (2003). Non-use of provided assistive technology devices, a literature overview. *Technology and Disability* 15 (4): 231–238.

Wilcock, A.A. (1999). Reflections on doing, being and becoming. *Australian Occupational Therapy Journal* 46 (1): 1–11.

World Health Organization (2001). *International Classification of Functioning, Disability and Health*. Geneva, Switzerland: World Health Organization.

12

Sociocultural considerations

Jacquie Ripat

Outline

Learning outcomes

After reading this chapter, you should be able to:

1. Describe how using a social constructionist perspective can provide a foundation for understanding TEI use and meaning.
2. Explain why sociocultural factors are important to consider in TEI assessment and procurement.
3. Discuss how the meaning of AT and TEI can relate to personal values, beliefs, and assumptions of a client/family/community.
4. Examine how a three-pronged approach may be used to provide socioculturally relevant TEI services.
5. Analyze the role that sociocultural factors have had in influencing the design and development of TEI.

Assistive Technologies and Environmental Interventions in Healthcare: An Integrated Approach, First Edition.
Edited by Lynn Gitlow and Kathleen Flecky.

Companion website: www.wiley.com/go/gitlow/assitivetechnologies

Active learning prompts

Before you read this chapter:

1. Consider a walker and the various meanings you might be able to ascribe to a walker (e.g. walker may indicate improvement in function or decline in function, represent aging, increase mobility or autonomy, or be a burden, or a symbol of a person with a disability). Which meanings do you most closely associate a walker with? What has contributed to this association (e.g. knew someone of a particular age who used a walker)? Ask someone else to tell you in one sentence what a walker symbolizes. Compare and contrast their responses with yours.
2. Consider the following statement: "The use of technologies is not a purely individualized activity: it always takes place in a sociocultural context that both shapes the meanings of technological artefacts and places limits on the extent to which such meanings can be transformed by users" (Lupton and Seymour 2000, p. 1852). What key ideas can you discern from this quote?
3. View the video "Disability Means Possibility" located at http://www.youtube.com/watch?gl=CA&hl=en&v=uhKMouRaWcY
   Use Figure 12.1 as a framework to discuss the actions and behaviors of each of the individuals shown in the video.
4. Amos Winter describes the development of a low-cost all-terrain wheelchair at http://www.ted.com/talks/amos_winter_the_cheap_all_terrain_wheelchair.html. What sociocultural considerations does he discuss?

Key terms

Culturally relevant service provision
Self-reflection
Social constructionism
Sociocultural factors
Three-pronged approach

Introduction

While assistive technology and environmental interventions (TEI) may be fit and matched to an individual user, it is essential that we recognize the interdependent relationship each person has with his or her social and cultural environment. While other chapters in this text have focused on person and environment elements that are interrelated to sociocultural factors, the aim of this chapter is to uphold that TEI must *always* be understood within a broader sociocultural context (Lupton and Seymour 2000) and to suggest ways to approach this understanding. In this chapter, you will be encouraged to understand how we might consider the effect of sociocultural influences and you will be asked to consider how the influence of the sociocultural context shapes the meaning a person may assign to a TEI. Later in the chapter, you will explore specific sociocultural influences on use and meaning of TEI that have been identified in current research. Next, you will be invited to examine how your own sociocultural factors may influence your interaction with TEI users, and how a sociocultural perspective of TEI can be assimilated into the context of TEI practice and service delivery. The chapter concludes with a review of how sociocultural factors have influenced the design and development of TEI over the years, and a prompt for you to consider how design might be influenced in the future.

Social constructionism

This chapter is founded on a social constructionism approach to understanding how sociocultural factors influence TEI use. Burr (2003) identifies four defining features of a social constructionism approach and it is useful to spend a few moments outlining each these features in order to understand how we might approach the topic of understanding different sociocultural factors influencing TEI users. Burr first explains that those adopting a social constructionist view must be willing to take a critical and reflexive stance toward our ways of understanding the world (our own worldview). This means that we need to identify and challenge the taken-for-granted assumptions that we hold, and recognize that there can be (and indeed are!) many divergent worldviews. Rather than passing judgment that a view is different from ours, and therefore erroneous, we need to respect and appreciate how others may view their world. The second feature of social constructionism outlined by Burr suggests that the way that we view the world, and what we believe to be true, is historically and culturally framed, in what she refers to as "historical and cultural relativism" (p. 6). This idea implies that the set of beliefs we hold about a phenomenon is influenced by current cultural and societal beliefs and values. Furthermore, this set of beliefs is not a fixed entity, but rather it changes over time. For example, we can consider how the concept of aging-in-place can be used as an example of historical and cultural relativism at work. At one point in time, institutionalized living (personal care home; nursing home) was viewed as the most probable method of providing care as people aged. However, over the past several decades there has been a substantial "paradigm shift" to focus on aging-in-place as the preferred way of addressing the housing needs and wishes of older adults, their family members, and policy-makers (Vasunilashorn et al. 2011). Burr (2003) proposes that knowledge, or what one believes to be true, is a product of an ongoing process of interaction between people within their social contexts. Through social interactions such as communication and language, people reinforce, challenge, and modify their knowledge (their "truths") on an ongoing basis. Finally, Burr identifies that knowledge and action are linked, such that current knowledge and understanding of a phenomenon will lead to the action that one (or society) takes to work with that knowledge, i.e. as understanding of a phenomenon shifts, the subsequent actions and activities related to that understanding will also change. We can use these interrelated ideas about social constructionism as a framework to explore what we know about sociocultural influences on TEI.

Sociocultural factors

Each of us holds knowledge, attitudes, and values that have been shaped by our unique, and our shared, social, historical, and cultural experiences and opportunities. For example, consider how three different students attending their first year of university might view the concept of *post-secondary education*. The first student may view post-secondary education as an opportunity to develop advanced knowledge and explore an area of his particular interest; the second may see post-secondary education primarily a means to future employment; and for the third, it may be symbolic as she represents the first of her family to attend a post-secondary institution. Each of these experiences is valued and "real" for the individual student, and none of these perspectives can be judged as better or right. Rather, each is different, and the individual meaning ascribed was likely influenced by sociocultural factors such as family conventions and expectations, socioeconomic factors, and past academic experiences and opportunities.

Fitzgerald (2004) defines culture as "the learned, shared, patterned ways of perceiving and adapting to the world around us (our environment) that is characteristic of a population or society" (p. 494). In this regard, sociocultural factors may include "age, ability status, gender, race, ethnicity, religion, social class, sexual orientation, citizenship status and so on" (Canadian Association of Occupational Therapists [CAOT] 2014), as well as the political, historical, geographical, and economic experiences and opportunities experienced by people (Browne 2005). It is important to recognize that the term culture is a much broader concept than the term ethnicity, and thus the terms are not interchangeable (although ethnicity may be one sociocultural influence) (Hunt 2007). Thus, the term sociocultural refers to the numerous social and cultural factors that influence the way one views and experiences the world, and the factors are shaped by broader family, community, and societal beliefs, values, and assumptions (CAOT 2014; Fitzgerald 2004; Iwama 2003).

Returning to the features of social constructionism outlined by Burr (2003) (including societal context, interaction, historical and cultural relativism, dynamic and changing nature, and knowledge-action link), we can ponder an example of how a sociocultural factor such as the concept of age can be considered. While we may agree that a person is a particular biological age based on date of birth, for example 18 years old, whether or not that 18-year-old individual is considered to be an adult or a child is less clear. Age is often used as a determining factor in societal decisions regarding whether one is considered an adult or child, and these decisions are dependent on contextual views and expectations that are socially constructed. These views are then conveyed into policies, rules, and laws that are context specific. For example, determining whether an 18-year-old might be considered a child or an adult, and thus eligible for a particular service (such as funding for school-related technology) or opportunity (such as the right to vote in municipal election), is dictated by regional policy or law. However, whether that 18-year-old considers him or herself an adult or a child may also be influenced by family and community expectations (e.g. living with parents, or parenting own child), and current roles (e.g. attending high school, or working fulltime).

How is disability viewed as a sociocultural factor by TEI users?

TEI users, as people with various abilities, may hold differing worldviews on the meaning of disability (Lovern 2008), and thus may have a different response to TEI use, dependent on their held definition and explanation of disability. Armstrong and Fitzgerald (1996) provide us with a set of questions that can be useful as a thinking frame to help us understand the meaning that disability has for different people and their response to it, in different sociocultural contexts (Figure 12.1). Through the questions they pose, they help us to realize that there are many diverse ways in which a concept such as disability may be understood. However, there are two points of caution required as you seek to develop an understanding of the meaning that people place on disability and their response to TEI. First, there is risk in assigning common characteristics to a group that is most likely quite heterogeneous in terms of any of the other sociocultural factors or influences (age, gender, sexual orientation, socioeconomic status (SES), etc.) (Harry 1992). While broad generalizations may be useful in developing a cursory understanding (Lovern 2008), the generalizations can result in oversimplification. Second, any understanding and meaning will be further shaped by historical and sociopolitical experiences and opportunities that individuals have (or have not) endured (Browne 2005; Stedman and Thomas 2011). Some groups of people have historically experienced (and continue to experience) discrimination, colonization, disempowerment, deprivation, restricted rights, and inequality based on sociocultural factors such as gender, ethnicity, sexual orientation, ability status, and religious beliefs. These experiences and (lack of) opportunities will shape the interaction one has within society, and influence ones response to health or rehabilitation services. Overall then, we must recognize that we cannot consider meaning and understanding of disability ascribed by an individual or family without contextualizing that meaning within broader historical and social constructs. Figure 12.1 depicts these ideas as they might be used to consider how one views the concept of disability. Try to use Figure 12.1 to make sense of the following description provided in a research report of

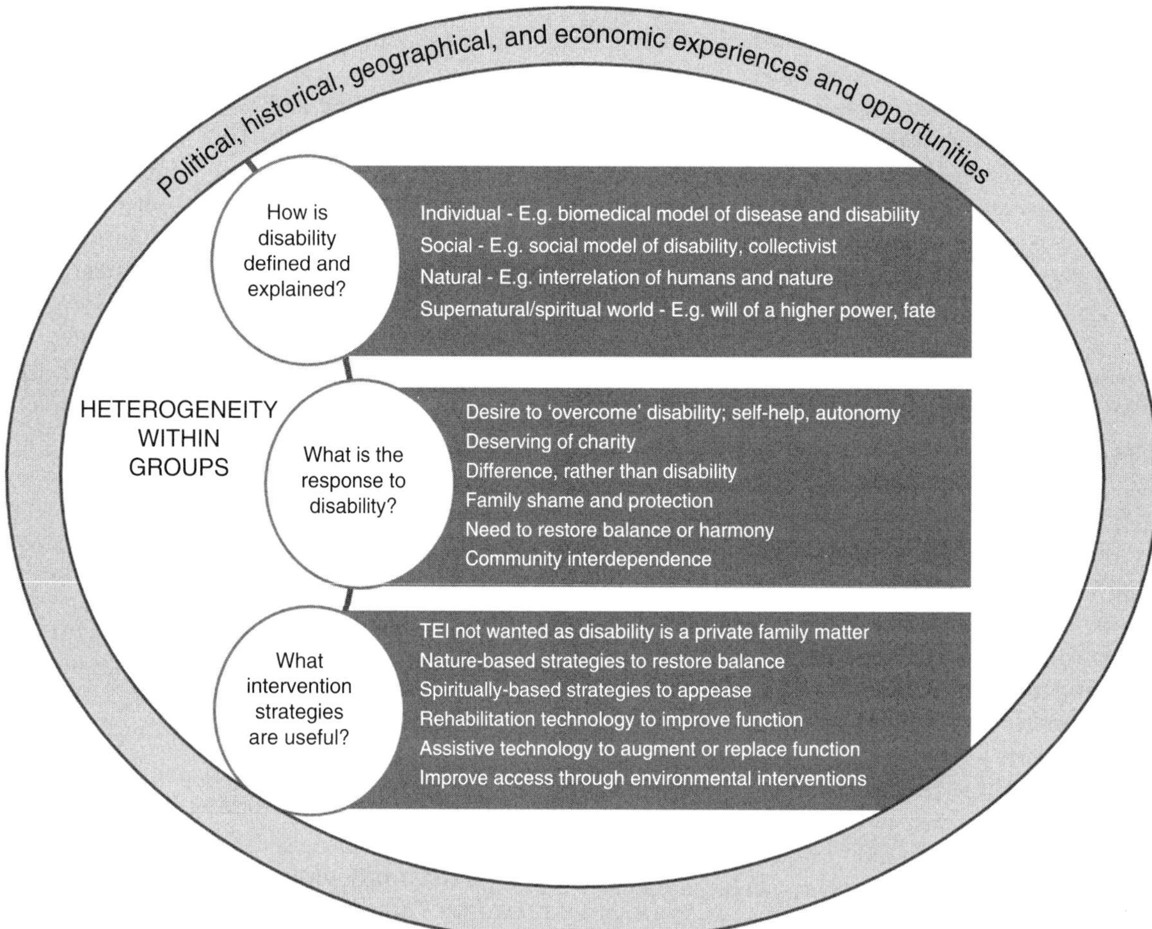

Figure 12.1 Framework for understanding the meaning and response to TEI taken by different people in different sociocultural contexts. Based on Armstrong and Fitzgerald (1996), Browne (2005), Burr (2003), Fitzgerald (2004), Harry (1992), Lovern (2008), Parette and Brotherson (2004), Thomas (2009).

prosthetic and orthotic service provider interviews in Sierra Leone (Magnusson and Ahlström 2012), which identified one of several social responses to disability as follows:

> A common perception was that a disabled child was being punished for being a witch or for the parents' bad behaviour. Some families did not want to maintain contact with a disabled family member, and there were instances where neighbours and society encouraged the family not to support their disabled child. People with disability were also neglected by their families because they could not contribute to the household. It was difficult to provide rehabilitation services when parents perceived the cause of their child's disability as witchcraft and refused such services. (p. 2114)

How might this description compare to a description of the societal response to children with disabilities you might construct in your own context?

Sociocultural influences on TEI use and meaning

In various studies, sociocultural factors have been examined as ones that might influence TEI use: age, gender, social supports, education, SES, ethnicity, location of residence, and ability status have all been identified as influences in various studies. Age as a influencing factor has been identified as an influence related to particular types of devices; for example, older age has been associated with increased use of walking aids, wheelchairs, bathrooms aids, hearing aids, and assistive listening devices (Edwards and Jones 1998; Hartley et al. 2010; Van der Esch et al. 2003). However, people who were older when they had an upper limb amputation were more likely to reject their upper limb prosthesis (Østlie et al. 2012), less likely to use memory tools as cognitive aids for multiple sclerosis (Johnson et al. 2009), and less likely to drive a modified vehicle post spinal cord injury (Norweg et al. 2011) than their younger counterparts. Social supports have been identified as an influence on device use; for instance, living alone has been identified as a factor in predicting assistive technology (AT) use in frail elders (Tomita et al. 2004), likelihood of using bathroom equipment for older adults (Hoffmann and McKenna 2004), and use of mobility and communication devices for young adults (Lindsay and Tsybina 2011). Gender has also been examined as an influence; for example, being male was found to predict increased use of a modified vehicle after spinal cord injury (Norweg et al. 2011). While some studies have reported no gender difference (Şimşek et al. 2012), the interaction between gender and age may complicate any conclusions. For example, in a study of older adults living in the community, males were more likely than females to use a wheelchair (Clarke and Colantonio 2005), while in a study of young adults, females were more likely than males to use mobility devices (Lindsay and Tsybina 2011).

A few studies have investigated socioeconomic influences on use; for example, lower education and household income were found to be a factors in explaining differences in access and use of AT (Kaye et al. 2008), higher education was associated with possession and use of a walking aid among people with arthritis (Van der Esch et al. 2003), and young adults who reported a higher income were more likely to use a mobility device (Lindsay and Tsybina 2011). Ethnicity has been identified in several studies where, generally, researchers found that people who identified as minority status were less likely to have access to (Kaye et al. 2008) or use (Kaye et al. 2008; Lindsay and Tsybina 2011; Norweg et al. 2011; Tomita et al. 2004) a TEI. A few studies have examined geographic location of residence as an influential factor on use: Veehof et al. (2006) established that people in the Netherlands were more likely to possess AT than those in Germany, and Goins et al. (2010) reported that members of one federally recognized American Indian tribe had a greater odds of AT use when compared to a peer reference group. Finally, ability status influences AT access and use, and many researchers have suggested that there are unmet AT needs among individuals with disabilities (see for example, Edwards and Jones 1998; Hartley et al. 2010; Johnson et al. 2009; Kaye et al. 2008; Lindsay and Tsybina 2011; Spiliotopoulou et al. 2012).

Overall, these studies confirm that sociocultural factors play a role in influencing TEI access, use, and likelihood of use. However, it is difficult to draw any broad conclusions as there is a complicated relationship between these factors that is likely further confounded by the local practices, context, and societal norms of the setting in which the study occurred. This literature gives us some indication of patterns and predictors of TEI use, and suggests issues of disparity in TEI access and service provision. However, the aim of these studies was not to examine the personal experience and meaning that individual users assign to TEI, and the role that meaning may play in TEI use: exploration of meaning as determined by qualitative methods of inquiry will be the focus of the next section.

Earlier, we established a basic understanding of social constructionism, defined sociocultural factors, and examined how one sociocultural factor (understanding and social response to disability) might take on different meanings, and now we can consider how these ideas might come together in influencing ones' perceived

Box 12.1 Here's the evidence

Lee, C. and Coughlin, J. F. (2015). Older adults' adoption of technology. *Journal of Product Innovation Management* 32: 747–759. doi:https://doi.org/10.1111/jpim.12176

Key Words: elders, stereotyping, technology adoption and use

Purpose: The purpose of this article is to identify and define factors that affect how technology is adopted and used by older adults.

Sample: The authors reviewed 59 articles describing older adults' technology adoption in a variety of fields including information technology, gerontology, human factors, and design. The study was done to identify common themes and important concepts that influence adoption.

Method: Articles were identified using a variety of search engines which included Google scholar, Thompsons Reuters, and more using the terms older adults and technology adoption or acceptance.

Findings: Results revealed 10 factors that can be used to provide a better understanding for "making decisions, strategies, and design specifications as a technology is planned, designed developed produced and distributed to older adults." (p. 749). Additionally, adoption of technology is influenced not only by the technical aspects of the product but by physical design, individual characteristics, social settings, and delivery channels as well. Understanding these multiple factors can reduce the stigma associated with AT use.

Critical Thinking Questions:

1. After reading this research article, what do you understand to be the limitations of this research? Are there any limitations not stated?
2. If you were to replicate this study using a different method or design, what designs would you use to increase the rigor and why?
3. Based on the findings of this study, what additional research do you consider is needed that is not addressed in the discussion section?

meaning of TEI. Hocking has suggested that: "the recipient's values and emotional responses to using assistive devices may be more potent factors in surviving, or flourishing with assistive devices than the occupational opportunities they enable" (1999, p. 6). In advancing this idea, she proposed that service providers move beyond considering only the functions enhanced through AT use, toward a thorough understanding of the sociocultural factors influencing TEI meaning and use. Since the time Hocking wrote that statement, researchers have begun to develop just this understanding (Box 12.1).

Self-identity and social reception

Self-identity, and the importance of considering the impact of AT on one's self-identity, has been described in the previous chapter. Self-identity is irrefutably linked with social perception and reaction, and thus it is worthy of touching on how one shapes one's identity in a social context. This link is clearly described in a study by Larsson Lund and Nygard (2003), where the use of AT to achieve a particular function was interpreted by users in different ways, and the researchers identified three types of AT users: "pragmatic user, ambivalent users, and reluctant users" (p. 70). In this study, *pragmatic users* were able to use the AT to maintain their self-identity through participation in occupations, while *ambivalent* users were hesitant to use AT despite the positive opportunities afforded by use, and *reluctant* users viewed AT use as an affront to their self-identity as the sociocultural meaning of being an AT user overrode the enjoyment they may have received by participating in occupations through the use of their AT. The researchers interpreted that these participants selected one or the other approach in an attempt to maintain congruence with their self-identity and image.

Recalling social constructionism, we must remember that devices themselves hold symbolic meaning, and thus it is not surprising that social reaction has been described as having influence on TEI use and personal acceptance. For some, the social reaction is perceived as negative, for example when they feel others treat them differently when they are using an AT. McMillen and Söderberg (2002) interviewed 15 mobility device users who described a "changed reception" (p. 181) from others when they began using a mobility device; for instance, participants in that study reported feeling stared at, or ignored. Other TEI users who have reported similar negative social reactions include people using augmentative and alternative communication devices (Iacono et al. 2013), prosthetics (Murray 2009; Murray and Forshaw 2013), hearing aids (Kent and Smith 2006), and wheelchairs (Korotchenko and Clarke 2014; Ripat and Woodgate 2012). For new device users, the social reception to device use may be most prominent and influential. Some people may consider a "hierarchy" of assistive devices related to social acceptance of disability: for example, one person may consider a cane to look less disabling-looking than a wheelchair, and a manual wheelchair less disabling in appearance than a power wheelchair (with all types of variations on this hierarchy possible and likely based on sociocultural meaning assigned). This perception of hierarchy may influence initial device selection and use. It is worth considering though, that as one becomes accustomed to TEI use, the social response to device use could become less of a consideration, and that other individual or personal factors take precedence. For some people, as self-identity and confidence as a TEI user develops, it might be more important for the person to consider the function that it promotes, comfort of the device, or feelings of safety. Consider the story told by Andrew, who, following a spinal cord injury, initially chose to use a manual wheelchair and, after a few years, decided to use a power wheelchair: "When I was first in a wheelchair everybody says 'oh you never want to go into a power chair'. And uh so the first couple of years I didn't, and just living in the country and going out on the lawn you know I had to get my wife to push me out here and you know I couldn't move around on the lawn after a couple of years of that I had it, I said enough of this, just because uh you know and I mean now I can go where I want. When I want" (Ripat and Woodgate 2012, p. 174). In your opinion, what balance of social and individual factors might Andrew be negotiating?

Thus, while TEI users' individual responses to negative social reactions may be different, it is clear that social response will affect patterns of and decisions about use (e.g. use, non-use, inconsistent use, reluctant use, selective use) of a device (Larsson Lund and Nygard 2003; Pape et al. 2002). It is further important to consider the potential duality that assistive devices may create for individuals (Gudgeon and Kirk 2015; Häggblom-Kronlöf and Sonn 2007; Korotchenko and Clarke 2014; Ripat et al. 2018). While TEI may indeed promote a sense of competence, empowerment, and autonomy, they can just as easily create a sense of embarrassment, shame, restriction, and inadequacy. At times, the positive and negative feelings about a device may co-exist, in what Lupton and Seymour (2000) described as a "love/hate relationship" (p. 1860) of feelings about an assistive device. Therefore, it is essential that TEI providers strive to understand and appreciate the meaning placed on the devices to best meet their clients' needs (Parette and Scherer 2004).

Family and TEI meaning

Families may be considered the most immediate social system that the TEI user will interact with: Fitzgerald (2004) states that "families provide the context for learning the beliefs, values, attitudes, and customs that guide much of our lives" (p. 489). The role of social supports and relationships as "prerequisites" (Petersson et al. 2012, p. 798) to technology use was emphasized in a study on how technology use and home adaptations influenced the experience of safety of older adults in Sweden. These authors found that a sense of safety in the home could not be established through technical device and home modifications in the absence of social supports. The introduction of TEI into one's home and family environment requires various adaptations take place for all family members. Individuals with high-level spinal cord injuries reported a sense of lessened burden on family members when using their environmental control systems (Myburg et al. 2017; Verdonck et al. 2018). Pettersson et al. (2005) interviewed spouses of individuals who had had a stroke and who used AT in their homes. She proposed that the presence of assistive devices and their use by an individual also required adaptation on the part of the spouse, who needed to develop and assign their own meaning to the devices, such as a tool that required mediation between themselves, their spouses, and society in general (p. 167). Correspondingly, mothers discussed how the introduction of a hoist lift for their children represented a change in the physical interactions they had with their children, and also needed to be accommodated within the physical and social structure of their families (Shepherd et al. 2007).

Family patterns, habits, and roles are altered by TEI, and families will respond differently to the introduction of TEI. In a study of 80 mothers of children with disabilities, Mayes et al. (2011) explored how the mothers organized and assigned meaning to spaces within the home. Different strategies were used, including shared spaces where they could simultaneously address home maintenance and childcare needs, working to avoid "medicalization" (p. 18) of a space filled with equipment and devices, and creating private, inaccessible spaces in the home that excluded their child. Choices are made by families in terms of how they will incorporate AT into their lives and homes. Parents of Mexican-American augmentative and alternative communication (AAC) users discussed their preferences for non-use of the AAC at home, due to the disruption the device placed on established and preferred ways of communicating within the family (McCord and Soto 2004). Likewise, Huang et al. (2009) found parents reported limited TEI use by their children at home, where the "social characteristics" (p. 136) of the home, such as parenting style, expectations, and habits influenced choice of use. In both of these studies (Huang et al. 2009; McCord and Soto 2004) parents reported that, while the devices were valued and used in schools and unfamiliar environments, they preferred not to use TEI-assisted function in the privacy of their own homes and within their families.

Social and community participation

The opportunity to use TEI to promote participation in everyday life is an emerging theme in the literature (e.g. Batorowicz et al. 2014; Fomiatti et al. 2014; Pettersson et al. 2012; Ripat and Woodgate 2012; Ripat et al. 2018; Verdonck et al. 2011; Woodgate et al. 2012). In these studies, participation has been self-perceived, defined by a sense of social inclusion, ability to engage in social relationships, and opportunity to interact within one's broader community. While negative social reactions to TEI use have been discussed in the literature, positive social opportunities, social relationships, and social participation have been reported by TEI users. Verdonck et al. (2011) interviewed users of electronic aids to daily living (EADLs) in Ireland: EADL users reported that use of the TEI decreased the users' sense of burden and dependence on family members. Social inclusion and acceptance have also been examined in the context of the built environment. For instance, Pettersson et al. (2012) identified that housing adaptations were understood to contribute to a sense of connectivity and community participation for older adults in Sweden, and Ripat and Becker (2012) found that accessible playgrounds were seen as the creation of a space that promoted a sense of social inclusion and peer acceptance for children with disabilities.

Social and political influences

Thus, there is a growing understanding of the varied meanings assigned to, and influences on, TEI use within the immediate (family) and near (community) social and physical/built environments. However, even when an interest in or desire to use TEI exists, opportunity may be limited by broader social and political forces such as funding policies and practices, and some research has considered how the opportunity to use AT may be thwarted by broader political, fiscal, geographic, and cultural structures (Wearmouth and Wielandt 2009; Woodgate et al. 2012). For example, despite having been provided with a wheelchair, people with spinal cord injuries living on a reserve in Canada described the barriers to community and cultural participation they experienced, attributed in part to the lack of government priority on infrastructure (Wearmouth and Wielandt 2009). In another study, parents of children who were assistive and medical device users were often unable to "harness" the social, physical, institutional, and economic resources needed for meaningful participation in their lives (Woodgate et al. 2012, p. 1916). Lastly, in a study exploring older adults' use of a power wheelchair, the participants are described as experiencing "marginalization through the disabling organization of public space" (Korotchenko and Clarke 2014, p. 441).

Returning full circle, consider the following proposition offered by Pape et al. (2002): "successful integration of AT into daily activities requires potential device users to explore: (1) the meanings they assign to devices; (2) their expectations of AT; (3) the anticipated social costs; and (4) ways to come to terms with disability as one, but not the defining, feature of oneself" (p. 18). Recognizing the importance of each of these factors, we are now in a position to address how one might support this as a TEI service provider.

Providing culturally relevant services

While the TEI service provider is considering how sociocultural factors might be influencing the TEI user, he or she must simultaneously be conscious of the sociocultural factors that influence his or her own actions or inactions, choices and decisions, and communications (Fitzgerald 2004; McCord and Soto 2004). Indeed, Western-held ideas and assumptions about people's desire for independence, reduced dependence, equality, individualism, competence, mastery, and productivity may be inconsistent with the values held by the others (Hocking 2000; Iwama 2003; McCord and Soto 2004). TEI practitioners may have been indoctrinated in these Western values through their family, educational, and professional teachings and experiences (Fitzgerald 2004). However, when there are differing or incongruent values of practitioners and TEI users, there may be misunderstandings, misinterpretations, and miscommunications (Fitzgerald 2004; Parette and Brotherson 2004). Consider how the three examples of TEI shown in Table 12.1 may have had differing values attached, depending on the perspectives.

As service providers, how can we address this apparent incongruence in the perspectives of the provider and end user? In the following section, a three-pronged approach to providing culturally relevant TEI services in proposed: self-reflection, understanding the TEI user, and measuring outcomes of relevance to the TEI user (Figure 12.2).

Self-reflection

The first step in providing socioculturally relevant TEI services is to gain an understanding of one's own values. Hitlin and Piliavin (2004) suggest that values "serve as standards for judging others' (and one's own) behaviour" (p. 361). As the values that one holds are not always articulated or conscious (McCord and Soto 2004), consideration of our "unexamined assumptions" is imperative so that we avoid making assumptions about the behaviors of others (Browne et al. 2009, p. 171). The challenge then, is to

Table 12.1 Value Placed on Technology and Environmental Interventions (TEI) by Different Stakeholders.

Technology and environmental interventions (TEI) provided	Potential value promoted by TEI provider	Alternate value/perspective
Low-technology device: independent feeding device	Reduced dependence on caregivers	A father chooses to feed his son rather than promoting independent feeding (Halderman and Springer 2007, personal communication)
High-technology device: augmentative or alternative communication device	Independence in communication	For some families, use of an augmentative and alternative communication (AAC) device precluded the families' ability to communicate in a more "intimate and interdependent" manner (McCord and Soto 2004, p. 220)
Environmental adaptation: access and equality	Accessible home environment	Some mothers of children with disabilities describe their intentional decision to maintain some areas of the home as inaccessible to their children to allow for privacy (Mayes et al. 2011)

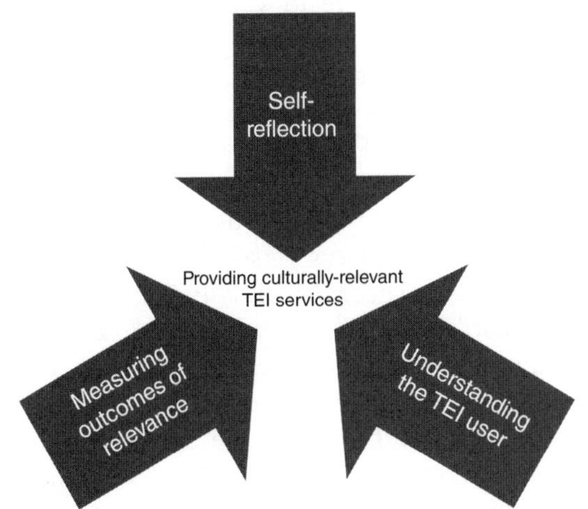

Figure 12.2 Three-pronged approach to providing culturally relevant technology and environmental interventions (TEI) services.

understand one's own values, to clarify how ones' values influence ones beliefs and assumptions, and to consider how they may be similar or different from those of others (McCord and Soto 2004).

> Values: "principles or standards of behaviour; one's judgement of what is important in life"
> Belief: "an acceptance that something exists or is true, especially one without proof"
> Assumption: "a thing that is accepted as true or as certain to happen, without proof"
> Behaviour: "the way in which one acts or conducts oneself, especially towards others"
>
> Source: oxforddictionaries.com

Examining our own values, beliefs, and assumptions is one way that we can intentionally work toward becoming a reflective practitioner (Fitzgerald 2004; Kinsella 2001). We all enter situations carrying assumptions about others, perhaps based on superficial characteristics, such as what we believe we know about the sociocultural indicators of a person's ethnicity, age, gender, SES, etc., or by comparing others' behavior to that of our own (Harry 1992). Kinsella challenges us to "unpack the suitcase" (p. 197) of beliefs and assumptions that we all carry in order to better understand how the assumptions guide our actions and behaviors. We can begin to do this by clarifying our own values and beliefs (articulating them, and bringing them to our consciousness) and considering the role that our own experiences and opportunities have had in shaping our assumptions and behaviors (CAOT 2014; Harry 1992; McCord and Soto 2004). The term cultural humility has been used as an expression for a process of self-reflection on one's own values, beliefs, and assumptions as the foremost activity, prior to focusing on those of others (California Health Advocates 2007). Cultural humility has been described as moving beyond cultural sensitivity and competence toward a process of self-reflection and increasing self-awareness of power differentials that practitioners in an increasingly globalized context are encouraged to embrace (Miller 2009).

Self-reflection involves "purposeful critical analysis of knowledge and experience, in order to achieve deeper meaning and understanding" (Mann et al. 2009, p. 597). Kinsella (2001) describes how one can become a reflective practitioner by engaging in a deliberate process of reflecting on our experiences, practice contexts, and examination of assumptions. Reflection can have a "vertical dimension" where there are deepening levels of critical reflection on an experience and/or an "iterative dimension" where the practitioner reflects on, and develops new ways of thinking about, that experience (Mann et al. 2009, p. 597).

With respect to sociocultural influences on TEI, self-reflection involves a desire and conscious decision to better understand the perspective and worldviews of the AT user. Self-reflection involves the AT provider thinking deeply about his or her own values, beliefs, and assumptions. It requires openness to other ways of understanding and knowing and not expecting that others' will merely be a mirror of his or her own. It requires the provider to stay attuned to his or her own feelings about a client, interaction, or decision, and to critically explore those feelings. It requires a provider to identify, explore, and discuss when his or her ideas seem to be in conflict with those of others, rather than jumping to fast conclusions.

Understanding the TEI user

The second prong is a deliberate focus on gaining an understanding of the TEI user (Gramstad et al. 2014). Client-centered practice is an approach to working with clients founded on principles of collaboration and partnership, respect for the individual, shared and informed decision-making, client empowerment, and acknowledgement of the client as the expert in his or her own life (Law et al. 1995; Sumsion and Law 2006; Townsend and Polatajko 2007). Practitioners who use a client-centered approach uphold the dignity, individuality, and sociocultural factors that are an inherent and central part of that person (Stedman and Thomas 2011). A client-centered practitioner will consider how to facilitate his or her interactions with the client at the individual practitioner-client/family level, within his or her practice setting, and at broader community and societal levels (Restall and Ripat 2008; Restall et al. 2003).

At the individual practitioner-client/family level, communication that demonstrates a clear interest in understanding the meaning placed on TEI by the user is paramount (Hunt 2007). Providers that have well-developed communication styles will demonstrate respect for the values and beliefs held by the TEI user and will avoid making assumptions that presume they know better or more than the TEI user. Focusing on the TEI user (and family) as the expert in his or her own life shows the importance you place on developing this understanding.

Instruments that allow the TEI user to identify their own issues and desired outcomes, in their own words, may be a useful place to start to develop this understanding. Some instruments have been developed with the intent of understanding issues and goals of importance and meaning as self-identified by the user. While not specifically designed for TEI use, the Canadian Occupational Performance Measure (COPM) (Law et al. 1990) is a standardized measure that allows users to self-identify their issues in self-care, productivity, and leisure. The COPM has been used to identify goals and evaluate outcomes in areas such as the use of personal digital assistants as aids to support cognitive functioning (Gentry et al. 2010), use of pushrim activated power-assist wheelchairs (Giesbrecht et al. 2009), and the use of high-technology vision aids (Petty et al. 2005). Developed specifically for use in the AT realm, the Individually Prioritised Problem Assessment (IPPA) (Wessels et al. 2000) is based on a similar construct of self-identification of issues and goals, and is purported to be able to be used to determine the extent to which the identified issues are reduced related to the TEI intervention (see for example, Pettersson et al. 2006; Wessels et al. 2004). The Wheelchair Outcome Measure (Mortenson et al. 2007) was designed for people to self-identify outcomes of importance that may be affected by wheelchair use, and to rank importance and rate satisfaction with performance in those outcome areas. Matching Person and Technology (MPT) (Scherer and Craddock 2002) is an individualized assessment process designed to select the best AT match for the TEI user through thorough consideration of the user's personal characteristics and contexts of use. The MPT has undergone extensive development and is well-referenced in the TEI literature as a client-centered assessment instrument. Thus, a client-centered approach, based on the user-identified outcomes of importance, can be promoted through selection of these types of individualized instruments.

To augment the use of standardized client-centered instruments, creative ways of learning about users' issues, goals, and desired outcomes may also be useful. For example, AT users have been asked to photograph aspects of their environment that supported or facilitated their community participation, and the photographs used as a catalyst for discussion about the role of AT in their community participation (Ripat and Woodgate 2012, 2017). In a study of children with disabilities' perspective on playground use, Ripat and Becker (2012) asked child participants to depict their desired playground in drawings, through crafts, or with miniaturized playground components, to better understand their perspectives. The ability to explore TEI meaning is bounded only by our imaginations, and continued research into ways to draw on constructed meaning is required.

Within the practice setting, the TEI practitioner may consider ways in which client-centered service can be delivered. Practice-setting examples that would address and respect the unique needs of individuals include ensuring: accessible and convenient service availability; consistent access to interpreters and translators; written materials and instructions available in a wide variety of formats; recognition and respect for the inherent power differential between practitioners and clients, and work to reduce that differential; opportunity for clients and families to provide feedback on service provision; and consideration of family needs such as making childcare available for siblings or children of the TEI user, or ensuring meeting space is large enough to accommodate extended family (Law et al. 2003; McCord and Soto 2004; Parette and Brotherson 2004; Restall et al. 2003). Overall, the intent is to create and cultivate a respectful, flexible, welcoming, accommodating, and responsive service provision environment.

At a community and societal level, the client-centered TEI practitioner can work to address the broader needs of TEI users. For example, the practitioner may choose to collaborate with other community organizations to advocate for services and funding that respect the sociocultural needs of their clients. The practitioner might draw awareness to inequities that exist related to sociocultural factors (e.g. discriminatory or inequality in service delivery or access to TEI), or partner with community groups to address community-level needs such as development of inclusive public spaces for TEI users.

Measuring outcomes of relevance to the TEI user

The final prong in the suggested three-prong approach is to measure outcomes of relevance to TEI users. However, with the provision that the TEI user is not the only stakeholder in our interaction, the focus here is not on an exhaustive examination of the many TEI outcome measures available for their sociocultural relevance. It is recognized that many stakeholders are interested in the assessment and outcomes of TEI, including funders, employers, and other organizations. Many well-developed measures are in existence to address these stakeholder needs. Rather, the intent of this section is to provide broader assistance to the reader in recognizing that outcome measures are also socioculturally derived, and to equip the reader to examine existing measures with a sociocultural lens during selection.

Some existing instruments focus on examining the influence of TEI on some of the sociocultural variables discussed earlier in this chapter. For example, the Family Impact of Assistive Technology Scale was developed "to detect the multidimensional effect of assistive device use on families who have young children with disabilities" (Ryan et al. 2007, p. 1436). Another instrument, the Psychosocial Impact of Assistive Devices Scale (Jutai and Day 2002), examines the influence of TEI on subjective well-being, and some of the instrument's items are closely connected to sociocultural influences discussed (e.g. effect on embarrassment, ability to participate). Recently, instruments have been developed to address the impact that AT use has on family and informal caregivers (e.g. The Power Mobility Caregiver Assistive Technology Outcome Measure [Mortenson et al. 2017]). While all of these instruments address the impact of TEI on sociocultural factors, it is important to remember that the instruments themselves are developed within particular contexts where particular broad sets of societal values are held.

With this in mind, perhaps the question we can consider then is: What sociocultural assumptions are made in the development of instruments that focus on measuring use, usability, effectiveness, or satisfaction with a particular TEI? Outcome measures are based on the idea that we can measure some construct, provide an intervention (e.g. TEI), re-measure that outcome, and attribute the change in measurement to the intervention. However, the basic premise of this assumption is rooted in Western positivistic ways of thinking about and understanding cause and effect. As Harry (1992) cautioned, measures developed with the Western-held belief that variables can be measured void of context and explanation, may be "incongruous with the task of gleaning information about a family's values and needs" (p. 344). Deconstructing aspects of the instrument may give us some insight into the assumptions used to guide the development. What assumptions might have been made if the ability to independently perform an activity using an AT was the desired outcome (i.e. the highest score was assigned if someone was independent)? What if speed of performance is an outcome of interest? The type of item response may also be influenced by sociocultural factors. For example, the use of rating scales assumes that people can consistently assign value in some numerical or hierarchical fashion – an assumption that may not be universal, as some have suggested that there may be sociocultural differences in the way that various groups of people respond to a standardized numerical scale (Lee et al. 2002).

There is a substantial challenge in creating TEI instruments that hold sociocultural relevance across all populations. When instruments are developed in a particular context with a particular set of assumptions, they run the risk of being less applicable to our own context and population. One option practitioners sometimes select is to develop a local, context-specific measure. However, this is not easily done. The development of a reliable and valid measure is an extensive undertaking that often requires years of research. A second option when a well-established instrument exists is translation for use into another context. Again though, there are challenges with this approach if cross-cultural considerations beyond language are ignored. For example, Mao et al. (2010) described their study exploring cross-cultural adaptation of the Quebec User Evaluation of Satisfaction with Assistive Technology in Taiwan. In their study, these researchers highlighted the need to consider context of use (e.g. different policies regarding service delivery or access to AT), terminology (e.g. cultural differences in terms of the meaning and ranking of satisfaction), and relevance of items, and suggested that "instruments used for the evaluation of user satisfaction with AT should be adapted to the society in terms of language, policy and sociocultural aspects, and the validity and reliability should be established" (p. 413). Thus, as conscientious TEI practitioners focused on evidence-based practice, the advice is to clearly understand the context and assumption under which a tool was developed, to explore the usefulness for the populations you work with, and to maintain a level of cautious and contextualized interpretation of results.

Design and development

Just as use of TEI is influenced by sociocultural factors, we can also consider how the design and development of AT has been influenced by sociocultural factors. Taking a historical view of the economic, technological, political, socioeconomic, and social forces over time that have influenced the design, development, meaning, and use of various AT reminds us of the powerful sociocultural influences at play. For example, writers have reviewed the development of wheelchairs (Woods and Watson 2003, 2004), wheelchair seating and positioning (Watson and Woods 2005), use and acceptance of hearing aids or cochlear implants (Pray and Jordan 2010), and augmentative communication and computer access (Vanderheiden 2002), each providing a captivating analysis of the various factors that have guided the development and uptake of AT. To illustrate, Woods and Watson (2004) trace the meaning ascribed to wheelchairs throughout their history, identifying that the meaning ascribed to wheelchairs in the early 1900s represented "the failure of medicine to find a cure and/or that the wheelchair user had given up on rehabilitation" (p. 407). With widespread availability of lightweight materials and the development of the folding wheelchair in the 1950s, the wheelchair became transportable. Woods and Watson describe the emergence of the wheelchair as a symbol of independence due to the convergence of social (disability movement, de-institutionalization), medical (production of penicillin and resultant diminished mortality, emphasis on rehabilitation), and political (demand from disabled veterans) movements of the time. Thus, it is clear that the intersection of many sociocultural factors had, and will continue to have, an influence on the development and design of AT such as wheelchairs. Consider the future: How might sociocultural factors associated with an aging population influence wheelchair design over the next two decades?

The importance of design for sociocultural context has been outlined; for instance, Lysack et al. (1999) describe a wheelchair development project for women with mobility impairments in India, explaining how often AT development is "based on Western designs which are expensive, elaborate, require a great deal of maintenance, and are generally not suited to the physical or economic environment in which they are used" (p. 2). They set out to design and develop a mobility device by establishing design criteria that considered the unique environmental context (physical, sociocultural, economic), functional needs, and roles of the women-users and incorporated a cycle of development that relied on input and evaluation from the end users (Lysack et al. 1999).

Some developers have focused on the social acceptability of AT, recognizing the social nature of AT use, and proposing that integration and unification of mainstream and assistive technologies is necessary, in an approach Shinohara and Wobbrock (2011) call "design for social acceptance" (p. 712). In his book *Design meets Disability* (2009), Graham Pullin weaves together his ideas of how disability can influence design and vice versa and challenges classification of persons based on disability, claiming that:

> design for disability has paid more attention to the clinical than the cultural diversity within any one group. The same prostheses, wheelchairs, and communication devices are often offered to people with a particular disability, whether they are seventeen or seventy years old, and regardless of their attitudes, toward their disability or otherwise (pp. 89–90).

Pullin (2009) provides numerous examples of products inspired by the interaction of design and disability that are simple in use, appealing to different people, and, at times, controversial to evoke emotion and confront and challenge stereotypes. Similar ideas were explored by Gardner (2017) in a study of older adults who modified and personalized their mobility devices as a way of preserving self-identity, addressing social stigma, and promoting social roles. It is clear that the future of design and development of AT will need to consider the dynamic and evolving sociocultural contexts in which we live.See Box 12.2 for a case study.

Box 12.2 Case study

Belinda is a TEI specialist at an urban center that provides rehabilitation services to children. She received a referral to complete an assessment for Phoenix, a six-year-old girl who had flown in with her family from a remote First Nation reserve in Canada, located 500 miles north of the center, for her appointment. Belinda worked quickly to complete the assessment and paperwork to order the equipment, access approval for the funding, and organize the delivery of several devices (including a standing frame, bath seat, toilet seat, and wheelchair lap tray) to the airport in time for the family's departure, scheduled 24 hours after the appointment. The day after the family left, Belinda received a phone call from an airport supervisor who informed her that the equipment, labeled with the rehabilitation center's contact information and the name *Phoenix*, had been left in the terminal. Belinda was frustrated as she arranged to have the equipment returned to the center – why would this equipment have been seemingly left behind by the family?

- What values/beliefs/assumptions did Belinda seem to hold as a TEI provider?
- What sociocultural factors might have influenced Belinda's values/beliefs/assumptions?
- What sociocultural factors (historical/socioeconomic/political/contextual) might have influenced Phoenix's family's decision to leave the equipment at the airport? Which of these factors would you want to learn more about?

Summary

Meaning and use of TEI is influenced by numerous intersecting, complex, and dynamic sociocultural factors. TEI use by an individual cannot be considered to the exclusion of the social and cultural influences that affect the ways that one views the world. These influences are most often tacit and unspoken and yet have a powerful effect on values, beliefs, assumptions, and behaviors. Part of the challenge is to elucidate those sociocultural influences and factors that affect how a user perceives their TEI, the perspectives TEI service providers take, the measurement of TEI outcomes, and the development of TEI. It is an exciting yet arduous journey to take as a TEI provider, as you begin to unravel the various influences in an attempt to understand how TEI use is perceived by the individual user. Adopting a three-pronged approach to culturally relevant TEI practice involves a combination of self-reflection, seeking ways to understand the TEI user, and identifying outcomes that matter to the TEI user. Combining this approach with your skills and knowledge of TEI devices and service delivery will contribute to your development as a competent, client-centered, and socioculturally sensitive TEI practitioner.

References

Armstrong, M. and Fitzgerald, M. (1996). Culture and disability studies: an anthropological perspective. *Rehabilitation Education* 10 (4): 247–304.

Batorowicz, B., Campbell, F., von Tetzchner, S. et al. (2014). Social participation of school-aged children who use communication aids: the views of children and parents. *Augmentative and Alternative Communication* 30 (3): 237–251.

Browne, A. (2005). Discourses influencing nurses' perceptions of First Nations patients. *Canadian Journal of Nursing Research* 37 (4): 62–87.

Browne, A., Varcoe, C., Smye, V. et al. (2009). Cultural safety and the challenges of translating critically oriented knowledge in practice. *Nursing Philosophy* 10 (3): 167–179. https://doi.org/10.1111/j.1466-769X.2009.00406.x.

Burr, V. (2003). *Social Constructionism*. Hove, UK: Psychology Press.

California Health Advocates (2007). Are you practicing cultural humility? – The key to success in cultural competence. Retrieved from https://cahealthadvocates.org/are-you-practicing-cultural-humility-the-key-to-success-in-cultural-competence/.

Canadian Association of Occupational Therapists (2014). Joint position statement on diversity. Retrieved from http://caot.ca/site/pt/caot_posn_stmt?nav=sidebar.

Clarke, P. and Colantonio, A. (2005). Wheelchair use among community-dwelling older adults: prevalence and risk factors in a national sample. *Canadian Journal on Aging* 24 (2): 191–198.

Edwards, N. and Jones, E. (1998). Ownership and use of assistive devices amongst older people in the community. *Age and Ageing* 27 (4): 463–468.

Fitzgerald, M. (2004). A dialogue on occupational therapy, culture, and families. *American Journal of Occupational Therapy* 58 (5): 489–498.

Fomiatti, R., Moir, L., Richmond, J., and Millsteed, J. (2014). The experience of being a motorised mobility scooter user. *Disability and Rehabilitation: Assistive Technology* 9 (3): 183–187. https://doi.org/10.3109/17483107.2013.814171.

Gardner, P. (2017). MAPx (Mobility Aid Personalization): examining why older adults "pimp their ride" and the impact of doing so. *Disability and Rehabilitation: Assistive Technology* 12 (5): 512–518. https://doi.org/10.3109/17483107.2016.1158327.

Gentry, T., Wallace, J., Kvarfordt, C., and Lynch, K. (2010). Personal digital assistants as cognitive aids for high school students with autism: results of a community-based trial. *Journal of Vocational Rehabilitation* 32 (2): 101–107. https://doi.org/10.3233/JVR-2010-0499.

Giesbrecht, E., Ripat, J., Quanbury, A., and Cooper, J. (2009). Participation in community-based activities of daily living: comparison of a pushrim-activated, power-assisted wheelchair and a power wheelchair. *Disability and Rehabilitation: Assistive Technology* 4 (3): 198–207. https://doi.org/10.1080/17483100802543205.

Goins, R., Spencer, S., Goli, S., and Rogers, J. (2010). Assistive technology use of older American Indians in a southeastern tribe: the Native Elder Care Study. *Journal of The American Geriatrics Society* 58 (11): 2185–2190. https://doi.org/10.1111/j.1532-5415.2010.03140.x.

Gramstad, A., Storli, S.L., and Hamran, T. (2014). Exploring the meaning of a new assistive technology device for older individuals. *Disability and Rehabilitation: Assistive Technology* 9 (6): 493–498. https://doi.org/10.3109/17483107.2014.921249.

Gudgeon, S. and Kirk, S. (2015). Living with a powered wheelchair: exploring children's and young people's experiences. *Disability and Rehabilitation: Assistive Technology* 10 (2): 118–125. https://doi.org/10.3109/17483107.2013.870609.

Häggblom-Kronlöf, G. and Sonn, U. (2007). Use of assistive devices – a reality full of contradictions in elderly persons' everyday life. *Disability and Rehabilitation: Assistive Technology* 2 (6): 335–345.

Harry, B. (1992). Developing cultural self-awareness: the first step in values clarification for early interventionists. *Topics in Early Childhood Special Education* 12 (3): 333–350.

Hartley, D., Rochtchina, E., Newall, P. et al. (2010). Use of hearing aids and assistive listening devices in an older Australian population. *Journal of The American Academy of Audiology* 21 (10): 642–653. https://doi.org/10.3766/jaaa.21.10.4.

Hitlin, S. and Piliavin, J. (2004). Values: reviving a dormant concept. *Annual Review of Sociology* 30 (1): 359–393. https://doi.org/10.1146/annurev.soc.30.012703.110640.

Hocking, C. (1999). Function or feelings: factors in abandonment of assistive devices. *Technology and Disability* 11 (1/2): 3–11.

Hocking, C. (2000). Having and using objects in the Western world. *Journal of Occupational Science* 7 (3): 148–157.

Hoffmann, T. and McKenna, K. (2004). A survey of assistive equipment used by older people following hospital discharge. *British Journal of Occupational Therapy* 67 (2): 75–82.

Huang, I., Sugden, D., and Beveridge, S. (2009). Assistive devices and cerebral palsy: factors influencing the use of assistive devices at home by children with cerebral palsy. *Child: Care, Health & Development* 35 (1): 130–139. https://doi.org/10.1111/j.1365-2214.2008.00898.x.

Hunt, M. (2007). Taking culture seriously: considerations for physiotherapists. *Physiotherapy* 93 (3): 229–232.

Iacono, T., Lyon, K., Johnson, H., and West, D. (2013). Experiences of adults with complex communication needs receiving and using low tech AAC: an Australian context. *Disability and Rehabilitation: Assistive Technology* 8 (5): 392–401. https://doi.org/10.3109/17483107.2013.769122.

Iwama, M. (2003). Toward culturally relevant epistemologies in occupational therapy. *American Journal of Occupational Therapy* 57 (5): 582–588.

Johnson, K., Bamer, A., Yorkston, K., and Amtmann, D. (2009). Use of cognitive aids and other assistive technology by individuals with multiple sclerosis. *Disability and Rehabilitation: Assistive Technology* 4 (1): 1–8. https://doi.org/10.1080/17483100802239648.

Jutai, J. and Day, H. (2002). Psychosocial Impact of Assistive Devices Scale (PIADS). *Technology and Disability* 14 (3): 107–111.

Kaye, H., Yeager, P., and Reed, M. (2008). Disparities in usage of assistive technology among people with disabilities. *Assistive Technology* 20 (4): 194–203.

Kent, B. and Smith, S. (2006). They only see it when the sun shines in my ears: exploring perceptions of adolescent hearing aid users. *Journal of Deaf Studies and Deaf Education* 11 (4): 461–476.

Kinsella, E.A. (2001). Reflections on reflective practice. *Canadian Journal of Occupational Therapy* 68 (3): 195–198.

Korotchenko, A. and Clarke, L. (2014). Power mobility and the built environment: the experiences of older Canadians. *Disability & Society* 29 (3): 431–443. https://doi.org/10.1080/09687599.2013.816626.

Larsson Lund, M. and Nygard, L. (2003). Incorporating or resisting ADs: different approaches to achieving a desired occupational self-image. *OTJR: Occupation, Participation and Health* 23 (2): 67–75.

Law, M., Baptiste, S., McColl, M.A. et al. (1990). The Canadian Occupational Performance Measure: an outcome measure for occupational therapy. *Canadian Journal of Occupational Therapy* 57 (2): 82–87.

Law, M., Baptiste, S., and Mills, J. (1995). Client-centred practice: what does it mean and does it make a difference? *Canadian Journal of Occupational Therapy* 62 (5): 250–257.

Law, M., Rosenbaum, P., King, G. et al. (2003). 10 things you can do to be family-centred. Retrieved from https://www.canchild.ca/system/tenon/assets/attachments/000/001/270/original/FCS5.pdf.

Lee, J.W., Jones, P.S., Mineyama, Y., and Zhang, X.E. (2002). Cultural differences in responses to a Likert scale. *Research in Nursing & Health* 25 (4): 295–306.

Lindsay, S. and Tsybina, I. (2011). Predictors of unmet needs for communication and mobility assistive devices among youth with a disability: the role of socio-cultural factors. *Disability and Rehabilitation: Assistive Technology* 6 (1): 10–21. https://doi.org/10.3109/17483107.2010.514972.

Lovern, L. (2008). Native American worldview and the discourse on disability. *Essays in Philosophy* 9 (1): 14.

Lupton, D. and Seymour, W. (2000). Technology, selfhood and physical disability. *Social Science & Medicine* 50 (12): 1851–1862.

Lysack, J., Wyss, U., Packer, T. et al. (1999). Designing appropriate rehabilitation technology: a mobility device for women with ambulatory disabilities in India. *International Journal of Rehabilitation Research* 22 (1): 1–9.

Magnusson, L. and Ahlström, G. (2012). Experiences of providing prosthetic and orthotic services in Sierra Leone – the local staff's perspective. *Disability and Rehabilitation* 34 (24): 2111–2118. https://doi.org/10.3109/09638288.2012.667501.

Mann, K., Gordon, J., and MacLeod, A. (2009). Reflection and reflective practice in health professions education: a systematic review. *Advances in Health Sciences Education* 14 (4): 595–621.

Mao, H., Chen, W., Yao, G. et al. (2010). Cross-cultural adaptation and validation of the Quebec User Evaluation of Satisfaction with Assistive Technology (QUEST 2.0): the development of the Taiwanese version. *Clinical Rehabilitation* 24 (5): 412–421. https://doi.org/10.1177/0269215509347438.

Mayes, R., Cant, R., and Clemson, L. (2011). The home and caregiving: rethinking space and its meaning. *OTJR: Occupation, Participation & Health* 31 (1): 15–22. https://doi.org/10.3928/15394492-20100122-01.

McCord, M. and Soto, G. (2004). Perceptions of AAC: an ethnographic investigation of Mexican-American families. *AAC: Augmentative & Alternative Communication* 20 (4): 209–227.

McMillen, A. and Söderberg, S. (2002). Disabled persons' experience of dependence on assistive devices. *Scandinavian Journal of Occupational Therapy* 9 (4): 176–183.

Miller, S. (2009). Cultural humility is the first step to becoming global care providers. *Journal of Obstetric, Gynecologic, & Neonatal Nursing* 38 (1): 92–93. https://doi.org/10.1111/j.1552-6909.2008.00311.x.

Mortenson, W.B., Demers, L., Rushton, P.W. et al. (2017). Psychometric properties of a Power Mobility Caregiver Assistive Technology Outcome Measure. *PLoS One* 12 (6): 1–9. https://doi.org/10.1371/journal.pone.0178554.

Mortenson, W., Miller, W., and Miller-Pogar, J. (2007). Measuring wheelchair intervention outcomes: development of the Wheelchair Outcome Measure. *Disability and Rehabilitation: Assistive Technology* 2 (5): 275–285.

Murray, C. (2009). Being like everybody else: the personal meanings of being a prosthesis user. *Disability and Rehabilitation* 31 (7): 573–581. https://doi.org/10.1080/09638280802240290.

Murray, C. and Forshaw, J. (2013). The experience of amputation and prosthesis use for adults: a metasynthesis. *Disability and Rehabilitation* 35 (14): 1133–1142. https://doi.org/10.3109/09638288.2012.723790.

Myburg, M., Allan, E., Nalder, E. et al. (2017). Environmental control systems – the experiences of people with spinal cord injury and the implications for prescribers. *Disability and Rehabilitation: Assistive Technology* 12 (2): 128–136.

Norweg, A., Jette, A.M., Houlihan, B. et al. (2011). Patterns, predictors, and associated benefits of driving a modified vehicle after spinal cord injury: findings from the national spinal cord injury model systems. *Archives of Physical Medicine and Rehabilitation* 92 (3): 477–483. https://doi.org/10.1016/j.apmr.2010.07.234.

Østlie, K., Lesj, I., Franklin, R. et al. (2012). Prosthesis rejection in acquired major upper-limb amputees: a population-based survey. *Disability and Rehabilitation: Assistive Technology* 7 (4): 294–303. https://doi.org/10.3109/17483107.2011.635405.

Pape, T., Kim, J., and Weiner, B. (2002). The shaping of individual meanings assigned to assistive technology: a review of personal factors. *Disability and Rehabilitation* 24 (1/3): 5–20.

Parette, H. and Brotherson, M. (2004). Family-centered and culturally responsive assistive technology decision making. *Infants & Young Children: An Interdisciplinary Journal of Special Care Practices* 17 (4): 355–367.

Parette, P. and Scherer, M. (2004). Assistive technology use and stigma. *Education and Training in Developmental Disabilities* 39 (3): 217–226.

Petersson, I., Lilja, M., and Borell, L. (2012). To feel safe in everyday life at home – a study of older adults after home modifications. *Ageing & Society* 1 (1): 791–811.

Pettersson, I., Berndtsson, I., Appelros, P., and Ahlström, G. (2005). Lifeworld perspectives on assistive devices: lived experiences of spouses of persons with stroke. *Scandinavian Journal of Occupational Therapy* 12 (4): 159–169.

Pettersson, C., Löfqvist, C., and Fänge, A.M. (2012). Clients' experiences of housing adaptations: a longitudinal mixed-methods study. *Disability and Rehabilitation* 34 (20): 1706–1715.

Pettersson, I., Törnquist, K., and Ahlström, G. (2006). The effect of an outdoor powered wheelchair on activity and participation in users with stroke. *Disability and Rehabilitation: Assistive Technology* 1 (4): 235–243.

Petty, L., McArthur, L., and Treviranus, J. (2005). Clinical report: use of the Canadian Occupational Performance Measure in vision technology. *Canadian Journal of Occupational Therapy* 72 (5): 309–312.

Pray, J. and Jordan, I. (2010). The deaf community and culture at a crossroads: issues and challenges. *Journal of Social Work In Disability & Rehabilitation* 9 (2–3): 168–193.

Pullin, G. (2009). *Design Meets Disability*. Cambridge, MA: MIT Press.

Restall, G. and Ripat, J. (2008). Applicability and clinical utility of the client-centred strategies framework. *Canadian Journal of Occupational Therapy* 75 (5): 288–300.

Restall, G., Ripat, J., and Stern, M. (2003). A framework of strategies for client-centred practice [corrected] [published erratum appears in Canadian Journal of Occupational Therapy 2003, 70(3): 169]. *Canadian Journal of Occupational Therapy* 70 (2): 103–112.

Ripat, J. and Becker, P. (2012). Playground usability: what do playground users say? *Occupational Therapy International* 19 (3): 144–153. https://doi.org/10.1002/oti.1331.

Ripat, J., Verdonck, M., and Carter, R. (2018). The meaning ascribed to wheeled mobility devices by individuals who use wheelchairs and scooters: a metasynthesis. *Disability and Rehabilitation: Assistive Technology* 13 (3): 253–262. https://doi.org/10.1080/17483107.2017.1306594.

Ripat, J. and Woodgate, R. (2012). The role of assistive technology in self-perceived participation. *International Journal of Rehabilitation Research* 35 (2): 170–177.

Ripat, J. and Woodgate, R. (2017). The importance of assistive technology in the productivity pursuits of young adults with disabilities. *Work* 57 (4): 455–468. https://doi.org/10.3233/wor-172580.

Ryan, S., Campbell, K., and Rigby, P. (2007). Reliability of the Family Impact Of Assistive Technology Scale for families of young children with cerebral palsy. *Archives of Physical Medicine and Rehabilitation* 88 (11): 1436–1440.

Scherer, M. and Craddock, G. (2002). Matching Person & Technology (MPT) assessment process. *Technology and Disability* 14 (3): 125–131.

Shepherd, A., Stewart, H., and Murchland, S. (2007). Mothers' perceptions of the introduction of a hoist into the family home of children with physical disabilities. *Disability and Rehabilitation: Assistive Technology* 2 (2): 117–125.

Shinohara, K. and Wobbrock, J.O. (2011). In the shadow of misperception: assistive technology use and social interactions. In *Proceedings of the SIGCHI Conference on Human Factors in Computing Systems*, Vancouver, Canada (7–12 May). New York: ACM.

Şimşek, T., Yümin, E., Sertel, M. et al. (2012). Assistive device usage in elderly people and evaluation of mobility level. *Topics in Geriatric Rehabilitation* 28 (3): 190–194. https://doi.org/10.1097/TGR.0b013e3182581d72.

Spiliotopoulou, G., Fowkes, C., and Atwal, A. (2012). Assistive technology and prediction of happiness in people with post-polio syndrome. *Disability and Rehabilitation: Assistive Technology* 7 (3): 199–204. https://doi.org/10.3109/17483107.2011.616921.

Stedman, A. and Thomas, Y. (2011). Reflecting on our effectiveness: occupational therapy interventions with indigenous clients. *Australian Occupational Therapy Journal* 58 (1): 43–49. https://doi.org/10.1111/j.1440-1630.2010.00916.x.

Sumsion, T. and Law, M. (2006). A review of evidence on the conceptual elements informing client-centred practice. *Canadian Journal of Occupational Therapy* 73 (3): 153–162.

Thomas, D.M. (2009). Culture and disability: a Cape Verdean perspective. *Journal of Cultural Diversity* 16 (4): 178–186.

Tomita, M., Mann, W., Fraas, L., and Stanton, K. (2004). Predictors of the use of assistive devices that address physical impairments among community-based frail elders. *Journal of Applied Gerontology* 23 (2): 141–155.

Townsend, E.A. and Polatajko, H.J. (2007). *Enabling Occupation II: Advancing an Occupational Therapy Vision for Health, Well-being and Justice Through Occupation*. Ottawa, ON, Canada: CAOT Publications.

Van der Esch, M., Heijmans, M., and Dekker, J. (2003). Factors contributing to possession and use of walking aids among persons with rheumatoid arthritis and osteoarthritis. *Arthritis & Rheumatism: Arthritis Care & Research* 49 (6): 838–842.

Vanderheiden, G. (2002). A journey through early augmentative communication and computer access. *Journal of Rehabilitation Research and Development* 39 (6): 39–53.

Vasunilashorn, S., Steinman, B.A., Liebig, P.S., and Pynoos, J. (2011). Aging in place: evolution of a research topic whose time has come. *Journal of Aging Research* 2012: https://doi.org/10.1155/2012/120952.

Veehof, M., Taal, E., Rasker, J. et al. (2006). What determines the possession of assistive devices among patients with rheumatic diseases? The influence of the country-related health care system. *Disability and Rehabilitation* 28 (4): 205–211.

Verdonck, M., Chard, G., and Nolan, M. (2011). Electronic aids to daily living: be able to do what you want. *Disability and Rehabilitation: Assistive Technology* 6 (3): 268–281. https://doi.org/10.3109/17483107.2010.525291.

Verdonck, M., Nolan, M., and Chard, G. (2018). Taking back a little of what you have lost: the meaning of using an environmental control system (ECS) for people with high cervical spinal cord injury. *Disability and Rehabilitation: Assistive Technology* 13 (8): 785–790.

Watson, N. and Woods, B. (2005). The origins and early developments of special/adaptive wheelchair seating. *Social History of Medicine* 18 (3): 459–474.

Wearmouth, H. and Wielandt, T. (2009). "Reserve is no place for a wheelchair": challenges to consider during wheelchair provision intended for use in First Nations community. *Disability and Rehabilitation: Assistive Technology* 4 (5): 321–328. https://doi.org/10.1080/17483100902807120.

Wessels, R., de Witte, L., Andrich, R. et al. (2000). IPPA, a user-centred approach to assess effectiveness of assistive technology provision. *Technology and Disability* 13 (2): 105–115.

Wessels, R., de Witte, L., Jedeloo, S. et al. (2004). Effectiveness of provision of outdoor mobility services and devices in the Netherlands. *Clinical Rehabilitation* 18 (4): 371–378.

Woodgate, R., Edwards, M., and Ripat, J. (2012). How families of children with complex care needs participate in everyday life. *Social Science & Medicine* 75 (10): 1912–1920. https://doi.org/10.1016/j.socscimed.2012.07.037.

Woods, B. and Watson, N. (2003). A short history of powered wheelchairs. *Assistive Technology* 15 (2): 164–180.

Woods, B. and Watson, N. (2004). The social and technological history of wheelchairs. *International Journal of Therapy and Rehabilitation* 11 (9): 407–410.

13

Technology and environmental interventions for cognition

Tony Gentry

Outline

Assistive Technologies and Environmental Interventions in Healthcare: An Integrated Approach, First Edition.
Edited by Lynn Gitlow and Kathleen Flecky.

Companion website: www.wiley.com/go/gitlow/assitivetechnologies

Learning outcomes

After reading this chapter, you should be able to:

1. Identify everyday functional challenges faced by people with cognitive impairment.
2. Describe the difference between remediative and compensatory cognitive rehabilitation strategies.
3. Identify low-tech strategies for managing memory impairment.
4. Identify mobile technology-based strategies for managing everyday functional challenges related to cognitive impairment.
5. Compare mobile apps intended to address cognitive disability.
6. Identify home-based environmental modifications that can promote safety and functional independence for people with cognitive impairment.
7. Identify low/mid/high-tech assistive technologies that may be used as cognitive aids at home.

Active learning prompts

Before you read this chapter:

1. Consider your home and workspace. What environment, surroundings, and tools make it easier to concentrate and stay on task?
2. If you use a cell phone or tablet computer, list the apps and features that you use every day. Do you know how to access other features? What features of the device are easy to use? Which ones are frustrating?
3. If your handheld device has accessibility features, explore them one by one. If you have an Apple iOS device, use the website http://www.apple.com/accessibility to guide your exploration. If you have an Android OS device, use the website http://www.google.com/accessibility/products/.

Key terms

Assistive technology for cognition (ATC)
Cognitive impairment
Compensatory technologies
The Functional Assessment Tool for Cognitive Assistive Technology
Smart home adaptations

Introduction

Assistive technology for cognition (ATC) has evolved alongside the revolution in desktop and portable computers over the past 40 years, providing cognitive rehabilitation clinicians with an ever-changing variety of adaptive tools. The first use of the term cognitive rehabilitation in a scientific journal is believed to have been in 1980 (Parente and Herman 1997). This is the same year in which the IBM desktop computer was released, rapidly spreading to offices and workplaces worldwide, and marking the dawn of the personal computer age.

Cognitive rehabilitation clinicians were quick to find uses for personal computers as cognitive aids, developing computerized assessment and training tools designed to foster the *remediation* of process-specific impairments such as attention, concentration, memory, and executive function. At the same time, others began to use computers as *compensatory* technologies, creating software intended to assist in task and time management, both for busy office workers and for people with cognitive challenges (IOM 2011). In many instances, these compensatory programs were simply computerized versions of low-tech pen-and-paper reminders. Electronic sticky notes and onscreen calendars and alarm clocks are the most prevalent of these early tools. The ability to append a reminder alarm to a calendar entry and to automatically create repeating alarms for medications, chores, and appointments held promise, but because these programs resided on a desktop computer, they were not portable, as were the pocket calendars, paper sticky notes, and battery-powered alarm clocks they complemented.

It was not until the emergence of handheld personal digital assistants (PDAs) in the late 1990s that computers began to come into their own as ATC, providing users with pocket-sized devices that could help them manage appointments, contacts, and tasks wherever they might need such assistance. The dream of healing brains with computers has not yet come to fruition, and a growing body of research suggests that *remediative* computer programs are not successful in improving the everyday functioning of people with cognitive impairments (Cicerone 2007). The use of computers as *compensatory* cognitive aids does not heal underlying cognitive processes, but does appear to help people with conditions ranging from intellectual disability and autism to brain injury, multiple sclerosis, and Alzheimer's disease to function more successfully in everyday life (O'Neill and Gillespie 2015; Sohlberg and Mateer 2001).

Electronic devices or environmental interventions that make homes safer and more accessible also hold promise for people with cognitive disability. This is a perfect example of how future technology and/or environmental interventions can increase the participation of people with cognitive problems. Mid-tech tools include alarm clocks, automatic coffee pots, and automated thermostats, for instance; high-tech devices include computerized smart home suites that automatically control lighting and appliances. Today, the same smartphone that provides cognitive assistance in the community can access and manage smart home apps as well, providing a supportive web of technological aids for people with cognitive impairment wherever they may be.

In this chapter, I will explore a range of mobile technologies and environmental interventions (TEI) that support everyday function among people with cognitive-behavioral challenges, including low-tech, mid-tech, and high-tech solutions. Because evidence of efficacy is slim for computer programs designed to *remediate* cognitive function, these products will not be discussed. My focus is on *compensatory* tools, intended to support people with cognitive impairment in functioning more safely and independently in their everyday lives. Cognitive disability is a global term that may include people who require total assistance in performing basic activities of daily living and people who function independently with very little support. The ATC discussed in this chapter works most readily for people with mild to moderate cognitive impairment, who can learn to interact with device reminders and other supports. Those with more severe cognitive challenges, and those with profound sensorimotor deficits, may require additional accommodations in order to benefit from the technologies discussed herein.

Cognitive impairment in everyday life

Cognitive impairment is an umbrella term that covers an array of mental processes, typically categorized under the headings of attention, perception, concentration, memory, problem-solving, and executive functioning, among several others (Ponsford 2004; World Health Organization 2017). All of these processes work together to allow us to sense, think, and act in everyday life, and the failure of any of them can cause significant functional disability. In treating cognitive impairment, our primary goal is to improve everyday functional performance. It can be helpful, then, to consider what tasks are typically impacted by cognitive challenges.

Over the past dozen years, I have conducted a series of studies with over 300 people who have conditions including autism (Gentry et al. 2010, 2012, 2015), brain injury (Gentry et al. 2008), and multiple sclerosis (Gentry 2008) that have impacted their cognitive function. Their seven most prevalent functional complaints have been: (i) remembering to do things, (ii) medication management, (iii) memory for names and faces, (iv) task-sequencing, (v) multi-tasking and switching between tasks, (vi) communication difficulties, and (vii) coping with frustration. These problems impact every aspect of a person's life, from work and school to health maintenance, recreation, and social interaction. ATC that addresses these problems can be life-changing.

Clinicians typically aim to address functional difficulties related to cognition by utilizing a variety of assessment and treatment paradigms that may include elements of process-specific training, the teaching of cognitive strategies, and the use of ATC (LoPresti et al. 2008; Sohlberg and Mateer 2001). The practical approaches discussed in this chapter can be part of the treatment arsenal of any cognitive rehabilitation therapist. The following section examines each of the seven problems my study participants listed, offering a range of assistive technologies that may help. A subsequent section will discuss strategies for deploying ATC in a systematic and individualized way to promote improved everyday function. The chapter concludes with a review of home and office-based environmental adaptations and smart home technologies that can promote safety and functional independence in those settings (see Box 13.1).

Remembering to do things

In our fast-paced world, entire industries have grown up around helping us meet the many demands of our calendars. Often, the same tools designed for the busy office worker can assist a person with a memory

Box 13.1 Here's the evidence

Gillespie, A., Best, C., and O'Neill, B. (2011). Cognitive function and assistive technology for cognition: a systematic review. *Journal of the International Neuropsychological Society* 18(1): 1–19.

Key Words: self-help devices, delirium, dementia, amnesic, cognitive disorders, neuropsychology

Purpose: This systematic review examines the relationship between assistive technology for cognition (ATC) and cognitive function.

Method: A systemic review of relevant literature was completed using narrative synthesis, which is based on textual synthesis. Additionally, an analysis of methodological quality of the studies was done using the Scottish Intercollegiate Guidelines Network levels of evidence

Findings: The article finds that there is support for the effectiveness of ATC in clients with a variety of cognitive functional needs such as organization, planning, and reminding. The article has three recommendations. First it suggests using the International Classification of Functioning, Disability and Health (ICF) for evaluating and prescribing ATC. Second, it recommends classifying ATC on cognitive function based on the ICF cognitive functions. Finally, it recommends increasing research efforts to study ATC that focuses on more areas than those which support reminding and prompting interventions.

Critical Thinking Questions:

1. After reading this article, what do you understand to be the limitations of this research? Are there any limitations not stated?
2. How can the results of the review be useful to your practice?
3. Based on the findings of this study, what additional research is needed?

impairment to successfully manage a day's tasks. In order to avoid confusion, however, it is essential to provide a simple, reliable, and efficient technology that provides the reminding support needed without unduly taxing the user's cognitive reserve. Pen-and-paper-based notes may serve that purpose as low-tech solutions. Day planners, wall calendars, and address books are, of course, designed as basic memory aids. If a person can consistently use such a tool to remember, then no further intervention is required. Unfortunately, when a person has cognitive impairment, this is rarely the case.

Often, when I meet a client for the first time, they show me the tools they have been striving to use to stay on task. These typically include a mish-mash of low-tech reminders: wall and pocket calendars, address books, and refrigerators stuccoed with sticky notes. In my experience, people rarely can keep all of these materials straight, since items on one calendar may not migrate to another and sticky notes eventually drift onto the floor. Appointments are missed, bills go unpaid, chores are left undone, friends are left waiting at the coffee shop: Frustration swells.

The purpose of ATC is to substitute for human support, but paper-based reminders often fail to do so. For instance, when I worked on a locked brain injury unit, I dutifully taught patients (as their memory emerged from a post-coma state of disorientation) to use memory notebooks to keep track of their schedules on the ward. I assumed, foolishly, that they would continue to use these day calendars when they returned home, so I taught caregivers how to assist them in logging daily tasks in their notebooks. It was only when I began serving clients with brain injury in the community that I realized my folly: Memory books only work when you remember to look at them. My clients still needed a caregiver to tap them on the shoulder and remind them to look at their schedules. I had done nothing to make them more independent, since they still relied on a loved one to stay on task (and this constant nagging often led to family discord). Clearly, what was needed was a *talking* memory book, one that provided an automated alert for each of a day's events. I found that solution in the early *Palm Pilot* PDAs, and since then that useful feature has migrated to every cell phone and tablet computer on the market.

PDAs, tablets, and smartphones – no matter whether they run operating systems from Apple, Google, or Microsoft – come bundled with reminder alert apps. Apple apps include the *iCal* calendar, *Clock* (which offers a variety of sounds for different alarm messages), and *Reminder* (a to-do list that allows the setting of reminder alarms). Google's Android devices include *Google Calendar*, a rich reminder solution that can send text message reminders to any phone or personal computer. Microsoft's portable devices run the *Office Outlook* task management programs familiar to most personal computer users. Thousands of add-on apps are available for these products as well. A table with some information about the apps mentioned in the chapter is included in the Toolbox at the end of the chapter.

With so many low-tech and high-tech reminder choices, it can be easy to succumb to a clutter of solutions that only confuse matters more. The goal, then, is to settle on a single platform where all of these snippets of vital information can be housed and easily accessed. Ideally, this will be a portable solution, one that includes an option for a just-in-time reminder alert, as needed, and one that includes a safe backup copy stored elsewhere, in case the original device is lost. In some cases, a cell phone fills the bill. Even the cheapest cell phone includes an electronic address book, a calendar with options for reminder alerts, and a still camera. (The camera can be used to photograph the location of a car in a mall parking lot, a particular food package for purchase in the store, and other things that may be easy to forget.) Many cell phones include digital recorders, as well, allowing the voice recording of to-do lists, grocery lists, and other "notes to self." Basic cell phones can be difficult to navigate, however, requiring a user to thumb through a series of menus in order to record or access a note or calendar item. Most smartphones and tablets, however, are readily navigable. Each of these devices offers the safeguard of automatic backup to a computer or offsite cloud server, as well, so that if the device itself is lost or stolen, the information onboard can be retrieved for a replacement device.

Learning to operate a handheld device as a memory aid can be challenging for many people. Because the procedure required to record a message is the same every time, however, the repetitive effort can aid in the learning process. Another enabling and motivating feature of these devices is what I call the "nag factor." People who learn to program and respond to their own reminder messages may no longer need prompts from a caregiver to complete their chores. That is a signal achievement, and one all parties cheer. In some cases, however, a person with a cognitive impairment has difficulty learning to program a handheld device. In these cases, I recommend a daily or weekly planning meeting with a caregiver, in which reminders and other information are logged onto the device. The user, then, is required only to respond to the device when an alarm reminder sounds. This procedure works well for many people who have moderate cognitive impairment. I have used it successfully in a vocational training research trial among people with autism. In this trial, job coaches programmed workday schedules onto the workers' mobile devices, and these prompts were then followed independently on the job (Gentry et al. 2015).

Specialized reminder apps are sometimes necessary. For instance, the iOS app *PhotoMind* and the Android app *RePic Picture Reminder* are good reminder options for non-readers. The iOS app *Reminder* and the Android app *Voice Reminder* offer self-recorded verbal prompts for non-readers and the visually impaired.

People who have difficulty managing data entry on reminder programs may also benefit from the voice-controlled interfaces on advanced smartphones. Apple's *Siri* feature, for instance, launches at a tap or voice prompt. The user then verbally instructs *Siri* to post a reminder message, which chimes at the appropriate time.

In cases where a person is uncomfortable using a computerized device and in cases where there is no caregiver to provide assistance in programming reminders, a specialized cell phone can help. The *Jitterbug* cell phone, available online from a variety of sources, is designed to be simple to use and allows one-touch communication with a human operator, who can place calls and even phone a customer with a reminder message when scheduled. All interaction with the *Jitterbug* operator is managed in a phone call, requiring no technological literacy. *Jitterbug* monthly payment plans are competitive and lower than many smartphone plans. The *Jitterbug* works well for non-readers, too, since reminder messages are delivered by a human voice.

The strategies discussed here can work well for people with memory impairment, helping them remember important everyday events. Clinicians are encouraged to experiment with the various app options in order to effectively match user needs to the proper solution.

Medication management

Many people with cognitive impairment take powerful medications that modulate neuronal functions, and it is essential that these medications be dosed correctly. It is easy, however, to forget a pill or to take a second pill, having forgotten taking the first. These mistakes can have devastating health effects. For that reason, clinicians are advised to work closely with clients and caregivers to ensure timely medication management.

People who can consistently respond to the types of reminder alarms discussed in the previous section can probably benefit from reminder alerts for medications. These alerts may be programmed into generic reminder apps, into medication apps, or into specialized pillboxes with onboard alarm clocks. The iOS app *Pillboxie*, for instance, offers reminder alerts that display a picture of the pill to be taken and a check-off box to record that the pill was taken. The online store epill.com sells a wide variety of reminder pillboxes, ranging from simple weekly divider trays to purse-sized versions and even an Internet-linked pill dispenser (the *MD2*) that sends a text message to a caregiver if a scheduled dose is not taken.

Because medication management is essential to good health, caregivers are advised to check in on a regular basis to make sure an automated reminder system works for the user. Devices may fail, cognitive status may change, pillboxes may be left behind when a user goes into the community. Troubleshooting these issues can assure more consistent dosing.

Memory for names and faces

Many people have difficulty remembering the names of acquaintances, but this can be especially troubling for people with cognitive impairment, who may forget important information about close friends. The low-tech solution of keeping an address book with photographs and snippets of key information (job, names of spouse and children, etc.) has been made much easier by smartphone apps. Apps like *Contacts* for iOS allow a user to take a photograph of an acquaintance, append that photograph to an alphabetized list of names, and type in notes about the user for future reference. Contacts can be saved in contextual folders to make searching easier (for instance, you may have folders for people you know at "work," "the gym," "church," etc.).

Task-sequencing

Complex, multi-step tasks may pose special challenges for people with cognitive impairment. Low-tech solutions such as step-by-step tasks lists or picture sequences in task notebooks are appropriate for some people, though task notebooks can grow bulky, unwieldy, and stigmatizing. App-based versions are available for smartphones and tablets, offering options ranging from to-do lists and picture-sequence prompts to instructional video clips. Because the variety of task supports available is so large, it is important to analyze whether the user is best served by a written list, an auditory prompt, a picture-based task sequence, an instructional video, or some combination of these.

To-do lists and sequential photographic prompts can be created in the iOS app *Notes* or the Android app *Google Keep*. Picture and text-based task-sequencing slide shows can be built and accessed in apps such as *The Functional Planning System* or *Plan it, Do it, Check it Off!* Non-readers and the visually impaired may prefer task-sequence support offered by voice recording. The app *Voice Memo* packaged with iOS devices may be used for this purpose.

The use of instructional videos to model task behaviors is a heavily researched teaching strategy, with over one hundred research articles published on this topic over the past decade (Baker et al. 2009; Buggy and Ogle, 2011; McCoy and Hermansen 2007). Evidence supports using this strategy with people who have significant cognitive impairment and those who are non-readers and visual learners. Sigafoos et al. (2007) authored an instructional manual that I have followed successfully. They recommend a stepwise strategy that includes: (i) identifying a complex task that is difficult for a user to perform independently, (ii) making a brief video clip showing that task being performed successfully (either by the user or by another actor), and (iii) offering the video clip as an instructional tool. Ideally, the user then follows a rehearse-perform-review strategy, initially with caregiver support. The user watches the video before attempting the identified task, has the video available while performing the task for play-and-pause support, and reviews the video upon completion of the task to compare actual performance to that shown on the video. The authors recommend frequent repetition in varied settings to reinforce learning. Over time, I have found that many people are able to reduce their need for video support, relying on occasional video review or the use of picture prompts or a task list instead, while no longer needing human supervision to perform the task.

Previously, producing video clips was an unwieldy process that involved a handheld camera, video transfer to a computer, and the use of computer-based software for editing and playback. Now most tablets and smartphones have an onboard video camera and playback capability, so the production and use of an individualized video library is not so cumbersome. The iOS apps *CanPlan* and *Functional Planning System* allow the creation and playback of photographic slide shows or instructional videos within their apps, along with reminder prompts linked to media support. On *CanPlan*, for instance, a user can set a tooth-brushing reminder alert that immediately opens an instructional video showing how to do so, providing just-in-time support for everyday tasks.

Multi-tasking and switching between tasks

Cognitive rehabilitation therapists often discourage multi-tasking. We advise our clients to do one thing at a time and to work in non-distracting environments, turning off telephones and televisions while cooking or paying bills. We recommend simplifying the workspace, so that it is uncluttered, and following the adage "a place for everything and everything in its place" to make everyday tasks less cognitively challenging. Unfortunately, in many situations that advice cannot be easily followed. Students undertaking a laboratory experiment in a busy classroom, workers negotiating the distractions of a factory floor, shoppers in a mall, and parents with small children must find ways to manage distractions while multi-tasking and switching successfully between activities, at least some of the time.

Environmental management, to the extent it is possible, can lessen the cognitive load of these situations. Having distinct workplaces for each activity, and moving back and forth from one to the other, can reduce confusion. It can be helpful to monitor the sensory distractors in the environment and address them as well, by seeking quiet, well-lit, and uncluttered workspaces. Ear plugs, portable lamps, and workspace dividers can be used to set up provisional workspaces that meet these requirements. I often recommend setting an empty placemat on a workplace table. Whenever a distraction occurs, the worker is advised to place the tool being used at the time on the placemat, so they can remember where to resume work later. Scribbling a "note to self" or digitally recording a message on a cell phone can serve as a reminder of what to do next. Task-sequencing checklists can be helpful, too, showing what steps have been completed and what comes next.

It is important to allow enough time for the work being done. Hurry is a great thief of cognition and robs us of much of the pleasure that performing a task methodically and well affords. Planning ahead, making a task schedule, and sticking to it can provide the time needed for an activity. This same strategy works well for people who sometimes become so absorbed in a task that they forget to stop at an appropriate time. Reminder alarms, especially those linked to a to-do list, can help in assuring the timely switching from one task to another.

Multi-tasking often leads to cognitive fatigue, the exhaustion that comes from working our brains too hard. Learning the early warning signs of cognitive fatigue – anxiety, frustration, tired eyes – and having a plan for taking rest breaks when needed, can improve functional independence and self-efficacy. Relaxation apps such as *Simply Being* and *Breathe-2-Relax* provide guided meditation routines that can ease a cluttered mind.

Communication difficulties

Cognitive impairment may be accompanied by communication challenges that include aphasias and other language processing difficulties, dysarthria, sensory issues (complete or partial deafness or blindness), intellectual deficits in understanding conversation and body language, and a range of executive functioning-related issues that impact social interaction. Assistive technologies that promote communication are intended primarily to compensate for communication issues, not to remediate organic injury. The most common ATC tools of communication include portable computers that generate speech based on a screen-tap on an icon or picture, or typing on a keyboard. Free-standing speech-generation devices range from highly programmable portable computers from *Tobii Dynavox* and *Zygo-USA* that may cost several thousand dollars to inexpensive digital recorders with icon-based touch screens that can generate a few verbal commands.

A number of mobile apps generate speech from text or picture input. They range from the expensive and fully programmable icon-based *Proloquo2Go* to free apps that translate text to spoken words (*Speak*). In selecting a device or app, it is important to seek the consultation of a speech-language pathologist, who can assess communication strengths and needs and offer an individualized approach to this very complex problem and provide ongoing training to optimize communication successes.

A few developers are exploring mobile apps intended to address the difficulties in social interaction experienced by many people with cognitive impairment. The iOS app *Conversation Builder*, intended primarily for children, offers video-based social situations and quizzes users on strategies for communicating appropriately in those settings. The video modeling strategy previously discussed can be leveraged to model appropriate social interactions.

Coping with frustration

The challenges of everyday life can be frustrating for anyone, and for those with cognitive impairment, these frustrations are often magnified, sometimes leading to emotional exhaustion, behavioral outbursts, or social withdrawal. Therapists are advised to work closely with clients and caregivers to examine daily activities and environments in order to pinpoint situations that may lead to frustration and collaborate on plans to reduce frustration-building stressors, while enabling a more fulfilling engagement in favored activities. It can be useful to keep a one-week activity log that records work, recreation, diet, pain, and sleep in order to capture variables that offer especially frustrating cognitive challenges. Mobile apps can assist in this effort. *MoodTracker* for iOS devices, for instance, alerts the user to note levels of stress, anxiety, and general well-being up to three times a day, generating a graphical record over time that can be used to monitor the success of behavioral interventions and activity adaptations.

Mobile apps may be used to treat stress and frustration as well. *Simply Being* and *T2TB* (the Tactical Breathing Trainer) provide meditation routines for relaxation, and *Moodkit* encourages users to substitute positive affirmations for thoughts or feelings that impact a sense of well-being. Assurances or suggestions by a loved one, recorded and played back on video clips as needed, can provide emotional support and behavioral guidance. These clips of clients or loved ones reciting advice for managing stressful situations or simply offering a kind work of encouragement can be calming and instructive. Any strategy or tool that affords improved everyday functioning may serve to reduce anxiety and frustration. People who make use of the recommendations in this chapter may find that they are doing more, functioning more independently, and facing less frustration, because of the assistance provided by these tools.

Matching device and user

Handheld computers grow more versatile and powerful each day, and with over two million downloadable apps available, the devices themselves can eventually become cluttered and hard to navigate, making a cognitively impaired user's life more confusing instead of less. It is important to carefully assess each user's needs, preferences, and goals, carefully matching these to a small suite of apps and strategies that provide exactly the support needed to function more independently. The Functional Assessment Tool for Cognitive Assistive Technology (FATCAT) (Gentry 2012) is one tool that can assist in making these decisions. (See Table 13.1 for a copy of this assessment tool.) Clients (sometimes accompanied by caregivers) self-rate their performance on everyday tasks, prioritize their needs, and describe their familiarity with electronic devices. The *FATCAT* can also guide a clinician's choice of mobile devices and apps, including determining whether a client can navigate a particular device, respond to a reminder alarm, enter data successfully, and manage other user-interface activities. The *FATCAT* is not intended as an all-in-one assessment system; rather, it provides information and insight for the clinician who seeks to match client and device. The *FATCAT* can also be used as an outcome measurement tool, with clients self-rating functional performance after intervention for comparison with pre-treatment self-ratings.

In most cases, to reduce the risk of confusion, I encourage people to use only three or four apps as cognitive aids. Most people will need reminder alerts for everyday tasks, and it is usually best to select a single app for programming these messages. In cases where clients have difficulty completing multi-step tasks, one of the task-sequencing apps discussed previously can help. In consultation with a speech-language pathologist, a communication app may be helpful. A stress management app or a behavioral video can be included for review as needed in times of frustration or distress. Having selected appropriate tools, the clinician should set about instructing the client in their use one by one. For instance, during the first week of use, it can be helpful to program only four or five daily reminder alarms (focusing on the important tasks that the user most often forgets). As the client demonstrates success in attending to these alerts, more can be added, as needed. Once a client has demonstrated success in using the device as a memory aid, the other strategies can be addressed in a stepwise fashion, depending on the goals of each user.

Portable computers come in a wide variety of sizes, though their functionality is not size-dependent. For instance, the 3.5-in. Apple *iPod Touch* has all the functionality of a full-size 10-in. *iPad* tablet. Many workers prefer using a smaller device as a cognitive aid, because it can be worn on a belt clip or carried in a shirt pocket, allowing full use of one's hands for work tasks. Students, office workers, and those with impaired vision or dexterity problems may prefer a larger tablet, which can readily double as a word processor, sometimes with the addition of an add-on keyboard.

Clinicians must consider protecting the device and its information as well. Insulating cases, like those from *OtterBox*, can provide shock and water resistance. People who use their devices as speech production tools may benefit from a belt-clip or pocket speaker, connected wirelessly to their device via Bluetooth. It is important to teach the user and/or a caregiver how to save information from the device onto a personal computer or a cloud server, as well, so that vital information is preserved in case the mobile device is lost. See Box 13.2 for a case study.

Environmental and smart home adaptations

People with cognitive impairment are often excellent candidates for environmental modifications that make homes and workplaces safer, and that promote functional independence. A well-organized, clutter-free living area and workspace reduce the cognitive load involved in performing any task; inexpensive low- and mid-tech devices may be readily deployed to address safety and task management; and computerized systems may be utilized to automate some home and office functions, interact with tablets and smartphones for reminder cueing, and offer non-intrusive passive monitoring solutions. The needs and goals of each individual must drive decisions in this area, and in many cases a judicious combination of low-, mid-, and high-tech ATC will be appropriate.

Low-tech home and workspace recommendations

Clutter is a great enemy of anyone with a cognitive impairment, making it hard to find things and keep track of activities. I have often heard tales of clients spending hours searching for car keys or a wallet, losing track of hand tools in the garage or kitchen, and feeling frustrated and confused amidst a pile of bills. Taking the time to organize the home or office, reducing clutter,

Table 13.1 Functional Assessment Tool for Cognitive Assistive Technology

(FATCAT) (revised 2017)

Client:____________________________________ Identifying No.________________

Assessment Date:____________________________

Please ask client to rate independent performance on the following cognitive tasks, on a 1 to 10 scale, with 1 being *very poor* and 10 being *excellent*.

Home and Community Tasks	Performance									
Home safety	1	2	3	4	5	6	7	8	9	10
Community mobility	1	2	3	4	5	6	7	8	9	10
Performing routine activities	1	2	3	4	5	6	7	8	9	10
Keeping track of appointments	1	2	3	4	5	6	7	8	9	10
Taking medications on schedule	1	2	3	4	5	6	7	8	9	10
Performing multi-step tasks (cooking, shopping, etc.)	1	2	3	4	5	6	7	8	9	10
Multi-tasking (doing two or more things together)	1	2	3	4	5	6	7	8	9	10
Following through on plans	1	2	3	4	5	6	7	8	9	10
Remembering important events	1	2	3	4	5	6	7	8	9	10
Remembering everyday events	1	2	3	4	5	6	7	8	9	10
Managing frustration	1	2	3	4	5	6	7	8	9	10
Staying focused on a project	1	2	3	4	5	6	7	8	9	10
Remembering facts (names, passwords, phone numbers)	1	2	3	4	5	6	7	8	9	10
Keeping track of keys, wallet, other items	1	2	3	4	5	6	7	8	9	10
Learning new information	1	2	3	4	5	6	7	8	9	10
Dealing with distractions	1	2	3	4	5	6	7	8	9	10

Access to Device:

Device used:______________________________________

Yes	No	Client demonstrates:
		Ability to read information on screen
		Ability to hear device alarm when 5 feet away
		Sufficient dexterity to hold device and navigate screen interface and buttons
		Responds to an alarm reminder and performs task as reminded

Needs and Preferences (Basic Functions):

Check	Function	Check	Function
	Reminder alerts App:		Medication alerts App:
	Calendar App:		Web-surfing App:
	Task List App:		Phone

(*Continued*)

Table 13.1 (*Continued*)

Needs and Preferences (Advanced Functions):

Check	Function	Check	Function
	Task-Sequencing cues Modality & app:		Health tracking App:
	Video Chat App:		Person tracking App:
	Way-finding App:		Stress management App:
	Behavioral coaching* App:		Communication App:
	Behavioral plan App:		Augmentative Communication App:

* If checked, determine modality of cues needed (text, graphics, video, etc.)

Needs and Preferences (Peripherals):

Check	Function	Check	Function
	Belt clip case		Vision access settings Apps:
	Arm strap case		Hearing access settings Apps:
	Lanyard case		Tactile access settings:
	Outboard speaker		Switch control Device:
	Keyboard		Cellular access
	Stylus		Other:

Intervention Plan:

Device Used & OS:

Case/peripherals:

Applications:

Training sequence:

Follow-up:

Box 13.2 Case study – Johnathan – college senior and Iraq war veteran

Johnathan is a hard-working Army Staff Sergeant and pre-medical student at Virginia Commonwealth University, who faces everyday functional challenges related to a blast-related concussion and post-traumatic stress disorder (PTSD) suffered while deployed to Operation Iraqi Freedom in Iraq. Johnathan uses a variety of *iPad*-based tools to help with his schoolwork. Because he tends to forget assignments, appointments, contact information, and medications, he has learned to enter all of this information as it comes to him in a trio of iOS apps. He keeps track of National Guard work and other appointments using the onboard *iCal* calendar app, always including a reminder alarm for every event. He tracks schoolwork using an add-on app called *iStudiezPro*. This academic scheduling app is designed to manage courses and assignments, automatically entering all scheduled activities on the device's *iCal* calendar app as well. Because Johnathan takes numerous medications, he relies on the dedicated medication app *Pillboxie* for reminders that include onscreen displays of the pills due at a particular time. Because he tends to forget whether he has taken a pill or not, he trusts *Pillboxie* to automatically track whether he has done so.

Johnathan finds note-taking difficult, because of slowed information processing and because his attention tends to wander amidst classroom distractions. He digitally records lectures with the *Notability* app, using a Bluetooth keyboard to take notes within the app. *Notability* links Johnathan's typed notes to a recording of the professor's spoken words, so he can quickly review the lecture after school, tapping on a note and hearing exactly what the professor was saying when that note was typed. Johnathan uses the *iPad* camera to photograph the professor's notes from the blackboard, to capture the location of his parked car, and to include head shots of acquaintances in the *Contacts* app. He stores personal information about these acquaintances in notes attached to each person's *Contact* entry.

Johnathan uses a pair of apps to track and manage PTSD-related anxiety. The *MoodTracker* app cues him three times a day to self-rate his mood and stress. When he goes to see his doctor and is asked how he has been doing, rather than responding, "Okay, I guess," he can whip out his *iPad* and provide a graphical representation of health fluctuations over time. Johnathan finds this information enriches health care interactions, helping the medical team titrate treatments more effectively. When feeling anxious, Johnathan finds a quiet place on campus and spends a few minutes wearing earbuds and performing either a deep-breathing routine using the *Breathe-2-Relax* app or a calming meditation using *Simply Being*. He reports turning to these apps several times a day and finds they help him stay "centered" despite school-day challenges.

Altogether, Johnathan uses eight *iPad* apps, his *iPad* camera, and a Bluetooth keyboard to manage his busy schedule. Since developing this routine, he reports consistent medication adherence, reduced anxiety, and improved grades. He says, "This *iPad* is the best therapy I've had since Iraq, and I couldn't do what I do without it."

assuring a "place for everything and everything in its place," and planning periodic (as often as weekly) reorganization days, is an essential early step in addressing cognitive disability.

Clutter is a problem for many people, of course, so much so that the profession of "home organizer" has emerged, and bookstores display entire bookshelves of home organization guidebooks. Though the effort involved in conducting a home organization makeover may be daunting, the recommended process is straightforward. A classic self-help text on this subject, Morgenstern's *Organizing from the Inside Out* (1998) recommends the following five-step strategy:

1. Sort: In this step, the organizer examines everything in the home, separates what is important and what can be discarded, and groups similar items that are considered important in one place (for instance, all spices go in a spice rack, all socks in a single sock drawer).
2. Purge: In this step, everything deemed unimportant is sold, given away, thrown out, or stored in an out-of-the-way storage space not used for everyday living.
3. Assign a home: Each item deemed important is assigned one place (and one place only) to be kept.
4. Containerize: In this step, similar items deemed important are organized in appropriate labeled containers or baskets and placed in the one place assigned to them.
5. Equalize: This step follows a couple of weeks after the initial home organization; it involves evaluating whether the organization process worked and resolving any issues that are still bothersome.

Following this process successfully requires time and often a team, but can result in time saved and frustration averted. Anyone serious about taking on the task of home organization is advised to consider the help of a professional or the recommendations of a self-help text such as Morgenstern's. As an initial step toward home organization, I suggest setting a small table by the front door, then forming a habit of emptying one's pockets of wallet, cell phone, and keys upon entering the house. This one small step can save hours of searching when it's time to go outside again. (While developing the habit, it may help to put a reminder sign, "Empty your pockets," by the door.)

Other important areas to consider in organizing the home include: (i) drawer dividers for cutlery, clothes, etc.; (ii) a filing system for bills and records (and a reminder alert for bills that are due); (iii) a dedicated shelf in the refrigerator for leftover food; and (iv) hanging hand tools on a garage wall where they can be easily located (using a felt tip pen to outline the shape of a tool on the wall helps in returning it to the right place).

Low-tech reminders in the form of hand-written signs can be placed, as needed, in the home. For instance, a sign in the kitchen reading, "Turn off the stove," one in the bathroom that reads, "Turn off the faucet," and another by the front door that reads, "Lock me when you leave!"

Mid-tech solutions

In many cases, low-tech home organization and reminder strategies work well, but many consumer devices can offer additional assistance for the cognitively impaired. Alarm clocks, automatic shut-off coffee pots, smoke alarms, kitchen timers, and automated plant and pet feeders are some of the mid-tech devices that can promote function and safety in the home. An additional recommended device is an inexpensive water leak alarm, sold at many hardware stores. Placed near a bathtub, these devices sound a loud siren if the water overflows after someone forgets to turn off the faucet. A similar device, the iGuard-Stove (https://iguardfire.com), connects to the kitchen stove and monitors movement in the kitchen, shutting down the stove if it is left alone too long. A digital recorder incorporated into a movement monitor (https://www.maxiaids.com/motion-sensor-alarm-systems) that incorporates a movement monitor can be stationed by the front door. This recorder turns on when the door opens and may be programmed to say, "Turn off the lights and lock the door" or offer other guidance a user may need. It can be useful, too, to install motion-detecting lights, especially on stairwells, for people who may forget to flip a light switch, risking a fall.

High-tech smart home solutions

A judicious mix of low- and mid-tech home management solutions can go far in helping many people with cognitive impairment manage home life more safely and independently. Additional support may be provided by a range of high-tech products designed to automate home functions or provide non-intrusive, passive safety monitoring. These may include remote-controlled or computer-mediated electronic aids to daily living (EADL) and other smart home technologies.

The earliest form of EADL – the *X10* environmental control unit – was introduced in the 1960s (www.x10.com), allowing remote control of lights and appliances via portable modules that communicate via a home's electrical wiring. *X10* modules may be attached to any lamp or tabletop appliance and readily programmed to accept on/off commands from a wireless remote control device. The remote control communicates with these modules via a radio-frequency pulse that is sent to a module plugged into a vacant wall outlet. *X10* products have evolved over the years, now including modules for overhead and outdoor lighting, video cameras, home thermostats, and remotely controlled window shade and door openers. Computer software packages are available that allow the programming of timed actions, so that module-mediated home functions operate on an automatic schedule. Basic X10 packages cost less than $100 and can be installed by a consumer.

EADL has long been used by people with mobility impairments, and a wide variety of switches are available that allow voice, sip-n-puff, or muscle twitch remote control of home operations. EADL use by people with cognitive impairment is emerging, however, as a strategy for facilitating safety and functional independence in the home. In the past decade, new appliance control technologies have emerged, designed to address perceived weaknesses of the *X10* products. Because *X10* units utilize a home's electrical wiring for transmission, malfunctions can occur. *Insteon* (www.insteon.net) modules communicate via home wiring as well, but add radio frequency-based signal transmission, and this redundancy can make the *Insteon* modules more reliable. Other emerging EADL technologies include General Electric's *Z-Wave* (www.z-wave.com) and Phillips's *ZigBee* (www.zigbee.org) (which operate via radio frequency waves).

People with cognitive impairment may benefit from remote-controlled or automated home systems in a number of ways. The ability to control lighting using a remote control switch, a smartphone app, or a voice-activated home assistant such as Amazon's *Echo* or Google's *Home* appliance, for instance, can make a home safer. Automated appliance schedules can be especially useful. For instance, an *X10* or *Insteon* software, linked to modules in the home, can automatically manage indoor and outdoor lighting, a thermostat, even a coffee pot, for improved safety and energy conservation. Some people program a living room lamp to blink on and off several times as a reminder cue for bed times or chores.

Passive safety monitoring

Over the past decade, computerized programs that allow remote monitoring of human activity in the home have become popular. In the United States, solutions such as

Rest Assured (www.rescare.com/rest-assured), *Night Owl Support Systems, LLC* (www.nossllc.com), and *QuietCare* (www.careinnovations.com) offer sensor-based offsite monitoring and response systems for a monthly fee. The various approaches these companies use illustrate the opportunities and obstacles involved in the offsite support of cognitively impaired individuals in the home. For instance, Rest Assured relies on video observation cameras. Observers stationed at remote offices monitor and query residents by phone or contact first responders when unsafe behavior is noted. Many people, however, refuse to be video monitored in their own homes. *Night Owl Support Systems* addresses this personal privacy concern by eliminating video cameras and offering passive monitoring options that use motion detectors and door and window security switches set up at key locations in the home. This information is monitored by a central dispatcher, who queries the resident or sends a helper if a problem is detected. *QuietCare* eliminates human observation entirely, relying on motion detector sensors linked to an offsite computer server. The computer compares a resident's observed activities to their typical routine, triggering a caregiver text message or phone alert if the resident deviates greatly from that routine.

Some consumer-level smart devices can be configured to provide passive home monitoring. For instance, Samsung SmartThings (www.smartthings.com) motion detectors and door monitors can be linked to a smartphone app and programmed to send an offsite caregiver a text message when a monitor is activated, thus providing some insight into the activities of people at home. Person-tracking apps for smartphones can be useful for people at risk for wandering and getting lost, assuming the person takes their phone with them on their walk. A variety of wrist-worn, keyfob, and even shoe-imbedded GPS tracking devices are available from various sellers.

These person-tracking systems are designed to reduce the need for onsite human supervision, but weaknesses include gaps in observed data (the systems can only monitor some activities in some home locations), historically slow response times by first responders nationwide, and inherent challenges of the systems themselves (for instance, *QuietCare* uploads data every two hours and the other systems rely on human observers, who may miss or misinterpret unsafe behavior). Because home-based monitoring systems rely on the electrical grid, they may shut down during power outages, unless a battery system or generator is deployed. Clearly, passive monitoring systems are not yet fail-safe substitutes for people who need ongoing supervision, but they may work well for those with mild cognitive or physical conditions that warrant less intensive attention.

Assuring the just-right fit

As with any recommendation for a behavioral change or assistive technology, therapists must always work collaboratively with clients in a respectful, problem-focused way to help them function more safely and independently at home and in the community. Often it is the small changes – an automated medication alert or a table by the front door for keys and wallet – that make the biggest difference. People may be especially reluctant to accept changes to their home environments, so it can be helpful to offer one or two suggestions at first, try them out on a trial basis, and then move forward with additional adaptations as the client becomes comfortable with the changes already put in place. This approach takes time, patience, and a recognition that no strategy will work unless the client sees the need for it and wants to use it, but following this model is more likely to lead to acceptance of the adaptations recommended. As client needs change over time and as helpful technologies evolve, it is important to check in periodically to tweak adaptations. In this way, client and technology can be assisted in maintaining their just-right fit. See Box 13.3 for a case study.

Box 13.3 Case study: Practical, affordable smart home and tablet solutions

Mary is a 53-year-old crafter who operates a handmade miniature figurine business from her suburban home, where she lives alone. Diagnosed with relapsing–remitting multiple sclerosis at age 29, she has learned to manage chronic fatigue and dysesthesia (especially a numbness and tingling in her fingers that makes detail work challenging), but over the past year her memory impairment has worsened, impacting both work and home management. She has been relying on a kitchen calendar and a system of sticky notes to keep track of activities, but she has fallen behind in her work, missing mailings and losing clients. Mary takes immunity modulating medications that are prescribed on a strict schedule, but she sometimes forgets to take her medications. On one particularly harried day, she forgot the soup heating on the stove and burned a pot so badly that it melted to the stovetop. She feels frustrated, anxious, and worried that something worse might happen.

Working with a home care occupational therapist (OT), Mary prioritized her most important goals, which included home safety, her medication routine, keeping track of appointments and bills, and home management. They decided to follow a plan that included a gradual introduction of low-, mid-, and high-tech assistive technologies to help her manage these situations, and over the course of six weekly visits instituted the following adaptations:

Home safety

Mary had motion-controlled lighting installed on her front and back porches and on her stairway. She placed battery-operated water leak alarms beneath sinks, next to toilets, and by her bathtub. Because of her sensory impairment, she turned down her water heater, to avoid the possibility of burning herself if water was too hot while bathing. She added a *Stoveguard* monitor to her stove. Mary designated the middle shelf of her refrigerator for food with an expiration date, and put a laminated sign on the shelf reminding her to "check expiration tag."

Medication management

Mary purchased an *Apple iPad mini* tablet and set reminder alarms for medications using the pre-installed *Reminder* application. The mini tablet, she decided, was large enough to make navigation easy despite her tactile sensory impairment, but small enough to carry in the pocket of her smock or in her pocketbook, so she could have it with her at all times. She added alerts to remind her to plug the device in for charging at bedtime and a monthly alert to check the batteries of her water leak alarms. Uncomfortable with the idea of saving data using a cloud-based server, she set a *Reminder* alarm to back up her data onto her home computer weekly using a USB-cord.

Appointments and bills

Mary set up automated bill paying with her bank for most of her monthly bills. She spent a day boxing up old bills and storing them, then set up a file box with a folder for each month of the year. Though she cannot afford to hire an accountant to manage her finances, she decided to set aside money for an annual tax accounting that includes the extra duty of sorting through her files. Working with the OT, Mary collected all of her sticky notes and calendars, separated tasks with due dates from those without, and transferred them to the *iPad* mini tablet. Those with due dates, she added to the *Reminders* app, including an alert reminder. Those without due dates, she saved as text messages in the pre-installed *Notes* app. She was elated to see that she could use the *Siri* voice control feature of the tablet to speak this information, which was then automatically saved as text to her *iPad*. She began to use the *voice recorder* on the tablet to record requests made by telephone, so she remembered them for later entry as reminders.

It took about an hour a day for two weeks, but Mary built address entries for each of her clients using the *Contacts* app on her *iPad*. Using the *iPad* camera, she has begun to snap photos of miniatures she has made for each client, and adds that item to the appropriate contact entry, along with a note about the client's preferences and interests, so she can refer to this information when talking with a client by phone.

Home management

Mary bought a Roomba robotic vacuum cleaner (www.irobot.com) as an energy-saving appliance, and set its onboard reminder to clean her living space once each week. The Roomba device, she learned, docks itself in its charger and beeps when its dust bag is full, so she does not need to set other reminders to take care of it. Mary decided to use the Roomba as a cue to clean her home. She goes to work cleaning when the Roomba turns on. She dusts and does her laundry at that time, typically finishing her work about the time the Roomba finishes vacuuming. Like many people, she has named her robot, choosing the name *Rosey*, borrowed from the name of the housekeeping robot from the old *Jetsons* television show.

Mary added repeating periodic reminders on her *iPad* to have her home appliances and car inspected and maintained. She made a list of food staples that she has asked a local grocery store to deliver automatically every week, and lists other needed items using the *iPad's* voice recorder app. Mary is most rested and cognitively sharp in the morning, so she has set an alert that reminds her to check her reminders and voice recorder after breakfast. She placed a table with a lockable cabinet by her front door, and makes a habit of leaving her purse and keys in the cabinet when she comes in the house. She wears the cabinet key on a lanyard around her neck.

When cooking, Mary learned to set out a pair of placemats on her counter. She reads through her menus before cooking, making sure to put all ingredients on one placemat before they are used. She then puts their containers on the other placemat after they have been used, so she remembers whether she has included a cooking ingredient or not. In addition to her *Stoveguard*, she relies on the oven timer, an automatic shut-off coffee pot, and a whistle-spout teapot as well. Mary follows a similar strategy at her work table. She sometimes fashions several miniature tableaux at once, waiting for glue to dry on one piece while sewing another, sometimes having to wait for an item to arrive in the mail before finishing a tableau. She places each piece on its own placemat and makes a note on an index card about the next step needed, which she leaves on the placemat as a reminder.

The OT discussed implementing a passive monitoring system in the home, linked to an app on Mary's daughter's cell phone, as a support in case of a fall or other problem when Mary might not be able to reach the phone herself. Mary felt that this was not yet necessary, but said she would keep it in mind for later.

With these strategies and tools in place, Mary finds she is less anxious, healthier, has more energy, and is more financially stable than before. She trusts herself to get her work and housekeeping done, to satisfy her clients, to take her medications on time, and to get through her day without nagging worries about tasks not completed. For the first time in years, she plans to set up a vendor table at a conference of miniature hobbyists and is baking holiday cookies for a church bake sale, confident that she now has the tools to do these things successfully.

References

Baker, S., Lang, R., and O'Reilly, M. (2009). Review of video modeling with students with emotional and behavioral disorders. *Education and Treatment of Children* 32 (3): 403–420.

Buggy, T. and Ogle, L. (2011). Video self-modeling. *Psychology in the Schools* 49 (1): 52–70.

Cicerone, K.D. (2007). Cognitive rehabilitation. In: *Brain Injury Medicine* (ed. N.D. Zasler, D.I. Katz and R.D. Zafonte), 765–778. New York: Demos.

Gentry, T. (2008). PDAs as cognitive aids for individuals with multiple sclerosis. *American Journal of Occupational Therapy* 52: 444–452.

Gentry, T. (2012). The Functional Assessment Tool for Cognitive Assistive Technology (FATCAT). Retrieved from http://itaalk.com/images/FATCAT-revised.pdf.

Gentry, T., Wallace, J., Kvarfordt, C., and Lynch, K.B. (2008). Personal digital assistants as cognitive aids for individuals with severe traumatic brain injury: a community-based trial. *Brain Injury* 22: 19–24.

Gentry, T., Wallace, J., Kvarfordt, C., and Lynch, K.B. (2010). PDAs as cognitive aids for high school students with autism: results of a community-based trial. *Journal of Vocational Rehabilitation* 32: 101–108.

Gentry, T., Lau, S., Molinelli, A. et al. (2012). The Apple iPod Touch as a vocational support aid for adults with autism: three case studies. *Journal of Vocational Rehabilitation* 37: 75–85.

Gentry, T., Kriner, R., Sima, A. et al. (2015). Reducing the need for personal supports among workers with autism using an iPod Touch as an assistive technology: delayed randomized control trial. *Journal of Autism and Developmental Disorders* 45 (3): 669–684.

IOM (Institute of Medicine) (2011). *Cognitive Rehabilitation Therapy for Traumatic Brain Injury: Evaluating the Evidence.* Washington, DC: National Academies Press.

LoPresti, E.F., Bodine, C., and Lewis, C. (2008). Assistive technology for cognition: understanding the needs of persons with disabilities. *IEEE Engineering in Medicine and Biology Magazine* 27: 29–39.

McCoy, K. and Hermansen, E. (2007). Video modeling for individuals with autism: a review of model types and effects. *Education and Treatment of Children* 30 (4): 183–213.

Morgenstern, J. (1998). *Organizing from the Inside Out.* New York: Holt.

O'Neill, B. and Gillespie, A. (eds.) (2015). *Assistive Technology for Cognition: A Handbook for Clinicians and Developers.* New York: Psychology Press.

Parente, R. and Herman, D. (1997). History and systems of cognitive rehabilitation. *NeuroRehabilitation* 8: 3–11.

Ponsford, J. (2004). *Cognitive and Behavioral Rehabilitation: From Neurobiology to Clinical Practice.* New York: Guilford Press.

Sigafoos, J., O'Reilly, M., and De la Cruze, B. (2007). *How to Use Video Modeling and Video Prompting.* Austin, TX: Pro-Ed.

Sohlberg, M.M. and Mateer, C.A. (2001). *Cognitive Rehabilitation: An Integrative Neuropsychological Approach.* New York: Guilford Press.

World Health Organization (2017). ICF Browser, b1, Chapter 1: mental functions. Retrieved from http://apps.who.int/classifications/icfbrowser.

Toolbox: Chapter apps

App name	Brief description of app
Remembering to do things	
iCal	This personal calendar application helps manage one's life and one's time, keeping track of appointments and events
Clock	This app offers a variety of sounds for different alarm messages
Reminder	A to-do list that allows the setting of reminder alarms
Google calendar	A rich reminder solution that can send text message reminders to any phone or personal computer
Office Outlook task management	Can be used to manage time and projects with tasks and to-do lists
PhotoMind	iOS – this app is a simple way to use pictures as reminders
RePic Picture Reminder	Android – good reminder option for non-readers
Reminder	iOS – offers self-recorded verbal prompts for non-readers and the visually impaired
Voice Reminder	Android – offers self-recorded verbal prompts for non-readers and the visually impaired
Siri	iOS – feature that allows users to speak natural language voice commands to operate mobile device

App name	Brief description of app
Medication management	
Pillboxie	iOS – offers reminder alerts that display a picture of the pill to be taken and a check-off box to record that the pill was taken
Memory for names and faces	
Contacts	iOS – allows a user to take a photograph of an acquaintance, append that photograph to an alphabetized list of names, and type in notes about the user for future reference. Contacts can be saved in contextual folders to make searching easier
Task sequencing	
Notes	iOS – to-do lists and sequential photographic prompts
Google Keep	Android – to-do lists and sequential photographic prompts
The Functional Planning System or *Plan it, Do it, Check it Off!*	Picture and text-based task-sequencing slide shows can be built and accessed
Voice Memo	Non-readers and the visually impaired may prefer task-sequence support offered by voice recording
CanPlan and *Functional Planning System*	These apps allow the creation and playback of photographic slide shows or instructional videos within their apps, along with reminder prompts linked to media support
Multi-tasking and switching between tasks	
Simply Being and *Breathe-2-Relax*	These provide guided meditation routines that can ease a cluttered mind
Communication difficulties	
Proloquo2Go	Symbol-based communication application
Speak	App that translates text to spoken words
Conversation Builder	iOS – This app, intended primarily for children, offers video-based social situations and quizzes users on strategies for communicating appropriately in those settings
Coping with frustration	
MoodTracker	iOS – alerts the user to note levels of stress, anxiety, and general well-being up to three times a day, generating a graphical record over time that can be used to monitor the success of behavioral interventions and activity adaptations
Simply Being and *T2TB* (the Tactical Breathing Trainer)	These apps provide meditation routines for relaxation
Breathe-2-Relax	Provides a deep-breathing routine
Moodkit	Encourages users to substitute positive affirmations for thoughts or feelings that impact a sense of well-being
Note-taking and student-specific apps	
iStudiezPro	This academic scheduling app is designed to manage courses and assignments, automatically entering all scheduled activities on the device's *iCal* calendar app as well
Notability	This app digitally records lectures

14

Assistive technology to support learning differences

Judith Schoonover

Outline

Assistive Technologies and Environmental Interventions in Healthcare: An Integrated Approach, First Edition.
Edited by Lynn Gitlow and Kathleen Flecky.

Companion website: www.wiley.com/go/gitlow/assitivetechnologies

Learning outcomes

After reading this chapter, you should be able to:

1. Describe learning disabilities, their causes and symptoms, and their impact on learning performance.
2. Summarize key US legislation related to learning disabilities.
3. Identify the three guiding principles of universal design for learning related to learning disabilities.
4. Explain the role of a full range of assistive technology in supporting students with disabilities in multiple learning environments.
5. List the impact of environment relating to assistive technology devices and services for students with learning differences.
6. Describe the roles and responsibilities of various assistive technology team members.

Active learning prompts

Before you read this chapter:

1. Describe your learning style and the tools and supports you use when learning and applying new information.
2. Define learning disabilities using two or more sources.
3. Complete a brief literature search using the following keywords: universal design, universal design for learning (UDL), and cognitive rescaling.
4. Using the website www.CAST.org, define the three principles of UDL.
5. Visit https://sites.google.com/view/freeudltechtoolkit/home?authuser=0 to explore a wealth of free, emerging technology resources, and think about the full range of tools you use or would like to have in your arsenal to address a variety of learning needs and styles.

Key terms

Invisible disability
Learning disability (LD)
Technology and environmental interventions (TEI)
Universal design (UD)
Universal design for learning (UDL)

Introduction

In this chapter, learning disabilities will be defined and described. Information regarding their causes and symptoms and the impact they have on student and adult participation in learning environments is presented. Key US legislation will be highlighted in relationship to learning environments. Universal design (UD) concepts will be presented as guiding principles for theory and practice in technology and environmental interventions (TEI) for students with learning disabilities. A full range of assistive technology (AT) supports and interventions will be discussed as part of a collaborative, team process to apply various theoretical frameworks to develop, implement, and evaluate technology supports for students with disabilities.

What is a learning disability?

The definition of learning disability continues to evolve (Atherton 2004). The *Diagnostic and Statistical Manual of Mental Disorders, Fifth Edition* (DSM-5) (American Psychiatric Association [APA] 2013) has renamed the diagnostic category of "Learning Disability" *Specific Learning Disorder* and placed it under the section titled "Neurological Disorders." Similarly, The National Joint Committee on Learning Disabilities (NJCLD 1994) defines learning disability (LD) as a "general term to refer to a heterogeneous group of disorders manifested by significant difficulties in the acquisition and use of listening, speaking, reading, writing, reasoning, or mathematical skills" (p. 65) and stresses that economic disadvantage, environmental factors, or cultural differences are not causes. According to the US Department of Education (2017) as many as one in five people in the United States have a learning disability, and one-third of all children who receive special education have a learning disability. Approximately 13% of public school students during the 2015–2016 school year received special education services, with about 34% of those students identified as having learning disabilities (US Department of Education 2017). Moreover, the highest prevalence of learning disabilities is reported by adults aged 18–24 (Cortiella and Horowitz 2014).

Research suggests that learning disabilities are the result of differences in how a person's brain works and how it receives, processes, analyzes, stores, or retrieves information, which can impact acquisition and application of information and skills (Hudson et al. 2007; LD Online 2010, para 1; Norton et al. 2015; Learning Disabilities Association of America n.d.); however, understanding of learning disabilities continues to evolve (Scanlon 2013).

Causes and symptoms of a learning disability

There is no one specific cause of learning disabilities; multiple factors appear to contribute to learning disabilities, which might include brain injury, irregularity in brain development, neuro-chemical imbalances, and heredity. Learning disabilities are not always identified strictly based on neurological findings (Fletcher 2008). The most common types of learning disabilities involve problems with reading, writing, math, reasoning, listening, organization, and speaking. Learning disabilities affect every person differently; however, the ability to learn, communicate with others, self-regulate, or organize oneself may be impacted (Fletcher et al. 2006; Scanlon 2013). Initial identification of learning disabilities is challenging because they are exhibited in so many ways. One person may struggle with math but be a skilled reader, while another may have difficulty connecting socially or find it difficult to initiate or complete tasks. Early indicators of potential learning disabilities might include uneven acquisition of developmental milestones such as delays in language and fine or gross motor skills, and/or problems with socialization (US Department of Education 2010).

Types of learning disabilities

As outlined in DSM-5 (2013) criteria, learning disabilities can be considered an umbrella term covering a variety of disorders that affect the ability to learn. Some examples include (but are not limited to):

- *Dyslexia*: a reading and language-based learning disability. The majority of students with learning disabilities receiving special education services experience difficulty in reading. Dyslexia is characterized by difficulties with accurate and/or fluent word recognition and impacts the development of reading skills, resulting in lower than expected reading levels despite normal intelligence. Reading difficulties arise when there is a problem understanding the relationship between sounds, letters, and words. Persons with reading disabilities may experience difficulty recognizing words that they already know, be poor spellers, and may have problems with decoding skills. An inability to grasp the meaning of words, phrases, and paragraphs may also exist. According to the International Dyslexia Foundation (2016), about 15–20% of people in the United States have a language-based disability, and of those, most have dyslexia.
- *Dyscalculia*: a learning disability related to math characterized by trouble with mathematical concepts such as counting and adding; trouble with reading, writing, and copying numbers; problems understanding math symbols and word problems; inability to line up numbers properly to add, subtract, or multiply; confusion with similar number (reversals); difficulty with money and time concepts and more.
- *Dysgraphia*: a learning disability related to handwriting as it relates to forming letters, writing within a defined space, and incorrect or odd spelling.
- *Information-processing disorders*: a learning disability related to a person's ability to use the information taken in through the sensory systems (seeing, hearing, tasting) and how that information is recognized, responded to, retrieved, and stored in the brain.
- *Language-related learning disabilities*: problems affecting age-appropriate communication, including speaking, listening, reading, spelling, and writing.

(Source: Eunice Kennedy Shriver National Institute on Child Health and Human Development 2018)

Is there a cure for learning disabilities?

There are no known "cures" for learning disabilities. Web searches may reveal claims of cures relating to dietary changes, megavitamins, eye exercises, eyeglasses, or vision training; however, it is generally believed that learning disabilities continue through a person's life span. For persons of school age, interventions for learning disabilities may include special education. Psychologists or trained educators may perform diagnostic evaluations and observations to assess academic and intellectual potential and level of academic performance. Once the evaluation is completed, depending on the environment and the impact of the disability on functional performance, the traditional approach has been to teach learning or compensatory skills by building on the person's abilities and strengths while correcting and accommodating for disabilities and weaknesses (Price and Cole 2009). Other approaches might include cognitive behavioral therapy, sensory integration, occupational therapy, speech and language therapy, social skills groups, and/or medications to enhance attention and concentration (Eunice Kennedy Shriver National Institute on Child Health and Human Development 2018).

An invisible disability

Learning disabilities have often been referred to as invisible or "hidden" disabilities. According to the US Department of Education Office for Civil Rights (1995), "hidden disabilities are physical or mental impairments that are not readily apparent to others. They include such conditions and diseases as specific learning disabilities, diabetes, epilepsy, and allergy." Persons with learning disabilities cannot be identified on the basis of visual or hearing acuity, a physical difference necessitating the need for specialized equipment to move or see, or other physical findings such as a missing limb or fluctuation in muscle tone. In other words, learning disabilities are not manifested as a physical difference, nor do they typically require visible devices (Fletcher et al. 2006). When a person uses a seeing-eye dog, wears a hearing aid, walks with a cane or walker, or uses a wheelchair for mobility, it is clear that he or she may require assistance to see, hear, or move.

Because of these cues, others in the environment might offer assistance or excuse behaviors such as difficulty complying with directions, problem-solving, or reading social cues. In contrast, others might misjudge a person with an invisible disability as being cognitively challenged, uncooperative, lazy, or aloof (Shapiro and Margolis 1988; Logsdon 2018). Do you know someone who is chronically late, disorganized, does not meet deadlines, is moody or unpredictable? It is possible they have a learning disability or difference. Because his or her disability is not visually evident, a person with a learning disability's actions and behavior might be misunderstood. As a result, those with learning disabilities may develop low self-esteem and/or other negative behaviors (Pandy 2012), compounding their initial difficulties. Concealment or hesitancy about disclosing an invisible identity perpetuates poor self-esteem, which can become a lifelong pattern (Nalavany et al. 2015).

Legislation and learning disabilities

The Human-Tech Ladder (Vicente 2006) reminds us that in making a good match between technology and its users, legislation and policy may need to be considered. In this case, considering legislation and policy is critical to providing those who have learning disabilities with the technology that they need. Viewed as variations of typical development, learning *differences* are only considered *disabilities* when they interfere significantly with school performance and adaptive functions. Interference with school performance and adaptive functions is described in The Individuals with Disabilities Education Act (IDEA 2004) definition of "specific learning disability":

> (10) *Specific learning disability* – (i) *General. Specific learning disability* means a disorder in one or more of the basic psychological processes involved in understanding or in using language, spoken or written, that may manifest itself in the imperfect ability to listen, think, speak, read, write, spell, or to do mathematical calculations, including conditions such as perceptual disabilities, brain injury, minimal brain dysfunction, dyslexia, and developmental aphasia.
>
> (ii) *Disorders not included.* Specific learning disability does not include learning problems that are primarily the result of visual, hearing, or motor disabilities, of intellectual disability, of emotional disturbance, or of environmental, cultural, or economic disadvantage.
>
> [34 CFR §300.8(c)(10)]

Additionally, IDEA 2004 refers to No Child Left Behind (NCLB), stating that an LD diagnosis cannot result from a "lack of appropriate instruction in reading," or if the determinant factor is diversity in a student's racial, cultural, and language background (614, b, 5, C). With the reauthorization of IDEA in 2004, a new process called early identification, known in some states as response to intervention (RtI) was advocated (please refer to Chapter 6 for the evolution of this legislation). IDEA encourages pre-referral interventions and supports initiatives such as RtI, positive behavioral interventions and supports (PBIS), and universal design for learning (UDL).

RtI is not mandated by IDEA or NCLB (2001), however, the 2004 reauthorization of IDEA included language about a process like RtI as an approach to determining whether a student has a learning disability. According to the National Center on Response to Intervention (American Institutes on Research n.d.), once a struggling student is identified, a variety of culturally and linguistically responsive instructional techniques are implemented to provide support or to help determine whether special education services are needed, including research-based classroom instruction, assessment of students with classroom focus, screening of academics and behavior of all students, continuous progress monitoring of students, and implementation of appropriate research-based interventions.

The most common model consists of three tiers. The first tier provides high-quality instruction to all students, with careful progress monitoring by educators in the classrooms. The second tier consists of the same high-quality instruction but with increased intensity students who are not making progress. If students fail to make progress with intensive instruction, they are identified for the third tier, which is targeted special education intervention. There is evidence that the IQ-discrepancy model normally used is ineffective in identifying all students with learning disabilities; therefore, many schools are implementing an RtI approach (Burns 2010). School districts have the option of using up to 15% of special education funding for students in the RtI program. The process has allowed some districts to cut down on the number of students enrolled in special education. When the Every Student Succeeds Act (ESSA) was signed into law in 2015, replacing NCLB, it included programs to improve reading and writing through the use of evidence-based instruction designed to support phonological awareness, phonic decoding, fluency, and comprehension. Other legislation supporting individuals with disabilities includes the Americans with Disabilities Act (ADA), which extends civil rights to people with disabilities. The ADA's most recent revision in 2008 included learning disabilities and specifically recognized dyslexia is a neurologically based impairment that causes individuals to use a "word-by-word and otherwise cumbersome, painful, deliberate and slow" reading process throughout their life (p. 17013) (Table 14.1).

Adults with disabilities

As mentioned above, learning disabilities are not "curable" and persist into adult life; the impact may resonate throughout the life span. Issues with self-regulation, time management, organization of information, and organization of materials can affect home life, higher education and job performance, and social relationships (Sharfi and Rosenblum 2014). Once the student transitions to higher education or the workplace, laws and programs which students are entitled to in K-12 no longer apply. However, legislation, such as the ADA and Section 504 of the Rehabilitation Act of 1973, protects these individuals from discrimination in these new environments. If qualified as an individual with a disability, he or she is entitled to reasonable accommodations under the law (DO-IT 2012), yet for some, fears of being "found out," failure, judgment, or rejection may prevent the individual from disclosing learning differences.

In summary, referring to the first rung of Vicente's (2006) Human-Tech Ladder, we described the legislative issues which must be considered when matching a person who has a learning disability with a TEI. In the next section, we will see how this legislation impacts practice.

UD: Creating accessible physical environments

As referred to in Chapter 7, the concept of UD has had an important impact on the learning as well as the physical environment. Gargiulo and Metcalf (2010) proposed considering the physical, academic, and social environments in order to produce a climate of learning. The late architect and visionary Ronald Mace, founder

Table 14.1 Legislation and (Learning) Disabilities.

	IDEA – mandates special education and related services based on identified needs	ESSA – seeks to improve the education of all children	Section 504 – prohibits discrimination on the basis of disability	ADA – prohibits discrimination against qualified individuals with disabilities
Defines legal rights for individuals with disabilities, which can include accommodations	X	X	X	X
Procedural safeguards to protect student rights during evaluation and service provision	X	X	X	
Prohibits discrimination at private schools receiving federal funding		X	X	X
Freedom from workplace discrimination				X

and program director of the Center for Universal Design pioneered the UD movement toward proactively creating accessible built environments based on first-hand experience with the barriers the physical environment imposed. Mace contracted polio at the age of nine years, and subsequently required AT in the form of a wheelchair for mobility purposes. As a wheelchair user, Mace found many of his surroundings inaccessible, and began designing tools and spaces that helped him do what he wanted to do (Ostroff et al. 2004). His experience with customizing tools and environments reiterates the philosophy of a client-centered approach, or the client as a partner and center for intervention and supports.

Mace was his own "client" and knew precisely what would work for him and what he was willing to use. As a result, he became a user-expert in designing assistive technologies and physical spaces that would provide him the access he desired and required to participate meaningfully in spaces and places that were important to him. Mace's work related to accessible design influenced the passage of national legislation prohibiting discrimination against people with disabilities. He created the term universal design to describe the philosophy of proactively making all products and the built environment physically pleasing and usable to the greatest extent possible by everyone, regardless of their age, ability, or status in life. UD is now a framework for the design of living and working spaces and products without special or separate design (Hillman 2011) and incorporates the following principles:

1. *Equitable Use*: The design is useful and marketable to people with diverse abilities.
2. *Flexibility in Use*: The design accommodates a wide range of individual preferences and abilities.
3. *Simple and Intuitive Use*: Use of the design is easy to understand, regardless of the user's experience, knowledge, language skills, or current concentration level.
4. *Perceptible Information*: The design communicates necessary information effectively to the user, regardless of ambient conditions or the user's sensory abilities.
5. *Tolerance for Error*: The design minimizes hazards and the adverse consequences of accidental or unintended actions.
6. *Low Physical Effort*: The design can be used efficiently and comfortably and with a minimum of fatigue.
7. *Size and Space for Approach and Use*: Appropriate size and space is provided for approach, reach, manipulation, and use regardless of user's body size, posture, or mobility.

(Center for Universal Design 1997)

Examples of UD in the built environment include: ramps, curb cuts, ground-level entrances, levered door handles, symbol signage, sensor-based flush toilets, and automated doors. Examples of universally designed products include flat light switch panels, flexible drinking straws, electric toothbrushes, closed captioning, accessibility features in software products, remote controls, and rubberized handles on kitchen tools.

UDL: Creating accessible academic and social environments

> Barriers to learning are not, in fact, inherent in the capacities of learners, but instead arise in learners' interactions with inflexible educational goals, materials, methods, and assessments.
>
> (Rose and Meyer 2002, p. vi)

Using the principles of UD as a foundation, the Center for Applied Special Technology (CAST), funded by the Office of Special Education Programs (OSEP), at the US Department of Education was established in the 1980s and originally committed itself to the use of technology, and with collaborating schools to adapt print-based curricula so these materials would be accessible to students with disabilities. It soon became evident that a proactive approach to designing educational materials would benefit all learners. Instead of blaming or labeling the learner when academic goals were not achieved, it became clear it was the curriculum that was "disabled" in its rigidity, and not the learner (National Center on Universal Design for Learning 2013).

Using UD principles, the UDL proactively designed and delivered a single curriculum, product, or environment from the beginning that was flexible enough to accommodate or be used by the widest range of learners. It "is really a merging of general education and special education, a sharing of responsibility, resources, and ownership. It gets away from the 'their kids-our kids' divide between general ed. and special ed." (Rose and Meyer 2006, p. 7).

From a foundation of brain-based learning research, three sets of broad teaching methods were developed and based on knowledge of how three distinct yet interrelated brain networks operate, the recognition, strategic, and affective networks. The works of Piaget, Vygotsky, Bloom, Gardner, and others who identified individual differences in the learning process and proposed educational strategies to address them, are reflected in the fundamental principles of UDL, for example, both Box 14.2 and Table 14.2, advocate for providing multiple means of engagement, representation, and action and expression.

Consider the evidence in Box 14.1.

Table 14.2 Universal Design for Learning (UDL) Principles and Guidelines.

Provide Multiple Means of **Engagement** in order to acquire and maintain learner interest so that they can relate to *why* the information is important	Provide Multiple Means of **Representation** With regards to content (the *what* of learning)	Provide Multiple Means of **Action and Expression** relating to *how* the learner will access learning activities and demonstrate what they know
Options for recruiting interest	Options for perception	Options for physical action
Options for expression and communication	Options for language, mathematical expressions, and symbols	Options for expression and communication
Options for self-regulation	Options for comprehension	Options for executive function

Source: From Meyer et al. (2014).

Box 14.1 Here's the evidence

Kennedy, M.J., Thomas, C.N., Meyer, J.P., et al. (2014). Using evidence-based multimedia to improve vocabulary performance of adolescents with LD: a UDL approach. *Learning DisabilityQuarterly*37(2):71–86.doi:10.1177/0731948713507262.

Key Words: access to education, adolescents, educational principles, educational technology, instructional effectiveness, learning disabilities, vocabulary development

Purpose: This article investigates the use of a UDL multimedia-learning tool called content acquisitions podcasts (CAPs), which presents vocabulary along with an instructional method.

Sample/Setting: Students both with and without disabilities in world history classes.

Method: Students in sections of world history were randomly assigned to alternating treatment (CAPs and business as usual) groups.

Findings: Results indicated that both groups of students exposed to this UDL strategy (CAPs) performed significantly higher on vocabulary posttests.

Critical Thinking Questions:

1. After reading this research article, what do you understand to be the limitations of this research? Are there any limitations not stated?
2. If you were to replicate this study using a different method or design, what designs would you use to increase the rigor and why?
3. Based on the findings of this study, what additional research is needed that is not addressed in the discussion section?

Box 14.2 Active learning: Providing multiple means of engagement, representation, and action and expression

Referring to the Universal Design Guidelines represented by Table 14.2, and reflecting on your own learning preferences, read the following scenarios and think about how you might answer the questions:

Scenario 1	Questions
Juanita sits in the back of Ms. Teacher's classroom. She twists her hair, fidgets with her water bottle, and slumps sideways in her chair as Ms. Teacher stands in the front of the room and lectures on the three states of matter in a low voice for 30 minutes. By the time Ms. Teacher is finished, Juanita is nearly asleep.	What might you suggest to *engage* Juanita? • How would you recruit her interest? • Can you think of any options for sustaining effort, or self-regulation?
Scenario 2	**Questions**
Eddie squints as he copies the 30 multiplication problems from the board. The glare from the window makes them hard to see, and he loses his place and copies the same problem twice. When he begins to solve the problems, he counts on his fingers. He has difficulty lining up his answers and soon his paper is a jumble of numbers and erasures. He has not been able to memorize the multiplication tables, so he makes frequent mistakes.	What might you suggest to *represent* the math problems in another manner? • What are some options for helping Eddie "see" or understand the math problems more easily? • Can you think of other options for mathematical expressions? • Can you suggest ways to help Eddie understand multiplication?

Scenario 3	Questions
It's St. Patrick's Day, and Ms. Teacher has just read a story to the class about two children who built a trap to catch a leprechaun. Now it's time for science and she reviews simple machines (pulleys, levers, ladders, etc.) and announces that there will be a simple machines essay test the following day. Davis clutches his stomach and begins to panic. He *knows* how simple machines work, but it is hard to organize and get his thoughts down on paper, and he can't spell the words he would like to use. Ms. Teacher complains that his handwriting is hard to read. Davis puts his head down on his desk.	Can you think of other *actions and expressions* Davis might use to show what he knows about simple machines as an alternative for writing an essay? • What are possible options for physical expression? Expression and communication? Executive function? • HINT: Think leprechaun trap!

Setting appropriate learning goals, selecting and/or creating effective teaching methods and instructional materials, and establishing accurate methods to assess learner progress are hallmarks of UDL (Rose and Meyer 2002). Information is presented in a manner that is easily perceptible, requires low physical effort, and provides a "just right" challenge. Barriers that impede access to the physical, educational, and social environment are broken down or circumvented through proactive and flexible planning. For example, students for whom writing is a challenge may flourish when given other options for engagement, representation, and action and expression, such as multimedia or the arts.

While the central practical premise of UDL is that a curriculum should include alternatives to make it accessible and appropriate for individuals with different backgrounds, learning styles, abilities, and disabilities in widely varied learning contexts, it is still possible to individualize learning experiences when presenting within a flexible curriculum (Hitchcock et al. 2002) using a variety of teaching methods. Even though digital technology is one means of changing instruction and engaging students, it is not necessary to create UDL lessons. The term technology may imply to some that solutions require complicated and expensive devices, or online resources or software. But as we emphasize throughout this text, it actually represents a full range of no-tech to high-tech *tools*. Implementation of UDL requires well-designed lessons constructed to offer sufficient options in terms of both challenges and supports so that all of its learners meet with success (Rose et al. 2012), and there are a variety of ways that UDL can be incorporated into education, such as the following:

- *Building accessibility into design* helps to ensure that features meeting the needs of the widest range of students are incorporated integrally into the curricula. Such designs can prevent the need for adaptations or retrofitting. For example, electronic curricular material that is designed to be compatible with assistive technology devices allows paraprofessionals, parents, or teachers to more easily program these devices with appropriate content.
- *Providing adaptable materials and media* allows students to choose and customize formats suited to their learning needs. For example, using digitized text, students can change text to speech, speech to text, font size, colors, and highlighting. Digitized materials also can support students through built-in scaffolding to assist with activities such as word recognition, decoding, and problem-solving. There also are non-digitized materials, such as highlighted passages or overheads that can provide support to students.
- *Using multiple media*, such as video and audio formats, provides a variety of ways to represent a concept and allows students to access the materials through different senses. For example, computer-based simulations that include video description can help students with and without disabilities to visualize difficult concepts. A more low-tech example might be using a book with large print or providing books on tape for students.
- *Providing challenging, salient, and age-appropriate materials* to all students motivates students who may not otherwise be able to access curricular content they need given their age and developmental level. For example, a student with a learning disability can use decoding supports and text-to-speech features incorporated into digitized history or science books, enhancing his or her ability to access grade-level content.
- *Presenting information in multiple, parallel forms* helps to accommodate diverse learning styles. For example, information can be presented orally in a lecture, visually through pictures or readings, kinesthetically through a model demonstration, and using technology based programs that further allow students to interact with the concepts. (US Department of Education 2008, pp. 4–5)

Assistive technology

UD, UDL, and AT share a common goal of reducing barriers and facilitating participation, yet UD and UDL do not replace AT either in terms of the *device*, or most especially in terms of the *service*. Specific AT devices such as communication supports, visual aids, wheelchairs, orthoses, and adapted toys will still be needed by some in order to

Box 14.3 Active learning: Enhancing a client-centered approach

Scenario	Question
A six-year-old boy appears to become distracted easily during whole-group instruction. The AT team recommends he use a gel cushion to sit on during class to help him focus on his work. He loves to use the cushion at home but refuses to use it in the classroom.	How might you adapt the boy's physical environment in the classroom and provide tools such as the gel cushion to decrease distractibility and improve academic success, yet keep him from "standing out" as one with an LD?

interact more fully with their environment. While AT has been defined in both legal and descriptive terms in other chapters, reciprocity with the environment is evident in the description offered by Blackhurst and Lahm (2000):

> ...mechanical, electronic, and microprocessor-based equipment, non-mechanical and non-electronic aids, specialized instructional materials, services, and strategies that people with disabilities can use either to (a) assist them in learning, (b) make the environment more accessible, (c) enable them to compete in the workplace, (d) enhance their independence, or (e) otherwise improve their quality of life. These may include commercially available or "homemade" devices that are specially designed to meet the idiosyncratic needs of a particular individual. (p. 7)

It is important to note that "homemade" devices are mentioned. In reflecting back to Mace's work with UD, it was perhaps those homemade devices that had the most meaning and were the most functional because they were created from personal experience. Consider the scenario in Box 14.3. A client-centered approach with emphasis on fulfilling roles that are meaningful and life sustaining can be found in Stoller's (1998) description:

> Assistive/Adaptive Equipment refers to the provision of special devices or structural changes that promote a sense of self-competence, the further acquisition of developmental skills into occupational behaviors and/or an improved balance of time spent between the occupational roles in an individual's life as determined by the individual's goals and interests and the external demands of the environment.
>
> (Stoller 1998, p. 6)

According to the Center for Universal Design, the goal of UD is to integrate persons with disabilities into mainstream environments, while AT attempts to meet the specific needs of individuals, but the two fields actually meet in the middle. The point at which they intersect is where products and environments are not clearly "universal" or "assistive," but have characteristics of each type (Center for Universal Design 2008).

AT and diversity

> We need to be clear that diversity is an essential part of the human condition and needs to be anticipated and celebrated.
>
> (Edyburn as quoted in Alberta Education 2010, p. 116)

With innovations in technology, changes in educational philosophy, advocacy groups, and federal mandates determining what should be taught and how the effectiveness of instruction is measured, schools are rapidly changing and educators and policy-makers are running to catch up. More than ever before, students with disabilities are being educated with their typically developing peers, necessitating a change in educational approaches and environments for all learners. Accessible, practical, and researched-based teaching methodologies must be employed for the benefit of all learners, considering the diverse needs they exhibit, and not their label or lack thereof (Meo 2008). Today's diverse educational and work environments include an ever-increasing number of persons with a variety of learning styles, requiring educators and employers to adjust to and embrace their unique learning needs and be willing to plan for and create optimal learning and work conditions, embedding supports throughout the day and relating to all tasks.

There are challenges and opportunities for persons working in educational and work environments to assist in the development of accessible academic, physical, and social environments by determining the strategies, supports, and tools that facilitate meaningful engagement for all learners. In terms of the classroom, the traditional one-size-fits-all approach to reading, writing, and 'rithmatic will not meet the continuum of needs and strengths this population represents. For educational settings in particular, demands and expectations of student performance are on the rise, with a shift from acquiring knowledge to integrating and applying it in authentic and meaningful situations relating to real-world experiences (Partnership for 21st Century Skills n.d.). Edyburn (2009) proposes a blueprint for diversity (Figure 14.1) as a launching point for designing accessible curriculum, stressing that instructional designers must understand and consider the social, cultural, physical, and academic

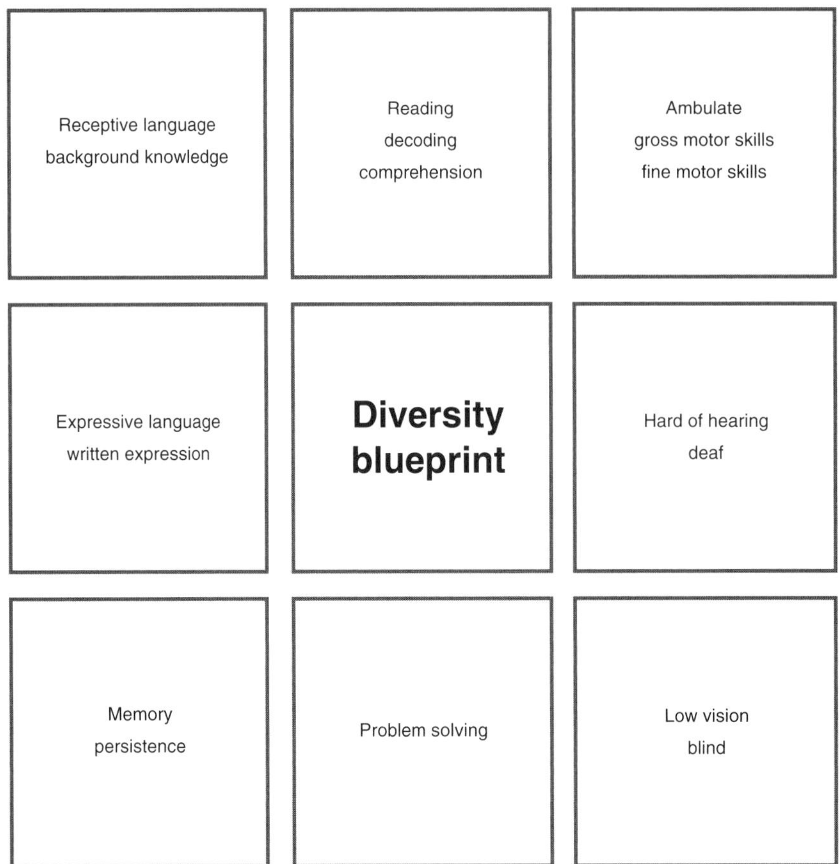

Figure 14.1 Diversity blueprint. Source: Reprinted with permission of Dave Edyburn.

diversity of the class and proactively build supports that will ensure that individual differences do not create barriers to access and engagement. He suggests that without a blueprint recognizing the full array of diversity including cognitive, language, motor, and visual differences, it will be difficult for instructional designers to design curricula that will meet the needs of all students. Establishing a supportive, caring learning and working community, including positive relationships with educators or employers, is as important as the physical setup and tools of the school and work setting and promotes an environment in which learning differences are not just tolerated, they are expected and valued.

Consider the questions in Box 14.4.

> **Box 14.4** Active learning prompt: Review the demographics of students in k-12 over the past decade
>
> What sorts of challenges do you notice that may not be evident in the diversity plan presented in Figure 14.1? Do you notice any trends? Would you add any other sections to the diversity blueprint to accommodate changes in the needs of the student population?

The right tool for the job

> Without ownership, people don't value the tools as they should – and that applies to both students and classroom teachers. It makes much more sense for the tools to live in the classrooms in which they are needed. They are available for instant use by students with special needs as well as other students who might benefit from them.
>
> (Sweeney 2007)

The right of individuals to have power and control of their lives regardless of disability is referred to as self-determination and "encompasses concepts such as free will, civil and human rights, freedom of choice, independence, personal agency, self-direction, and individual responsibility" (Bremer et al. 2003). All individuals, including those with disabilities, can achieve greater control over their lives if they are provided with the supports and accommodations they need for greater independence, and increased participation (Wehmeyer 2002). It should be the goal of every intervention to build opportunities for self-determination to begin the first time it is used. Since no one tool system or approach works for everyone, it is important that a full range of tools be explored until learners find one that they like and works for them. Examples of these free downloadable tools are highlighted in Table 14.3.

Table 14.3 Free Downloadable Tools Centered on Assistive Technology and Self-Determination.

Tool	Description	Website
Bowser, G. and Reed, P. (2007). Hey Can I Try That? A Student Handbook for Choosing and Using Assistive Technology.	Provides students with a variety of technology choices based on client-centered questions about the student's individual needs and capabilities.	http://www.wati.org/free-publications/other-materials/
Colorado State University: Access to Postsecondary Education/Student Self-Advocacy Module	*Handbook* looks at transition from high school to college, with three sections corresponding to the definition of self-advocacy: "Know yourself," "Know what you need and want," and "Know how to get what you need and want." Each section includes a worksheet, checklist, suggested activities, and links to additional resources.	http://accessproject.colostate.edu/sa/
Diablo Valley College Learning Style Survey	The DVC Learning Style Survey is designed to help students become more successful by identifying their learning style, and includes a set of recommended learning strategies to help them study in a productive manner.	http://www.dvc.edu/enrollment/counseling/lss
Student Resource Guide on Transition/Student Transition Portfolio (includes Transition Planning Checklist; My Desired Post-School Outcomes; Self-Determination and AT Management; AT Emergency Plan)	Two-part portfolio system to assist students as early as middle school in managing materials they need to transition from high school to a post school education or work setting.	http://www.wati.org/free-publications/other-materials/
Exploring learning styles:	Site contains a number of free online learning style inventories.	http://www.studygs.net/teaching/learningstyles.htm
Sweeney, J. (2009) *Organizational Inventory*. In: *Assessing the need for Assistive Technology* (ed. J. Gierach), 29–30. (ASNAT)	Inventory suggests sensory processing plays a role in technology tool selections depending on the student's preferred learning style.	http://www.wati.org/free-publications/assessing-students-needs-for-assistive-technology/page/2/
Sweeney, J. (2003) *Personal Choices: Finding Low and Mid Tech Tools That Work for You*	The purpose of this packet is to help students find which low- and mid-tech tools best match their interests, needs, tasks, and abilities.	http://assistedtechnology.weebly.com/uploads/3/4/1/9/3419723/personalchoices.pdf
Thoma, C. and Wehman, P. (2010). Getting the Most Out of IEPS: An Educator's Guide to the Student Directed Approach, 149. Paul H. Brookes.	A self-assessment inventory.	http://www.ttacnews.vcu.edu/wp-content/uploads/sites/2795/mt/thingsineedtoknowaboutmyselfandat.doc
Quality Indicators for Assistive Technology Post-Secondary Education	QIAT-PS for Students are indicators directed at K-12 transition teams and students with disabilities. The self-evaluation matrix is intended to measure and improve assistive technology transfer to higher education.	http://qiat-ps.org/

Selecting the right tool for the job necessitates involving the user, and determining tools that are intuitive and easily accessible with a minimal amount of setup for the maximum amount of effectiveness in most situations. Best practice when choosing specific AT devices and services involves collaboration between the student, when appropriate, school personnel, and parent/caregiver to ensure it will do the job for which it is intended, be accepted by the user, and be consistently used. Knowledge of the environment in which the tool is needed may lead to interventions and resources already available and accessible to all students in the classroom, and so consideration must be given to what already exists and what supports may need to be put in place for the student with LD to use their accommodation. Finding the "just right" match between a person and the most appropriate tool for the job involves task analysis and identifying the attributes or features of specific tools. This process of feature matching requires asking and answering pertinent questions about the student, the environment, and the tasks the student needs to accomplish.

With advances in technology and the lure of the "latest and greatest," it is easy to come up with "solutions" without thoroughly analyzing the problem. For example, a recent post on the Quality Indicators for Assistive Technology (QIAT) listserv queried, "What kind of assistive technology should I buy for high school students?" The individual posting did not say, "I have a student who struggles with the motor aspect of writing," or "converting measurement," or "turning assignments in on time." Dozens of responses flooded in listing the pros and cons of iPads versus other tablet forms before someone dared to ask what issues were impacting the student's performance. Because of the misconception that technology itself will level the playing field (rather than the right application of the right technology at the right time), there is a tendency to choose a tool based on what an item is advertised to do. Moreover, there can be suspicion that a high-tech solution has not been recommended "because the (school, insurance, employer) does not want to pay for it," and a climate of mistrust and resentment is created. It is important to understand the organizational level of the Human-Tech Ladder and how this can influence the human-tech interaction (Vicente 2006). Therefore, it is imperative to perform a feature match looking at the needs and abilities of the student and the attributes of the tool, and to implement trials and collect data on the effectiveness of suggested interventions while perpetuating the stance that the process is an ever-changing one, based on the need, the response to the intervention, the passage of time, user growth and change, and the development of more suitable tools (QIAT Leadership Team 2015).

AT theories related to learning disabilities

Modifying the environment and providing UDL supports or specific AT requires a systematic process. In terms of matching a person with TEI, there are a number of models that provide a framework for decision-making regarding the selection, implementation, and evaluation of AT, including: EASY approach (Sweeney 2007) Human Activity Assistive Technology (HAAT) model (Cook and Polgar 2015), Student, Environments, Tasks, and Tools (SETT) framework (Zabala 1995, 2010), and the Matching Person and Technology (MPT) assessment process (Scherer and Craddock 2002), all of which follow the person-environment-occupation (PEO) model (Law et al. 1996) and emphasize a client- and occupation-centered approach to service provision. These theoretical approaches are presented in Table 14.4 and in more depth in other chapters of this textbook.

It is important to start with the tools that are readily available in the learner's environment and those consistent with their needs. The drawbacks to bringing in novel tools include the need for additional training, difficulty with replicating or substituting if the tool fails, and so on when there might already be tools in the environment that may work. Copley and Ziviani (2007) determined barriers to implementation and integration of AT in the educational setting included lack of appropriate staff training and support, negative staff attitudes, inadequate assessment and planning processes, insufficient funding, difficulties with procuring and managing equipment, and time constraints. When the tools that are already available in the client's customary environment do not meet the client's needs despite customization, then the process would continue by introducing new tools. In addition to using the SETT framework, or other relevant model, to make decisions for individual ATs for a specific need and individual, framework- or model-based key questions can be can be applied to assist collaborative teams in designing UDL environments (Zabala 2010). Strategies to support specific areas of need can be found in a number of UDL toolkits found online (see Toolbox for web addresses). Two such resources are the UDL Guidelines, as displayed in Figure 14.2, an online interactive collection of instructional suggestions and resources for each UDL principle, and the UDL Toolkit. Consider the scenario in Box 14.5.

What a difference the environment makes: The role of environment in AT

Twenty-first-century learning environments are "support systems that organize the condition in which humans learn best – systems that accommodate the unique learning needs of every learner and support the positive

Table 14.4 Assistive Technology (AT) Processes, Models, and Frameworks to Guide how We Think about Assistive Technology.

Economy Additional use Standards-based Yours	Consideration of Economy of cost and time; Additional (or Adapted) use of familiar tools; tool selection based on Standards that are already a part of what must be taught; and ownership, telling the student and teacher (or parent) "the tool is Yours" may make the difference between acceptance and rejection of a suggested tool.	Sweeney (2007)
Human Activity Assistive Technology	Three factors – the human (including physical, cognitive, and emotional elements), activity (self-care, work, play leisure), and AT (device and/or service) – form a collective whole that is then placed within the context of participation.	Cook and Polgar (2015)
Matching Person and Technology	The MPT model and assessment process are designed to help individualize the process of matching each person with the most appropriate AT by considering *milieu* (i.e. characteristics of the environment and psychosocial setting in which the person uses the technology), *personality* (i.e. temperament and preferences), and *technology* (i.e. functions and features).	Scherer and Craddock (2002)
Person Environment Occupation	Emphasizes the interaction between the person, environment, occupation is interdependent.	Law et al. (1996)
Student Environments Tasks Tools	The SETT framework is designed to develop good decision-making. SETT includes a series of questions that are designed to guide discussion, evaluation, and intervention. The process promotes collaboration, communication, sharing of knowledge and perspectives, and flexibility among educational team members, resulting in student-centered, environmentally specific, and task-focused tool systems.	Zabala (1995)

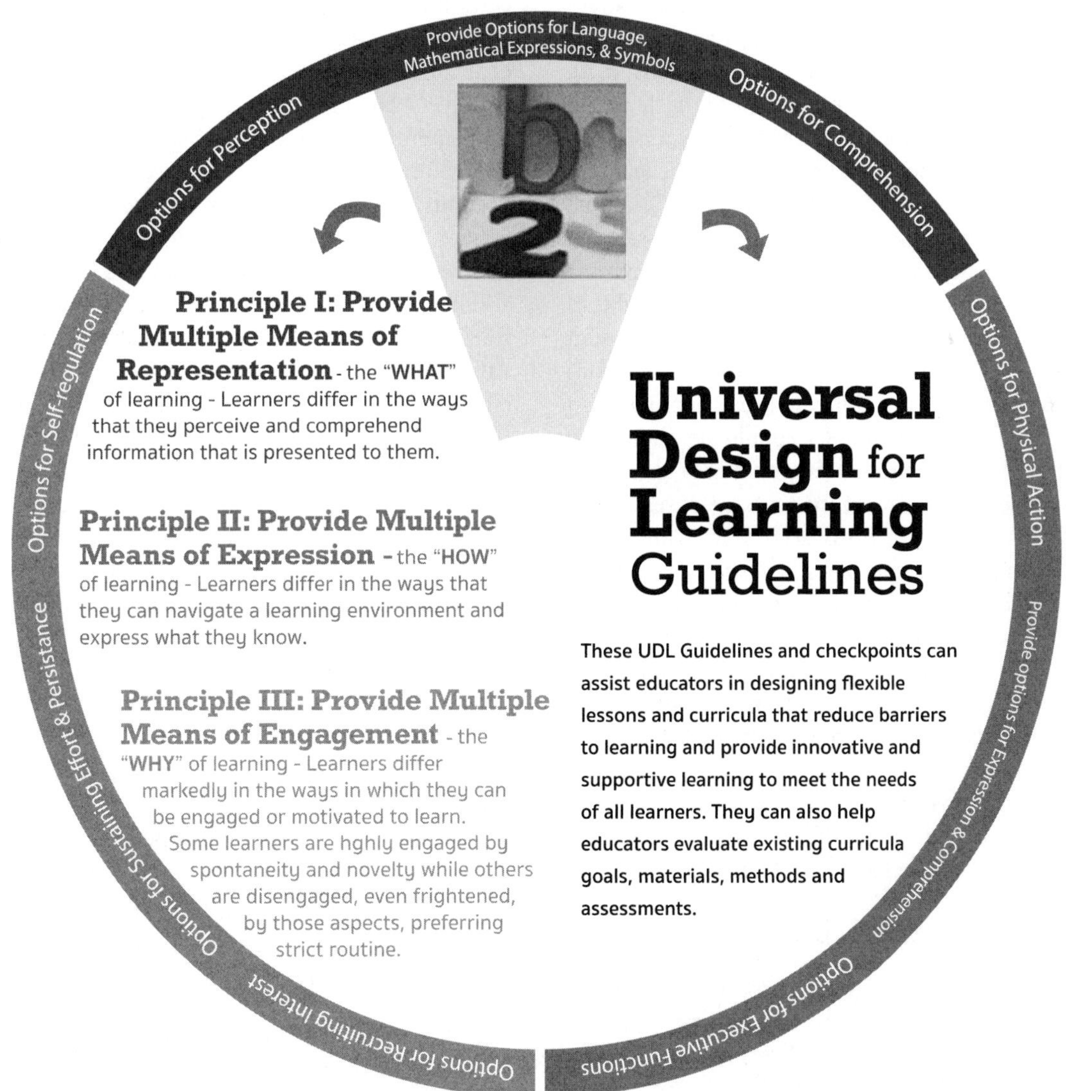

Figure 14.2 UDL Guidelines. Source: http://udlguidelines.cast.org/. Reprinted with permission, courtesy of David Gordon.

Box 14.5 Active learning: Applying the UDL guidelines and UDL toolkit

Situation	Questions
Jamal is a 15 year-old eighth grader who was "held back" in elementary school. While his verbal expression is good, he currently reads at the fourth grade level. He is embarrassed by the "baby books" his remedial reading teacher uses. Jamal's handwriting is difficult to read, and his writing is disorganized with poor spelling and grammar. He excels at sports, but is not allowed to play on the school teams because of his low grades. He has accommodations of having tests read aloud and dictation to a scribe, but he is rude and uncommunicative to the teaching assistant when he is pulled from class to do so. In addition, Jamal has been cutting class and getting into fights with classmates.	1. What do you think might happen to Jamal if he does not receive help at this crucial time in his education? 2. What alternatives to handwriting might be suggested? 3. How can grade level reading materials be scaffolded for Jamal? 4. What are the alternatives to a person reading to Jamal or having him dictate to a scribe? 5. Can you think of ways to recruit Jamal's interest when school is so difficult?

human relationships needed for effective learning. Learning environments are the structures, tools, and communities that inspire students and educators to attain the knowledge and skills the 21st Century demands" (21st Century Learning Environments White Paper 2009, p. 3). Based on white paper recommendations, the learning space should be configured to allow the educator(s) to move between the students easily and allow the learners to move around if they need to. TEIs are equally important in making the learning environment accessible to learners. Learners need to feel comfortable in the environment so they can concentrate on what is being taught. In addition to the role the physical aspects of the classroom environment (desk and chair heights, computer workstations, etc.) have in students' ability to learn, lighting, temperature, noise, and their impact should be taken into consideration. When the room temperature is too warm, learners may become sleepy or inattentive (Jensen 2005). Learners can be taught to dress according to the room temperature and be given permission to slip on or remove an outer garment for comfort. Noise within and outside of the classroom can also impact learning. Studies (Irlen.com 2015) have shown that color can have an impact on learning as well. Color filters are no-tech tools, which may help some students view text more clearly, focus for longer periods of time, and copy more accurately (Sweeney 2007). Additional environmental processes and strategies are available through a variety of AT initiatives and centers throughout the United States and globally.

Behavioral cultural tools – psychosocial interventions

PBIS is a proactive approach to establishing the non-physical supports and culture needed for learners to achieve social, emotional, and academic success by embedding them directly in authentic contexts. This school-wide system of support includes proactive strategies for defining, teaching, and sustaining appropriate behaviors to create positive school environments (Horner et al. 2015). Much like RtI, PBIS includes a continuum of positive behavior support for all students within a school implemented in areas including the classroom and non-classroom settings (such as hallways, the cafeteria, playgrounds, and restrooms) that (i) teaches students skills to behave appropriately, (ii) positively acknowledges students engaging in those behaviors, and (iii) provides consistency and stability in interactions among students and staff members (McKevitt and Braaksma 2008, p. 735). Attention is focused on creating and sustaining primary (school-wide), secondary (classroom), and tertiary (individual) systems of support that promote positive interactions by making identified misbehavior less effective, efficient, and relevant, and desired behavior more functional. Strategies and tools for self-regulation are integral for the success of PBIS. In terms of an approach that considers the physical, academic, and social environment, Gargiulo and Metcalf (2010) modeled and embedded a learning strategy in the form of an acrostic in their ACCESS approach:

- **A**pplicable – is the environment useful, accessible, and learner centered?
- **C**apability – is the design flexible?
- **C**larity – are the tools and materials flexible?
- **E**xpression – is essential information communicated via the environment or materials?
- **S**afety – are there any hazards? Is there tolerance for errors?
- **S**ize and Space – furniture/materials/group size proportionate to all users?

Use whatcha got: Use a full range of technology

Reading and writing are foundational productivity areas that need to be addressed when supporting persons with LD. These are the channels through which most academic and business information is provided, although the use of multimedia to exchange information is rapidly increasing. Specific tools and supports can be an effective intervention for persons with LD. For example, a person with a print disability who struggles with the decoding and word recognition aspect of reading, but who has good listening skills, might benefit from print information in an audio format. Additionally, there are inexpensive, readily available low-tech devices such as color highlighters readers can use to identify easily confused words that may appear similar, such as *their* and *there*, to help differentiate between the words (Raskind and Stanberry 2006).

Other low-tech supports might include the use of visual representation to assist with comprehension and sequencing of details. Adapting books with tangible supports and/or electronic methods can provide print access following the (UDL) framework. Books can be stabilized using book holders, rubberized shelf-liner, Dycem®, Velcro®, and magnets. Pages can be made easier to turn by stabilizing them with stiff textures (FabricATe 2018) and "fluffing" them with weather stripping, clothespins, craft sticks, cotton balls, or beads (Purcell and Grant 2004).

Moreover, outlining, removing background, adding texture, or changing colors can add definition and clarity to picture support. Content or key concepts can be emphasized with color, changes in font, tangible items, and sounds. Page appearance and text can be simplified by reducing words on pages, increasing margins and reducing number of words on each line can assist with visual tracking, and words can be supplemented with Widgit Symbols (Figure 14.3).

Books can also be adapted and viewed on computer, tablets, or smart devices by scanning the pages or finding comparable clip art and assembling in a multimedia slide show. Standard computer features can be employed to add sound, to read a story, to add animation, to change the visual contrast, to slow down, to speed up, or to alter the story to improve comprehension (Norton-Darr and Schoonover 2012).

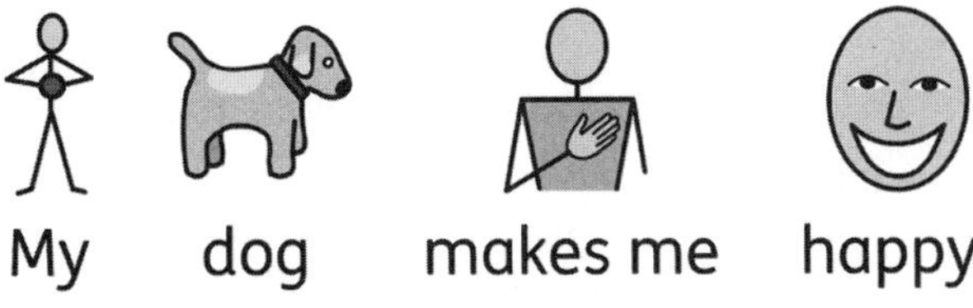

Figure 14.3 Widgit Symbols © Widgit Software 2002–2018 www.widgit.com.

Producing written text (writing) is a demanding task that requires motor skills and cognitive processes. Writing is a form of communication tool that puts ideas, information, knowledge, and feelings into a text format that can be read by others. Traditionally, learners have demonstrated their knowledge of what has been taught through writing (journaling, fill-in-the blank, worksheets, and so on). Handwriting instruction used to begin in kindergarten or first grade, although many preschools emphasized printing in their curriculum as well. Now, children often have exposure to technology tools at a very young age and can be found swiping and poking at screens even while strapped in their car seats. Handwriting instruction has fallen by the wayside as educators scramble to find room in the class schedule to teach the content students will be tested on to pass local and state standards of learning (Saperstein Associates 2012).

The good news is that technological advances have made numerous alternatives to handwriting available, including keyboarding, devices and software with record features, word prediction, handwriting recognition, and voice recognition. Most schools have computer labs, or technology on carts, but also a number of device choices within the classroom that might include computers, tablet technology, interactive whiteboards, and so on. The bad news is that for some learners, the interactivity of seeing, touching, feeling, and hearing the production of letters and their sounds, and relating them back to the acquisition of reading and writing skills, may be based less on manipulatives and guided practice and more on "screen time" (Saperstein Associates 2012). Students who experience difficulty with written language expression struggle to access and interact with academic material and cannot always demonstrate their knowledge. There are many ways to support struggling writers, depending on which aspects of the writing process they find problematic. Assessment tools such as the Writing chapters of the Assessing Student's Need for Assistive Technology (Gierach 2009) and the School-Based Assistive Technology Writing Evaluation: An Interdisciplinary Approach (Visvader et al. 2014) may help guide the process of selecting writing supports and alternatives. Please review Table 14.5 for strategies.

Visual thinking and learning strategies increase academic and work performance for everybody, and allow the viewer to "see" what the writer is thinking. The use of graphic organizers, from a folded piece of paper divided into quadrants to graphic organizer software, provides multiple mediums for engagement, representation, and action and expression, allowing persons to

Table 14.5 Low-Tech Tools and Solutions to Support Strategies for Writing.

Environment	Strategy
Seating	For those struggling with letter formation and spacing, it is essential to begin with the proper tools and strategies, which includes positional ergonomics so that the writer is sitting in a comfortable, stable position with feet resting on the floor and the writing surface at a level that allows the forearms to be supported and the writing surface to be viewed optimally.
Stabilization	Something as simple as a binder with a 3–4-in. spine serving as a less expensive version of a commercially purchased slant board can assist with the viewing of reading and writing materials. The addition of a binder clamp or chip bag clip at the top of the notebook can be used to secure materials.
Visual cues	Having a letter strip and/or number line in close proximity can cue the user with regards to letter formation, and paper with shaded or colored lines, including graph paper (which can be made using the Table features of MSWord, or downloaded from any number of free handwriting and graph paper websites) can assist with letter alignment, size, and spacing.
Writing tools	Pencil grips can ease the tendency of an anxious writer to squeeze the pencil tool tightly, causing discomfort, and can guide the fingers and thumb into a more functional gripping pattern to support the flow of letter formation. In addition to alternative pencils and pens, use of a word processor or writing app, word prediction, and voice dictation can result in a uniformly legible and spaced product.
Online tools	For struggling students who do not produce their best work on paper and pencil tasks. Interactive websites and apps can be used instead of, or addition to, traditional learning materials because of the immediate feedback and support that is provided. Websites such as Understood.org and CALL Scotland (https://www.callscotland.org.uk/information/) contain constantly updated resources and tutorials about apps, websites, and accessibility features.

(re)present information in an organized manner. Information can be visually arranged and ideas outlined to structure writing and improve communication and expression. With these tools, individuals can brainstorm using symbols and images to represent and sort their ideas, and create diagrams and graphic organizers to break work down into manageable sections.

A no- or (very) low tech-tool suggested by the AT team members of Loudoun County Public Schools is a "story rope," which provides both a visual and a kinesthetic "road map" to follow when writing or retelling a story (Moss 2005). Story ropes can be personalized to capitalize on an individual's interest. For example, a sports fan might relate to and enjoy using the football story rope displayed in Figure 14.4.

The stadium represents the setting, the players represent the characters, the kick-off represents the action, and so on. For an individual who enjoys cooking, one can see how to apply the same ideas to the start-to-finish process of following a recipe. Another no-tech graphic organizer that has gained popularity in recent years is paper that is folded and cut to separate, represent, and organize information. Educator Dinah Zikes has registered the term Foldable® to describe what she originally called 3D interactive graphic organizers as displayed in Figure 14.5. Foldables can be created with or without computers to produce a paper-based manipulative to display and organize information.

Clearly, visual representations can take place in many forms, from a simple folded sheet of paper to build vocabulary and teach critical thinking skills called the Frayer Model to free and for purchase only graphic organizer software programs. The Frayer Model is a concept development tool formed by folding a piece of paper into quadrants (Adlit.org. 2016). This no-tech approach helps to develop a better understanding of complex concepts by having students not just identify what something is, but also consider what something is not. The center of the diagram shows the concept being defined, while the quadrants around the concept are used for providing the details, such as characteristics, definitions, examples, and non-examples.

Other easy ways to access organizers include using the Outline Form and SmartArt in MS Word, taking advantage of free websites such as ReadWriteThink.org, or purchasing graphic organizer products that allow customized organizers to be produced that might include pictures, audio, and videos. Applications that enhance thinking and innovation skills include the Internet and the vast world of information to which this gives access, electronic databases, simulations, and educational games (Microsoft 2019; Apple 2019).

The computer's role as an AT power tool

The judicious use of computers and selection of appropriate software can help compensate for reading and writing difficulties and develop or strengthen skills. "Teaching is all about responsiveness, adaptability, and multiple strategies and resources, so the computer's flexibility – rather than any one particular feature – is

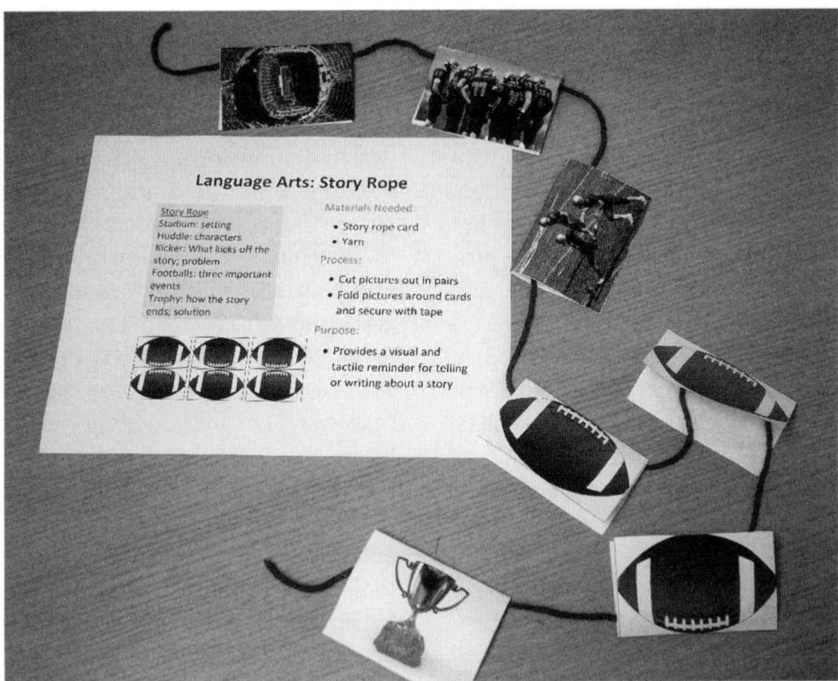

Figure 14.4 Story rope.

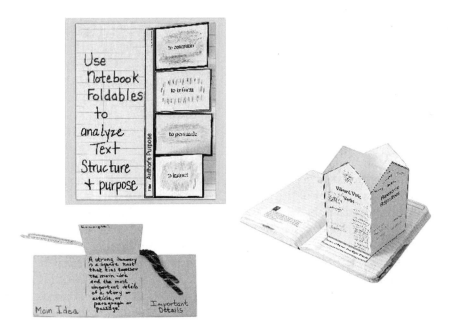

Figure 14.5 Foldable organizers. Source: Foldable is used by permission and those interested in learning more should visit www.dinah.com.

what gives it so much potential as a teaching tool" (Meyer and Rose 1998, p. 83). Computer simulations and virtual environments can provide preparation for social situations, academic tasks, pre-vocational training, and driver education. The multimedia features of the computer can support learning rules, turn taking, and social skills (Schoonover and Feist 2007). For persons with print disabilities, software and online supports such as screen readers and speech-to-text applications can decrease dependence on the support of others in the environment to read or write for them. For persons challenged to produce designs, art products, or written work as a result of motor, emotional, or attentional difficulties, the computer can assist in generating digital artwork or text that is neat and uniform in appearance (Schoonover and Argabrite Grove 2014; Microsoft 2019; Apple 2019).

Production of accurate, legible, or attractive work can increase self-esteem and self-expression and decrease frustration. UDL challenges educators to break out of the one-size-fits-all mentality of curriculum, instruction, and assessment by using digital technologies that alter the cognitive difficulty of information in order to provide multiple means of engagement, representation, and action and expression (CAST 2010).

Literacy, or lack thereof, impacts the likelihood of successful competitive or supported employment (Koppenhaver et al. 1991). In today's print-based society, those with print disabilities may experience challenges managing information and succeeding academically, which in turn may impact their quality of life. "The application of literacy skills and the use of a variety of literacy tools (such as listening and technology) to accomplish daily tasks in the home, school, community, and work settings" can be used to achieve functional literacy (Koenig and Holbrook 2000, p. 265). Most schools, starting in K-12 and continuing through college, use specialized services to provide alternative texts to replace print textbooks. While early reading experiences can be easily scaffolded with props and simplified language, print alternatives may be necessary for older children, adolescents, and college students. The IDEA requires school districts to provide accessible versions of instructional materials including textbooks and related core materials such as workbooks to students who are blind or otherwise unable to use printed materials. Accessible formats such as Braille, large print, audio, and digital text provide flexibility to meet a wide variety of needs. Digital text can be read with text-to-speech, modified in terms of font size, and navigated by unit, chapter, section, and page number. Options such as screen masking, changing color of text or background, synchronized highlighting with speech, dictionary, note-taking capabilities, and voice recording should be considered on an individual basis. Resources for educators and instructors on best practices to ensure the accessibility of self-created educational materials using MS Word, PowerPoint, Excel, PDF, websites, tablets, mobile phones, Windows, AT, and more can be found on the National Center on Accessible Instructional Materials website (aem.cast.org). In higher education, common services for text alternatives are AccessText, and Learning Ally. Kindle or other e-reader devices may be used as accommodations; while they are not fully accessible, individual students may find them useful.

Edyburn (2002) coined the term cognitive rescaling to define "a process of altering the cognitive difficulty of information." While reading has historically been a visual/perception cognitive process completed "within one's head" (Edyburn 2007, p, 151), with the influx of a vast variety of productivity tools, it is now possible to design or transform curriculum or instructional methodology with the scaffolds and supports needed to ensure that all learners have access to knowledge.

The cognitive difficulty of information can be scaled, engaging students and resulting in higher levels of academic achievement. For those operating with little to no budget for what has been generally considered as "assistive technology" or specialized software, multiple ways of representing traditionally print-based information can be achieved using commonly found features of Microsoft Office and Google Chrome in novel ways. Every educator can produce technology-enhanced digital text with readily available software tools and free Internet downloads. Students can also be taught to alter the amount, cognitive challenge, and appearance of text as a form of self-advocacy (Crouse 2009).

Using Microsoft Office or Google Docs, it is possible to create and customize an onscreen learning environment for students at a variety of developmental levels, as well as produce paper documents and products that can appeal to a variety of learning styles. By using a familiar software application that is typically available on most computers, learners are provided access to what they need in a variety of environments (Microsoft 2019). Tools for differentiating instruction and providing flexible means of accessing and applying information using multiple means of engagement, representation, and action and expression are displayed in Table 14.6.

For some persons, specific instructional software may be too fast-paced, complex, or made up of too many distracting "bells and whistles." With Microsoft PowerPoint or similar multimedia authoring programs, including free web-based applications, it is possible to create and individualize learning experiences and tools. Desirable applications are those that can be geared to any age level, are used by peers as well as adults, and can be applied to teach skills that extend into play, leisure, and work occupations (Microsoft 2019).

Some individuals may benefit from additional hardware, such as switches, trackballs, touch windows or interactive whiteboards, and alternative keyboards, to fully access or author activities. Presentations supplemented with graphics, digital pictures, sound effects, narration, and animation can be used to tailor instructional text to individual reading levels, motivate reluctant readers, reinforce and integrate curriculum content, teach social skills, provide a leisure time activity, support students' individualized education plan (IEP) objectives,

Table 14.6 Computer Software Applications for Learning.

Software feature	Description
Accessibility	*Accessibility Features* can make use of the computer easier for all individuals. There are a number of ways operating systems such as Windows can make it easier to see what is displayed on the screen, including making everything appear larger by adjusting the screen resolution, using the built-in Magnifier, enlarging the mouse pointer (cursor), personalizing the color theme, or selecting a High Contrast Theme. Microsoft Office applications can assist educators incorporate accessibility features into instructions and students to customize their computing environment. Font size, titles, menus, buttons, icons, scrollbars, mouse cursors, etc., can be adjusted for optimal viewing and efficient access. High-contrast options, captions with sounds/warnings, and special keyboard options are also available.
Shortcuts	*Keyboard Shortcuts* can increase access to and efficiency of commonly used buttons and icons for those who experience difficulty controlling a touchpad or mouse.
Templates and Forms	*Templates and Forms* can be created incorporating text boxes, check boxes, radio buttons, fill-in-the-blank, and drop-down menus to produce worksheets, tests, multiple-choice questions, letters, and reports that can be completed in Word. Forms can be locked, or protected, to prevent accidental deletion or modification of contents.
Table Tools	*Create Ruled and Graph Paper* using the Tables and Borders toolbar. Paper can be customized to the needs of specific students, with lines and spaces drawn or shaded in different colors and thicknesses.
Print Screen or Snipping Tool	*Print Screen or Snipping Tool* function to take "snapshots" of images on the computer monitor to document onscreen student work; and to customize pictures used for instructional purposes, communication boards, PowerPoint slides and more.
Readability	Microsoft Word can scan a document and provide with readability statistics, including *Counts, Averages*, and *Readability Scores*. When enabled, this proofing tool will review document and provide with a Flesch Reading Ease and Flesch-Kincaid Grade Level Score.

or document student learning as an alternative assessment. Multimedia presentations can be viewed and manipulated online, or printed with a variety of print and assembly options to provide tangible learning tools such as interactive talking storybooks, social situation stories, quizzes for classroom use, and digital portfolios (CAST n.d.).

There seem to be a limitless number of free and low-cost web-based tools and apps to support all areas of learning. Examples to investigate include: the Free Technology Toolkit for UDL in All Classrooms (https://sites.google.com/view/freeudltechtoolkit/home?authuser=0), the CAST Book Builder, UDL Curriculum Self-Check, a UDL Lesson Builder, UDL Science Writer, Strategy Tutor, and UDL Studio http://www.cast.org/whats-new/learning-tools.html#.XPudZlPRB0s.

Technology and environmental competencies needed for UDL implementation and assessment

Educational tools, from pencil grips and slant boards to tablet computing and apps as described earlier in this chapter, are only as effective as the environment in which they are implemented. Technology competencies should not be limited to teaching keyboarding as an alternative to handwriting, but rather encompass the accessibility features of computer operating systems and networked software; an awareness of the attributes available in instructional tools such as overhead projectors, interactive whiteboards, digital cameras, and tablet computing; an ability to use the Internet, connect with others electronically, and more (Schoonover and Argabrite Grove 2014; ISTE 2016).

Engineering of the environment goes beyond recommending desk heights and ergonomic computer workstations. The US Department of Education National Education Technology Plan (US Department of Education, Office of Educational Technology 2017) calls for schools to infuse curriculum and teaching methodology with technology skills. Additionally, school districts are challenged to redesign pre-service education programs to increase technology proficiency, promote equal access to technology, increase connectivity, adopt high-quality textbook alternatives, implement UD principles, and improve technology-based assessments. Competencies required include an understanding of no-tech and low-tech tools and materials that are readily available in the environment, as well as the accessibility features of computer operating systems and networked software. According to Don Knezek (Knezek cited in Pullen et al. 2010, p. 11), International Standards for Technology in Education (ISTE) CEO, "The digital-age teaching professional must demonstrate a vision of technology infusion and develop the technology skills of others. These are the hallmarks of the new education leader." The reader should be aware of the National Educational Technology Standards (NETS), which are standards of excellence and best practices for learning, teaching, and leading in the digital age and are widely recognized and adopted worldwide. They include: NETS for Students (NETS•S), NETS for Teachers (NETS•T), NETS for Administrators (NETS•A), NETS for Coaches (NETS•C), and NETS for Computer Science Teachers (NETS•CSE). One of the many goals (and benefits) of NETS is designing student-centered, project-based, and online learning environments to meet the learning styles and needs of a wide range of students. For more information, see http://www.iste.org/standards.

AT challenges

Despite the promise of UD, UDL, and AT, implementation is not without challenges. It should be noted that these frameworks provide access and serve as door-openers; however, they do not replace the need for training and support once the threshold has been crossed. These interventions require collaboration and time: time to observe and learn, time to plan, time to implement, and time to evaluate the effectiveness of the curriculum and teaching methods. Paradigms must be shifted with regards to traditional roles of teachers as "sages on stages" and related service providers as unilateral decision-makers about interventions. The shift from reliance on print-based media requires creativity, as well as an understanding of the different ways individuals learn (Rose and Meyer 2002; National Center on Accessible Educational Materials 2015). Additionally, this shift necessitates acquisition and mastery of new technologies with a critical eye toward matching the learner's needs with the right attributes offered by the technology (QIAT Leadership Team 2015).

Technology can be employed to bridge time and distance gaps, from use of an electronic survey to determine a time that works best to meet in real time, to posting planning documents online in order for all shareholders to contribute their thoughts and ideas (Schoonover and Argabrite Grove 2014). While meeting in person may be preferable, use of conference calls, multimedia, video conferencing, email, cloud storage of non-confidential documents, chat rooms, and more can allow participation if there is a comfort level with the chosen method (Schoonover 2014).

AT takes a team

AT teams take many forms, and currently there is no legislation determining their composition. In some school districts, no one is responsible for AT provisions, while in others, one or more employees may provide AT services in addition to other responsibilities. Some school districts employ transdisciplinary teams at the district level responsible for AT, either with some reduction in other responsibilities, or strictly as AT providers, and they are designated with specific responsibilities related to AT and given the necessary training, resources, and support to carry out those responsibilities (Bodine and Melonis 2005; Decoste et al. 2005). The ideal AT team would consist of "a knowledgeable, supportive network of people working together to help every IEP Team choose and provide appropriate AT devices and services" (Gierach 2009, p. 4) collaboratively. A collaborative model assumes "that no one person or profession has an adequate knowledge base or sufficient expertise to execute all the functions (assessment, planning, and intervention) associated with providing educational services for students. All team members are involved in planning and monitoring educational goals and procedures, although each team member's responsibility for the implementation may vary" (American Speech-Language-Hearing Association 1991). AT assessments commonly used do not tend to "belong" to any specific discipline, although discipline-specific assessment might be used as part of the process of determining the student's strengths and needs. Table 14.7 describes a sample of assessments that might be considered.

Productivity tools from pencils to computers are only as effective as the environment in which they are implemented. Training others to understand and use a continuum of tools is an essential part of proactively designing an environment that emphasizes the acquisition and application of knowledge via flexible instruction and assessment modalities following the principles outlined in a UDL approach. *The Assistive Technology Trainer's Handbook* (Reed et al. 2009) suggests that even when the selected tools are intuitive and easy to understand, users of the tools and those who may support the users may require training to help them plan for appropriate times and places to use the technology and to develop strategies to increase its usefulness (QIAT Leadership Team 2015). Effective training for service providers (e.g. teachers, related service providers, paraprofessionals, and administrators) and parents or other caregivers who support a person with a disability begins by identifying factors that need to be considered during the planning stage, moves to strategies and techniques to use during the training, and concludes with strategies

Table 14.7 A Sampling of Assistive Technology (AT) Assessments.

Assessment	Description	Reference
The DeCoste Writing Protocol	Formative assessment tool that helps identify factors affecting an individual student's ability to produce writing. The Writing Protocol compares individual performance across handwriting and keyboarding tasks. It examines spelling performance and writing skills so informed decisions about instructional strategies and the appropriate use of technology to meet classroom demands can be made.	DeCoste, D. (2014). http://donjohnston.com/decoste-writing-protocol/#.VKGQ2V4CA
Functional Evaluation for Assistive Technology (FEAT)	Five scales are completed by members of the AT team to allow for an ecologic assessment of needs: • *Contextual Matching Inventory* (information about setting-specific demands) • *Checklist of Strengths and Limitations* (gathers data about person-specific characteristics) • *Checklist of Technology Experiences* (additional information about the person-specific characteristics relating to past/current use of technology) • *Technology Characteristics Inventory* (examines device-specific characteristics such as dependability, product support) • *Individual-Technology Evaluation Scale* (determines whether proposed AT offers legitimate potential for effectiveness)	Raskind and Bryant (2002)
PAR (Protocol for Accommodations in Reading)	Helps determine the most suitable reading accommodations for specific students by assessing their individual needs. Collects data to compare independent reading, reading with a human reader, and reading with a text reader.	DeCoste and Wilson (2012)
Assessing Students' Needs for Assistive Technology (ASNAT)	Not designed as a test protocol but provides a process-based, collaborative systematic approach to assessment. Package includes WATI Assessment forms; the Consideration Guide, Student Information Guide, Environmental Observation Guide, Decision-Making Guide, AT Checklist, and Trial Use Guide	Gierach, J. (2009). Assessing Students' Needs for Assistive Technology. http://www.wati.org/free-publications/assessing-students-needs-for-assistive-technology/.

for follow-up after the training is over (Reed et al. 2009). Refer to Box 14.6 for AT Team members' roles and perspectives.

As indicated previously, there still may be a need for ATs based on distinct and individual needs. Those responsible for assessing individuals, making recommendations, and assisting with the implementation of strategies and application of tools have a responsibility to users and those who support them to help them understand how technology works. Training may take many forms. An excellent guide for training is *The Assistive Technology Trainer's Handbook* (Reed et al. 2009), which asserts training may or may not be a part of a larger professional development plan, and suggests basic principles that can be applied to the provision of (assistive) technology training:

- helping people understand how the technology operates and what it can do;
- how and when to use technology to increase the independence and productivity of students with disabilities;
- how adults in the educational environment and parents can use technology for personal productivity and information gathering.

Consider the scenario in Box 14.7.

Summary

There is a distinct relationship between learners and their learning environments, and it is important to recognize how the environment – physical, academic, social, virtual – can contribute to functional performance. While they affect every person differently, learning disabilities can be considered an umbrella term covering a variety of disorders that affect the ability to learn. For persons of school age, one

Box 14.6 AT team roles and perspectives

Potential AT team members	Potential role(s) and perspectives
Student or client	Identifies wants, needs, preferences, and willingness to use recommended supports
Educator(s)	Provides insight relating to the student's abilities and opportunities for participation and identifies barriers to learning-based knowledge of the curriculum and what the student needs to accomplish
Paraprofessional	May be the individual who works most closely with the student, therefore may contribute information on environmental factors impacting performance
Occupational therapist	In addition to providing information regarding fine motor, visual perceptual motor, and sensory processing, are experts in task analysis and problem-solving
Physical therapist	Evaluates seating, positioning, and mobility and promotes access to the physical environment
Speech-language pathologist	Provides information on communication and language and assists in the development of augmentative communication systems
Transition teacher/vocational counselor/community services representative	During critical transition planning provides insight into employment, post-secondary education options, and community resources
School administrator/Special education supervisor	Responsible for management of educational programs, meeting timelines, authorizing staff training, and guaranteeing implementation in various educational settings
Family/caregiver(s)	Provides perspective on who the student is when not in school

Other team members could include an audiologist, computer specialist, rehabilitation engineer, social worker, Teacher of Hearing Impaired, and/or Teacher of Visually Impaired as indicated by the reason for the request for AT support.

Box 14.7 Case study: Richard

The bell rings and students file into the classroom. There is a flurry of activity as backpacks are hung up, homework assignments are handed in, the lunch count is taken, and morning work is initiated. After the Pledge of Allegiance, Ms. Teacher asks the students to take out their language arts books and turn to page 20. She stands at the front of the class and begins reading from the text. She calls on a student to continue the reading.

Just then, Richard bursts into the classroom. "I missed the bus" he announces as he dumps his backpack by the coat rack. "Again," a classmate mutters under their breath. Ms. Teacher sighs in exasperation. She asks Richard to take his seat and asks him to get out his language arts book. Richard sits down and without looking at the contents of his desk begins to fumble around inside. Bits of papers, scissors, and crayons are dislodged as he feels around for his textbook. Ms. Teacher helps him locate his book and asks him to turn to page 20. Richard flicks pages back and forth until the student sitting next to him reaches over and locates the correct page.

Ms. Teacher calls on him to read. Richard pulls his book close to his face and begins re-reading the passage that has just been read aloud until Ms. Teacher points to the place where she wants him to begin. Richard uses his finger to follow the text across the pages but stumbles over many of the words. A number of the students around him shuffle their feet impatiently and raise their hands to be called on next. Ms. Teacher then passes out a worksheet and asks that the class get out their pencils. Richard can't find his and has to borrow from a neighbor.

Richard scrawls his name at the top of the page, pressing down so hard the paper tears. Ms. Teacher gives the class five minutes to complete the worksheet. Richard hunches over the page and begins to fill in the blanks, pausing frequently as he tries to recall how to spell the words in his answers. When the allotted five minutes are up, Ms. Teacher asks the students to exchange the papers so that they can be corrected in class. No one offers to exchange papers with Richard, so Ms. Teacher must intervene. Richard watches the student correcting his paper mark the incorrect answers with a red pen, neglecting to correct the paper he is supposed to correct. Next Ms. Teacher tells the students that they are allowed to find a partner to read the assigned pages from their social studies book and answer the questions at the end of the chapter. No one volunteers to partner with Richard. He puts his head down on his desk.

Case study questions

1. Have you met a student like Richard or have you been a student like Richard: late, disorganized, perhaps thought of by his classmates as slow because he just can't seem "to get it together"?
2. Have you had educators like Ms. Teacher who take a "sage on the stage" approach to education and are print or lecture dependent in the way they provide instruction?
3. How do you think Richard feels about school?
4. Do you have any ideas about what might help Richard based on what you have learned about him so far? What else would you want to know about him, and how might you find that information out?
5. Which disciplines or perspectives would you want to see contribute to determining supports for Richard?

traditional intervention for learning disabilities has been special education.

As the face of education changes, more emphasis has been placed on creating positive spaces, places, and techniques rather than labeling students. IDEA and other legislation encourages pre-referral interventions and supports initiatives such as RtI, PBIS, and UDL. Learning environments are the structures, tools, and communities that inspire students and educators to attain the knowledge and skills the twenty-first century demands. UDL, as a pedagogical framework that goes beyond technology, focuses on changes in school environments in order to make schooling a better experience for all children. UDL can be implemented without battery-operated, plugged in, online, or app-driven device technology.

At the college level, this is called Universal Design of Instruction (UDI). Note the difference in focus – learning versus instruction, highlighting the differences between K-12 and college. K-12 is focused on the student and how they learn. At the higher-education level, the focus is on the instructor and how they teach. Hopefully, the outcome is the same, but in higher education, the student is more responsible for the learning than the instructor. In college, a professor will hopefully (but not necessarily) instruct in a way that meets a variety of learning styles at least some of the time, but instruction is not individualized.

While the term technology implies solutions that are complicated and expensive, it actually represents *tools*. Effective tools and learning environments should be proactively planned and designed to support diversity in learning styles as well as the intended learning activities. UDL does require well-designed lessons constructed to offer sufficient options in terms of both challenges and supports so that all of its learners meet with success (Rose et al. 2012). An accessible learning environment supports and challenges students while minimizing barriers through highly flexible teaching strategies, materials, and technology. Ideally, a range of options should be available so that students can make choices to support their learning.

The National Technology Plan for Education 2017 calls for schools to infuse curriculum and teaching methodology with technology skills. One of the many goals (and benefits) of National Technology Plan for Education is designing student-centered, project-based, and online learning environments to meet the learning styles and needs of a wide range of students. Proactively initiating changes that make the physical, academic, and social environment more accessible for all may eliminate the need for so many individual accommodations that are burdensome for all. Introducing, modeling, and embedding low-tech solutions that are generally more available, easier to implement/use, and often found more acceptable by the learner and educational team can increase meaningful participation, and may serve as "door openers" to accepting more complex interventions when needed. Even simple adaptations to educational tools and materials can increase a learner's independent participation and their self-esteem, giving them a sense of control over their environment and a feeling of success.

References

21st Century Learning Environments White Paper (2009). Partnership for 21st century learning. Retrieved from http://www.battelleforkids.org/networks/p21/frameworks-resources.

Adlit.org (2016). Classroom strategies: the Frayer Model. Retrieved from http://www.adlit.org/strategies/22369.

Alberta Education (2010). *Making a Difference: Meeting Diverse Learning Needs with Differentiated Instruction*. Edmonton, Canada: Author Retrieved from https://education.alberta.ca/media/384968/makingadifference_2010.pdf.

American Institutes on Research (n.d.). Essential components of RTI. Retrieved from http://www.rti4success.org/essential-components-rti.

American Psychiatric Association (2013). *Diagnostic and Statistical Manual of Mental Disorders: DSM-5*, 5e. Washington, DC: American Psychiatric Association.

American Speech-Language-Hearing Association (1991). A model for collaborative service delivery for students with language-learning disorders in the public schools [Relevant paper]. Retrieved from https://www.asha.org/policy/rp1991-00123/.

Americans with Disabilities Amendments Act of 2008 (2008). Pub. L. No. 110-325 (S 3406). Retrieved from http://www.eeoc.gov/laws/statutes/adaaa.cfm.

Apple (2019). Accessibility. Retrieved from https://www.apple.com/accessibility.

Atherton, H. (2004). A history of learning disabilities. In: *Learning Disabilities toward Inclusion*, 5e (ed. B. Gates), 43–65. Edinburgh: Elsevier, Churchill Livingstone.

Blackhurst, A.E. and Lahm, E.A. (2000). Foundations of technology and exceptionality. In: *Technology and Exceptional Individuals*, 3e (ed. J. Lindsey), 3–45. Austin, TX: Pro-Ed.

Bodine, C. and Melonis, M. (2005). Teaming and assistive technology in educational settings. In: *Handbook of Special Education Technology Research and Practice* (ed. D. Edyburn, K. Higgins and R. Boone), 209–227. Whitefish Bay, WI: Knowledge by Design.

Bowser, G. and Reed, P. (2007). *Hey! Can I Try That? A Student Handbook for Choosing and Using Assistive Technology*. Oshkosh, WI: Wisconsin Assistive Technology Initiative.

Bremer, C., Kachgal, M., and Schoeller, K. (2003). Self-determination: supporting successful transition. *Research to Practice Brief: Improving Secondary Education and Transition Services through Research* 2 (1): 1–6. Retrieved from http://www.ncset.org/publications/researchtopractice/NCSETResearchBrief_2.1.pdf.

Burns, M.K. (2010). Response-to-intervention research: is the sum of the parts as great as the whole? Retrieved from http://www.rtinetwork.org/learn/research/response-to-intervention-research-is-the-sum-of-the-parts-as-great-as-the-whole.

Center for Applied Special Technology (n.d.). About CAST. Retrieved from http://www.cast.org/about/index.html.

Center for Applied Special Technology (2010). 2020's learning landscape: a retrospective on dyslexia. Retrieved from http://aem.cast.org/w/page/2020learning/l3.

Center for Universal Design (1997). About universal design. Retrieved from http://www.ncsu.edu/ncsu/design/cud/about_ud/udprinciples.htm.

Center for Universal Design (2008). Universal design history. Retrieved from https://projects.ncsu.edu/www/ncsu/design/sod5/cud/about_ud/udhistory.htm.

Cook, A. and Polgar, J. (2015). *Cook & Hussey's Assistive Technologies: Principles and Practice*, 4e. St. Louis, MO: Mosby.

Copley, J. and Ziviani, J. (2007). Use of a team-based approach to assistive technology assessment and planning for children with multiple disabilities: a pilot study. *Assistive Technology* 19 (3): 109–125.

Cortiella, C. and Horowitz, S.H. (2014). *The State of Learning Disabilities: Facts, Trends and Emerging Issues*. New York: National Center for Learning Disabilities.

Crouse, S. (2009). Uncovering the mysteries of your learning disability. Retrieved from http://www.ldinfo.com/self_advocacy_manual.htm.

DeCoste, D. (2014). DeCoste writing profile. Volo, IL: Don Johnston, Inc. Retrieved from http://donjohnston.com/decoste-writing-protocol/#.VKGQ2V4CA.

DeCoste, D.C., Reed, R. and Kaplan, M. (2005). *Assistive Technology Teams: Many Ways to Do It Well*. National Assistive Technology in Education Network Monograph Series. Roseburg, OR: NATE.

DeCoste, D.C. and Wilson, L. (2012). *PAR Protocol for Accommodations in Reading*. Volo, IL: Don Johnston Incorporated http://donjohnston.com/par.

DO-IT (2012). Working together: faculty and students with disabilities. University of Washington. Retrieved from https://www.washington.edu/doit/sites/default/files/atoms/files/Working-Together-Faculty-Students-Disabilities.pdf.

Edyburn, D.L. (2002). Cognitive rescaling strategies: interventions that alter the cognitive accessibility of text. *Closing The Gap* 1: 10–11, 21.

Edyburn, D.L. (2007). Technology-enhanced reading performance: defining a research agenda. *Reading Research Quarterly* 42 (1): 146–152.

Edyburn, D.L. (2009). Response to intervention (RtI): is there a role for assistive technology? *Special Education Technology Practice* 11 (1): 15–19.

ESSA (2015). Every Student Succeeds Act of 2015, Pub. L. No. 114-95 § 114 Stat. 1177 (2015–2016).

Eunice Kennedy Shriver National Institute on Child Health and Human Development (2018). About learning disabilities. Retrieved from https://www.nichd.nih.gov/health/topics/learning/conditioninfo/Pages/default.aspx.

FabricATe (2018). Page turners. Retrieved from https://www.fabricate4all.org/wp-content/uploads/2018/04/BD1_Page-Turners.pdf.

Fletcher, J.M. (2008). *Identifying Learning Disabilities in the Context of Response-To-Intervention: A Hybrid Model*. New York: RTI Action Network.

Fletcher, J.M., Lyon, G.R., and Fuchs, L.S. (2006). *Learning Disabilities: From Identification to Intervention*. New York: Guilford Press.

Gargiulo, R.M. and Metcalf, D. (2010). *Teaching in Today's Inclusive Classrooms: A Universal Design for Learning Approach*. Belmont, CA: Wadsworth, Cengage Learning.

Gierach, J. (ed.) (2009). *Assessing Students' Needs for Assistive Technology: A Resource Manual for School District Teams*, 5e. Milton, WI: Wisconsin Assistive Technology Initiative.

Hillman, C.N. (2011). The issue is: advocating for universal design in today's home market. Master's and Doctoral projects. Paper 83. Retrieved from http://www.utoledo.edu/library/projects/OccTherCP_Hillman_Corrie.pdf.

Hitchcock, C., Meyer, A., Rose, D., and Jackson, R. (2002). *Access, Participation, and Progress in the General Curriculum*. Wakefield, MA: National Center on Accessing the General Curriculum.

Horner, R.H., Sugai, G. and Lewis, T. (2015). Is school-wide positive behavior support an evidence-based practice? Retrieved from http://www.pbis.org/research.

Hudson, R.F., High, L., and Al Otaiba, S. (2007). Dyslexia and the brain: what does current research tell us? *The Reading Teacher* 60 (6): 506–515.

Individuals With Disabilities Education Act (IDEA) (2004). Retrieved from http://idea.ed.gov/explore/view/p/%2Croot%2Cstatute%2C.

International Dyslexia Foundation (2016). How widespread is dyslexia. Retrieved from https://dyslexiaida.org/how-widespread-is-dyslexia/.

Irlen.com (2015). Where the science of color transforms lives. Retrieved from http://irlen.com/published-research.

Jensen, E. (2005). *Teaching with the Brain in Mind*, 2e. Alexandria, VA: Association for Supervision and Curriculum Development.

Koenig, A.J. and Holbrook, M.C. (2000). Literacy skills. In: *Foundations of Education, Volume II: Instructional Strategies for Teaching Children and Youths with Visual Impairments*, 2e (ed. A.J. Koenig and M.C. Holbrook), 264–312. New York: American Foundation for the Blind.

Koppenhaver, D.A., Evans, D.A., and Yoder, D.E. (1991). Childhood reading and writing experiences of literate adults with severe speech and motor impairments. *Augmentative and Alternative Communication* 7: 20–33.

Law, M., Cooper, B., Strong, S. et al. (1996). The person-environment-occupation model: a transactive approach to occupational performance. *Canadian Journal of Occupational Therapy* 63 (1): 9–23.

LD Online (2010). What is a learning disability? Retrieved from http://www.ldonline.org/ldbasics/whatisld.

Learning Disabilities Association of America (n.d.). Retrieved from https://ldaamerica.org/.

Logsdon, A. (2018). How to help people cope with learning disabilities. Retrieved from https://www.verywellfamily.com/how-to-help-people-with-invisible-disabilities-cope-2162455.

McKevitt, B.C. and Braaksma, A. (2008). Best practices in developing a positive behavior support system at the school level. In: *Best Practices in School Psychology V*, vol. 3 (ed. A. Thomas and J. Grimes), 735–747. Bethesda, MD: National Association of School Psychologists.

Meo, G. (2008). Curriculum planning for all learners: applying universal design for learning (UDL) to a high school reading comprehension program. *Preventing School Failure* 52 (2): 21–30.

Meyer, A. and Rose, D.H. (1998). *Learning to Read in the Computer Age*. Cambridge, MA: Brookline Books.

Meyer, A., Rose, D.H., and Gordon, D. (2014). *Universal Design for Learning: Theory and Practice*. Wakefield MA: CAST.

Microsoft (2019). Accessibility. Retrieved from https://www.microsoft.com/enable/education.

Moss, B. (2005). Making a case and a place for effective content area literacy instruction in the elementary grades. *The Reading Teacher* 59: 46–55.

Nalavany, B.A., Carawan, L.W., and Sauber, S. (2015). Adults with dyslexia, an invisible disability: the mediational role of concealment on perceived family support and self-esteem. *British Journal of Social Work* 45 (2): 568–586. https://doi.org/10.1093/bjsw/bct152.

National Center on Accessible Educational Materials (2015). *Connecting Accessible Educational Materials and Learning.* Wakefield, MA: National Center on Accessible Educational Materials for Learning.

National Center on Universal Design for Learning (2013). What does it mean to say that curricula are disabled? Retrieved from https://udlguidelines.wordpress.com/introduction/what-does-it-mean-to-say-curricula-are-%E2%80%9Cdisabled%E2%80%9D/.

National Joint Committee on Learning Disabilities (1994). Learning disabilities: issues on definition. In: *Collective Perspectives on Issues Affecting Learning Disabilities: Position Paper and Statements*, 61–66. Austin, TX: Pro-Ed.

No Child Left Behind (NCLB) Act of 2001 (2002). Pub. L. No. 107–110, § 115, Stat. 1425.

Norton, E.S., Beach, S.D., and Gabrieli, J. (2015). Neurobiology of dyslexia. *Current Opinion in Neurobiology* 30: 73–78.

Norton-Darr, S. and Schoonover, J. (2012). Spreading "the word" about cognitive rescaling as a tool for inclusion. *Solutions Magazine*, (August/September): 7–13.

Office for Civil Rights (1995). *The Civil Rights of Students with Hidden Disabilities Under Section 504 of the Rehabilitation Act of 1973.* Washington DC: Office of Civil Rights.

Ostroff, E., Limont, M., and Hunter, D. (2004). *Building a World Fit for People: Designers with Disabilities at Work.* Boston, MA: Adaptive Environments.

Pandy, R.I. (2012). Learning disabilities and self-esteem. Capstone Projects. Paper 133. Retrieved from http://opus.govst.edu/capstones/133.

Partnership for 21st Century Skills (n.d.). Framework for 21st century learning. Retrieved from http://www.battelleforkids.org/networks/p21/frameworks-resources.

Price, A. and Cole, M. (2009). *Best Practices in Teaching Students with Learning Disabilities.* Calgary, Canada: Calgary Learning Center, Department of Education, Nova Scotia.

Pullen, D.L., Gitsaki, C., and Baguley, M. (2010). *Technoliteracy, Discourse, and Social Practice: Frameworks and Applications in the Digital Age.* Hershey, PA: Information Science Reference.

Purcell, S. and Grant, D. (2004). *Assistive Technology Solutions for IEP Teams.* Verona, WI: Attainment Company.

QIAT Leadership Team (2015). *Quality Indicators of Assistive Technology: A Comprehensive Guide to Assistive Technology Services.* Wakefield MA: CAST Professional Publishing.

Raskind, M.H. and Bryant, B.R. (2002). *Functional Evaluation for Assistive Technology: FEAT.* Austin, TX: Psycho-Educational Services.

Raskind, M. and Stanberry, K. (2006). Assistive technology for kids with LD: an overview. Retrieved from https://www.greatschools.org/gk/articles/assistive-technology-for-kids-with-learning-disabilities-an-overview/.

Reed, P., Kaplan, M., and Bowser, G. (2009). *The Assistive Technology Trainer's Handbook.* Roseburg, OR: National Assistive Technology in Education Network Retrieved from https://www.natenetwork.org/wp-content/uploads/at-trainers-handbook.pdf.

Rose, D.H., Gravel, J.W., and Domings, Y. (2012). UDL unplugged: applying universal design for learning in low-tech settings. In: *Universal Design for Learning in the Classroom: Practical Applications* (ed. T.E. Hall, A. Meyer and D.H. Rose), 120–134. New York: Guilford Press.

Rose, D.H. and Meyer, A. (2002). *Teaching Every Student in the Digital Age: Universal Design for Learning.* Alexandria, VA: Association for Supervision and Curriculum Development.

Rose, D.H. and Meyer, A. (eds.) (2006). *A Practical Reader in Universal Design for Learning.* Cambridge, MA: Harvard Education Press.

Saperstein Associates 2012. Handwriting in the 21st century? Research shows why handwriting belongs in today's classroom: a summary of research presented at Handwriting in the 21st Century? An educational summit. Retrieved from https://www.hw21summit.com/media/zb/hw21/H2948_HW_Summit_White_Paper_eVersion.pdf.

Scanlon, D. (2013). Specific learning disability and its newest definition: which is comprehensive? And which is sufficient? *Journal of Learning Disabilities* 46 (1): 26–33.

Scherer, M.J. and Craddock, G. (2002). Matching person & technology (MPT) assessment process. *Technology and Disability* 14: 125–131.

Schoonover, J. (2014). Interdisciplinary collaboration with assistive technology in schools. *School System Special Interest Section Quarterly* 24 (2): 1–4.

Schoonover, J. and Argabrite Grove, R.E. (2014). Influencing participation through assistive technology. In: *Occupational Therapy for Children*, 7e (ed. J. Case-Smith and J. O'Brien). St. Louis, MO: Elsevier Mosby.

Schoonover, J.W. and Feist, C. (2007). Using computers to design accessible learning environments. *School System Special Interest Section Quarterly* 14 (1): 1–4.

Section 504 of the Rehabilitation Act of 1973(1973). Pub. L. No. 93–112, 87 Stat. 394.

Shapiro, A. and Margolis, H. (1988). Changing negative peer attitudes towards students with learning disabilities. *Reading, Writing, and Learning Disabilities* 4: 133–146.

Sharfi, K. and Rosenblum, S. (2014). Activity and participation characteristics of adults with learning disabilities – a systematic review. *PLoS ONE* 9 (9): e106657. https://doi.org/10.1371/journal.pone.0106657.

Scherer, M.J. and Craddock, G. (2002). Matching Person & Technology (MPT) assessment process. *Technology and Disability, Special Issue: The Assessment of Assistive Technology Outcomes, Effects and Costs* 14 (3): 125–131.

Stoller, L.C. (1998). *Low-Tech Assistive Devices: A Handbook for the School Setting.* Framington, MA: Therapro.

Sweeney, J. (2007). Getting assistive technology into the mainstream the EASY way. *Closing The Gap* 25 (6): 7–8.

Thoma, C. and Wehman, P. (2010). *Getting the Most Out of IEPS: An Educator's Guide to the Student Directed Approach.* Baltimore, MD: Paul H. Brookes.

US Department of Education (2008). Tool kit on universal design for learning. Retrieved from https://osepideasthatwork.org/sites/default/files/intro.pdf.

US Department of Education (2017). Office of Special Education Programs, Individuals with Disabilities Education Act (IDEA) database. Retrieved from: https://www2.ed.gov/programs/osepidea/618-data/state-level-data-files/index.html#bcc.

US Department of Education, Office of Educational Technology (2017). *Reimagining the role of technology in education: 2017 National Education Technology Plan update.* Washington, DC: US Department of Education Retrieved from https://tech.ed.gov/files/2017/01/NETP17.pdf.

Vicente, K. (2006). *The Human Factor: Revolutionizing the Way People Live with Technology.* New York: Routledge, Taylor & Francis Group.

Visvader, P., Leonesio, J., Brandstatter, E. et al. (2014). *School-Based Assistive Technology Writing Evaluation: An Interdisciplinary Approach.* Boulder, CO: Boulder Valley School District.

Wehmeyer, M.L. (2002). Promoting the self-determination of students with severe disabilities. ERIC Digest. Retrieved from https://files.eric.ed.gov/fulltext/ED470522.pdf.

Zabala, J.S. (1995). The SETT framework: critical areas to consider when making informed assistive technology decisions. ERIC Document Reproduction Service No.ED381962. Houston, TX: Region IV Education Service Center.

Zabala, J.S. (2010). The SETT Framework: straight from the horse's mouth. Retrieved from http://www.joyzabala.com/Handouts_for_Download.html.

Toolbox

Bowser, G. and Reed, P. (2007). *Hey Can I Try That? A Student Handbook for Choosing and Using Assistive Technology.* http://www.wati.org/free-publications/other-materials/.

DeCoste, D. (2005). Assistive Technology Assessment: Developing a Written Productivity Profile. Volo, IL: Don Johnston, Inc. In order to make decisions about a student's written language production and recommend appropriate interventions, data on handwriting and keyboarding must be collected, as well as assessment of spelling.

Foldables® are hands-on manipulatives that are used nationally and internationally by teachers, parents, and educational publishing companies: https://www.dinah.com/about/graphic-organizers.

Free technology toolkit for UDL in all classroom features a wide range of free technology tools that can support universal design for learning (UDL) and assistive technology efforts: https://sites.google.com/view/freeudltechtoolkit/home?authuser=0.

TechMatrix: Search a database of over 300 assistive and educational technology tools and resources to support learning for students with disabilities and their classmates using extensive criteria tailored to assistive and educational technologies, compare up to four products across search criteria, and read related research articles on the theory and practice of using technology to improve student learning. Search by content area, grade level, IDEA Disability Category, or instructional support: https://techmatrix.org/.

The Evaluation Tool for Children's Handwriting (ETCH) focuses on assessing a student's legibility and speed of manuscript and cursive handwriting tasks similar to those required of students in the classroom and includes alphabet and numerical writing, near-point and far-point copying, dictation, and sentence generation. Additionally, observations of pencil grasp, hand preference, manipulative skills with the writing tool, and the classroom are included. Amundson, S. J. (1995). Evaluation tool of children's handwriting. O.T. Kids, P. O. Box 1118, Homer, Alaska 99 603.

The PAR manual helps determine the most appropriate reading accommodations for individual students by assessing their specific needs, and outlines evidence-based practices that can be used to make decisions about suitable reading accommodations: https://ivweb.nwtoolbox.org/Sherwood/LinkClick.aspx?link=PAR_Manual.pdf&tabid=204&mid=664.

The WATI Assistive Technology Assessment is a process-based, systematic approach to providing a functional evaluation of the student's need for assistive technology in their customary environment using the SETT framework as a guide. It was most recently updated in 2017. This series of protocols and observation forms assist the school-based teams gather, analyze, and use information to make informed decisions in the selection and use of assistive technology. Each chapter guides teams through the evaluation process, explains each step, highlighting important considerations for each aspect of the assessment, and concludes with topic-specific lists of AT resources: http://www.wati.org/.

FabricATe is a national research program about AT and includes information about adaptations and devices for infants and toddlers, resource information, and links to many useful sites: https://www.fabricate4all.org/.

Zabala, J.S. (2005). Using the SETT Framework to level the learning field for students with disabilities. Retrieved from http://www.joyzabala.com/uploads/Zabala_SETT_Leveling_the_Learning_Field.pdf.

15

Seating and positioning factors in wheeled mobility

Lindsey Veety and Amy Baxter

Outline

Assistive Technologies and Environmental Interventions in Healthcare: An Integrated Approach, First Edition.
Edited by Lynn Gitlow and Kathleen Flecky.

Companion website: www.wiley.com/go/gitlow/assitivetechnologies

Learning outcomes

After reading this chapter, you should be able to:

1. Explain the importance of seating and positioning for a person using wheeled mobility.
2. Describe the human factors through common diagnoses, injuries, and disabilities that result in seating and positioning challenges for wheeled mobility.
3. Apply the Human-Tech Ladder (Vicente 2006) to persons who have seating and positioning needs and use wheeled mobility.
4. Specify assessment and evaluation strategies in technology and environmental interventions (TEI) for individuals with seating and positioning needs using wheeled mobility.
5. List what an evaluator would record during a TEI wheelchair seating and mobility evaluation.
6. Describe the roles of the client, family members, evaluator, and vendor during a complex TEI rehabilitation evaluation.

Active learning prompts

Before reading this chapter:

1. Define and locate these prominent body markers for seating and positioning: iliac crests, anterior superior iliac crests (ASIS), and posterior superior iliac crests (PSIS).
2. Define and demonstrate the following key movements related to seating and mobility: flexion, extension, lateral flexion, internal and external rotation.
3. Go to your local wheelchair vendor location and request to sit in and navigate a chair in the showroom. Try out a variety of chairs. Notice which movements and muscles you use in using the wheelchair. Reflect on how vision and cognition impact wheelchair use. What other body systems and abilities are used to navigate a chair? Think about having to perform typical tasks such as transferring in and out of bed, cooking a meal, getting something off a high shelf, going through a door, and performing tasks in the community such as getting groceries. What are your thoughts?
4. Using the Rehabilitation Engineering and Assistive Technology Society of North America (RESNA) website (www.resna.org), locate and read both the Wheelchair Service Provision Guide and their current position papers related to seating and wheelchairs.

Key terms

Wheelchair	Positioning	Power wheelchair
Seating	Manual wheelchair	TEI

Introduction

Seating and positioning is a complex, multidisciplinary technology and environmental intervention. When thinking about seating and positioning, an occupational or physical therapist, as a member of an interdisciplinary team, may immediately envision a person seated in a wheelchair or other piece of alternate positioning equipment designed for children or adults with disabilities. Alternatively, an ergonomist may see an individual seated at a computer or other workstation in a vocational setting. Moreover, a teacher may visualize a student seated at their desk at school. No matter what you think of when you hear the terms seating and positioning, the basic principles of seating and positioning are the same, and it is important to understand key concepts and definitions. The chapter will begin with a review of anatomical terms and definitions directly related to seating and positioning. These key terms/concepts are used when documenting evaluation findings and describing postural positions. Neutral position is presented for each body segment/region and is used as a baseline to describe movement and positions out of neutral alignment. The chapter will continue with a discussion of functional positioning and evaluation for wheelchair seating and positioning. It will continue with a basic introduction of wheelchair/seating components and their use, types of wheelchairs available, followed by a case study. The next chapter (Chapter 16) will build on the concepts presented in this chapter by presenting other mobility devices as well as other assistive equipment frequently utilized by wheelchair users.

Human factors and common conditions requiring wheeled mobility

In order to begin our discussion of technology and environmental interventions for seating and mobility, some terminology and positions of the body will be presented to set the stage for concepts that are discussed in the next two chapters (Waugh and Crane 2013).

Definitions and positions

Planes of the body

- Sagittal – vertical plane from front to back – divides the body into right and left sides
- Coronal – vertical plane from left to right – divides the body into front and back sections
- Transverse – horizontal plane dividing the body into top and bottom halves (Figure 15.1).

Neutral/anatomical seated position

The neutral/anatomical seated position is described as 90–90–90 with 90° angles at the pelvis, knees, and ankles (Figures 15.2 and 15.3).

The 90–90–90 position distributes body weight equally through the trunk and lower extremities (Hamm 2007).

Pelvis

Neutral pelvic alignment – pelvic alignment is measured by palpating or feeling several general landmarks on the body: the iliac crests, the anterior superior iliac spine (ASIS), and the posterior superior iliac spine (PSIS) (Figures 15.4–15.6).

Pelvic tilt – movement or position of the pelvis in the sagittal plane (Figures 15.7–15.10).

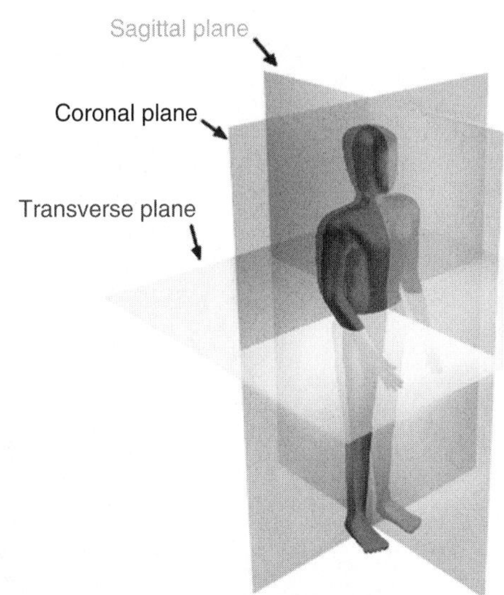

Figure 15.1 Planes of the body. Source: From https://en.wikipedia.org/wiki/Anatomical_plane.

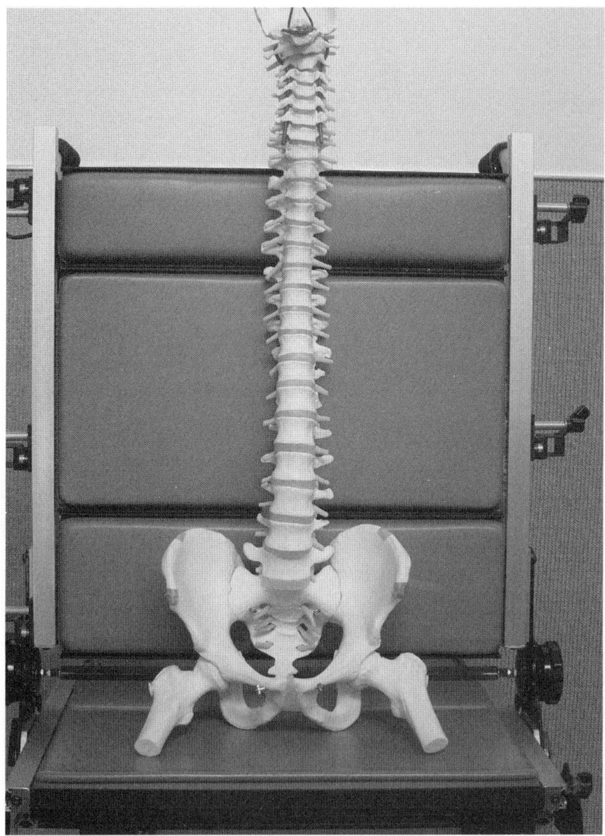

Figure 15.2 Neutral/anatomical seated position (front view).

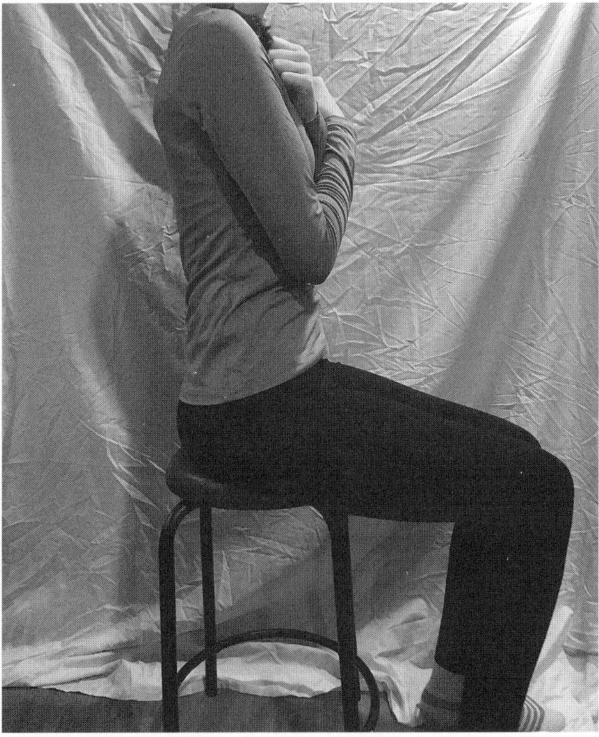

Figure 15.3 Neutral/anatomical seated position (side view).

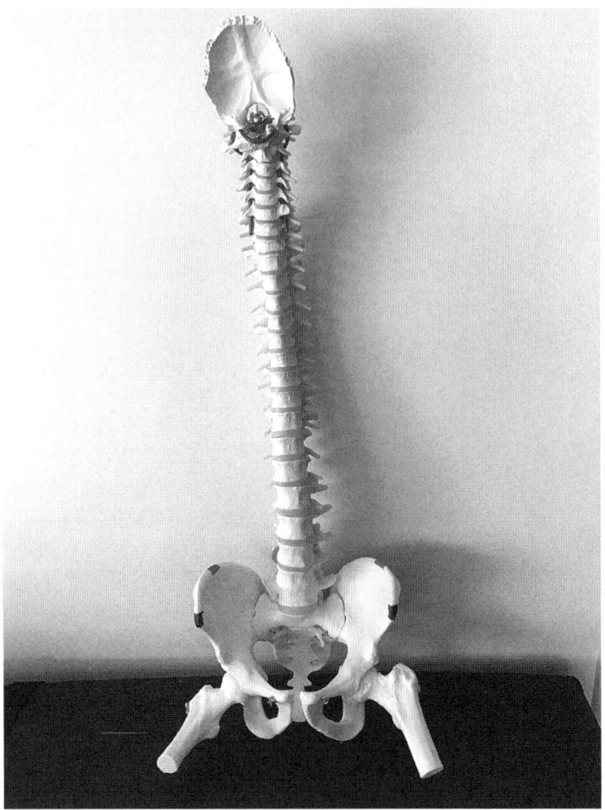

Figure 15.4 Neutral pelvic alignment – coronal plane – skeletal representation.

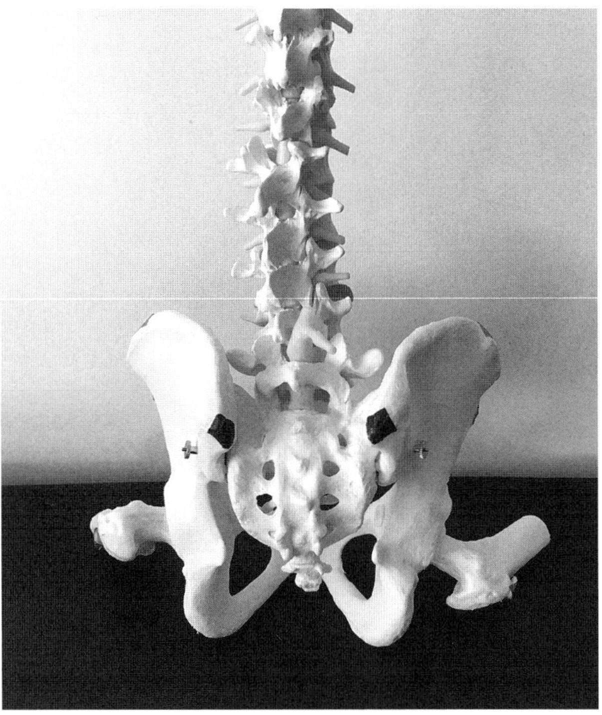

Figure 15.5 Neutral pelvic alignment – transverse plane – skeletal representation.

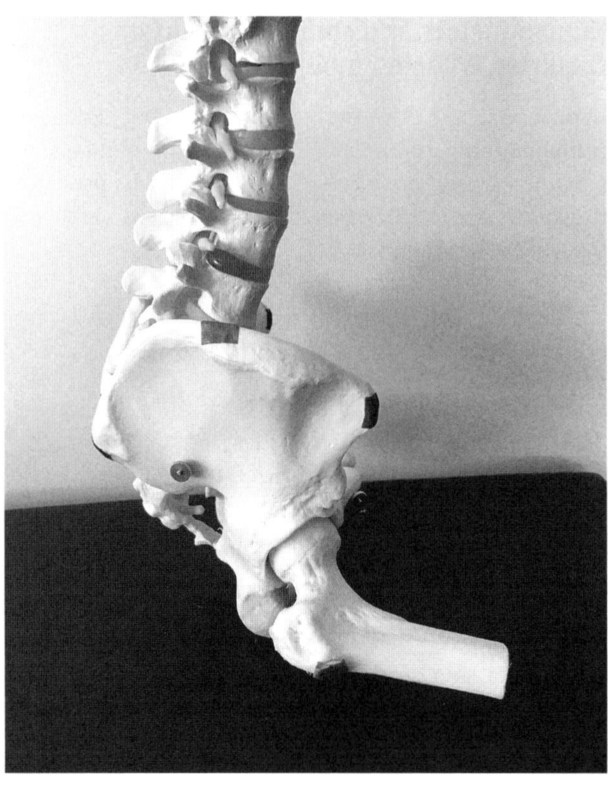

Figure 15.6 Neutral pelvic alignment – sagittal plane – skeletal representation.

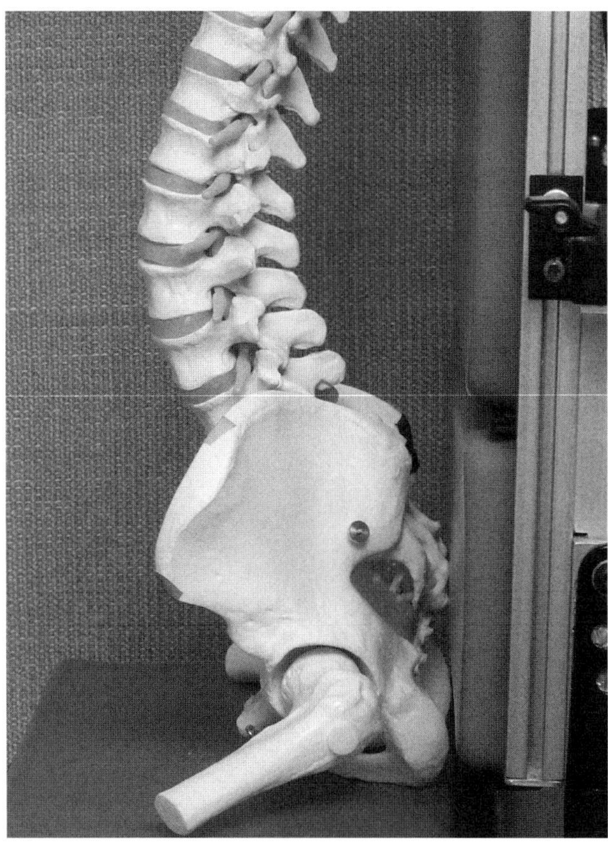

Figure 15.7 Anterior pelvic tilt – skeletal representation.

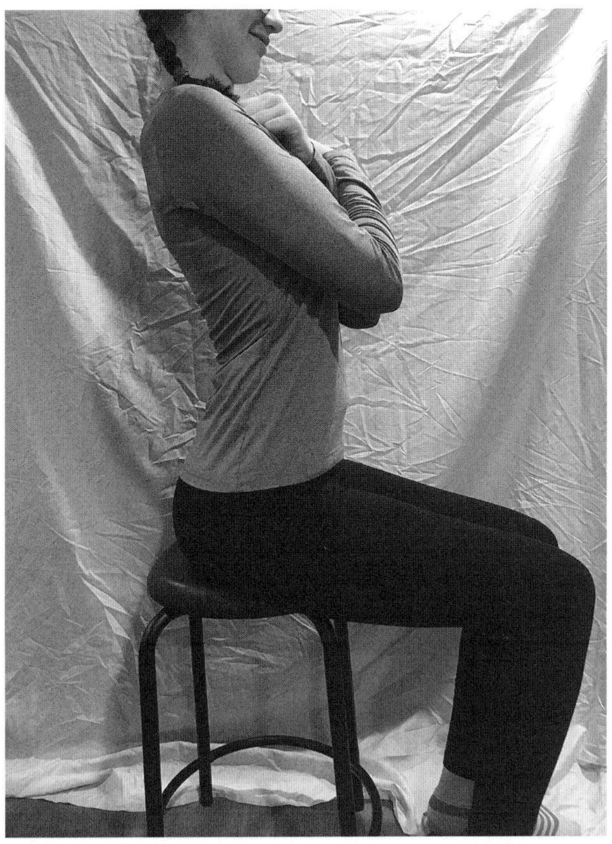

Figure 15.8 Anterior pelvic tilt.

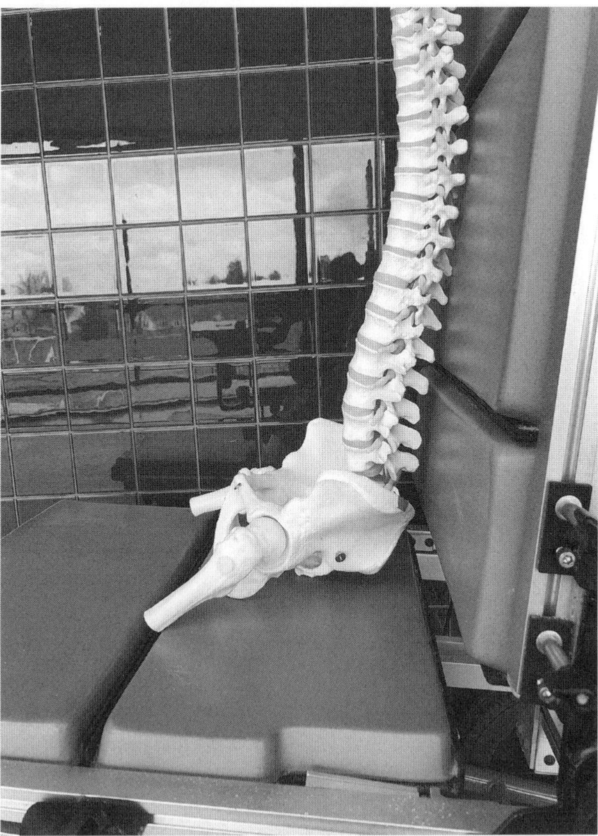

Figure 15.9 Posterior pelvic tilt – skeletal representation.

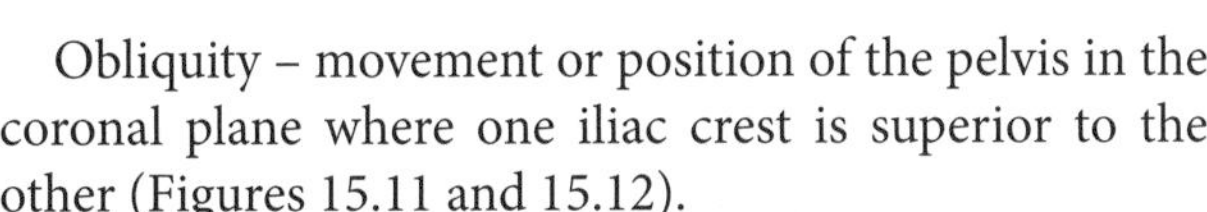

Obliquity – movement or position of the pelvis in the coronal plane where one iliac crest is superior to the other (Figures 15.11 and 15.12).

Pelvic rotation – movement or position of the pelvis in the transverse plane where one hemi-pelvis is anterior to the other (Figures 15.13 and 15.14).

Trunk

Neutral alignment – in the coronal plane, the lumbar spine has a slight inward curve, the thoracic spine a slight outward curve, and the cervical spine a slight inward curve. There should be no rotation and no curvature in the sagittal plane.

Common asymmetries of the spine include:

- Increased lordosis – spinal curvature beyond neutral in the coronal plane with increased extension (Figure 15.15)
- Increased kyphosis – spinal curvature beyond neutral in the coronal plane with increased flexion (Figure 15.16)
- Scoliosis – spinal curvature in the sagittal plane. Typically described as convex or concave to the right/left (Figure 15.17)

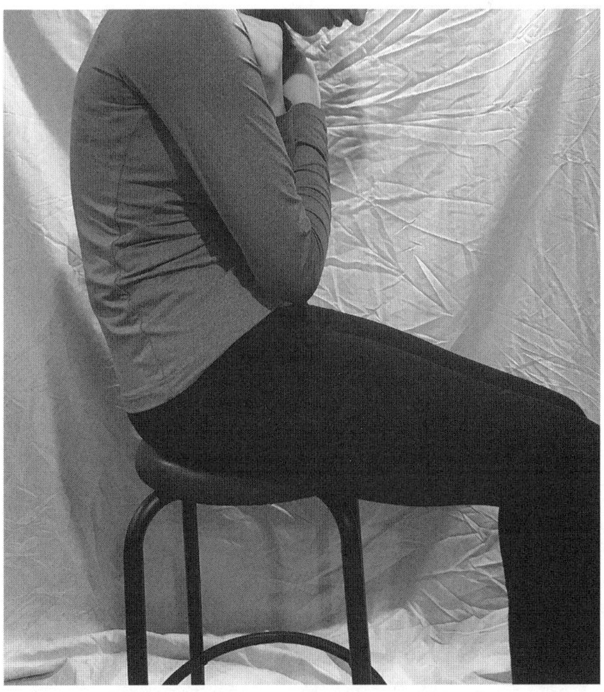

Figure 15.10 Posterior pelvic tilt.

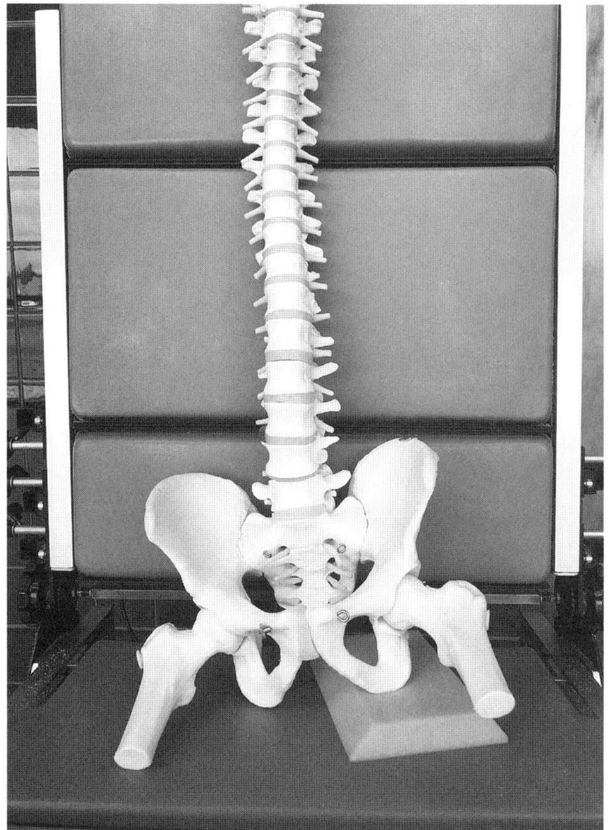

Figure 15.11 Pelvic obliquity – skeletal representation.

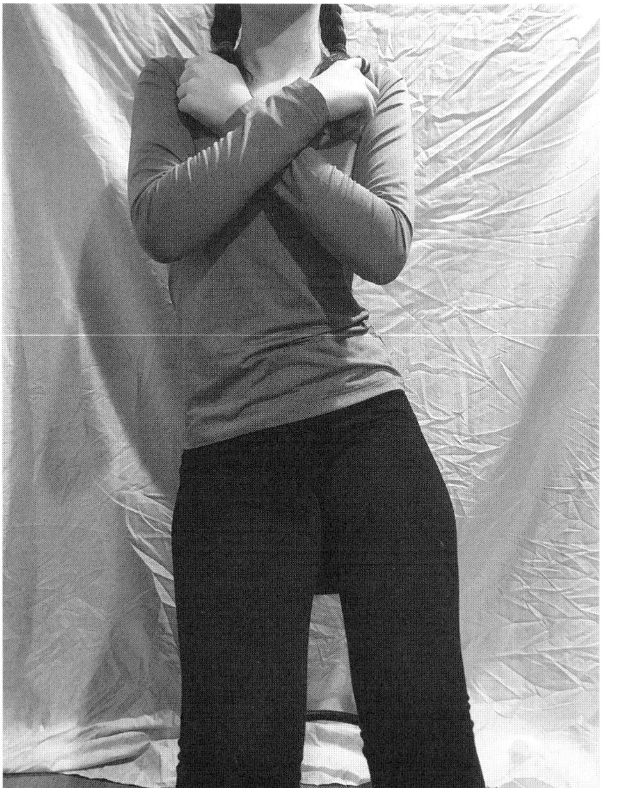

Figure 15.12 Pelvic obliquity.

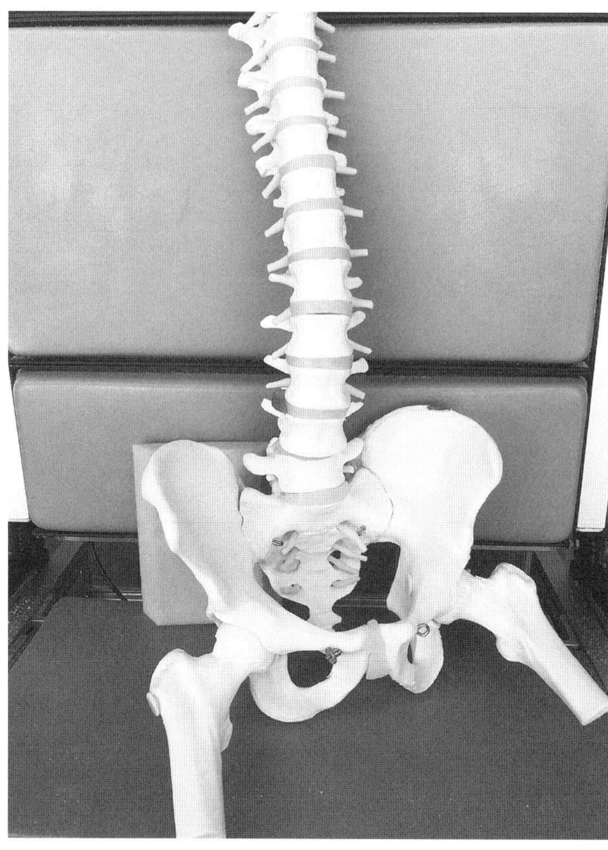

Figure 15.13 Pelvic rotation – skeletal representation.

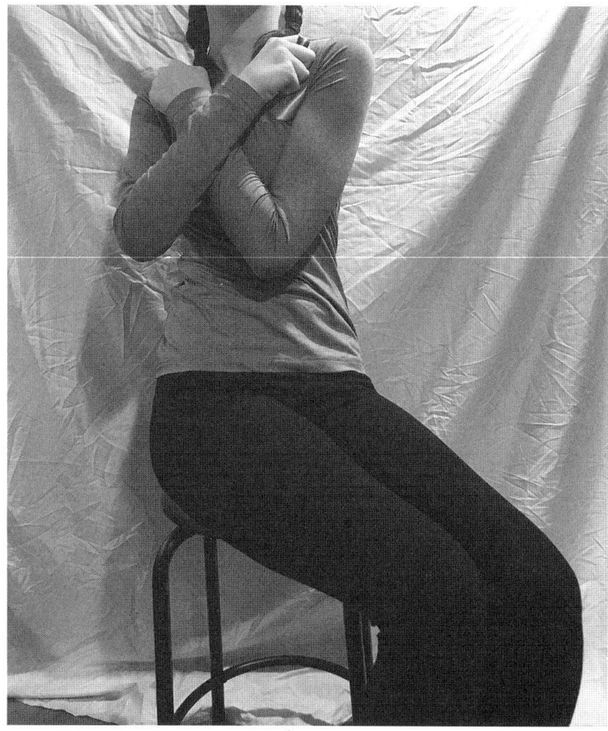

Figure 15.14 Pelvic rotation.

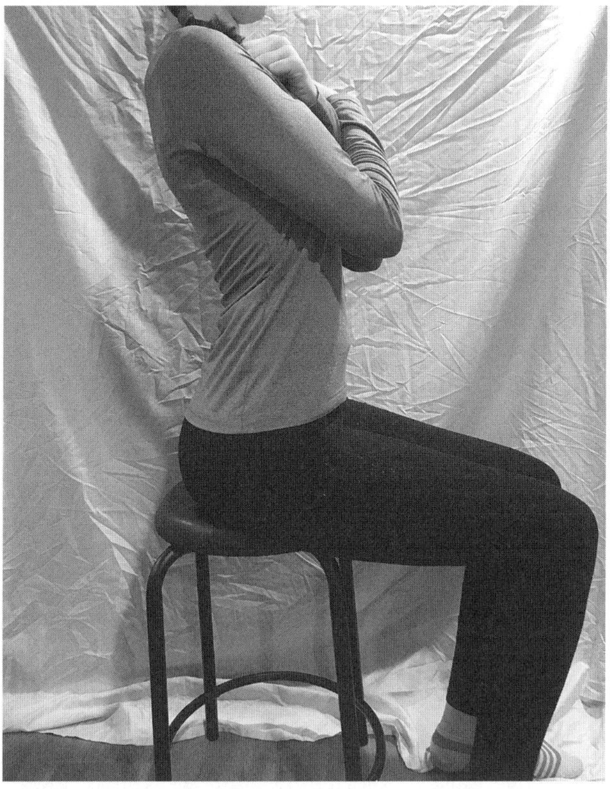

Figure 15.15 Spinal lordosis.

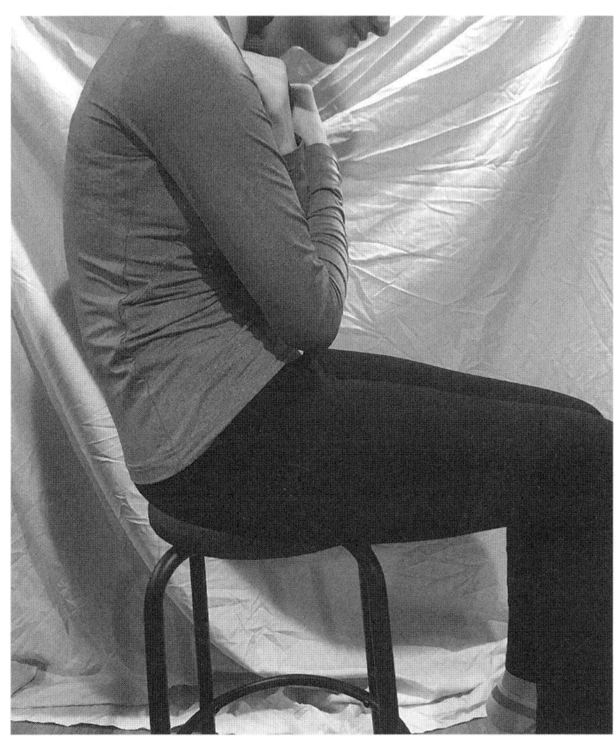

Figure 15.16 Spinal kyphosis.

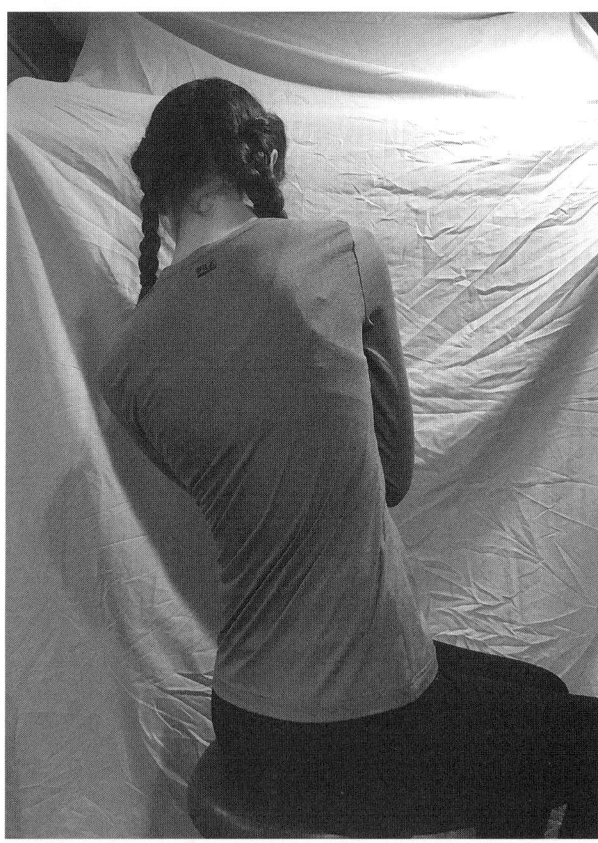

Figure 15.17 Spinal scoliosis.

- Rotoscoliosis – scoliosis with a rotational component labeled in the direction of rotation.

Head/Neck

Neutral alignment – the cervical spine has a slight inward curve in the coronal plane. The occiput or base of the skull sits upon the cervical spine. In a resting position, the head should not be flexed forward or back, and in a neutral alignment it is not rotated or laterally flexed.

Common postures that are seen can include increase cervical flexion or extension combined with capital extension, which is rotation of the occiput on the C2 vertebrae moving it into extension.

Hips

A freely moving hip joint should include motions into flexion, extension, abduction/adduction, and internal and external rotation.

Common asymmetries include:

- Windswept position – when in a seated position, one hip is abducted and the other is adducted. This is often paired with abnormal pelvic positions, including pelvic rotation and pelvic tilt (Figures 15.18 and 15.19).

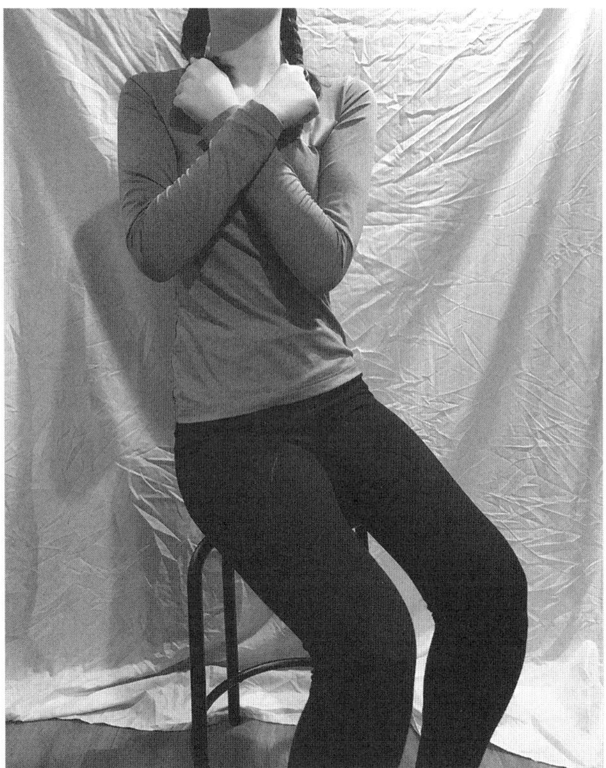

Figure 15.18 Windswept deformity.

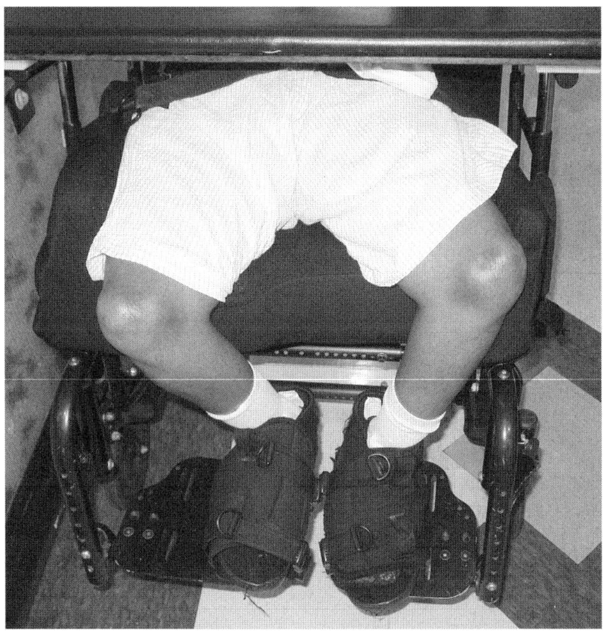

Figure 15.19 Abducted/externally rotated position.

Knees

The knees move into flexion and extension.

Common asymmetry:

- Contractures – flexion and extension.

Ankles/Feet

Neutral alignment – 90° between foot and leg, foot resting in subtalor neutral.

Common asymmetries include:

- Contractures plantarflexion/dorsiflexion/supination/pronation/inversion/eversion.

Functional positioning

Positioning refers to the alignment of body segments with respect to one another and to the environment (Jones and Gray 2005). The former standard for an optimal seated position was 90–90–90, representing 90° angles at the hips, knees, and feet, and represents an anatomical approach to seating (Costigan and Light 2011). This is a good guide and appropriate in some situations; however, humans are dynamic beings and it is widely discussed the 90–90–90 position is not ideal for active participation (Batavia 2010; Kangas 2016). We are constantly changing positions throughout the day to enable us to best participate and maximize our ability to perform the task at hand. Sustaining the same seated position throughout the day can cause musculoskeletal changes, including muscle shortening and weakness, lower-extremity edema, nerve impingement, and a particular concern for wheelchair users, pressure ulcers (Maltchev 2012; RESNA 2012; Taule et al. 2013). More currently, a functional approach to seating has been derived to assist people with disabilities in meeting their goals to participate in tasks that are meaningful to them, taking into account the environment in which those tasks are completed (Batavia 2010; Costigan and Light 2011; RESNA 2012). Selection of an optimal seated position is also based upon factors such as tonal influences and musculoskeletal limitations. While riding in a vehicle or dining, an individual may be best seated in a neutral position for safety or an improved alignment for swallowing. During a functional activity which requires use of the upper extremities and reaching, the seated individual may require a less rigid approach that will enable them, for example, to have greater hip and knee flexion to obtain the proximal stability required for distal control enabling them to perform their daily activities.

Often persons referred for an assistive technology evaluation, which may include accessing a computer or augmentative communication device, have seating challenges due to high or low tone. It is imperative to address their seating and positioning needs in order to effectively evaluate their other assistive technology needs. Consistent with the organizing framework of this book, seating and positioning goes beyond just the individual but must consider multiple levels including organization and invoke a team approach to problem-solving.

Wheelchairs

The RESNA Wheelchair Service Provision Guide defines a "wheelchair" as a "wheeled mobility device with a seating support system for a person with impaired mobility intended to provide mobility in a seated position as its primary function" (Waugh 2013). It is inclusive of all wheeled mobility devices including manual and powered wheelchairs, strollers, and powered scooters. "Complex Rehab Technology includes medically necessary and individually configured manual and power wheelchairs, seating and positioning systems, and other adaptive equipment such as standing devices and gait trainers" (Access2CRT 2019).

In this section, the different types of wheelchairs will be defined, along with how they can work together with the supports needed to promote an individual's participation.

Manual wheelchairs

Standard non-adjustable

The standard non-adjustable wheelchair is defined as a "standard upright manual wheelchair that does not have adjustability in frame and height" (Waugh 2013). It typically has a sling back, sling seat, swing away footplates, large rear wheel for upper extremity propulsion and standard 8″ front casters (Figure 15.20). The standard manual wheelchair is designed to be used for short distances for short periods of time (Cooper 1998; Batavia 2010). It is portable and may fold easily to fit into a vehicle. There are few external support options available for standard manual wheelchairs. This chair is best suited for a user who has good-to-normal head and trunk control and is able to sit upright independently.

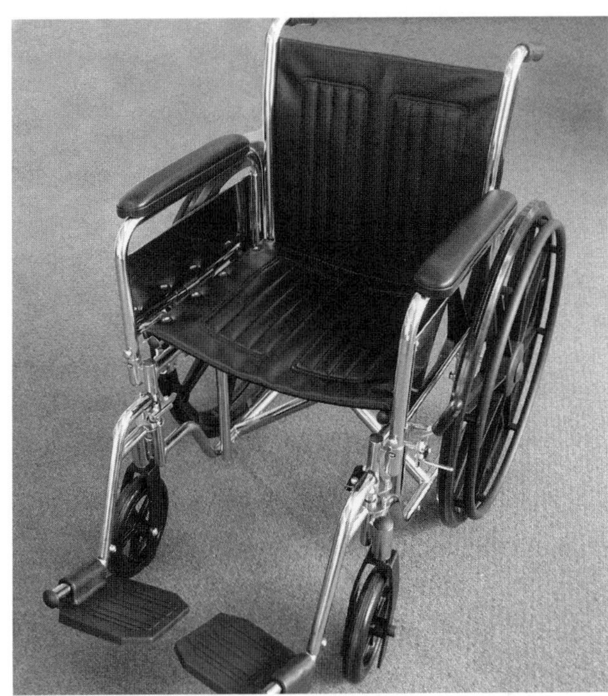

Figure 15.20 Standard manual wheelchair.

Standard adjustable

A standard upright manual wheelchair allows frame adjustments, which could include rear wheel axle and front casters to enable the clinician to adjust the front and rear seat-to-floor height, and back support angle and seat depth adjustment, as well as foot support options, to provide a custom fit to the user (Waugh 2013). This type of wheelchair gives the clinician more options by allowing for the addition of off-the-shelf seat and back supports.

Transport wheelchairs and strollers

A transport chair is similar to a standard non-adjustable wheelchair. A transport chair may have large wheels and small casters, or wheels that are the same size as or slightly larger than the front casters (Figure 15.21).

The user is unable to propel this type of chair with their upper extremities and must rely on a caregiver or use their lower extremities for movement. Another type of transport chair, an adaptive stroller, is often designed with upholstered seating for pediatric users (Figure 15.22). Any additional supports are specific to the stroller and added to the existing upholstered seating. The user is dependent upon others for mobility in a stroller.

Lightweight, ultra-lightweight

As the name implies, lightweight and ultra-lightweight wheelchairs (Figure 15.23) are often made of carbon fiber, titanium, or other lightweight materials and therefore are easier to propel than standard manual wheelchairs. Often these types of chairs have options for wheel type, caster type, and adjustment of seat and wheel position. Light and ultra-lightweight wheelchairs are important to users with reduced upper body strength and individuals who independently propel their wheelchairs greater distances throughout the day. Options for adjustments are important to enable the user to obtain optimal angles for propulsion to ensure greatest efficiency and the least amount of energy loss (RESNA 2012).

Frames

Rigid vs. Folding frames

Wheelchair frames are available as rigid and folding. There are many considerations when choosing a wheelchair frame and the type will vary for each user. A rigid frame is preferred by active users because they are more efficient to propel with the upper extremities.

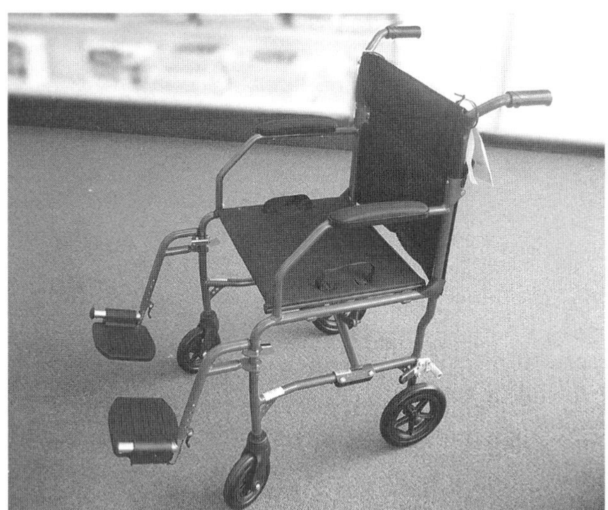

Figure 15.21 Transport wheelchair.

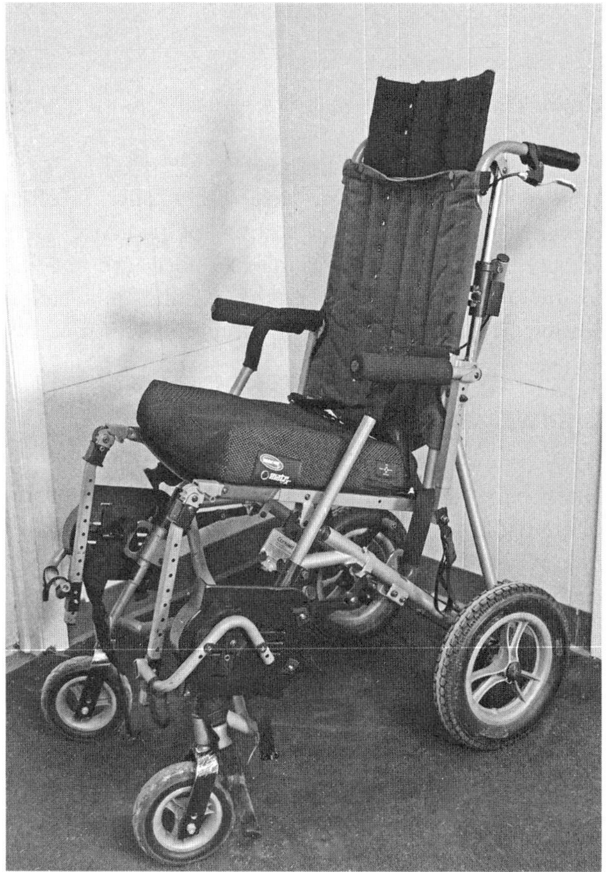

Figure 15.22 Stroller.

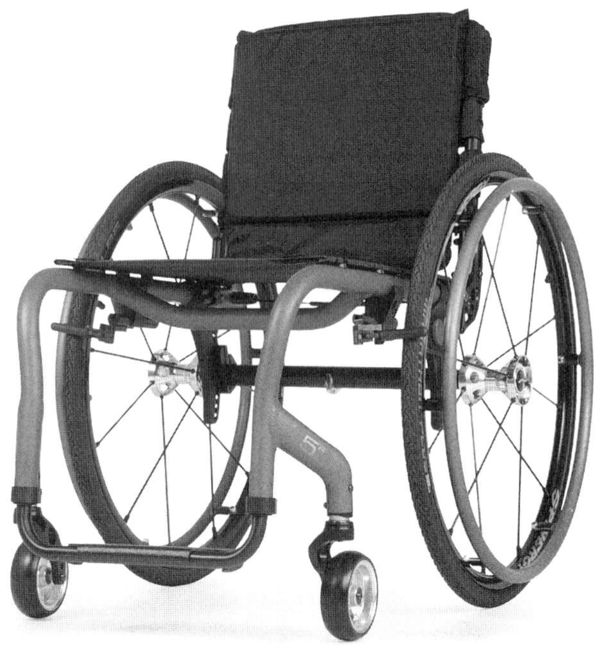

Figure 15.23 Ultra-lightweight wheelchair with rigid frame.

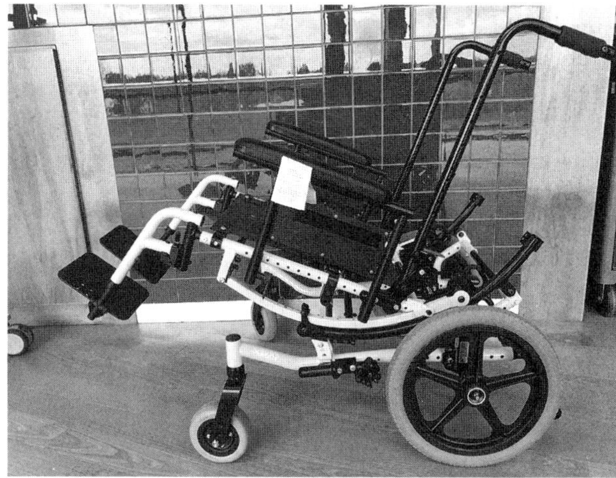

Figure 15.24 Manual wheelchair with tilt-in-space frame.

A significant amount of energy is lost with each stroke of propulsion through a folding frame, which results in decreased distance traveled with each stroke. On the other hand, a folding frame will absorb energy when the user is on uneven surfaces, with fewer and less forceful bumps felt by the user. If the user plans to transport the chair in a standard vehicle, a folding wheelchair may be preferred (Batavia 2010; Medola et al. 2014).

Tilt-in-space

Tilt- in-space is the ability to adjust the angle of the entire seating system in relation to the frame (Figure 15.24). In other words, the user can increase their tilt as they maintain the same seat-to-back angle; it is the seating that tilts on the frame. Altering the seating system on a wheelchair frame from an upright to tilted position shifts the user's center of gravity backward and shifts weight to the individual's trunk, thereby decreasing pressure on the buttocks. This feature may be beneficial for individuals who sit for long periods of time in their wheelchair and are unable to independently shift their weight (Groah et al. 2015). Tilting an individual can also help with trunk and head control and assist with managing secretions.

Recline

Recline is the ability to adjust the seat-to-back angle on a wheelchair, or in other words, open or close the seat in relation to the back. This is important for activities of daily living (ADLs) and position change; however, the individual must closely monitor the skin integrity of their back and buttocks as there is increased sheer during the recline process (Lange 2000). Newer technology is available that allows the back support surface to maintain contact with the individual while the chair is reclined, therefore reducing sheer. Please refer to Box 15.1.

Powered mobility

Power operated vehicles (POVs), also known as scooters (Figure 15.25), come in three- or four wheel-models with a variety of options. They typically have a captain's style seat with a swivel mount for easy transfers on and off the mobility device (Cooper 1998; Batavia 2010; Babinec 2018). Some break down into four or five components for transportation in a vehicle. Three-wheel POVs have a smaller turning radius than four-wheel scooters and are often better suited for indoor use.

Power assist systems can be added to a manual wheelchair to assist with wheelchair propulsion over long distances. They give the user the flexibility to have power-assisted mobility when needed, without the weight and bulk of a power wheelchair. These systems can be easily removed from the manual wheelchair, enabling the user to transport the system in a standard vehicle. Power assist may be a good option for individuals

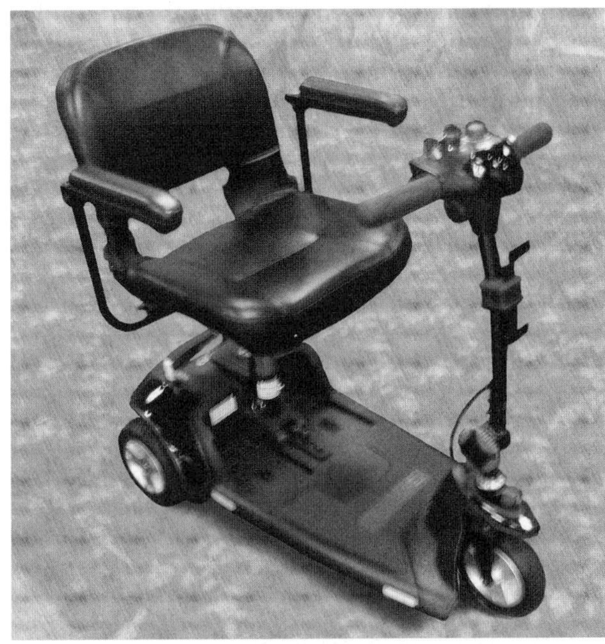

Figure 15.25 Three-wheel power operated vehicle (POV)/ scooter.

Box 15.1 Here's the evidence

Jan, Y.-K. and Crane, B.A. (2013). Wheelchair tilt-in-space and recline does not reduce sacral skin perfusion as changing from the upright to the tilted and reclined position in people with spinal cord injury. *Archives of Physical Medicine and Rehabilitation* 94(6): 1207–1210. doi: 10.1016/j.apmr.2013.01.004.

Key Words: tilt-in-space, recline, pressure ulcer prevention, skin, spinal cord injury (SCI)

Purpose: To investigate the effect of various wheelchair tilt-in-space and recline angles on sacral skin perfusion in wheelchair users with SCI.

Sample/Setting: Eleven power wheelchair users with spinal cord injuries were recruited to participate in this study, which took place in a university-setting laboratory.

Method: The research methodology used for this study was a repeated measures, intervention, and outcome measures design. Six randomly assigned protocols of tilt-in-space and recline angles were tested on participants. Each participant spent five minutes in an upright seated position and five minutes in the titled and reclined positions. Laser Doppler flowmetry was used to measure skin perfusion over the sacrum and right ischial tuberosity.

Findings: In all protocols, skin perfusion over the ischial tuberosity increased while remaining unchanged over the sacrum. These results indicate that tilt-in-space and recline protocols can enhance perfusion over the ischial tuberosity without decreasing perfusion over the sacral skin.

Critical Thinking Questions:

1. After reading this research article, what do you understand to be the limitations of this research? Are there any limitations not stated?
2. If you were to replicate this study using a different method or design, what designs would you use to increase the rigor and why?
3. Based on the findings of this study, what additional research is needed that is not addressed in the discussion section?

who occasionally need to propel longer distances, may fatigue quickly, need to conserve energy, or have limited upper extremity function or upper extremity pain. They are also often used when architectural barriers inhibit the use of a power wheelchair. There are several types available, including power assisting wheels or add-on modules which add power into each manual push of the wheel, meaning when the user pushes the wheel, their chair will go a longer distance (DiGiovine and Berner 2018). A joystick can also be added to fully convert a manual wheelchair to a power wheelchair.

A power wheelchair is a wheelchair that is propelled by means of an electric motor, often using a joystick for directional control. They are classified as front-, mid-, or rear-wheel drive, depending on the location of the drive wheels (Figures 15.26–15.28).

Many power wheelchairs have options for power seat functions, some of which include: tilt-in-space, recline, seat elevate, elevating footrest. With a power wheelchair, the user is able to independently control the power functions to enable them to perform weight shifts for pressure relief independently throughout the day. This can be critical to decrease the risk of developing a decubitus ulcer (Jan et al. 2010; Dicianno et al. 2015). Seat elevation can be used to assist with transfers as well as improve access to independence in activities of daily living (IADLs) such as reaching, dressing, and grooming.

Most individuals are able to drive a power wheelchair with a standard joystick or a joystick with an alternate grip such as a T handle (Figure 15.29).

If the user is not able to control a power wheelchair with a joystick, there are options for expanded electronics that will enable the user to drive with alternate controls such as a head array (Figure 15.30), switch array

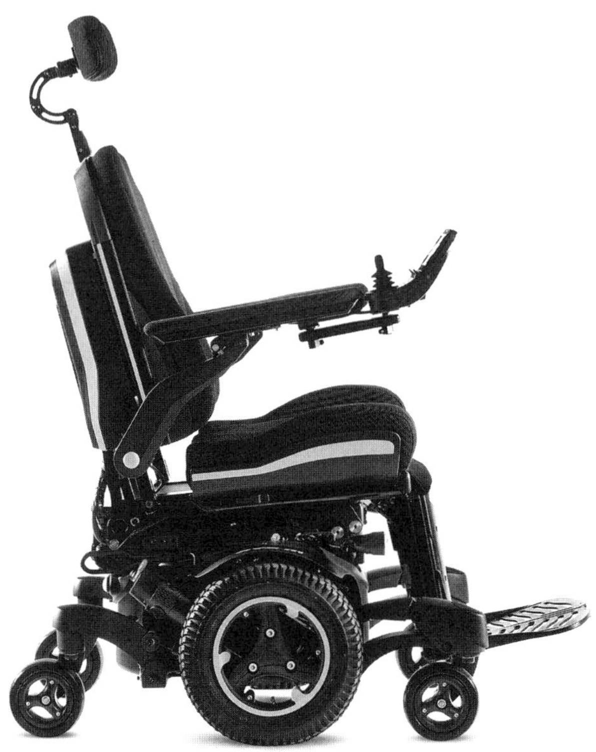

Figure 15.27 Mid-wheel drive power wheelchair.

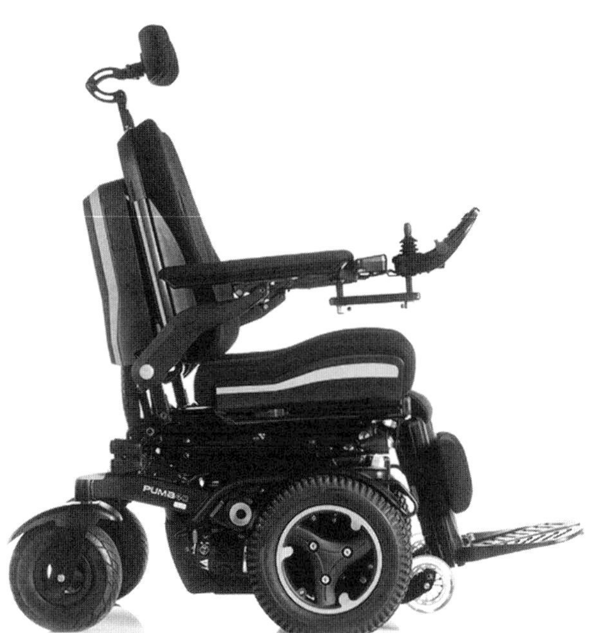

Figure 15.26 Front-wheel drive power wheelchair.

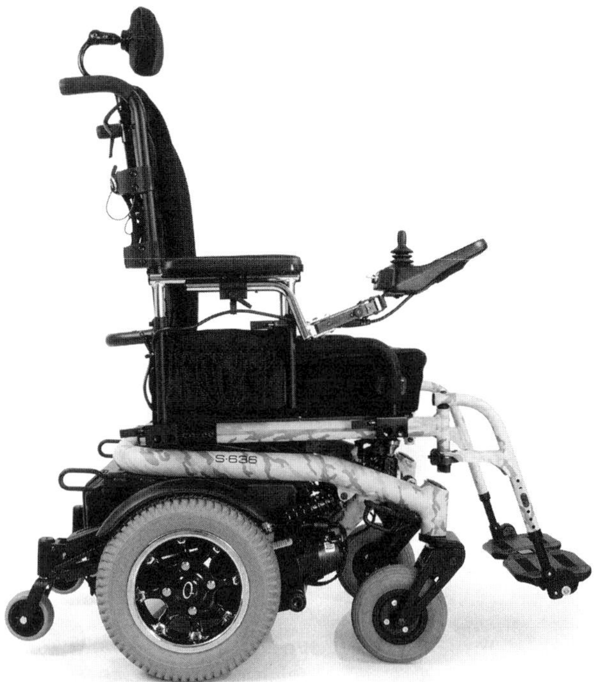

Figure 15.28 Rear-wheel drive power wheelchair.

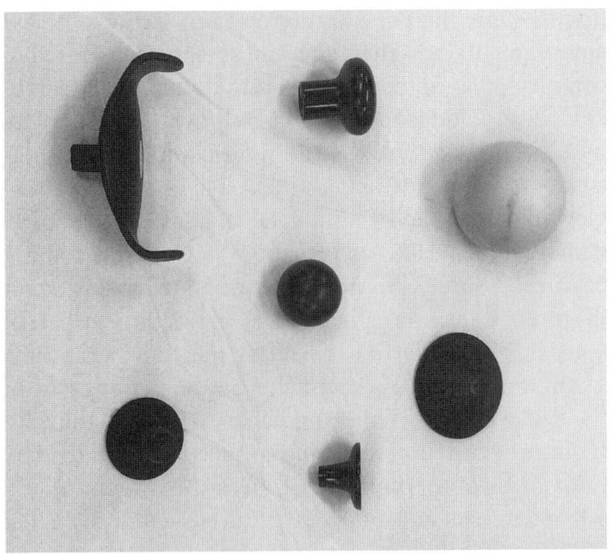

Figure 15.29 Variety of joystick knobs and handles for power wheelchair.

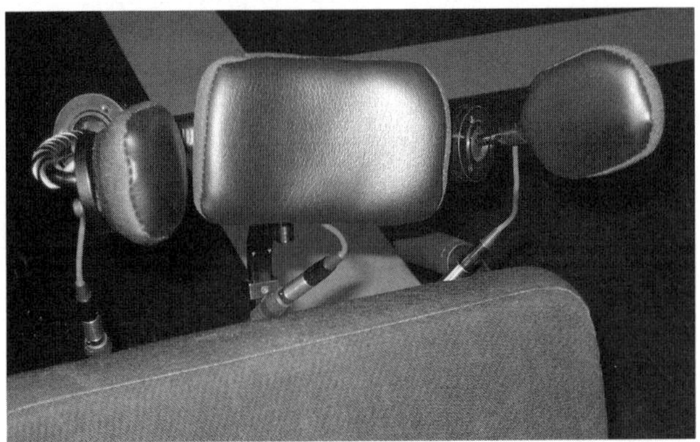

Figure 15.30 Head array alternate drive control for a power wheelchair.

(Figure 15.31), micro joystick (Figure 15.32), and sip and puff (Figure 15.33) (Lange 2018). A head array is typically set up to enable the user to locate their head on the back pad to drive forward and turn left and right with the two lateral pads. Reverse would be accomplished with a switch that would enable them to toggle between modes. The user would push the toggle switch and use the back pad (that was previously used for forward) for reverse. They would again push the toggle switch to return to forward mode.

A switch array can be set up with any type of switch or fiber optic cable located at any body part, depending on the user's ability. The switches can be programmed to perform any of the necessary drive/seat control functions. A micro joystick (Figure 15.32) is a joystick that takes minimal motion to operate and is often located

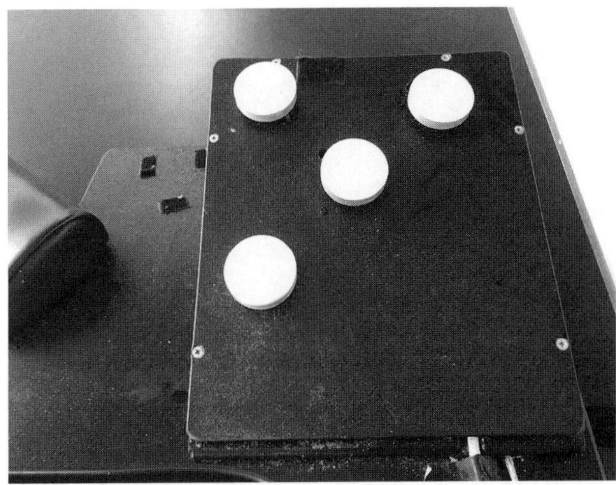

Figure 15.31 Switch array alternate drive control for a power wheelchair.

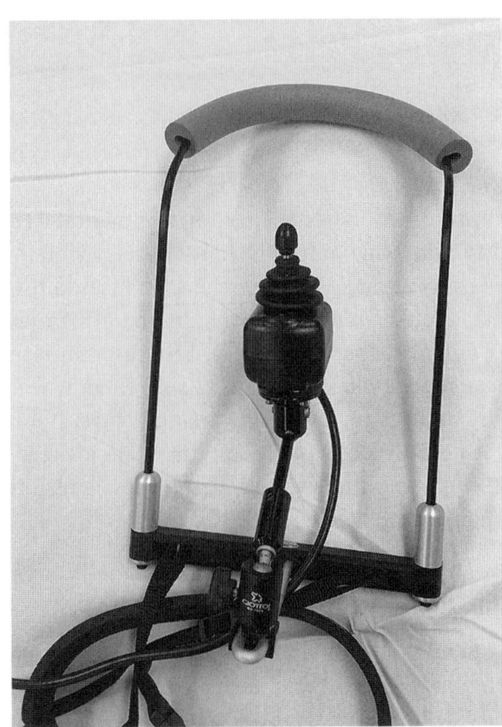

Figure 15.32 Micro-joystick/chin control alternate drive control for a power wheelchair.

at the hand or chin for persons with spinal cord injuries or muscle weakness disorders.

Sip and puff drive controls (Figure 15.33) use a blowing action, or puff, and a sucking action, or sip, into a straw in the user's mouth. By coordinating the sips and puffs the user can coordinate four different directions of movement or control the power seat functions (Waugh 2013).

In addition to alternate drive controls, expanded electronics can allow for access to a computer, use of a

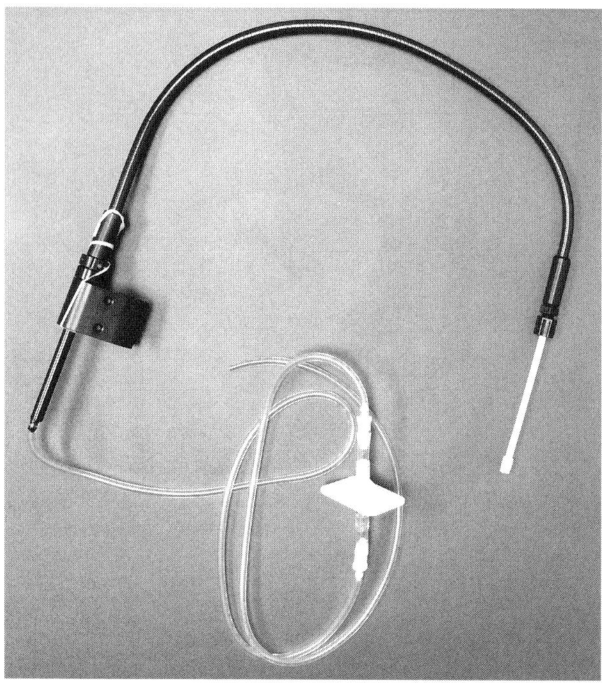

Figure 15.33 Sip and puff alternate drive control for a power wheelchair.

communication device, or environmental control functions that will control the lights or television in their home (Lange 2015). For example, with the addition of a wireless control interface box or Bluetooth module, a user would be able to move a computer mouse and perform mouse click functions using their wheelchair joystick or head array. Many manufacturers are now integrating Bluetooth function within the joystick electronics, enabling the user to integrate smart technology with their wheelchair Permobil 2018).

Wheelchair seating

Assessment of seating and positioning is a critical component when determining needs for a manual or power mobility device. The occupational and/or physical therapist who specializes in wheelchair seating, positioning, and selection must be able to perform a comprehensive evaluation taking into account the individual's medical, social, environmental, and transportation needs. Other team members, including caregivers and family members, equipment vendors, and rehabilitation engineers, to name a few, may be present at the assessment as well.

Assessment and evaluation

Use of any of the conceptual practice models presented in previous chapters (Chapter 2, for example) should be considered to guide the seating evaluation. As we will discuss here, the person, their current technology and environments, and their goals must all be considered to complete a comprehensive seating evaluation (Arledge et al. 2011; Dudgeon et al. 2014). When a client comes into the clinic for an evaluation for complex rehabilitation equipment, the appointment begins with an interview to gather background data. In addition to general demographic data, information regarding primary payment source, physician information, and current diagnosis should be gathered if it was not done as part of a general intake form supplied by the clinic. As a time saving measure, a questionnaire can be used as part of the pre-evaluation screening paperwork (Appendix A). If the pre-evaluation screening is mailed to the individual prior to their appointment, it gives them time to do a self-assessment and analyze their needs and goals. A list of current equipment, its age, serial numbers, and any upgrades should be recorded if possible, as this could affect funding of future equipment.

When the appointment begins, it is critical to start with a conversation to ensure the practitioner is fully aware of the client's goals as these will influence equipment choices such as postural supports and hardware components. The reason for the appointment should be clearly established, determining what equipment the client is seeking to obtain. A detailed history of any past or upcoming surgeries should be discussed as this could have a direct impact on the plan for complex rehabilitation equipment needs (Walls and Rosen 2008). Also, the use and management of the client's current and future equipment within their environment (house, day facility, school, day habilitation program, vehicle, or other) must be discussed.

The interview should continue by asking the client or caregiver about the client's level of independence at home regarding ADL's such as dressing, bathing, toileting, feeding, grooming, meal preparation, and other home management tasks. Also, the client's level of independence with bowel and bladder management should be recorded. Seat cushion choice later could be directly related to this (Walls and Rosen 2008). As presented in the Toolbox, there are standardized assessment tools available to determine level of function with ADLs, such as the Bathel Index (Mahoney and Barthel 1965) or Katz ADL scale (Katz 1983). Mobility skills should also be recorded, asking the level of assistance the individual requires to move in and out of bed, transfer on and off the commode or toilet, ambulate if possible, or propel their chair. This information will give critical feedback to the therapist and supplier as to the type and setup of the equipment.

Sensation of the extremities needs to be noted as intact, impaired, or absent. Again, this will guide your equipment choice. History of past skin breakdown or any present skin breakdown on the extremities or buttocks is also important to note. Skin breakdown or any color changes on the skin can (and must) also be observed for during the mat portions of the evaluation as well.

After the above information is gathered from the client and their caregiver, the therapist will then begin the mat evaluation (Cooper 1998; Batavia 2010). (See the Additional Learning Resources at the end of this chapter for sample mat evaluation videos.) It is important to have a form to follow when collecting data for the mat evaluation, both to record data and also to ensure the evaluation is organized and as efficient as possible (Appendix B). The mat evaluation should be done using a firm surface, preferably a mat table. When looking at body segments, the therapist should observe the client in both a seated and a supine position on the mat during the evaluation, as this will enable the clinician to determine origination of any deficits found. The mat evaluation is a critical component of the overall wheelchair evaluation.

Neuromuscular status can be observed throughout the duration of the evaluation. The modified Ashworth scale (Pandyan et al. 1999) can be used to note any abnormal tone within the trunk or extremities during movement. It is important to note if the individual has high, low, or fluctuating tone, as well as if there are differences within body sides, left versus right. This will have an impact on the seating and components that are chosen.

With the client in a supine position on a mat table, begin by looking at and palpating their pelvis. Observe the plane that the pelvis naturally rests in, remembering to take into account the three planes of the pelvis, anterior/posterior (in the sagittal plane – are the ASISs higher or lower than the PSIS?), left/right oblique (in the frontal plane – is one ASIS more elevated than the other?), and left/right rotation (in the transverse plane – is one ASIS more forward than the other?). Note if the movement in any of the three planes is non-correctable, meaning that it is unable to be moved, or correctable, or if it cannot be moved to neutral position. The movement can also be a combination of the above, meaning that the client's pelvis can move in only a certain direction, or in only one plane, and not others, or on only one side and not the other. It is important to remember that every patient is unique. The therapist should determine if they can position the client's pelvis into a neutral position, and if so, whether it is comfortable for the client. A correctable deformity that can be manually corrected and maintained with a small amount of force can often be maintained with appropriate support components. Non correctable or fixed deformities such as severe joint contractures must be accommodated (Kuchler O'Shea et al. 2006; Watanabe 2017).

After looking at the pelvis and spine, the therapist moves to the client's lower body and hips. Are the hips currently positioned in a neutral position beneath the pelvis? If not, the therapist should see if it is possible to move them into this alignment. If they cannot, then it should be documented where they rest, again noting if it is correctable or non-correctable. The therapist should look to see if the client is abducted or adducted, internally or externally rotating, and also note if their hips are subluxed or dislocated. Range of motion (ROM) should be recorded for the hips in supine, being sure to record a measurement for the hamstrings, as this two-joint muscle is often tight. One common deformity is called a windswept position (Figure 15.18). This is when one lower extremity is abducted and externally rotated and the other is adducted and internally rotated, making it look like both legs are sitting to one side or the other. It is named windswept to the left or right depending on which way the client's knees are oriented in relation to midline. ROM for the knees and feet can be measured in supine as well. Document any contractures at the knees; any positioning limitations at the feet into dorsiflexion, plantarflexion, inversion, or eversion should be noted as well.

After a thorough supine evaluation is completed, the client should be moved into a seated position at the edge of the mat table, being supported if necessary. After assessing their pelvis as noted above, the therapist will examine the trunk in sitting (Cooper 1998; Batavia 2010). The therapist will note the presence of a scoliosis, including direction and spinal region as well as presence of spinal rotation, as best as possible with observation and palpation as it relates to the position of the pelvis. They will also note increased or decreased thoracic kyphosis or lumbar lordosis. As above, the therapist will note if the spine is correctable or non-correctable. The therapist should also note the relationship of the pelvis to the spine.

The relationship of the head and neck to the spine should be documented next. If the client has cervical or capital hyperextension or flexion, is laterally flexed in one direction or another, or has rotation as a resting position, this should be noted. Also, the therapist should note the client's level of head control, and if the amount of head control is functional, limited (meaning that the client can maintain their head in an upright position for brief periods only – note for how long), or absent altogether.

Position of the shoulders and upper extremities in relation to the trunk can be documented. Shoulder position should be assessed, noting if the shoulders are elevated or depressed, protracted or retracted, or if they are subluxed and if there is a difference between the left and right sides. If there is any shortening at the elbow or wrist as well as functional contractures at the hand, these should be documented as well, as these will have an impact on mobility and positioning. If there are contractures, ROM measurements should be recorded.

A full inspection of the current seating system and chair should be done while the client is out of the chair as well. The therapist should look at the seat cushion to determine the integrity of the seating material, and have the seating vendor assist if needed to assess the overall integrity of the frame and other chair components. Visually inspecting and palpating for wear patterns on upholstery and in any foam surfaces can give a good indication of where the individual puts the most pressure or wear and tear on the seating system. It is easier to determine if seating hardware is loose or broken when the individual is not seated in their wheelchair. Once the client is back in the chair, appropriateness of fit and alignment of the current parts can be determined if this has not been done already.

Before the client moves back to their chair, the therapist can use the mat to trial a variety of positions with the client to determine which may be the best for them in their new seating system. A seating simulator is another tool that can be used within the clinic to do this (Sparacio 2018). If you have an individual whose lower legs are slightly windswept to the left and whose trunk is in a non-correctable position rotated to the right due to a scoliosis, the therapist may be tempted to position their lower legs and pelvis in a more forward facing position (Figure 15.34), as this is more typical.

By doing this, however, the client's trunk would be turned to the right, and they would then have to turn their head to the left to look straight. Instead, if it was trialed with the client's trunk facing forward, letting the legs and pelvis remain askew to the left (windswept), this may be a more functional position for the client (Figure 15.35).

A balance needs to be struck, however, between comfort and function, as the chair would still need to remain a reasonable width to ensure easy movement through doorways and into narrower spaces. This could all be tested and measured either on the mat or on a simulator.

After the ROM and musculoskeletal information is gathered, balance, transfers, ambulation, and use of the current mobility device should be assessed in order to

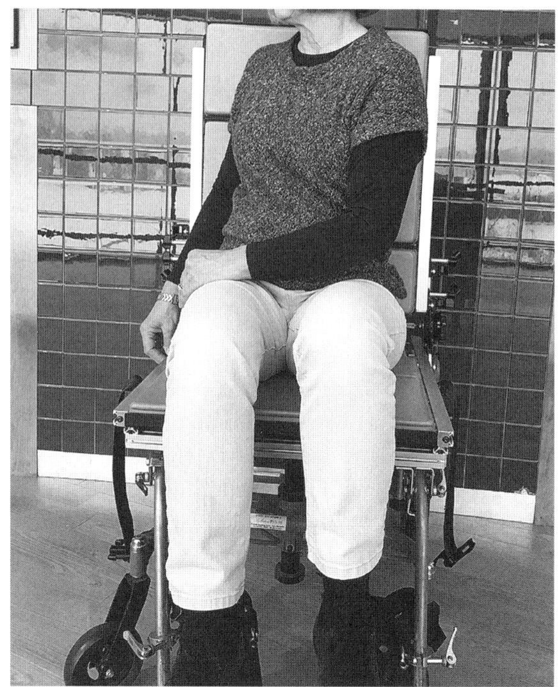

Figure 15.34 Simulation of seated position with individual with a pelvic/spinal rotation positioned with pelvis and legs facing forward and trunk rotated.

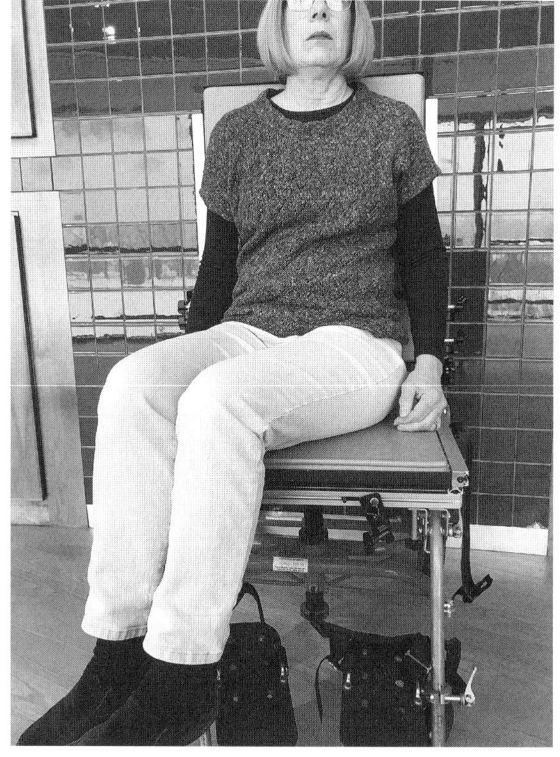

Figure 15.35 Simulation of seated position with individual with a pelvic/spinal rotation positioned with pelvis and legs windswept to the left and trunk facing forward.

appropriately determine correct fit and alignment for comfort, improved function, and pressure management. In addition, this information is required to determine wheelchair setup of seating components to facilitate independence with transfers and ADLs. Balance can be assessed in sitting and, if possible, standing. Note if the client is within normal limits, requires assistance, and if so, how much and what, or is unable to maintain balance. Observe and document how the client transfers. This could be noted when they move onto the mat table earlier in the evaluation. Is the client independent? Does she or he require assistance? Note how much and what type of assistance is needed or if the client is dependent on a caregiver or an external device such as a mechanical lift. The therapist should note if the client is able to ambulate, and if so, with what level of assistance, whether with or without a device, for what distance, and whether they are impacted by varying terrain or fatigue. Amount of caregiver assistance should also be reviewed and documented, as this is important to help both with justification and with determining which type of chair or piece of equipment will best meet the client's needs.

If it is decided that a seating system is required, basic measurements such as hip and trunk width, leg length, thigh length, and trunk height will need to be recorded (Appendix C) to determine the correct dimensions of the new equipment. Table 15.1 shows the basic measurements and the importance for different wheelchair users. Many clinics develop their own seating measurement forms based upon the clientele they serve. More comprehensive information on wheelchair seating and support measures is available for review (Waugh and Crane 2013).

Ideally, it is best to perform complex seating assessments in two (or more) sessions. The initial assessment would be considered the referral assessment where the therapists and family would meet and perform a therapy evaluation to determine needs and goals and perform a mat evaluation with ROM measurements. A second session for the purpose of equipment recommendation and selection would include a wheelchair vendor where equipment could be trialed and other measurements needed to order a wheelchair/seating system would be obtained. Two or more visits are not always possible. Individuals who live in rural areas and who travel long distance for services may only have one opportunity to meet at a seating clinic for evaluation. Funding may also often be a factor, as some insurance sources limit the number of visits available for wheelchair seating services.

Wheelchair seating components

Wheelchairs vary in size, style, function, and overall complexity and should be chosen based upon the individual's needs to enable the user to meet their functional goals. Common wheelchair seating components (Figure 15.36) and their function (Table 15.2) will be described, followed by a discussion of types of wheeled mobility devices and their use.

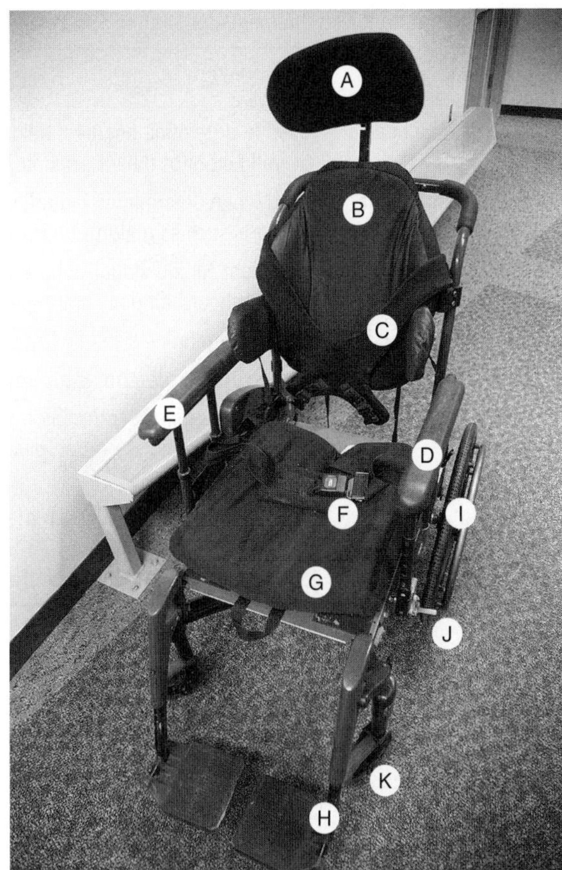

Figure 15.36 Labeled wheelchair components. A – head support; B – back support; C – anterior trunk support (chest harness); D & E – arm support; F – pelvic positioning belt; G – seat cushion; H – hanger and foot support; I – wheel; J – wheel lock castor; K – castor.

Seating surface/cushions

The seating surface may very well be considered the most critical component in a wheelchair seating system. It provides a base for stability and can impact the decision for all other positioning supports. There are many considerations when prescribing a seating system (and specifically a seat cushion), including: comfort, neuromuscular management, improvement of postural control, and maintenance of the integumentary system (Kuchler O'Shea et al. 2006; Kreutz 2018). Types of seat cushions include: foam, gel, viscous fluid, air, or a combination of materials. Each type of cushion has its own unique properties and is made to provide postural support, minimize risk for pressure ulcers, or both (Smith n.d.).

Table 15.1 Important Measurements for Seating and Positioning.

Measurement	Importance
Seat to top of the head	Used to determine headrest height. This can also be important when discussing transportation. The overall height of the wheelchair plus the user in a seated position must be able to fit into a vehicle.
Seat to shoulder height, shoulder width	Used when determining overall seat backrest dimensions for an individual who requires full trunk supports such as a high seat back and chest harness.
Seat to scapular angle	Important for individuals who self-propel, especially active users. It is necessary to be sure the backrest on the wheelchair does not impede the individual's ability to propel the wheelchair.
Chest depth, chest width	Used to determine size of extra supports such as trunk laterals
Seat to elbow	Can be used to determine armrest height
Seat depth	Used to determine seat/cushion size. For an individual with a pelvic rotation, windswept deformity, leg length discrepancy, or other lower-extremity anomalies, this measurement may be different on the right vs the left.
Leg length	Used to determine the length of the leg rest hanger and locate the footrest. This measurement can also help determine the overall seat height of the wheelchair. If the individual performs a stand pivot transfer, optimizing the seat height on the wheelchair is crucial for independence.

Table 15.2 Wheelchair Components.

Component	Types/features	Function
Foot supports/ footplates	Swing away, flip away, angle adjustable	1. Provide positive support to the lower extremities to help maintain positioning in the wheelchair 2. Prevent injury to the feet
Arm supports	Single point, two point, flip away, full length, desk length	1. Provide positioning support with upper extremity weight bearing 2. Used for weight bearing for transfers 3. Often hold Upper Extremity Support Surface (UESS), i.e. lap tray
Seat cushions	Foam, gel, air, combination	1. Provide pelvic support for positioning 2. Prevent pressure ulcers 3. Comfort
Pelvic positioning belt	2, 3, or 4 point, multiple closure/ buckle options	1. Provide pelvic support to maintain proper positioning 2. safety
Trunk supports/trunk laterals	Standard, swing away, removable	Provide lateral support for improved upright posture
Head support		Provide support for alignment for individuals with high and low tone

Despite postural support needs, special attention must be paid to ensure the individual user receives the appropriate seat cushion for their environment. A seat cushion that is too thick and making the seat-to-floor measurement too high can impact transfers and require increased caregiver assistance. If the user is an athlete, they may require a seating surface that is dynamic to allow position changes and decreased sitting forces while still providing adequate support to maintain trunk and upper extremity stability. If the user has continence issues, they would likely benefit from a cushion or cover that would deflect fluids. There are many off-the-shelf wheelchair seats and backs available and these are typically linear or have minimal ability to provide customization for the user. For individuals with more significant non-correctable deformities such as significant pelvic obliquities or rotations or spinal scoliosis, custom molded seating is an option (Sparacio 2018). With custom molded seating, the support surface is molded to the shape of the user's body (Figure 15.37).

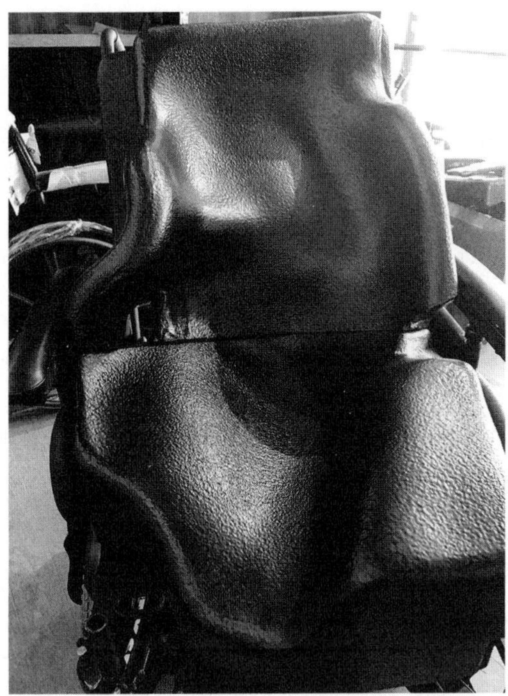

Figure 15.37 Custom molded seating system.

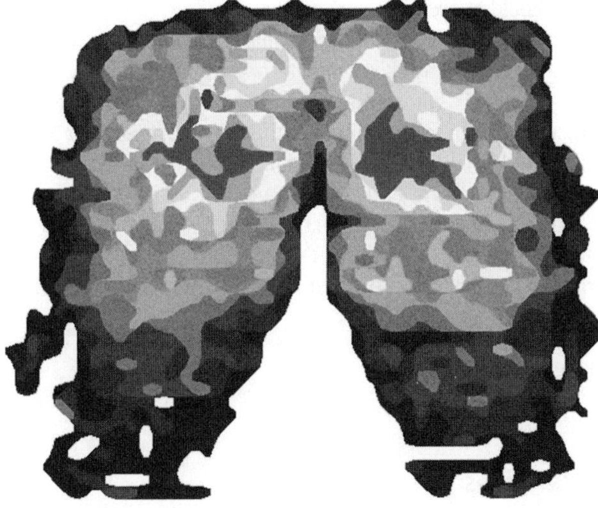

Figure 15.38 Sample diagram of pressure mapping data. Source: Photo used with permission of Tekscan's CONFORMat™ software.

Pressure mapping systems are valuable tools to provide the clinician with data regarding seat-to-user interface pressures. They are used in the seating clinic to assist with determining seat cushion selection (Chisholm and Yip 2018; Crawford et al. 2005). Pressure mapping systems are also often also used for patient education for individuals with impaired or absent sensation to enforce the need for frequent pressure-relieving measures. A sample pressure map is shown in Figure 15.38.

When reading a pressure map, it is important to be sure you have a clear understanding of the orientation of the user, which is not always easy when working with complex seating needs. Looking at this pressure map, the individual is seated with their legs facing forward (pointing toward the bottom of the screen) and the buttocks are approximately in the center. There is a clear outline of seating body shape. Measured pressure is displayed in colors from blue to red, with blue being the least amount of pressure and red the greatest. The red areas are showing large amounts of pressure at the region of the ischial tuberosities bilaterally.

Pelvic positioning belt

A pelvic positioning belt is used to help provide pelvic stability while seated in a wheelchair or other positioning devices (Cooper 1998). It can help a user maintain stability and position while shifting in their wheelchair to reach for objects. Pelvic positioning belts can also be used by individuals with high tone to assist in maintaining desired position for tone reduction or individuals with low tone to assist with sustaining pelvic alignment to facilitate active movement.

Back support

A back support can be basic, such as a standard sling with little support, or complex, such as a custom molded solution that provides maximal support, depending on the user's needs. An active manual wheelchair user may be prescribed a seat back that may stop at the mid-thoracic level to give them adequate upper body movement for efficient wheelchair propulsion. An individual who requires complex seating components may require a seat back that supports the user up to the shoulder level to provide adequate postural support to accomplish their functional goals (Cooper 1998; Batavia 2010).

Trunk support

Trunk support can be provided in many different ways, depending on the needs of the user. Lateral support pads can be placed on one or both sides (Waugh and Crane 2013). Considerations must be made to ensure adjustability for weight changes and clothing needs in colder climates. Anterior chest supports also help support the trunk. Chest straps provide added stability at the trunk and are often used by individuals with high and low tone as well as individuals with spinal cord injury. A chest harness can be custom designed to provide trunk support with a three- or four-point attachment, with special consideration for pressure management surrounding bony prominences and surgical sites (G-tubes, baclofen pumps, etc.).

Box 15.2 Case study

Mr. Smith is a 34-year-old man who was referred to the seating clinic by his primary care physician to have his seating system assessed, as he was getting breakdown over his sacrum that did not appear to be healing. Prior to the appointment, a chart review of medical as well as previous seating history was performed. It was determined his current wheelchair is two years old and there is no documentation of weight or medical changes. He came into clinic with his mother, who is primary caregiver.

The therapist began the appointment with a patient interview. During the interview, she learned that, five years prior, Mr. Smith was in a motor vehicle accident and as a result now has a complete C6-level spinal cord injury. He now lives at his mother's house with her. He stays at home during the day, with the assistance of an aide when available, while his mother works. He is able to operate the mechanical lift himself, but needs assistance with sling placement. He currently has a power wheelchair that has power tilt and recline functions; however, Mr. Smith reports that the tilt and recline haven't worked in several months. He has a catheter and requires assistance with bathing and other home skills. When the therapist asked about Mr. Smith's sensation, he reported that he did not have any feeling below his trunk and was unaware of where his legs where.

After gathering the information, the therapist then moved on to the mat evaluation. With assistance from a mechanical lift, she transferred Mr. Smith over to the mat table in the clinic space. She noted that Mr. Smith's lower body was flaccid, although clonus was noted in his left lower extremity. She moved his pelvis and noted that it was in a minimal posterior pelvic tilt, and not flexible. There was no other obliquity. His trunk was symmetrical, although he had a mild kyphosis, but could correct this with a cue. In sitting, his preferred position was with slight hip external rotation and abduction. He had notably tight hamstrings. She also noted that he had stage II wound to his sacrum.

The therapist also evaluated his current chair before moving him back to look for signs of wear to the cushion or any other issues. She noted that the foam was beginning to wear thin on the back of the seat. The therapist transferred Mr. Smith back into his seat and, while the seat and back were adjusted appropriately for him, she noted that the footplates were lower than they should have been.

Based on her clinical findings, the therapist concluded that the combination of the lowered footplates and tightened hamstrings had led to Mr. Smith sitting in an increased posterior pelvic tilt in a seated position on a daily basis. Since his tilt and recline functions were not working, he had not been changing positions during the day, and the foam in his seat was compromised. This was leading to his skin breakdown.

The seating vendor was contacted. The footplates were raised to the correct height. A pressure relief cushion was provided on loan while a new cushion was ordered through Mr. Smith's insurance. In addition, repairs to his tilt and recline were requested to bring his chair back up to working order. Mr. Smith and his mother were counseled regarding the importance of timely maintenance of his power chair and were provided with the contact information for the wheelchair vendor, in case his chair should break again in the future.

Seating and positioning needs vary from the user with good postural control who uses a manual or power mobility device to the individual with complex neuromuscular involvement requiring custom seating solutions that require a team approach (end user, family/caregivers, clinician, wheelchair vendor, physician, etc.) to ensure all needs are met for optimal functional outcomes. Obtaining a detailed history, performing a mat evaluation, and good knowledge of seating components and types of wheelchair available are essential to success in assisting the end user to meet their goals.

Hangers/foot support

The hangers provide the attachment site between the wheelchair and foot supports and come in many different designs and configurations (Cooper 1998; Waugh and Crane 2013). Some are elevating to accommodate for post-surgical users, amputees, and users who must elevate their extremities due to edema. Many hangers swing away or remove to provide clearance to facilitate transfers. Foot supports are not necessarily just a place for a wheelchair user to rest their feet. They provide a solid surface of support and can be an integral part in maintaining pelvic and thus whole-body positioning.

Please refer to Box 15.2 for a case study application.

References

Access2CRT (2019). Retrieved from http://www.access2crt.org.

Arledge, S., Armstrong, W., Babinec, M. et al. (2011). RESNA wheelchair service provision guide. Retrieved from https://www.resna.org/sites/default/files/legacy/resources/position-papers/RESNAWheelchairServiceProvisionGuide.pdf.

Babinec, M. (2018). Power mobility applications: mobility categories and clinical indicators. In: *Seating and Wheeled Mobility: A Clinical Resource Guide* (ed. M. Lange and J. Minkel). Thorofare, NJ: Slack.

Batavia, M. (2010). *The Wheelchair Evaluation: A Clinician's Guide*, 2e. Boston, MA: Jones and Bartlett.

Chisholm, J. and Yip, J. (2018). Pressure management for the seated client. In: *Seating and Wheeled Mobility: A Clinical Resource Guide* (ed. M. Lange and J. Minkel). Thorofare, NJ: Slack.

Cooper, R.A. (1998). *Wheelchair Selection and Configuration*. New York: Demos Medical Publishing.

Costigan, F.A. and Light, J. (2011). Functional seating for school-age children with cerebral palsy: an evidence-based tutorial. *Language, Speech, and Hearing Services in Schools* 42 (2): 223–236.

Crawford, S., Strain, B., Gregg, B. et al. (2005). An investigation of the impact of Force Sensing Array pressure mapping system on the clinical judgement of occupational therapists. *Clinical Rehabilitation* 19 (2): 224–231.

Dicianno, B., Lieberman, J., Schmeler, M. et al. (2015). RESNA position on the application of tilt, recline, and elevating legrests for wheelchairs: 2015 current state of the literature. Retrieved from https://www.resna.org/sites/default/files/legacy/resources/position-papers/RESNA%20PP%20on%20Tilt%20Recline_2017.pdf.

DiGiovine, C. and Berner, T. (2018). Alternative drive mechanisms for manual wheelchairs: bridging the gap between manual and power mobility. In: *Seating and Wheeled Mobility: A Clinical Resource Guide* (ed. M. Lange and J. Minkel). Thorofare, NJ: Slack.

Dudgeon, B.J., Deitz, J.C., and Dimpfel, M. (2014). Wheelchair selection. In: *Occupational Therapy for Physical 13 Dysfunction*, 7e (ed. M.V. Radomski and C.A. Trombly-Latham), 495–579. Baltimore, MD: Lippincott Williams & Wilkins.

Groah, S.L., Schladen, M., Pineda, C.G., and Hsieh, C.H. (2015). Prevention of pressure ulcers among people with spinal cord injury: a systematic review. *PM&R* 7 (6): 613–636.

Hamm, R. (2007). Tissue healing and pressure ulcers. In: *Physical Rehabilitation Evidence-Based Examination, Evaluation, and Intervention* (ed. M. Cameron and L. Monroe), 733–776. St. Louis, MO: Saunders Elsevier.

Jan, Y.-K. and Crane, B.A. (2013). Wheelchair tilt-in-space and recline does not reduce sacral skin perfusion as changing from the upright to the tilted and reclined position in people with spinal cord injury. *Archives of Physical Medicine and Rehabilitation* 94 (6): 1207–1210. https://doi.org/10.1016/j.apmr.2013.01.004.

Jan, Y.-K., Jones, M.A., Rabadi, M.H. et al. (2010). Effect of wheelchair tilt-in-space and recline angles on skin perfusion over the ischial tuberosity in people with spinal cord injury. *Archives of Physical Medicine and Rehabilitation* 91 (11): 1758–1764.

Jones, M. and Gray, S. (2005). Assistive technology: positioning and mobility. In: *Meeting the Physical Therapy Needs of Children* (ed. S. Effgen), 621–634. Philadelphia, PA: F.A. Davis.

Kangas, K. (2016). Beyond 90/90/90: seating & access to AT. Pre-Conference workshop presented at ATIA Conference, Orlando, FL.

Katz, S. (1983). Assessing self-maintenance: activities of daily living, mobility, and instrumental activities of daily living. *Journal of the American Geriatrics Society* 31 (12): 721–726.

Kreutz, D. (2018). Postural support and pressure management for hands-free sitters. In: *Seating and Wheeled Mobility: A Clinical Resource Guide* (ed. M. Lange and J. Minkel). Thorofare, NJ: Slack.

Kuchler O'Shea, R., Carlson, S., and Ramsey, C. (2006). Assistive technology. In: *Physical Therapy for Children* (ed. S. Campbell, D. Vander Linden and R. Palisano), 983–1024. St. Louis, MO: Saunders Elsevier.

Lange, M.L. (2000). Tilt in space versus recline – new trends in an old debate. *Technology Special Interest Section Quarterly* 10: 1–3.

Lange, M. (2015). Power wheelchairs: an overview of advanced features. Retrieved from https://www.occupationaltherapy.com/articles/power-wheelchairs-overview-advanced-features-2479.

Lange, M. (2018). Power mobility: alternative access methods. In: *Seating and Wheeled Mobility: A Clinical Resource Guide* (ed. M. Lange and J. Minkel), 179–198. Thorofare, NJ: Slack.

Mahoney, F.I. and Barthel, D. (1965). Functional evaluation: the Barthel Index. *Maryland State Medical Journal* 14: 56–61.

Maltchev, K. (2012). Preventing injuries in the workplace: ergonomics. In: *Work: Promoting Participation and Productivity Through Occupational Therapy* (ed. B. Braveman and J. Page). Philadelphia, PA: F.A. Davis.

Medola, F.O., Elui, V.M.C., Santana, C.d.S., and Fortulan, C.A. (2014). Aspects of manual wheelchair configuration affecting mobility: a review. *Journal of Physical Therapy Science* 26 (2): 313–318. https://doi.org/10.1589/jpts.26.313.

Pandyan, A.D., Johnson, G.R., Price, C.I. et al. (1999). A review of the properties and limitations of the Ashworth and Modified Ashworth Scales as measures of spasticity. *Clinical Rehabilitation* 13: 373–383.

Permobil (2018). Bluetooth iDevice Module. Retrieved from https://permobilus.com/product/bluetooth-idevice-module.

RESNA (2012). RESNA position on the application of ultralight manual wheelchairs. Retrieved from http://www.resna.org/sites/default/files/legacy/resources/position-papers/UltraLightweightManualWheelchairs.pdf.

Smith, M. (n.d.). SpinLife's guide to seat cushions. Retrieved from https://www.spinlife.com/buying-guide/seat-cushions.

Sparacio, J. (2018). Postural support and pressure management considerations for prop sitters. In: *Seating and Wheeled Mobility: A Clinical Resource Guide* (ed. M. Lange and J. Minkel), 73–84. Thorofare, NJ: Slack.

Taule, T., Bergfjord, K., Holsvik, E.E. et al. (2013). Factors influencing optimal seating pressure after spinal cord injury. *Spinal Cord* 51 (4): 273–277.

Vicente, K. (2006). *The Human Factor: Revolutionizing the Way We Live with Technology*. New York: Routledge, Taylor & Francis Group.

Walls, G. and Rosen, L. (2008). Wheelchair seating and mobility evaluation. *PT: Magazine of. Physical Therapy* 16 (1): 28–42.

Watanabe, L. (2017). Asymmetry in balance: do you intervene? Accommodate? Or do both? Mobility Management. Retreived from http://www4.mobilitymgmt.com/Articles/2017/09/01/Asymmetry.aspx.

Waugh, K. (2013). *Glossary of Wheelchair Terms and Definitions, Version 1.0*. Denver, CO: Paralized Veterans of America.

Waugh, K. and Crane, B. (2013). *A Clinical Application Guide to Standardized Wheelchair Seating Measures of the Body and Seating Support Surfaces*. Denver, CO: Paralized Veterans of America.

Additional resources

Mat Evaluation (RESNA) Part 1 – Presented by Jean Minkel: http://www.youtube.com/watch?v=yHjn4y9H-6M

Mat Evaluation (RESNA) Part 2 – Presented by Jean Minkel: http://www.youtube.com/watch?v=J04eKjR49fI

Wheelchair Seating Mat Evaluation: Part 1: http://www.youtube.com/watch?v=Is8WAT4i9ZU

Wheelchair Seating Mat Evaluation: Part 2: http://www.youtube.com/watch?v=Phy9p9J3SsY

Access to Independence: http://www.atilange.com/resources.html

Assistive Technology Partners – Colorado University School of Medicine: http://www.ucdenver.edu/academics/AssistiveTechnologyPartners/resources/Pages/Resources.aspx

AbleData https://abledata.acl.gov/

Digital reference

Alternate Drive Controls and ECU Interface companies
Adaptive Switch Labs: www.asl-inc.comAbledata
HMC: http://www.permobil.com/en/Corporate (click on products)
Stealth Products: http://www.stealthproducts.com

Toolbox: Resources

Law, M., & Letts, L. (1989). A critical review of scales of activities of daily living. *American Journal of Occupational Therapy*, 43(8):522–528. doi: 10.5014/ajot.43.8.522.

Mlinac, M. & Feng, M. (2016). Assessment of activities of daily living, self-care, and independence, *Archives of Clinical Neuropsychology*, 31(6) pp. 506–516, doi: 10.1093/arclin/acw049.

Katz Index of Independence in Activities of Daily Living (ADL) Katz, S. (1983). Assessing self-maintenance: activities of daily living, mobility and instrumental activities of daily living. *Journal of the American Geriatrics Society*, 31(12), 721–726. Available online at http://clas.uiowa.edu/socialwork/files/socialwork/NursingHomeResource/documents/Katz%20ADL_LawtonIADL.pdf.

Barthel Index of Activities of Daily Living Mahoney FI, Barthel, D. "Functional evaluation: the Barthel Index." *Maryland State Medical Journal* 1965;14: 56–61.Available online at http://www.strokecenter.org/wp-content/uploads/2011/08/barthel.pdf

Appendix A

Mobility Device Evaluation

Please complete questions below to the best of your knowledge.

What is the purpose of your visit today?______________________________

Does your current equipment meet your needs? ☐ Yes ☐ No

Why or why not?______________________________

List current equipment______________________________

Current day location:______________________________

Current therapies and frequencies:______________________________

Check all that you do: ☐ Healthcare appts. ☐ Work ☐ School ☐ Shopping ☐ Community events ☐ Vacation/Travel ☐ Access family dining room

ADLs	Independent	Min. Assist	Mod. Assist	Max assist	Dependent
Bathing	☐	☐	☐	☐	☐
Upper-body dressing	☐	☐	☐	☐	☐
Lower-body dressing	☐	☐	☐	☐	☐
Grooming	☐	☐	☐	☐	☐
Toileting	☐	☐	☐	☐	☐
Eating	☐	☐	☐	☐	☐
Transfers					
Bed	☐	☐	☐	☐	☐
Toilet	☐	☐	☐	☐	☐
Chair	☐	☐	☐	☐	☐
Wheelchair	☐	☐	☐	☐	☐

How do you transfer? ______________________________

Requires an assistive device for transfers:______________________________

Home environment

Environment	☐ House	☐ Apartment	☐ Assisted living	☐ ICF	☐ IRA
Entrance	☐ Level	☐ Stairs	☐ Ramp	☐ Lift	
Bathroom	☐ Accessible	☐ Inaccessible			
Living area	☐ Accessible	☐ Inaccessible			

Is the inside of the home wheelchair accessible? ☐ Yes ☐ No

Describe:______________________________

Wheelchair storage if not in residence: ______________________________

Transportation
Driving: ☐ Independent driver ☐ Independent driver from w/c ☐ Passenger in w/c ☐ Passenger transfers out of w/c
Vehicle: ☐ Car ☐ Mini van ☐ Full size van ☐ Truck ☐ Medical transport
☐ W/C school bus ☐ Public transportation
Lift/ramp: ☐Yes ☐ No ☐ Other: ____________________
Accessibility of w/c to vehicle: ☐ Side door ☐ Back door/trunk ☐ Ramp/lift
Safety: ☐ N/A – don't transport in w/c ☐Tie-downs in vehicle ☐ Other

Mobility – ambulation
☐ Non-ambulatory
☐Ambulates but speed/distance/endurance are not functional to complete ADLs
☐Ambulates with speed/distance/endurance to complete ADLs
☐ Without an assistive device
☐ With an assistive device:____________________________________
Ambulates on: ☐ Flat level surfaces only ☐ Uneven surfaces ☐ Stairs ☐ Inclines
Balance: ☐ Safe for ambulation without an assistive device ☐ Safe for ambulation with an assistive device
☐ Unsafe for ambulation

Mobility – manual wheelchair
☐ Unable to propel any kind of manual wheelchair
Caregiver is willing and able to push manual chair for all patients ADLs? ☐ Yes ☐ No
☐ Self-propels but speed/distance/endurance are not functional to complete all ADLs
☐ Self-propels but speed/distance/endurance are functional to complete all ADLs
Method of propulsion_________________________
☐ Needs specific seat-to-floor height for transfers, propulsion, ADLs, other:______________ (circle all that apply)

Mobility – power wheelchair
☐ Unable to operate a power wheelchair
☐ Able and willing to operate a power wheelchair to participate in ADLs using:
☐ Joystick ☐ Alternate control:_____________________________
☐Able and willing to operate a power scooter to participate in ADLs

Appendix B

Wheelchair/DME Evaluation Form

Wheelchair/Durable Medical Equipment Assessment

<table>
<tr><td>Name:</td><td>DOB:</td><td>DOE:</td></tr>
<tr><td>Insurance:</td><td>Date of script:</td><td># of approved visits and/or date new script is needed</td></tr>
<tr><td>PCP:</td><td>Physiatrist:</td><td>Vendor:</td></tr>
<tr><td>Diagnosis:</td><td colspan="2">Team members present at evaluation:</td></tr>
<tr><td colspan="3">Reason for evaluation:
_____ Power mobility assessment
_____ Manual wheelchair assessment
_____ Equipment fitting/delivery/training as needed
_____ Custom equipment modifications
_____ Mobility equipment evaluation
_____ ADL equipment evaluation</td></tr>
</table>

_____ Posture assessment _____ Pressure area or ulcer/pressure mapping (please state location): _____ Other:
Goals of client/family/team: If family not present, has family been contacted, and in agreement with plan?
List current equipment and age: Issues with current equipment:

Medical background

Cardiovascular history:	Respiratory history:
Integumentary history:	Overall health (explain):
Orthopedic history: __ Benign __ Osteoporosis __ Scoliosis – current degree and last MD visit: __ Spinal surgeries __ Hip dislocation/subluxation __ Muscle lengthenings __ Other orthopedic surgeries – list: __ Any planned procedures/surgeries and dates	Neuromuscular/tone __ Benign __ Currently utilizing tone management medications __ Baclofen pump __ Other:
Orthotics/positioning aids – list:	Will they use orthotics in w/c?

Pain __ No pain currently __ Impaired sensation – unable to report __ Pain – list location and level of pain:	Breakdown/open skin areas: __ No history __ Mild redness:_______________ __ Open area (location and stage)__________ __ Surgery:

Current level of function

Sitting
Sitting balance:
__ WFL
__ Min assist
__ Mod assist
__ Unable to sit without support
	Standing
	Standing balance:
	__ WFL
	__ Min assist
	__ Mod assist
	__ Unable to stand without support
		Transfers
		__ Independently mobile
		__ Min assist
		__ Mod assist
		__ Full assist
		  __ Uses lift assist
		  __ Gait belt
		  __ Pivot disk
		  __ Mechanical lift

Ambulation __ Able to ambulate without an ambulation aid __Requiresanambulationaid:__________________ Level of assistance: __ Independent __ Min Assist __ Mod Assist __ Max Assist __ Unable to ambulate	Describe (list things like max distances, falls, environmental barriers, pain, etc.)

Manual wheelchair mobility
__ Unable to propel – dependent on caregiver
__ Able to propel with assistance
__ Able to propel independently – short distances only
__ Able to propel independently
__ 1 arm drive chair
How do they propel currently:
  Left UE / LE
  Right UE / LE
	Describe: (List barriers such as asymmetries, environmental barriers, pain, etc.)

Power wheelchair mobility __ Unable/never attempted power mobility __ Requires verbal or physical prompting __ Independent __ Unsafe How do they drive currently? Joystick – right / left Head array Switches: Proximity switches: Other:	Describe: (List barriers such as asymmetries, environmental barriers, pain, etc.)

Evaluation for seating system/DME – Body should be aligned as well as possible and is comfortable for the client prior to performing measurements. Note if assessed in sitting or supine.

	Posture		
Pelvis	Anterior/posterior __WFL __Anterior tilt __Posterior tilt	Anterior/posterior: Mobility: __Fixed __Flexible __Describe:	Comments:
	Obliquity: __WFL __Right side lower __Left side lower	Frontal plane: Mobility: __Fixed __Flexible __Describe: Is obliquity caused from the pelvis or trunk?____________	Comments:
	Rotation: __Neutral __Left side forward __Right side forward	Rotation: Mobility: __Fixed __Flexible __Describe: Is rotation caused from the pelvis or trunk?____________ Can the pelvis be derotated and the trunk straightened? If so what is the resulting LE position?	Comments:
Trunk	__WFL __Scoliosis __Laterally flexed to __Left __Right __Rotated to __Left __Right __Rib cage deformity __Rib hump __Increased thoracic kyphosis __Increased lumbar lordosis __Decreased lumbar lordosis	Trunk mobility: __Fixed __Flexible __Describe Does Client utilize a TLSO?	Comments (Include tone, movement patterns, skin integrity, etc.):

Hips	__Neutral __Abducted__Adducted __IR __ER __Windswept to the left __Windswept to the right	Hip ROM: L: R: Flex:____ _____ Ext:_____ _____ IR: _____ _____ ER: _____ _____ ABD: _____ _____ ADD:_____ _____	Comments (Include tone, movement patterns, skin integrity, etc.):
Lower extremities/ feet	Knee: __Hamstring tightness __ROM/deformities __Tibial torsion __LLD Foot: __WFL __Right ankle __PF __DF __Inv __EV __Left ankle __PF __DF __ Inv __EV	Knee ROM Flex: Ext: Hamstring (90/90): Ankle: DF: PF: Does client wear orthotics in chair?	Comments (Include tone, movement patterns, skin integrity, etc.):
Head and neck	__Functional – able to keep upright on own __Flexed to _____ side __Rotated to_____side __Laterally flexed to _____ side __Cervical hyperextension	Head control: __Good for long periods __Good for short periods __Brief control __Absent – requires support at all times Are there concerns with secretions/ swallowing? Communication?	Comments (Include tone, movement patterns, skin integrity, etc.):
Upper extremities	Shoulders: Left: Prot/ret Abd/add IR/ER Elev/dep Right: Prot/ret Abd/add IR/ER Elev/dep Elbow: Left: Flex/ext. Right: Flex/ext.	Shoulder ROM: __WFL __Limited: Elbow ROM: __WFL __Limited:	Comments (Include tone, movement patterns, skin integrity, etc.):

Wrist/hand	Left: Flex/ext at wrist Ulnar/radial deviation Right: Flex/ext at wrist Ulnar/radial deviation	Wrist ROM: __WFL __Limited:	Comments (Include tone, movement patterns, skin integrity, etc.):

Seating measurements: See attached form for measurements

Recommendations:
Including information from above, including goals, making decisions with client on best options for optimal alignment, skin protection, and to maximize client function. This should be done in conjunction with a vendor for best options on available products.
Thoroughly list all recommendations here.

Plan: *Specifically list what will happen next (i.e. PT to obtain scripts, vendor to get orders, therapist to write letter, get trial equipment and reconvene with date,* etc.*)*

Clinician signature

Date

Appendix C

SEATING MEASUREMENT FORM

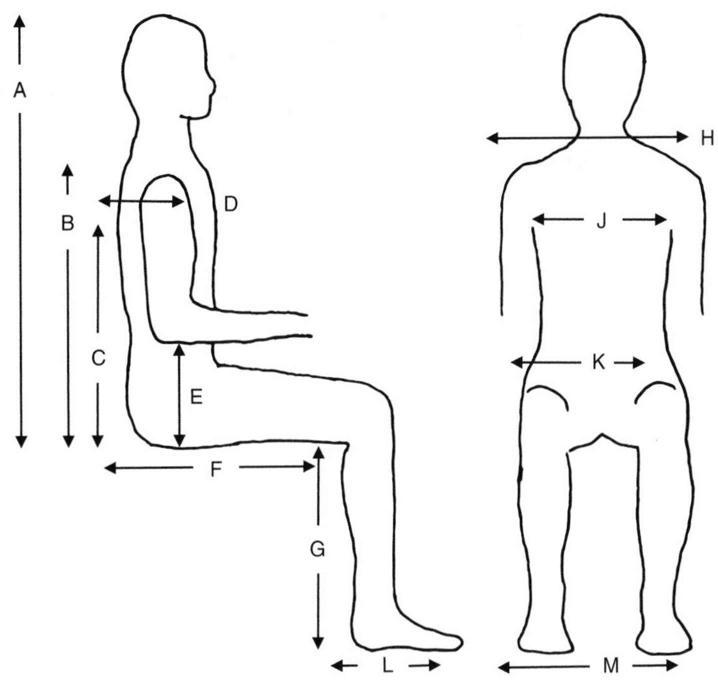

A __________ Seat to top of head
B __________ Seat to shoulder height
C __________ Seat to scapular angle
D __________ Chest depth
E __________ Seat to elbow
F __________ Seat depth – pop to post buttocks
G __________ Leg length – heel to pop
H __________ Shoulder width
J __________ Chest width
K __________ Hip width
L __________ Foot length
M __________ Feet width
__________ Elbow to wrist
__________ Elbow to tips fingers

Current Chair

☐ Manual ☐ Power
______ Seat Width
______ Seat Depth
______ Seat to floor without cushion
__________ Cushion type
______ Seat to floor with cushion
______ Legrest hanger angle
______ Seat to back angle

Seat to back angle: ______________
Popliteal angle (in sitting): __________

Weight: __________
Height: __________

16

Positioning and mobility technology and environmental interventions other than wheeled mobility

Amy Baxter and Lindsey Veety

Outline

Learning outcomes

After reading this chapter, you should be able to:

1. Delineate common diagnoses, injuries, and disabilities that result in positioning and mobility challenges.
2. Describe the purpose and range of positioning and mobility technology, other than wheeled mobility; for example, adaptive seating, positioning and transfer assistive technology, walking aids, standing technology, school chairs and tables, toileting and bathing positioning.
3. Describe the differences between positioning equipment systems, such as prone, supine, sitting, and standing systems for technology and environmental interventions (TEI).
4. Apply the Human-Tech Ladder (Vicente 2006) to persons in need of positioning and mobility TEI.
5. Identify relevant assessment tools related to positioning and mobility TEI.
6. Describe strategies for potential technology and environmental interventions for persons who use positioning and mobility TEI.

Assistive Technologies and Environmental Interventions in Healthcare: An Integrated Approach, First Edition.
Edited by Lynn Gitlow and Kathleen Flecky.

Companion website: www.wiley.com/go/gitlow/assitivetechnologies

Active learning prompts

Before you read this chapter:

1. Search for research articles documenting the benefits of standing.
2. Review the Rehabilitation Engineering and Assistive Technology Society of North America (RESNA) website (www.resna.org), discussed in Chapter 15.
3. Review the components of normal gait cycle and the position of the arms and legs during each phase of gait.
4. Review concepts for center of gravity and center of mass and where these points are in both a seated and a standing position.

Key terms

Seating and positioning other than wheelchairs
Adaptive seating
Positioning and transfer assistive technology
Walking aids, i.e. crutches, canes, and walkers
Standing technology, i.e. prone, supine, sitting, and standing
School chairs and tables
High tone
Low tone
Toileting and bathing positioning

Introduction

> Assistive Technology associated with seating, positioning and mobility can be as varied and complex as physical disabilities themselves. An interdisciplinary approach to the complex problems regarding seating, positioning and mobility yields the best solution. Attainment of appropriate assistive technology related to seating, positioning and mobility could mean increased independence and productivity.
>
> (Dubose and Nelson 2006)

Positioning and other mobility-related factors, including relevant assessment tools and interventions, are presented here. In this chapter, students will learn how to decide on and implement a full range of low- to high-tech interventions for individuals with mobility impairments. In addition to wheelchairs and seating systems, which were discussed in Chapter 15, a therapist can evaluate a client for many other pieces of rehabilitation equipment that can enhance independence and improve quality of life. These can include items as simple as canes or crutches, or more complex tools such as gait trainers, standers, or bathing equipment. These items all have an array of supports, options, and accessories and are designed to meet a variety of client needs. Similar to performing a wheelchair seating evaluation, a proper assessment is required when evaluating a client for these devices as well. The therapist should be sure to consider the multiple factors that a conceptual practice model guides them to think about, including the client's' pathology, impairments, functional limitations, goals, preferences, and environment (Cameron and Monroe 2007). Continued re-evaluation is also critical to be sure that the equipment continues to meet the client's needs. The therapist who works as part of an interdisciplinary team with the seating vendor needs to remain on top of the current products that are on the market as well as funding availability, as these numerous considerations discussed throughout the book will all play a role in the evaluation process and influence the person–technology match.

It cannot be emphasized enough that proper device selection must be part of a comprehensive evaluation guided by a conceptual practice model (see Chapter 2). If this does not occur and the evaluation is not comprehensive, that is, the client is not included in the evaluation process, or all environmental factors are not considered (i.e. whether equipment can fit into the space, storage, time needed to set up and use), or an adequate trial period is not provided, this could lead to abandonment of the equipment, or possibly further musculoskeletal or neuromotor compromise.

In this chapter we will present seating and positioning content relevant to situations that the TEI practitioner (TEIp) considers other than wheelchair seating and positioning. As mentioned in the previous chapter, seating and positioning is the basis to all functional activities. In this chapter we build on terms and information from Chapter 15 and discuss other situations and settings when seating and positioning might be considered.

Human-tech ladder

Policy and legislation

Numerous policy issues impact the extent to which the devices discussed in this chapter are available to the people who need them. While low-tech mobility devices such as crutches, canes, and walkers are often not a problem to obtain and are what we often think about when we think of mobility devices, other devices discussed in this chapter may be more challenging to fund. Please refer to the previous chapter and to Chapter 4 for more information on this topic.

Human factors and common conditions that challenge seating and positioning

Physical

There are a variety of reasons that people of all ages might need to use positioning and mobility devices. In many cases we need to consider physical positioning for those who do not have disabilities, as we will describe in the section on seating. The ergonomics of seating is an area of great concern, as many of us spend over half of our waking hours in a seated position (Matthews et al. 2008). Therefore, ergonomics of seating will be included in this chapter along with other TEI. In other cases, people may need seating and positioning options to compensate for or treat a variety of medical conditions. These conditions may be lifelong or temporary or acquired at different stages during the life span. They may be static or progressive and result from a variety of physical factors and conditions such as cerebral palsy, head injury or other neurologic injury, muscular dystrophy, cancer, and aging, to name a few (Trefler et al. 1993).

Psychological

In addition to the consideration of physical factors, which influence matching a person with a device, psychological factors must be considered as well. These include the individual's cognitive functioning, motivation, and willingness to use the device. These factors have been considered in other Chapters (13 and 15), but we mention it again as these factors may significantly influence whether or not an individual will accept and be able to use a device, no matter how well it may meet their physical needs. For example, we may all know older family members who could benefit from the use of a cane or a walker but will not use those devices because they don't want the stigma they feel may be associated with it, so the cane the therapist or doctor prescribed hangs on the doorknob. On the other hand, fear of falling and the need to be able to get around may be just what is needed for someone to incorporate a mobility device into their daily lives (Griffiths et al. 2015). As described in Chapter 11, numerous psychological factors influence one's decisions regarding whether or not to use TEI, and identifying these factors is part of the comprehensive evaluation the provider completes with the client. See Box 16.1 for an example of seating for function in a classroom.

Box 16.1 Seating for function: Using classroom seating as an example

Students sit in a wide variety of classroom chairs from grade school to college. They are either attached to or independent of the desk. Matching the appropriate desk to the student is often difficult. Each desk in a classroom is typically the same size regardless of the great variation in the height and physical characteristics of each student (Saarni et al. 2007). Ideally, the student should be seated with their pelvis positioned as close to the rear of the chair as possible. Thighs should be supported by the seat of the chair to within 1–2 in. of the back of the knee, with the feet in contact with the floor (Cornell University Ergonomics Web 2015). If the seat is too deep (or the student is too short for the seat), then they may slide forward off of the seat, and if the seat is too shallow (or the student is too tall for the seat), then pressure is on their bottom instead of equally distributed, making sitting for longer durations uncomfortable and inefficient.

In addition to comfort and efficiency, Wingrat and Exner (2005) found that students seated in smaller, better-fitting furniture were more on task than when seated in larger furniture. Another study showed the fit of furniture may have a significant impact on object manipulation skills of young children, with more complex hand skills requiring stabilization being most affected by the quality of the child's seated position (Smith-Zuzovsky and Exner 2004).

A chair that is too tall with a seat that is too deep often forces the student to sit in a posterior pelvic tilt with decreased lumbar lordosis, increased thoracic kyphosis, and capital extension (Figures 16.1 and 16.2)[1].

This position does not allow for positive support through the feet to assist with maintaining an erect posture. Students may then have difficulty reaching their desks. Poor positioning for students with neuromotor compromise would have greater impact, as seen in their inability to regulate their respiration efficiently, which would have an impact on their ability to speak effectively as well as remain alert and on task (Costigan and Light 2010).

A chair that is too small for a student causes increased hip and knee flexion resulting in hamstring shortening. Because the chair does not support the thighs, the student's weight is no longer distributed over a large surface area, which results in increased pressure at the ischial tuberosities and sacrum. This can then cause discomfort, which can lead to decreased ability to sit for long periods, as the student will be forced to repeatedly shift their weight off their overloaded ischial tuberosities and sacrum. These students often will frequently move in their chairs throughout the duration of a task (Box 16.2).

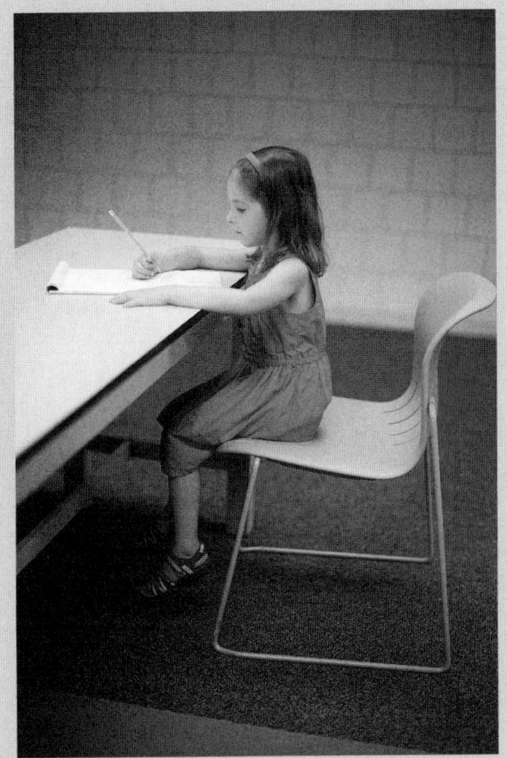

Figure 16.1 A chair that is too tall with a seat that is too deep.

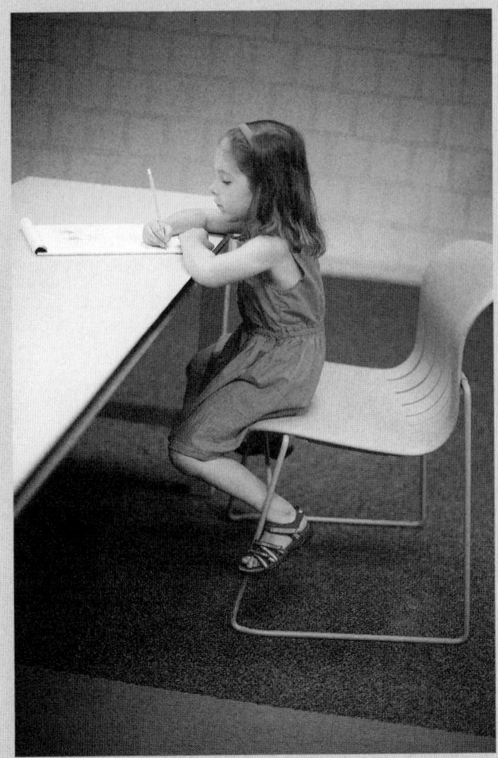

Figure 16.2 Student sitting in a posterior pelvic tilt with decreased lumbar lordosis, increased thoracic kyphosis, and capital extension.

Low Tone

Low tone can occur for a variety of reasons. Selection of a classroom chair for an individual with decreased tone and strength throughout their core may include a wedged seat that is high in the back to promote an anterior pelvic tilt position (Kim et al. 2014). The anterior pelvic tilt then creates and upright trunk with improved spinal, head, neck, scapular, and shoulder alignment. Foot support is required to sustain this position. This position is active and promotes increased attention (Kangas 2016). Placing the pelvis in a slight anterior pelvic tilt activates the core musculature and forces the student to work to maintain this position. A student with low tone would not be able to sustain this position throughout the day and still meet cognitive learning demands of the educational environment because these students inadvertently focus more on their positioning needs (through leaning on their arms, slouching, frequent repositioning, etc.) and end up missing content in the process (Stindt et al. 2009). The addition of a wedge may be beneficial for times when active participation is critical (Figure 16.3), with the wedge removed during less active periods such as leisure reading (Goncalves and Arezes 2012).

Students with low core strength who present with poor seated postures often show other subtle signs and have difficulty in other academic areas. For example, when a student is challenged academically or asked to perform a writing task, they may place the elbow of the hand opposite their writing hand on a support surface and hold their head. This student may also display poor handwriting and unwillingness to write more than a sentence or two. These signs are often misinterpreted as academic difficulties when in reality the student's low core strength may be a large contributing factor (Smith-Zuzovsky and Exner 2004). Students with low tone have difficulty

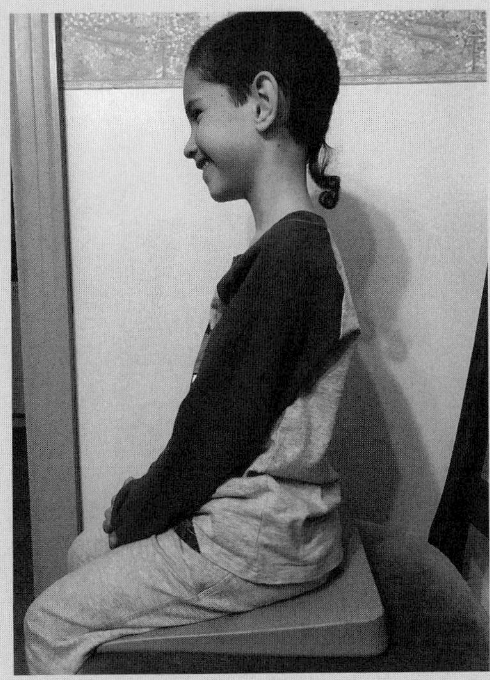

Figure 16.3 Use of a wedge for positioning.

activating the musculature around the trunk that is needed to remain in an upright position for the duration of an activity. These muscles need to remain active so that muscles around the shoulder and elbow and the hand muscles can then have a stable base to work off to do a task such as handwriting. When the student is unable to keep their trunk muscles active, they will often be seen leaning into the desk with their trunk, or laying on the table in an attempt to stabilize their trunk muscles (Stindt et al. 2009). Other students with low core strength prefer to lie on the floor where they are able to gain maximal stability when performing combined writing and cognitive tasks.

A challenge for these students as they age is that they are often less likely to accept and use additional seating supports so as not to stand out from their peers. As mentioned above, this is one of the psychological factors, which can impact the successful adoption of a TEI.

High Tone

For students with greater positioning needs, such as those with high tone, there are a variety of alternate seating systems available for use in a classroom (see Figure 16.4) (Furumasu 2018).

These systems are highly adjustable and have a variety of available positioning supports such as shoe holders, pelvic supports, trunk laterals, and head positioning supports (see Figures 16.5 and 16.6). In addition, alternate seating systems often include options for tilt and/or recline and height adjustment to enable young students to sit on the floor with their peers or at a table for a group activity. Options such as pistons to absorb extension forces are also available on certain models.

Similar to children's classroom seating, university and office seating or seating other functional tasks poses similar challenges for many individuals.

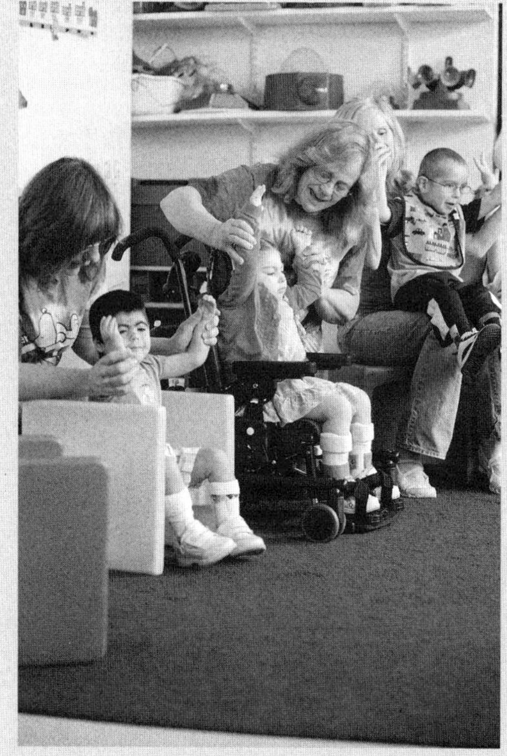

Figure 16.5 Seating options with positioning supports such as shoe holders. Source: Photos © 2017 by Rifton Equipment. Used by permission.

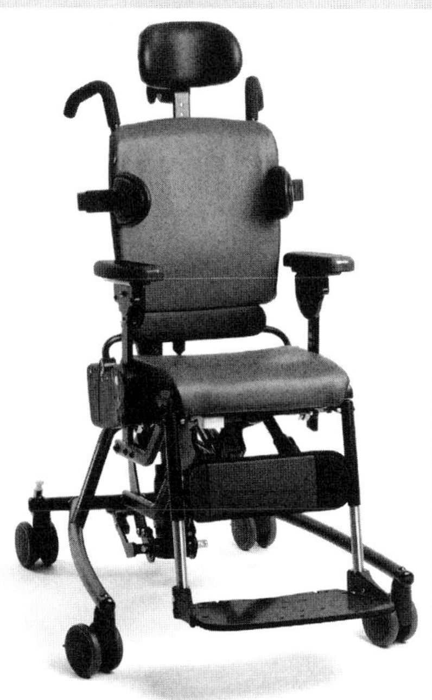

Figure 16.4 Alternate seating System. Source: Photo © 2017 by Rifton Equipment. Used by permission.

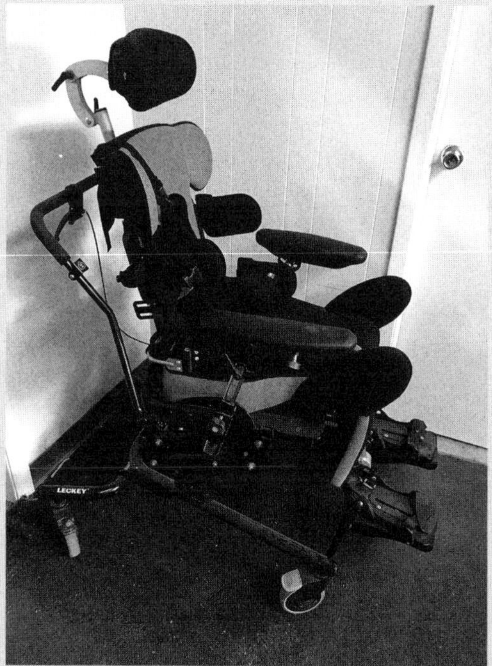

Figure 16.6 Seating options with positioning supports, pelvic supports, trunk laterals, and head positioning supports.

Box 16.2 Here's the evidence

Smith-Zuzovsky, N. and Exner, C. (2004). The effect of seated positioning quality on typical 6- and 7-year-old children's object manipulation skills. *American Journal of Occupational Therapy* 58(4): 380–388. doi: 10.5014/ajot.58.4.380.

Key Words: children, classroom furniture, fine motor skills development

Purpose: This study investigated the effect of seating in individually fitted seating vs. standard classroom furniture on the object manipulation skills of 6- to 7-year-old children measured by the In Hand Manipulation Test.

Sample/Setting: Forty students from an elementary school in Maryland participated in the study.

Method: An experimental research design was used for the study. IMT performance of two groups of 20 children was compared. One group was positioned in standard, too-large classroom furniture that did not support an optimal seated position, and one group was positioned optimally in furniture fitted to each child for tabletop activities, which allowed for hip flexion to 90°, foot placement on the floor, and the table to be at flexed elbow height.

Findings: Independent group's t tests indicated that children who were optimally positioned performed significantly better ($t = -2.77$, $df = 38$, $p < 0.01$) than children who were tested in the too-large standard classroom furniture. The study's results suggest that the fit of furniture relative to the child's size may have a significant impact on a young, typical child's object manipulation skills.

Critical Thinking Questions:

1. After reading this research article, what do you understand to be the limitations of this research? Are there any limitations not stated?
2. If you were to replicate this study using a different method or design, what designs would you use to increase the rigor and why?
3. Based on the findings of this study, what additional research do you think is needed that is not addressed in the discussion section?

Ambulation aids

Ambulation aids, much like standers, which will be discussed later in the chapter, come in a variety of types, with multiple supports and accessories. When selecting an ambulation aid, the function of the task should be considered. These functions may include to improve the client's balance, assist propulsion during gait, reduce weight or load on one or more of their extremities, improve posture, enable the client to access areas inaccessible to them when in a wheelchair, provide a safer means of ambulation, or provide a means of ambulation that may not otherwise be possible (Cameron and Monroe 2007). Low-tech basic ambulation aids include crutches and canes, which can come with a single tip or have a wider quadruped four-tipped base to add increased stability (see Figures 16.7 and 16.8).

Canes can be solid or folding and are usually height adjustable. The most commonly used types of crutches include axillary crutches and forearm or loft strand crutches. Axillary crutches can be wooden or metal and are adjustable (see Figure 16.9). Loft strand crutches are usually metal and have a forearm cuff (see Figure 16.10). These are typically height adjustable as well.

Walkers can also be considered a low-tech ambulation aid (Bolding et al. 2018). A basic walker can be used anteriorly or posteriorly. Walkers are lightweight, usually folding, and easily transportable. Their light weight and foldability make it easy to put them in a vehicle.

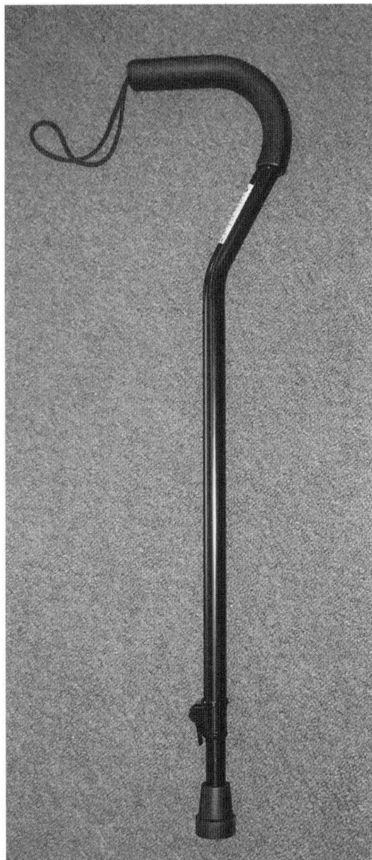

Figure 16.7 A single tipped cane.

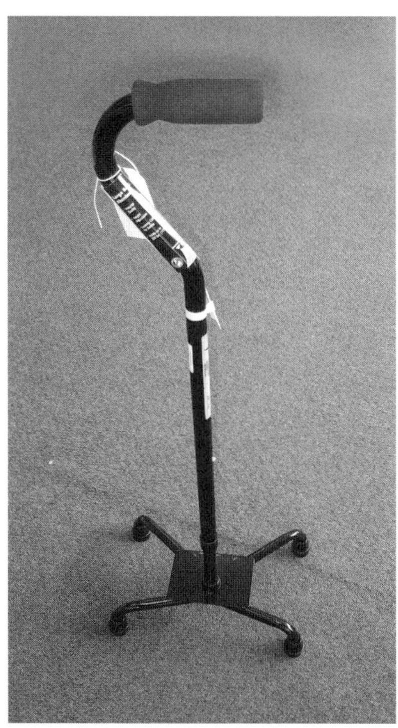

Figure 16.8 A cane with a quadruped four-tipped base.

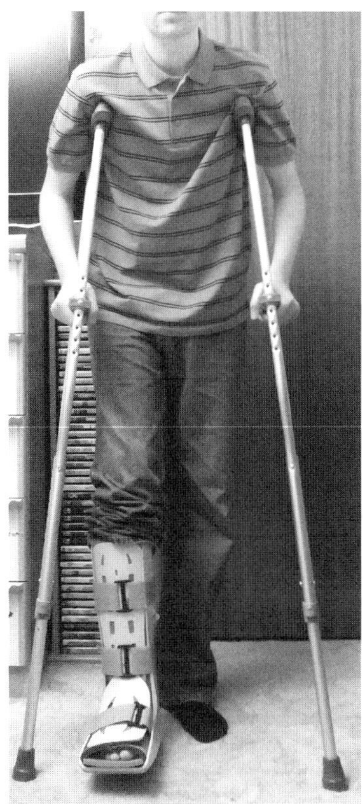

Figure 16.9 Axillary crutches. Source: https://commons.wikimedia.org/wiki/File:Axillary_(underarm)_crutches.JPG. Licensed under CC BY SA 4.0.

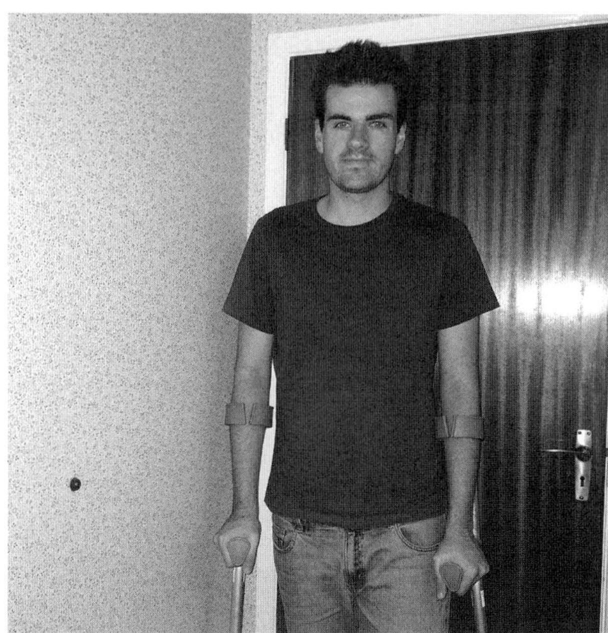

Figure 16.10 Loft strand crutches. Source: https://upload.wikimedia.org/wikipedia/commons/f/f6/Teenage_boy_on_crutches.jpg. Licensed under CC BY SA 4.0.

Because they are lightweight, if they are not used appropriately, they can tip easily. Walkers can have a standard tip bottom, glides, or be set up with two or four rolling wheels (Figure 16.11). A rollator walker has three or four wheels and usually includes a seat to enable the user to sit and rest when fatigued. Rollator walkers should never be used instead of a transport chair or wheelchair.

If an individual requires more support to walk, there are multiple models of basic gait trainers (see Figures 16.12 and 16.13). A standard gait trainer can be set up for use with the individual facing in an anterior or posterior direction. These devices have a wheeled base and can have a variety of supports, including trunk support, upper extremity supports, leg or thigh supports, and on some models, head support. They can include larger wheels for outdoors, and other wheel options such as drag, no-roll-back, or lock. The individual can require assistance from a caregiver to get into and out of a gait trainer and to fasten all of the accessories.

In addition to basic gait trainers, there are partial weight-bearing or weight assist models (see Figure 16.14). These generally work with a spring, hydraulic, or suspension action to help alleviate a portion of the user's body weight, making it easier for them to take steps.

The spring or hydraulic systems are set up similar to the basic gait trainers mentioned above. This type of gait trainer is useful not only for gait but also for working in a sitting-to-standing plane, as once the user is in, they can

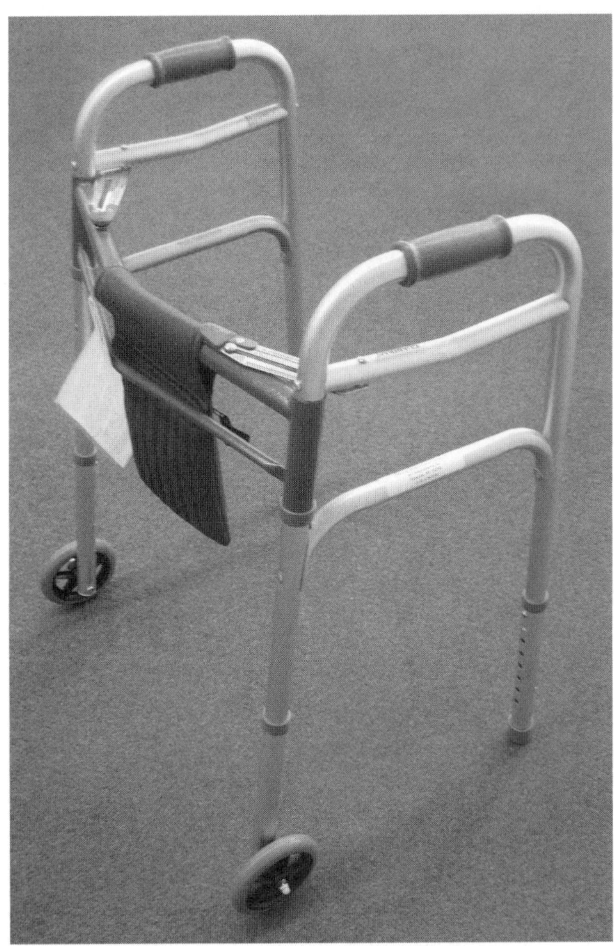

Figure 16.11 Walker – can have all four legs stationary, wheels on just the front two legs, or wheels on all four legs.

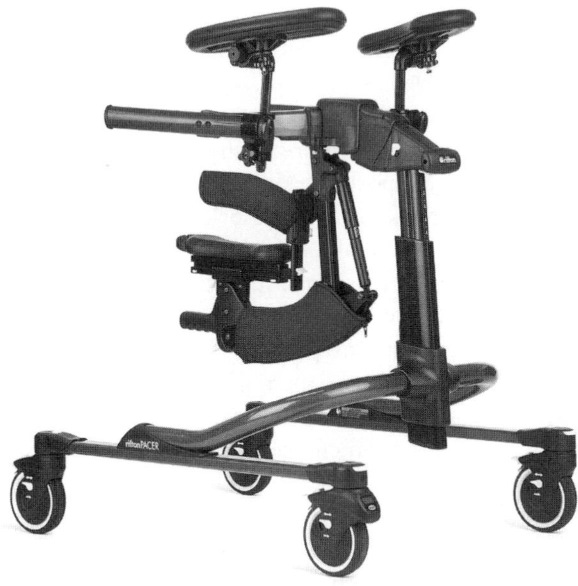

Figure 16.12 Gait trainer with a variety of supports. Source: Photo © 2017 by Rifton Equipment. Used by permission.

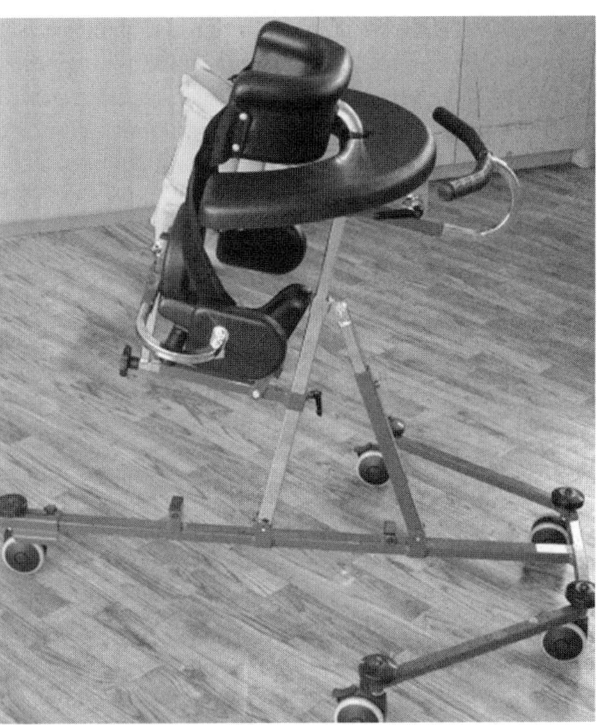

Figure 16.13 Gait trainer.

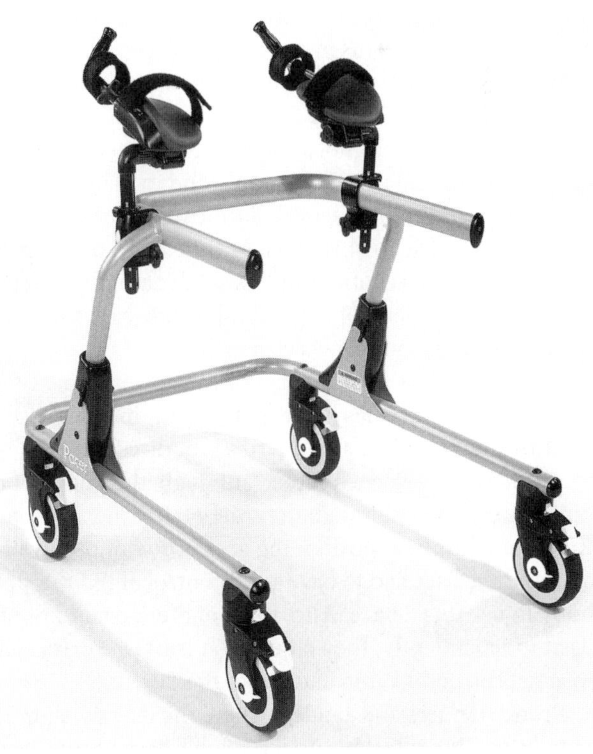

Figure 16.14 Gait trainer that allows for vertical movement.

easily move between the two positions. A standard gait trainer does not typically allow for practicing this transition if the user is using accessories such as a standard trunk support or a saddle. Some newer models combine side-to-side and vertical motion to allow the user to be suspended while focusing on the motions of the gait cycle. Suspension-based systems are often very large models where the user is in a harness and will gait train in one spot, usually over a treadmill. These are typically found in a physical therapy gym or rehab center (Gharib et al. 2011).

When deciding on a walker or gait trainer and their appropriate supports, selection will depend on what stage of rehabilitation the individual using the device is in, as well as where they will be using it. An individual may start with one type of gait device and then progress to another. As with standers, a vendor can assist with obtaining demonstration units for trial if a facility does not have ones available, so an individual can try out a variety of different types with supports to determine which will work best for them. As mentioned above, trialing the equipment is a critical part of a comprehensive evaluation, and neglecting the trial period can lead to inappropriate equipment being prescribed/purchased as well as equipment abandonment.

Standing

Standing has many benefits for an individual who would otherwise be exclusively using a wheelchair or have very limited mobility. Although many clinicians have been able to state the benefits of standing to their patients, this is an area of evidence-based practice that is continuing to evolve (Dicianno et al. 2013; Paleg et al. 2013). To stand alone is often impossible, as it can take multiple caregivers to stand up with an adult, and to maintain this standing position for a period of time would be very difficult. To assist with this, devices have been developed that can be either static standers or dynamic standers. There are a variety of types and some can even be integrated into a power wheelchair base.

A standing box or frame is the earliest example of a stander. These frames were easily and inexpensively built from home with a standard set of directions. They were often for small children, although they could be built in any size. Although they were fairly inexpensive, there were minimal positioning accessory options available and the user had to have good control of their upper body to use this device. Also, most of them could not be used independently; they required at least one caregiver to assist the person into and out of the device.

Prone standers are standers where the user's weight is mostly on the anterior surface of the user's body (see Figure 16.15). A prone stander has positioning accessories for the trunk and legs, and many have upper extremity support surfaces. They can be angle adjustable, moving from horizontal for easier loading to a vertical position for standing or not. This stander can be a good choice if you are working to promote extension through the body. If the user mildly lacks hip extension, you can use gravity to increase hip extension. Also, most prone standers allow for growth and are available in both pediatric and adult sizes. If a client is eliciting increased extension throughout his or her trunk, head, and neck, this stander may not be the best choice (Aubert 1999). Also, it is difficult to use a prone stander alone due to the strapping involved.

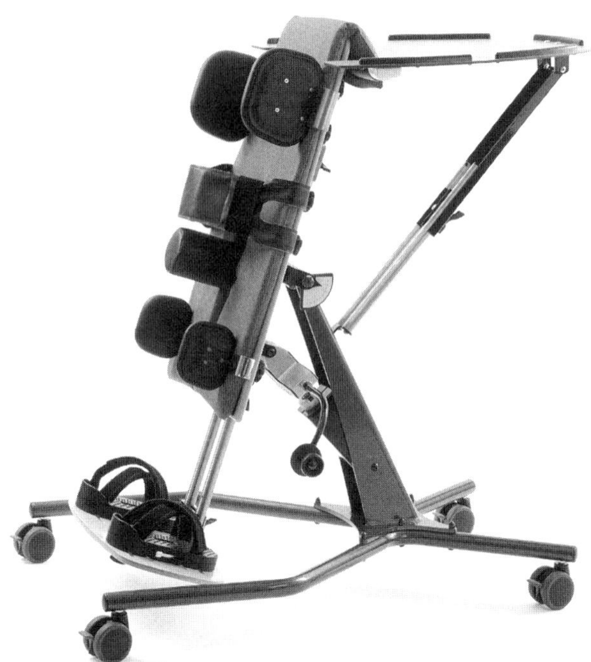

Figure 16.15 Prone stander. Source: Photo © 2017 by Rifton Equipment. Used by permission.

In a supine stander, the user's back is against the back of the stander, and they are facing out. They have full support along the posterior surface of their body. Supine standers have positioning accessories for the trunk, legs, and head. The position of the stander can be angle adjustable, similar to a prone stander, from horizontal to vertical. This allows the individual standing to be transferred over in a supine position, have all of the positioning straps secured, then moved into a standing position to an angle that is comfortable to them. This stander can be a good choice for individuals with poor head control, due to this adjustable angle. This stander often requires caregiver assistance, due to the strapping and adjusting the angle from horizontal to vertical. If you have a client who has increased upper trunk, neck, and head flexion, or an increased kyphosis, or muscle asymmetries, this stander may not be the ideal choice (Aubert 1999). There are also several standers that can

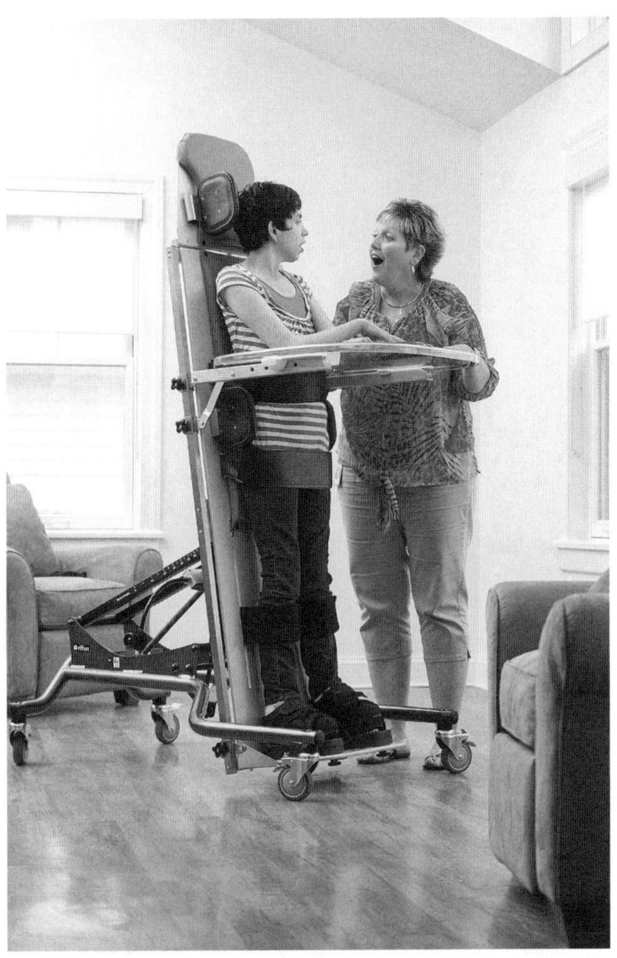

Figure 16.16 Multi-position stander. Source: Photo © 2017 by Rifton Equipment. Used by permission.

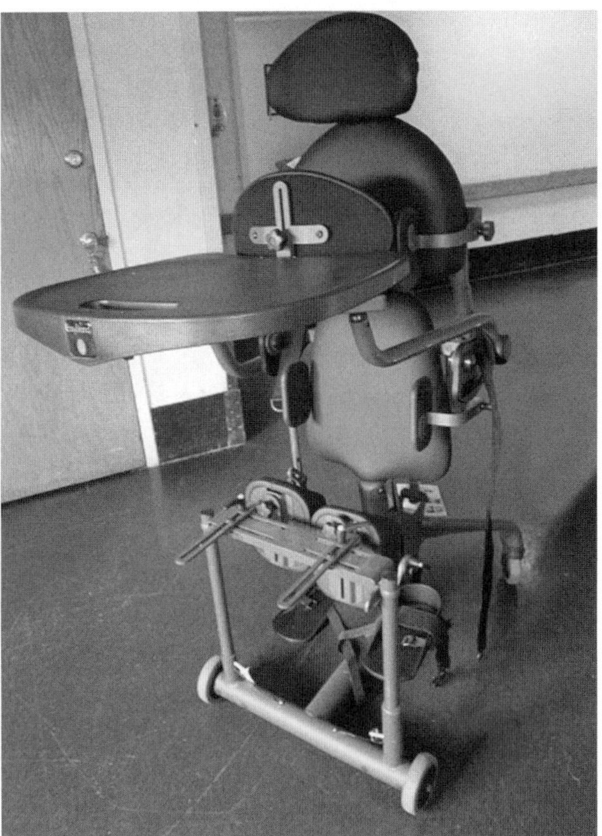

Figure 16.17 Sit-to-stand stander.

be used in multiple positions and switched between prone and supine to be used either way (Figure 16.16).

The final option of independent standing devices is a sit-to-stand stander. With this stander, the user can transfer into the device in a seated position, fasten the required supports, and then transition into a standing position. Similar to the supine stander, you can stop at any point on the way up through the transition for increasing incremental weight-bearing. The standing support and weight-bearing surfaces are through the feet, knees, buttocks, and trunk. There are additional positioning accessories available for the feet, trunk, and head. This stander can be used if the user does not have full knee or hip range of motion (ROM). Also, the user can use this stander more independently. If the user does not have full head control (the head falls into a flexed position), or if they are severely osteoporotic, this may not be an ideal choice (Figure 16.17). There is also a power option to assist with moving the user from a seated to standing position.

Both prone standers and sit-to-stand standers have mobile options. These are wheel attachments that allow the individual to make the stander move when they are in it. Another option that is available on the sit-to-stand style standing device is a glider option, which allows the individual, once they are standing, to unlock the stander and then to move their arms and legs opposite of each other in a walking pattern. All of these mobile options require the user to have good upper extremity and head control (Figure 16.18).

When recommending a stander for an individual, first, consult their primary care physician to be sure that standing is safe and recommended. There are reasons why standing may not be recommended (Paleg et al. 2013). Contraindication or precautions may include:

- Current bony or muscular contractures or deformities: If an individual has a fixed posture that they are unable to move out of and attempting to stand would cause pain, or if they have decreased sensation, this may cause harm. Change in alignment should be closely watched while moving into a standing position (Arva et al. 2009)
- Decreased bone mineral density (BMD): Although osteoporosis may be a precaution, a diagnosis such as osteogenesis imperfecta requires serious consideration (Campbell et al. 2000). Standing with low BMD can cause fractures and should be done with caution.

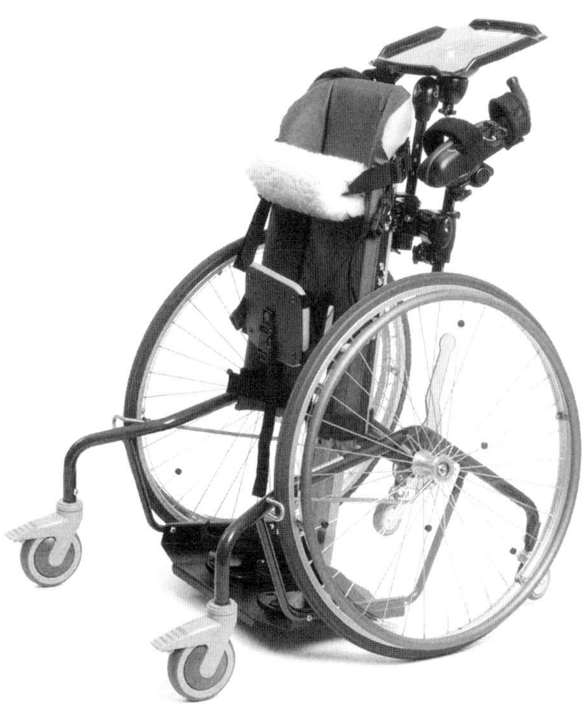

Figure 16.18 Sit-to-stand-style standing device with a glider option. Source: Photo © 2017 by Rifton Equipment. Used by permission.

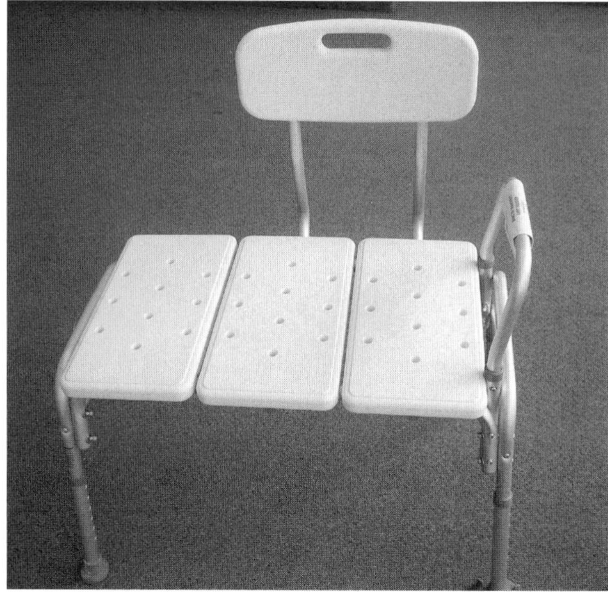

Figure 16.19 Long tub bench with back support.

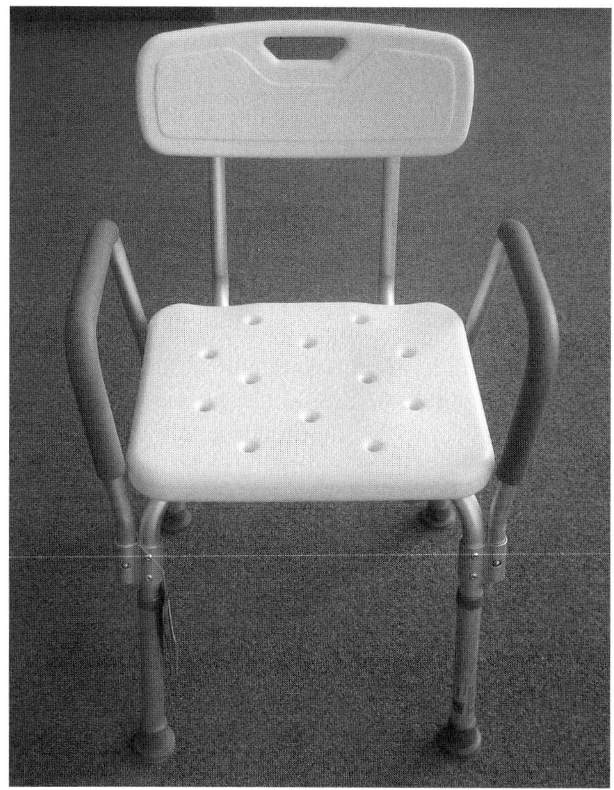

Figure 16.20 Shower chair with arm supports.

- Orthostatic hypotension, postural tachycardia syndrome, or orthostatic intolerance syndrome: Monitor patient's heart rate and blood pressure when standing and if the individual is able to tell you they are dizzy or lightheaded.

When selecting a stander for patient use or purchase, the factors above will all come into consideration. In addition, size of the device should be considered if it would be used in the home. Demonstration units can be obtained through vendors for trials prior to purchase to determine if the supports will be adequate and if the stander will meet the needs of the individual. These can be made available at the time of the evaluation.

Bathing and toileting equipment

There are a variety of supports available to assist individuals in the bathroom with the activity of daily living (ADL) of bathing and toileting. Supports in the bathroom can be required for individuals who have minor balance challenges. Such supports include tub benches, commode seats, or grab bars (Figures 16.19–16.21) for individuals post injury or surgery, such as a raised toilet seat, or for individuals with a more permanent level of need, such as an adapted shower chair (Figure 16.22). These supports range from very minimal to very high end. They can be separate items, such as a tub and toilet like in most homes, or can be one combined item to save space and money.

If an individual will require an adapted toileting system because they are unable to sit on a typical toilet, either

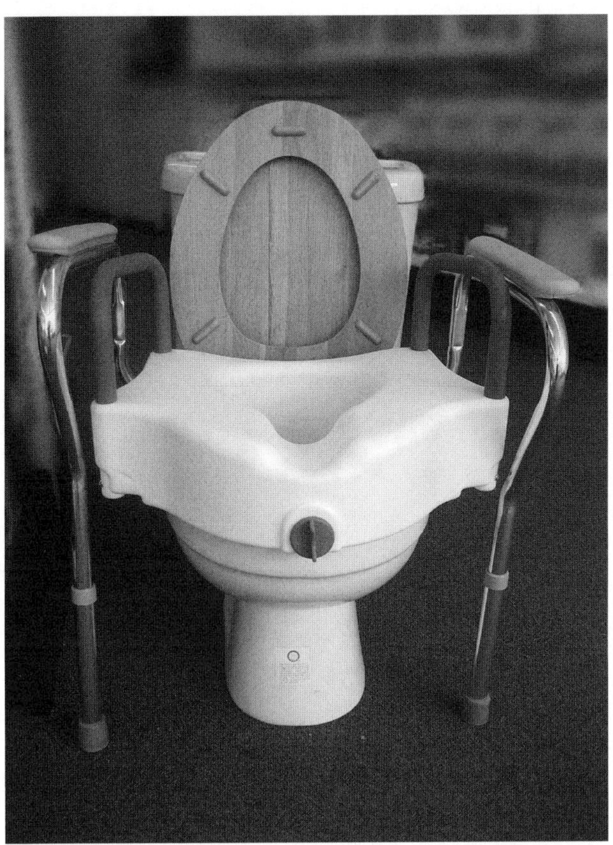

Figure 16.21 Raised commode seat and arm supports.

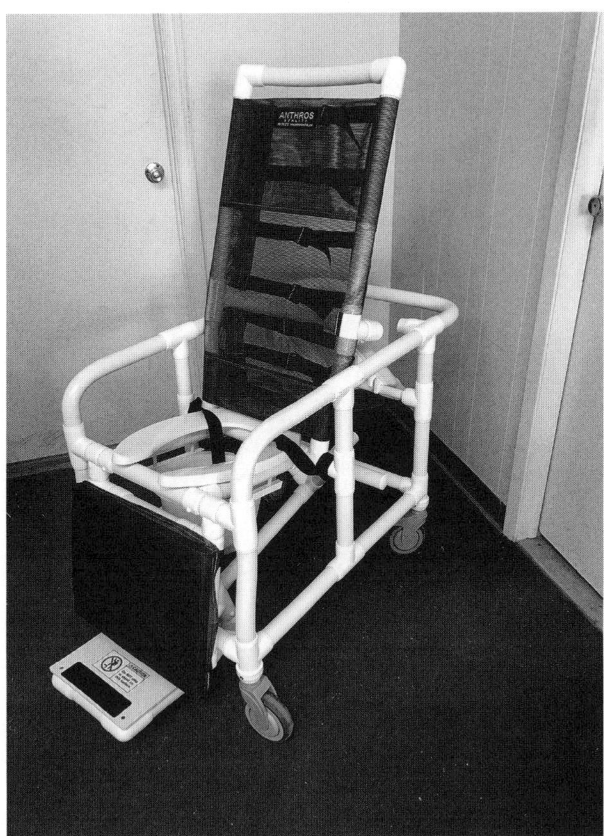

Figure 16.22 Adapted shower chair here.

due to injury or because they require an increasing level of support that a typical toilet will not provide, there are two main types. There are toileting systems/supports that can connect directly to the toilet or be used in conjunction with the existing toilet, and ones that are freestanding. Toileting systems that connect to the toilet can be mounted using a variety of methods, but generally are connected via the bolt that holds on the toilet seat. These can have a back with support and an alternate seat, and, depending on the model, some can be removable so others in the house can also use the toilet. The size also depends on the model (Figures 16.23 and 16.24). If the user is removing the system, there is the issue of storage.

Freestanding models are used with a bucket system and generally have additional levels of support. These models can come with positioning supports such as headrests, chest support, positioning belts, and foot rests. These toileting chairs may also have a tilt-in-space feature to assist with positioning. Due to this feature, there may be difficulty fitting it over a standard toilet, as the back of the toilet chair would interfere with the back of the toilet. There are several hybrid models on the market currently that provide increased supports such as chest and head support, belts, foot supports, and minimal tilt, and are able to be wheeled directly over the toilet for use there as well. These systems tend to have a large footprint, so storage of the item needs to be considered. Most are made of PVC or a rust-free metal with a mesh or other waterproof material and can also double as a showering/bathing chair to avoid adding further equipment to the house (Figures 16.25–16.29).

Showering or bathing equipment is also made out of a PVC or rust-free metal frame with a mesh, plastic, or waterproof material-based seat and back. They can be as simple as a shower bench or board that can be placed within a bathtub to assist an individual who has difficulty with sliding in and out of the tub or just to give a supported seating surface (Figure 16.30).

A lift-style system with hand control is another option, which a user would sit in and then be lifted from one side of a tub up and over into the bathtub. Simple manual wheelchair-style bath chairs are another option, as these can roll into a walk-in shower or can be a more complex support system, as mentioned above, similar to the toileting systems but with a solid seat. Tilt-in-space bathing systems often come with a high- or low-base option. The low-base option is used with smaller children in a bathtub, as they can be partially submerged

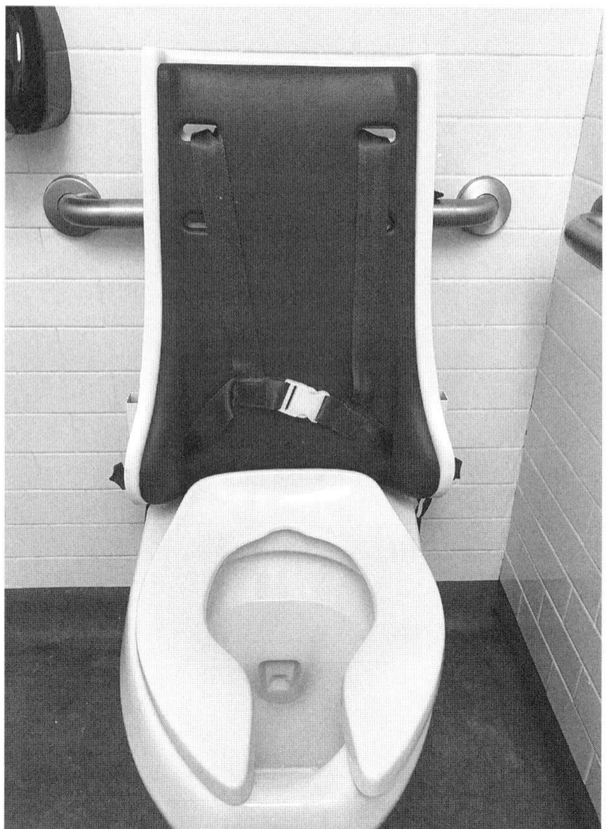

Figure 16.23 Toileting system with back support.

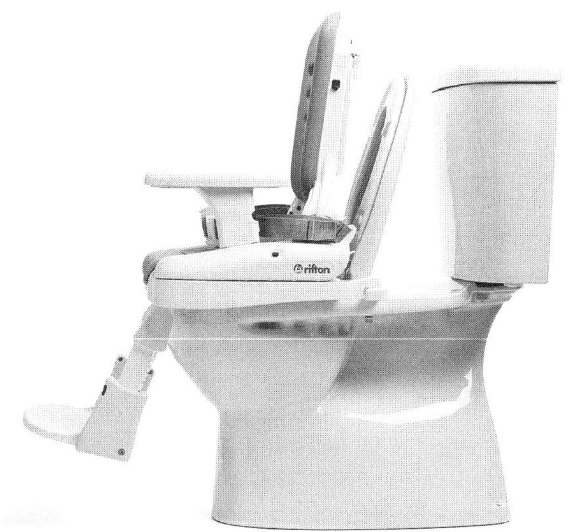

Figure 16.24 Toileting system. Source: Photo © 2017 by Rifton Equipment. Used by permission.

in the water but still have the required support of the bathing system. The higher, wheeled bases are used more often with older individuals, as these are easier to transfer in and out of. This style of chair works best in a roll-in shower-type bathroom.

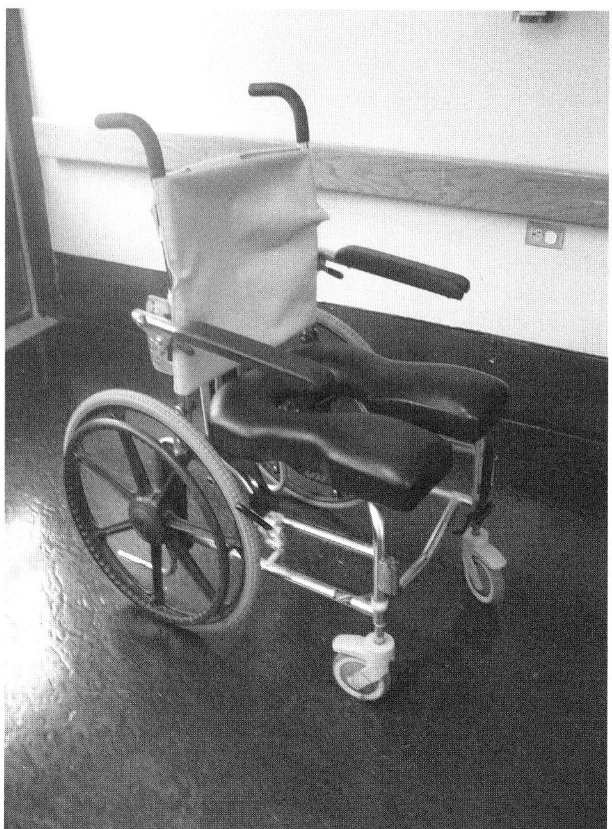

Figure 16.25 Wheeled toileting chair.

When evaluating an individual for a toileting or shower chair there are a few critical components to consider. First, the evaluator would need to interview the user regarding the setup of their current home, inquiring about the layout of their bathroom, storage needs, needs of other users, and ability for the equipment to be cleaned on a regular basis. When assessing the client, making an informed decision on factors such as patient tone (high or low), ability to assist with transfers, sitting balance and postural control for the duration of a bath/shower or while toileting, ROM, and the safety awareness of the patient should be considered. After all information is gathered, an informed decision can be made to determine which system would be the correct fit for the patient. Although it is optimal for a demonstration unit to be trialed, due to hygiene reasons this often is not possible with toileting and showering equipment. Vendors may allow a fitting with the clients clothing in place in the clinic setting to assess appropriate fit of the toileting or shower chair. If either a trial or a fitting is not possible, a correct size and type of device would have to be selected based on measurements provided from vendor literature.

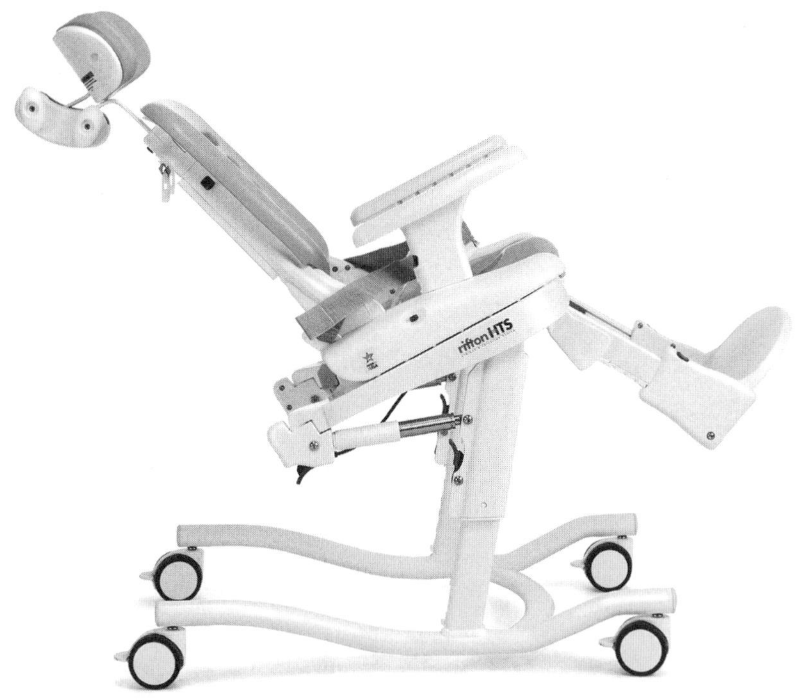

Figure 16.26 Mobile shower commode chair. Source: Photo © 2017 by Rifton Equipment. Used by permission.

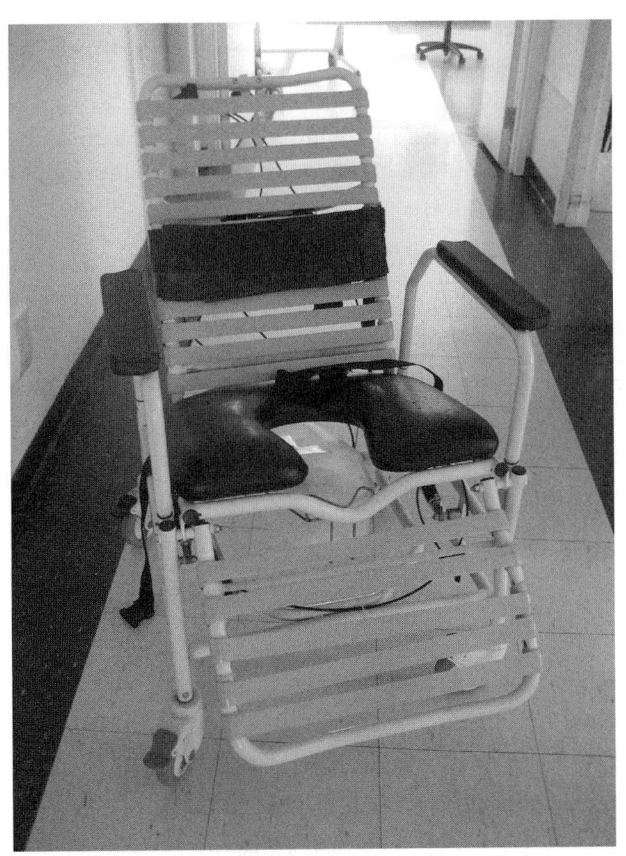

Figure 16.27 Waterproof shower commode chair.

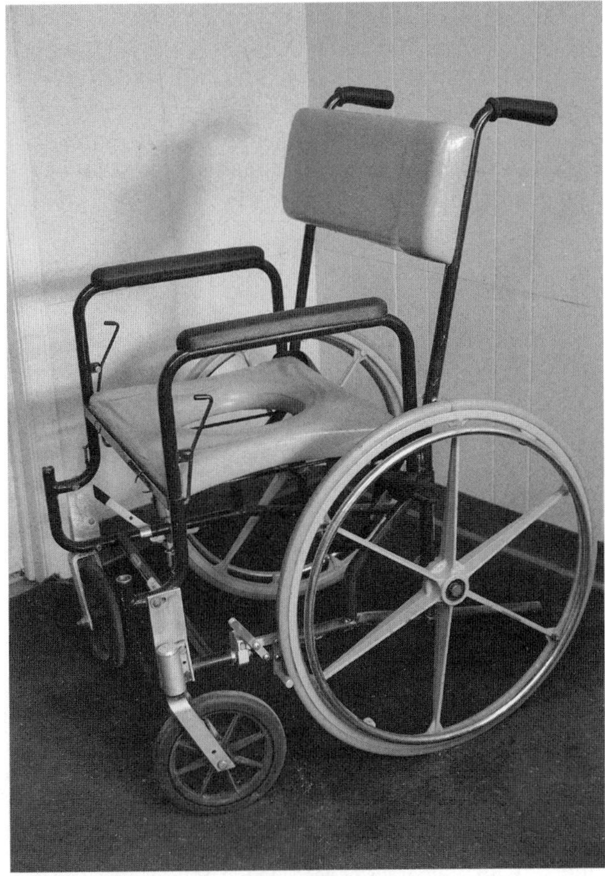

Figure 16.28 Wheeled commode chair.

Mechanical lift and transfer systems

There are three main types of mechanical lift systems: overhead, full assist floor or mobile lifts, and sit-to-stand lifts. There are accessories to go with each of these styles of lifts, such as batteries for the motorized lifts, and slings.

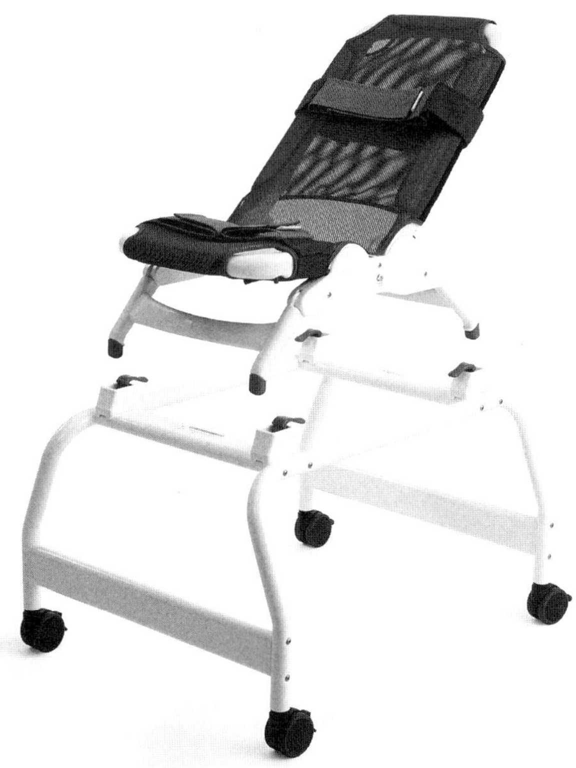

Figure 16.29 Mesh shower chair. Source: Photo © 2017 by Rifton Equipment. Used by permission.

There are two main types of overhead lift systems: ceiling-mounted and free-standing track lift. The ceiling-mounted system is installed on the user's ceiling in various rooms within their home (Figure 16.31). This system is popular within schools or residential facilities or in any setting where floor space is limited. The user requires a sling, which would be placed underneath their body and would attach to a bar on the lift that is lowered down. The bar then rises via a hand remote control to raise the user up off the surface; they can then move anywhere within the tracking system to the desired location. One of the benefits of this system is that it does not require any additional floor space within the user's dwelling, making it ideal for small spaces such as bathrooms. Slings for these systems come in various shapes and types, including anti-shear, bathing, and toileting styles. The free-standing system attaches to two or four posts and would go over the top of the user's bed (Figure 16.32). This is good for areas where you need the benefit of an overhead lift system but either the ceiling structure will not support the weight of the user or the individual is living in rental property and a more temporary solution is required.

A floor or mobile lift will also require the use of slings, similar to a ceiling-mounted lift. The difference with this lift is that it has a wheeled base and moves on the floor within the user's living space (Figure 16.33). These lifts can be a manual pump style, meaning the user has to pump a handle to raise an individual up or

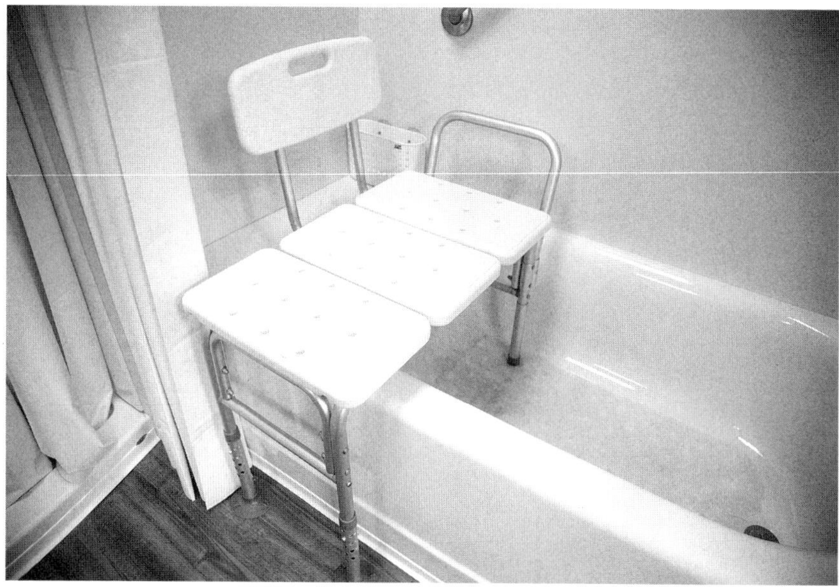

Figure 16.30 Tub transfer bench in tub. Source: https://en.wikipedia.org/wiki/Transfer_bench#/media/File:Transfer_bench.jpg. Licensed under CC BY SA 2.0.

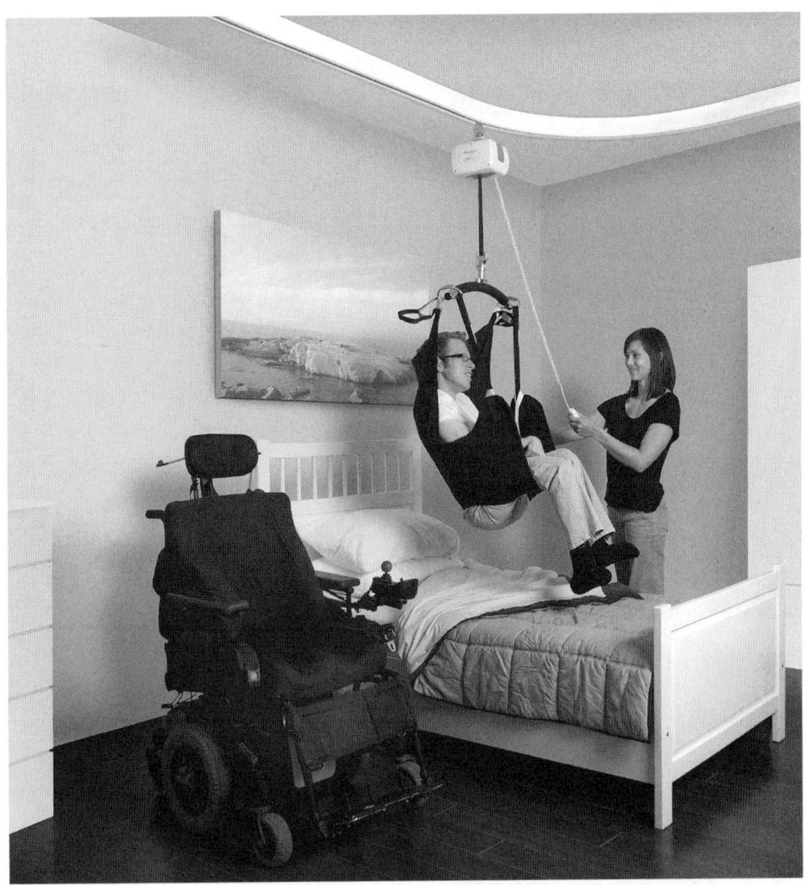

Figure 16.31 Ceiling-mounted lift system. Source: Permission to use photo granted by Handicare.

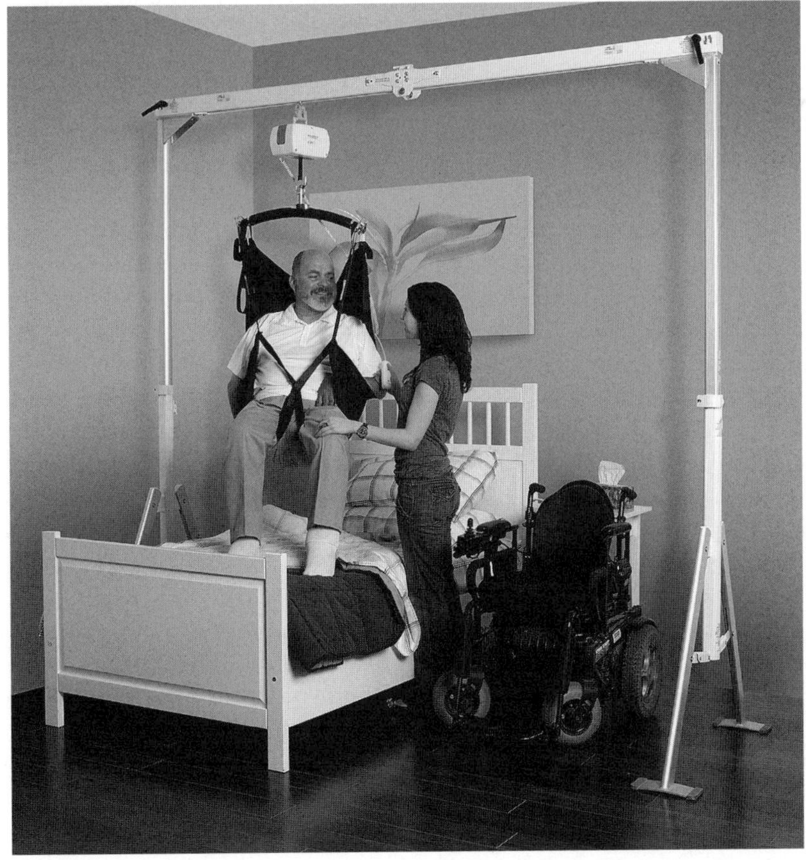

Figure 16.32 Free-standing lift system. |Source: Permission to use photo granted by Handicare.

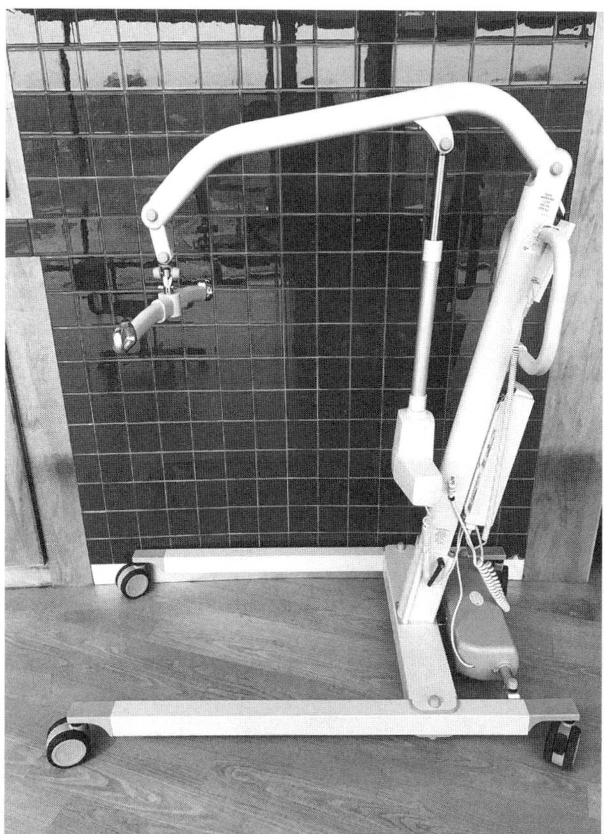

Figure 16.33 Floor-based mobile lift.

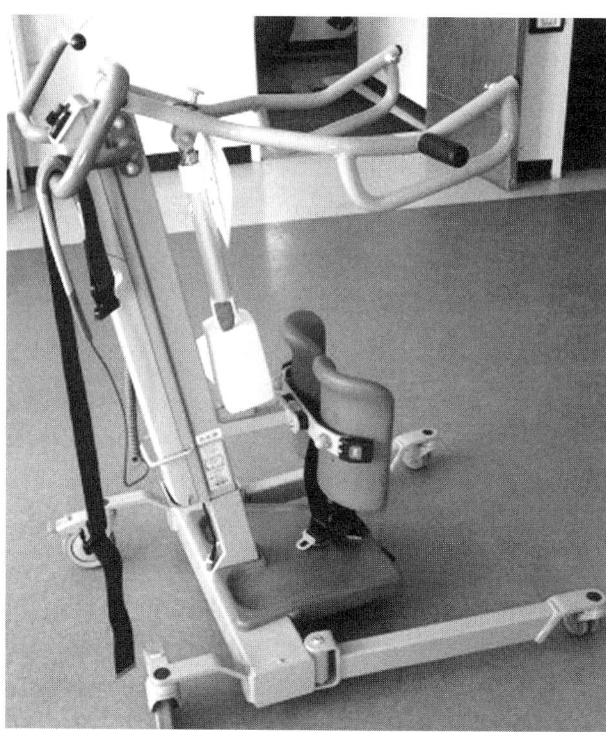

Figure 16.34 Sit-to-stand transfer system with wheeled base.

lower them, or can be battery operated and have a hand remote. One of the benefits of this system is that it is able to move freely within the user's living space; however, it has a large footprint, so this needs to be carefully considered. The large base may prevent its use in smaller spaces such as a small bathroom. Also, to keep the user's weight centered within the base of the system, the wheeled base needs to roll under or around objects such as beds, couches, and chairs. Vertical height measurements and horizontal width measurements should be taken to make sure that the lift will accommodate all living spaces and, if this is not currently the case, that simple modifications like bed raisers could be added.

Sit-to-stand transfer systems have a wheeled base similar to a floor lift, but these differ, as do ceiling-mounted and floor lifts, and these are fully dependent transfers. With a sit-to-stand transfer system, the lift system assists the patient to stand, partially taking their weight to assist with completing the transfer. The user either will have a sling around their trunk or a trunk support, depending on the style of lift. Their feet can be supported on a board so that the wheels can be moved to complete the transfer, or on some models their feet remain free so they can assist with stepping. With this style of lift, the patient must participate in the transfer. If they do not participate by actively bearing weight through their legs and holding their trunk erect, the lift could be dangerous and it would be advised to use one of the other styles of lifts. A vendor can assist with a demonstration unit for trial (Figure 16.34).

When evaluating a client for any rehabilitation device, whether a walker, shower chair, or stander, proper device selection must be part of a comprehensive evaluation guided by a conceptual practice model, as stated in previous chapters. To maximize equipment usage and further independence, re-evaluation should be performed on a regular basis to be sure that the current equipment continues to meet the client's needs. It is also critical that the therapist working within the complex rehabilitation field works closely with their vendors to remain up to date with current products, funding streams, and evidence-based practice in order to be as effective as possible and be able to deliver the best final product to their client. See Box 16.3 for a case study.

Box 16.3 Case study: Billy

Billy is a 13-year-old boy with hypotonic cerebral palsy. He comes into seating clinic with his mother and younger sister, seated in a two-year-old, well-fitting tilt-in-space wheelchair, equipped with a fully supported headrest, trunk support, pelvic belt, and foot sandals. His chair is in 10° of tilt and his head is positioned in cervical flexion with his arms positioned on his lap. His mother states that she is at the clinic because Billy's physical therapist wants him to have a stander at home, as currently he does not have one.

The evaluation begins with a family interview.[2] Billy is nonverbal but able to respond to yes and no questions when prompted. Mom states that Billy is not currently walking or standing for any transfers. His current height is 58″ and his current weight was 99 pounds at their doctor's appointment last month. She states that although she wants him to stand, she is concerned that she would not be able to lift him into or out of a stander as she has seen the staff at his school do, and she verbalizes that the school staff seemed "really big and strong." She also reports that Billy has gained about 15 pounds in the last year. The evaluator enquires about how Billy is currently bathing and toileting. Mom states that he has a toilet-mounted system that she is able to lift him on to and he is successful using that, and he has a PVC framed mesh system on a high frame that rolls into their walk-in shower. When asked about storage and if anyone else used the bathroom, she states that the chair is able to be stored in the shower when it is not being used, and that his sister shares the bathroom with him, so she does have to take the toilet system off and on. She says that they have had the system since he was six years old, and he seems to really be outgrowing it, and the mesh is in need of repair.

With this information, the evaluator moves Billy onto the mat for a mat evaluation. In a seated position, he requires a maximal amount of assistance to remain upright. He prefers to position his pelvis in a posterior pelvic tilt, with a decreased lumbar lordosis, an increased thoracic kyphosis, and a significant amount of cervical neck flexion. With assistance, however, this position can be corrected and he can be brought to neutral, but he is unable to remain there on his own. In supine ROM is taken. He has full hip range, with the exception of hip extension, which is only to neutral. He minimally lacks full knee extension, lacking only 5° of knee extension on both knees. His feet are typical, although he does wear orthotics. His hamstrings are tight, as his hamstring 90/90 measurement or knee extension hamstring flexibility test is only 120° before his pelvis begins to move. This is an important measure in seating to determine the relationship of the pelvis to the seated knee angle.

After gathering the information from the interview and the mat evaluation, the evaluator discusses her findings with Billy's mom and the local complex rehabilitation vendor, who has joined the appointment. The vendor brings knowledge of Billy's insurance coverage, what will be covered and current products on the market. Based on the interview it is clear to the evaluator that Billy needs more than a stander; the evaluator also wants mom to think about a mechanical lift for the home and a new bathing system for Billy. Both Billy and his mom are very open and excited about this and agree that to use both the stander and the larger bathing equipment the lift would be a necessity. The evaluator begins discussing types of lifts – specifically, would an overhead or floor lift best meet Billy's needs. After a thorough discussion, Billy's mom decides that a floor lift would be best and a handle pump style is the least costly alternative that would provide Billy with the ability to change positions.

Next the topic of standers is discussed. In his current school program Billy's physical therapist had been trialing both a supine and a prone stander, as she was working to promote improved active neck extension. Since Billy would be using the stander with the mechanical lift, the prone stander would not be a viable option. The supine stander is determined to meet his needs, as he could easily transfer into it using the mechanical lift, be positioned in a horizontal supine position, and then be moved into a vertical position, relying on gravity as needed to keep his head and neck in an upright position. The chosen supine stander has adequate trunk and lower-extremity supports to keep him safe and upright.

The discussion moves next to bathing equipment. Billy's current style of bathing system is working fine, it is just too small for him. The evaluator asks Billy's mother if she has considered an all-in-one bathing and toileting system, as this will not only provide Billy the postural supports needed for both bathing and toileting, but also eliminate the need for his sister to remove the current toileting system from their shared toilet repeatedly. Although this initially seems like a good plan, in further discussion, concerns arise, as Billy is very successful with his current toileting system. He uses the bathroom approximately every two hours. The concern is that if Billy was just bathed and the system was still wet, he may not be able to comfortably toilet. Therefore, as his current system is still adequate, it is decided to continue with that and to order the bathing chair he has in a larger version.

The request for equipment is processed through Billy's insurance and a short time later is received. All of the equipment was fit to Billy at the time of the delivery by the evaluator and participating vendor. Billy and his family were happy with the process and outcome and are currently using the new equipment in his home setting. As you can see, multiple factors depicted in Vicente's Human-Tech Ladder (2016), including those at the level of the individual and the family, both physical and psychological, had to be considered. Additionally, environmental factors regarding where the intervention was taking place (at home) and funding considerations all impacted the person–technology match that successfully worked for Billy.

Notes

1 Disclaimer: All figures/photos pictured are meant to be representations of the described products only. The authors do not have any associations or relationships with the manufacturers listed. There are many manufacturers of complex rehabilitation equipment and when considering any piece of equipment a thorough evaluation should be completed prior to selecting any piece of equipment.

2 Refer to Appendix A, B, and C from Chapter 15. These are the evaluation tools that should be used by the therapist when working with the DME vendor to evaluate the client for a specific piece of equipment.

References

Arva, J., Paleg, G., Lange, M. et al. (2009). RESNA position on the application of wheelchair standing devices. *Assistive Technology* 21: 161–168.

Aubert, E.J. (1999). Adaptive equipment for physically challenged children. In: *Pediatric Physical Therapy*, vol. 3 (ed. J.S. Tecklin), 423–460. Philadelphia, PA: Lippincott Williams & Wilkins.

Bolding, D., Hughes, C.A., Tipton-Burton, M., and Verran, A. (2018). Mobility. In: *Pedretti's Occupational Therapy Skills; Practice Skills for Physical Dysfunction* (ed. H.M.H. Pendleton and W. Schultz-Krohn), 230–288. St. Louis, MO: Elsevier.

Cameron, M.H. and Monroe, L.G. (eds.) (2007). *Physical Rehabilitation: Evidence-Based Examination, Evaluation and Intervention*. St. Louis, MO: Saunders Elsevier.

Campbell, S.K., Vander Linden, D.W., and Palisano, R.J. (eds.) (2000). *Physical Therapy for Children*. Philadelphia, PA: Saunders.

Cornell University Ergonomics Web (2015). Workstation ergonomics guidelines for computer use by children. Retrieved from http://ergo.human.cornell.edu/cuweguideline.htm.

Costigan, F. and Light, J. (2010). Effect of seated position on upper-extremity access to augmentative communication for children with cerebral palsy: preliminary investigation. *American Journal of Occupational Therapy* 64 (4): 596–604.

Dicianno, B., Morgan, A., Lieberman, J. and Rosen, L. (2013). RESNA position on the application of wheelchair standing devices: 2013 current state of the literature. Retrieved from https://easystand.com/research-and-articles/resna-position-application-wheelchair-standing-devices/.

Dubose, L. and Nelson, G. (2006). Seating, positioning and mobility. Retrieved from vats.org/downloads/attraining06.doc.

Furumasu, J. (2018). Considerations when working with the pediatric population. In: *Seating and Wheeled Mobility: A Clinical Resource Guide* (ed. M. Lange and J. Minkel). Thorofare, NJ: Slack.

Gharib, N., El-Maksoud, G.M., and Rezk-Allah, S.S. (2011). Efficacy of gait trainer as an adjunct to traditional physical therapy on walking performance in hemiparetic cerebral palsied children: a randomized controlled trial. *Clinical Rehabilitation* 25 (10): 924–934.

Goncalves, M. and Arezes, P. (2012). Postural assessment of school children – an input for the design of furniture. *Work* 41: 876–880.

Griffiths, F., Mason, V., Boardman, F. et al. (2015). Evaluating recovery following hip fracture: a qualitative interview study of what is important to patients. *British Medical Journal Open* 5: e005406. https://doi.org/10.1136/bmjopen-2014-005406.

Kangas, K. (2016). Beyond 90/90/90: seating & access to AT. Pre-conference workshop presented at ATIA Conference, Orlando, FL.

Kim, J.-W., Kang, M.-H., Noh, K.-H. et al. (2014). A sloped seat wedge can change the kinematics of the lumbar spine of seated workers with limited hip flexion. *Journal of Physical Therapy Science* 26 (8): 1173–1175.

Matthews, C.E., Chen, K.Y., Freedson, P.S. et al. (2008). Amount of time spent in sedentary behaviors in the United States, 2003–2004. *American Journal of Epidemiology* 167 (7): 875–881. https://doi.org/10.1093/aje/kwm390.

Paleg, G.S., Smith, B.A., and Glickman, L.B. (2013). Systematic review and evidence-based clinical recommendations for dosing of pediatric supported standing programs. *Pediatric Physical Therapy* 25 (3): 232–246.

Saarni, L., Nygård, C.H., Kaukiainen, A., and Rimpelä, A. (2007). Are the desks and chairs at school appropriate? *Ergonomics* 50 (10): 1561–1570. https://doi.org/10.1080/00140130701587368.

Smith-Zuzovsky, N. and Exner, C. (2004). The effect of seated positioning quality on typical 6- and 7-year-old children's object manipulation skills. *American Journal of Occupational Therapy* 58 (4): 380–388.

Stindt, K.J., Reed, P. and Obukowicz, M. (2009). AT for seating, positioning and mobility. Retrieved from http://www.wati.org/free-publications/assessing-students-needs-for-assistive-technology.

Trefler, E., Hobson, D.A., Taylor, S.J. et al. (1993). *Seating and Mobility for Persons with Physical Disabilities*. Tucson, AZ: Therapy Skill Builders.

Vicente, K. (2006). *The Human Factor: Revolutionizing the Way We Live with Technology*. New York: Routledge, Taylor & Francis Group.

Wingrat, J. and Exner, C. (2005). The impact of school furniture on fourth grade children's on-task behavior in the classroom: a pilot study. *Work* 25: 263–272.

Additional resources

www.abledata.com: http://Abledata.com is maintained for the National Institute on Disability and Rehabilitation Research of the US Dept. of Education and provides information and pictures for assistive technology and rehabilitation products.

https://law.resource.org/pub/us/code/ibr/ansi.a117.1.2009.pdf: https://codes.iccsafe.org/content/ICCA117_12017?site_type=public. Provides standards for accessibility throughout all living environments.

17

Communication-related factors

Tina N. Caswell

Outline

Learning outcomes

After reading this chapter, you should be able to:

1. Define augmentative and alternative communication (AAC).
2. Describe the candidates who might benefit from AAC.
3. Describe the significance of the Participation Model and feature matching in the AAC assessment process.
4. Identify no-, low-, mid-, and high-tech options and solutions.
5. Identify intervention strategies that contribute to an individual's communication success.

Active learning prompts

Before you read this chapter:

1. Describe a communication impairment by accessing the American Speech-Language Association (ASHA) website (www.asha.org).
2. Compare and contrast AAC and assistive technology (AT).
3. Complete a web-based search of AAC-related websites (www.isaac-online.org).
4. Observe adults and children utilizing AAC by accessing webcasts.
5. Review the history of the Americans with Disabilities Act (ADA) and its relevance to AAC (www.ada.gov).

Assistive Technologies and Environmental Interventions in Healthcare: An Integrated Approach, First Edition.
Edited by Lynn Gitlow and Kathleen Flecky.

Companion website: www.wiley.com/go/gitlow/assitivetechnologies

Key terms

Communication impairment
Augmentative and alternative communication (AAC)
AAC assessment
Participation Model
Communication partners
Feature matching
Speech-generating devices
Non-dedicated devices
Mobile devices and mobile applications (apps)
Multimodal communication strategies

Introduction

Augmentative and alternative communication (AAC): What and why

> If all my possessions were taken from me with one exception, I would choose the power of communication, for by it I would regain all the rest.
>
> Daniel Webster

The gift of communication, to share personal thoughts, ideas, opinions, and feelings, with family, friends, and colleagues is an essential human need. For most individuals, daily interactions are natural and easy; we don't think about how we engage socially or exchange information with one another. Interactions may take place through spoken or written language, by phone, face-to-face, or by email, text messages, or social media (e.g. Facebook). Communication is a basic human right, it is the gateway to personal relationships, self-advocacy, social acceptance, academic inclusion, and vocational success. We communicate to share stories, express dreams, argue, inquire, wonder, and say "I love you." Through communication we share who we are, our personalities, and what we know. Effortless communication, however, is not an option for all; some individuals are unable to rely on natural speech or written language to communicate ideas, values, or opinions. Williams (2000) states:

> The silence of speechlessness is never golden. We all need to communicate and connect with each other-not just one way, but also in as many ways possible. It is a basic human need, a basic human right. And much more than this, it is a basic human power. (p. 248)

The desire to communicate, to have a voice, leads us to the field of augmentative and alternative communication (AAC). Through the power of alternative communication one can enjoy the spirit of life. "Communication is what makes us uniquely human; all individuals have the right to communicate to their fullest potential. Communication is the 'essence of human life and a basic human freedom'" (Light 1997). The American Speech-Language Hearing Association (ASHA) Special Interest Division 12: Augmentative and Alternative Communication (AAC) defines AAC as follows: AAC refers to "an area of research, clinical, and educational practice. AAC involves attempts to study and when necessary compensate for the temporary or permanent impairments, activity limitations, and participation restrictions of individuals with severe disorders of speech-language production and/or comprehension, including spoken and written modes of communication" (2015, p. 1). Simply stated, AAC is using something other than speech to communicate; as the definition implies, "augment" means to supplement and "alternative" means to replace. Similar to speech, AAC transmits information from one person to another utilizing multimodal communication strategies, including vocalizations, verbal approximations, gestures, sign language, facial expressions, eye gaze, body language, objects, symbols (written or pictorial), and/or speech-generating devices (SGD). The primary goal of AAC is to support the communication and participation of persons with complex communication needs (Light and McNaughton 2015). These methods of communication represent ideas, thoughts, and events that occur in a person's life. The messages shared are frequently a combination of symbols governed by a set of rules, or language. Language as defined by the ASHA: "*is a* complex and dynamic system of conventional symbols that is used in various modes for thought and communication and is rule-governed." The rules of language correspond to form (e.g., syntax-grammatical structure), content (e.g., semantics-meaning) and use (e.g., pragmatics-social use). "Effective use of language for communication requires a broad understanding of human interaction including factors such as nonverbal cues, motivation, and socio-cultural roles" (ASHA 1982).

Language is the medium that allows us to talk, read, write, inquire about the world, and understand what others say. When an individual cannot produce sounds or words to communicate, it does not mean they lack language or desire to participate in a conversational exchange. AAC tools and strategies provide the individual an avenue to share ideas or express emotions with a communication partner, even if they can't access the spoken word. Communication is reciprocal; it takes at least two people, a dyad, to have a meaningful exchange or conversation. Prizant and Wetherby (1989) noted that children learn language involving people with whom they have meaningful relationships. Communication is the heart of any relationship, be it with family, friends, or colleagues for business, romance, or friendship; ultimately, communication is an interactive process where meaning is created in partnership with another (Teachman and Gibson 2014). "Just as a dance couldn't possibly be a dance unless people moved to it, so language doesn't become communication until people grow to understand and express it back. It has to be a two-way exchange. This is why 'communicating' is an action word" (Staehely 2000, p. 3). For individuals with complex communication needs, it is crucial to provide support for communication development, and access to the power of communication, so they can interact with others, participate fully in society, and influence their environment (Beukelman and Mirenda 2013). AAC is a journey to finding the best possible solutions for individuals with complex communication needs; as with all abilities and disabilities, it is not a one size fits, each individual is unique. With the advancement of technology, finding the key or solution continues to improve for individuals with complex communication needs. For example, the introduction of mobile applications (apps) and mobile devices has significantly impacted the field of AAC. The availability of touch screen tablet computers and apps has increased options for people with severe communication impairments. Research documents that the availability of mobile technology has resulted in an increase of consumer-driven AAC device selections (Costello, Shane, and Caron, 2013). The development of portable tablets, such as the iPad, has certainly changed the way we look at AAC technologies. The mobility and portability of these devices, as well as the user-friendly platform, has created a buzz in the AAC world. These new communication platforms have changed how professionals assist those with severe communication impairments. The attraction to these devices is affordability and personal appeal; they are widely accepted and mainstream, being utilized by the young and the old, for work, education, and leisure (Figure 17.1). Today, when participating in a public venue you may witness mobile devices being used as cameras, for checking email, obtaining the latest Facebook message, or viewing a personal video. There has been an explosion of tools that an individual with complex communication needs can access, such as social media applications, photos, and videos, and these have become broadly acknowledged modes of communication (Light and McNaughton 2012). Images, such as photos, that support communication have been long recognized in the field of AAC (Hanson et al. 2013). Individuals with complex communication needs may be more apt to use mobile technologies as AAC tools to enhance communicative competence: "… [the iPad] provides a rather elegant solution to the social integration problem. Kids with even the most advanced dedicated speech device are still carrying around something that tells the world 'I have a disability.' Kids using an iPad have a device that says, 'I'm cool.' And being cool, being like anyone else, means more to them than it does to any of us (Parent of a teenager who uses AAC, Rummel-Hudson 2011, p. 22).

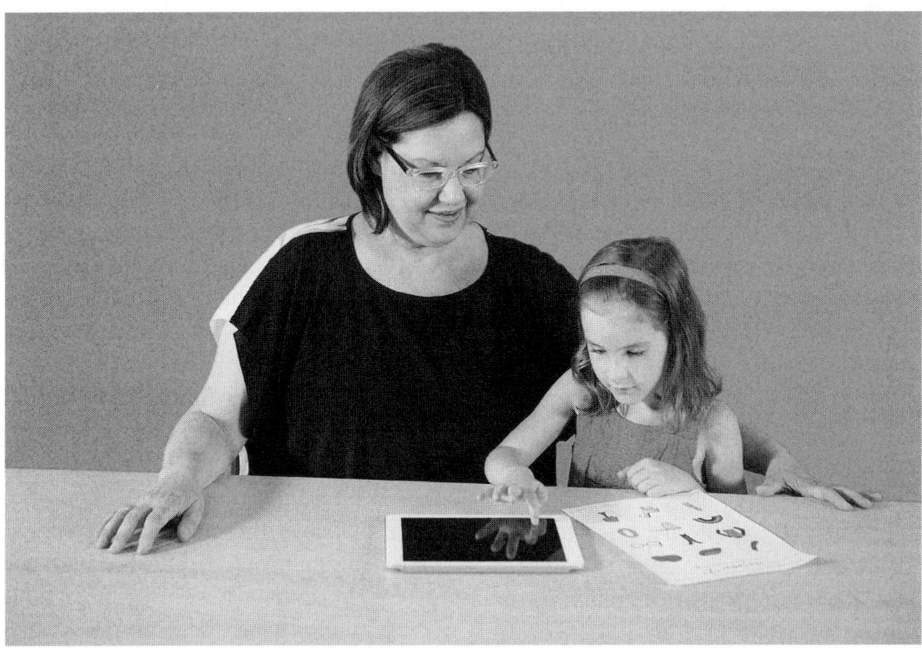

Figure 17.1 Using an iPad for communication.

> Functionally non-verbal was included in my diagnosis. It wasn't that I couldn't or didn't communicate verbally; I did and do. It was individuals beyond my family who didn't understand what I had to say. During my school years there was an occasional attempt to introduce me communication devices, which were primitive back then. I wasn't interested. I felt those clumsy-looking "voice boxes" were more difficult to understand than me. And during my years at university, my low tech, no batteries required alphabet card became my security blanket. I didn't leave my apartment without it. Fast forward to 2005. I had some communication success with the Libretto and adding a $15 roll-up keyboard made typing easier. The laptop, although useful for some purposes, wasn't really convenient for communication in the way I needed it to be. Fast forward again to April 2010. While in Chicago for a conference, I found my way to the Apple store and, after playing with an iPad for an hour, I pulled out my Visa to buy one, a month before the device was available in Canada. I also bought the Proloquo2Go (Assistiveware, 2009) app. Typing in Proloquo2Go came in handy. A combination of lip reading, American Sign Language, and typing on the iPad, now there's AAC on the fly! Being able to whip out my iPad from my handbag and having a choice of communication methods for when I'm on the go is life changing. Technology is finally catching up to my needs. The cool thing was, because the Holiday Inn and bar had WiFi, I had Internet access. When asked what I had been up to, I responded "problogging and ghost writing," and I was able to show what I had written. I also shared the video of me ziplining across Robson Square in downtown Vancouver during the Winter Olympics. The iPad allowed for a deeper level of communication that would not have been possible with a single-function AAC device.
>
> Hyatt (2011)

Legal and policy influences

As discussed in Vicente's (2006) Human-Tech Ladder, legal and policy factors can influence access to technology interventions and their use. Historically, AAC is considered part of assistive technology (AT). As defined by the Technology-Related Assistance for Individuals with Disabilities Act (PL-100-407, 1988), AT is "any item, piece of equipment, or product system, whether acquired commercially, off the shelf, modified or customized, that is used to increase, maintain or improve the functional capabilities of individuals with disabilities." As explained by King (1999), augmentative and alternative communication is a subset of AT that focuses on supporting and/or replacing one's natural speaking or writing abilities, or other communication functions that do not meet an individual's communication needs. AAC is considered to be multimodal in nature, encompassing gestures, eye gaze, facial expressions, body language, vocalizations, sign language, and needed speech-generating devices (e.g. voice output system). AAC is defined by ASHA (2015) as a "set of procedures and processes by which an individual's communication skills (i.e. production as well as comprehension) can be maximized for functional and effective communication." The field of AAC is relatively new and so does not have a long history. AAC strategies date back to the 1950s and 1960s, with research and academic coursework developing in the 1970s. Historically, many individuals with complex communication needs lived in residential institutions, separated from their families and communities, with little access to education or vocational options (Mirenda 2014). In recent years, individuals with complex communication needs live with their families, attend school, find employment, and actively participate in their communities (Calculator 2009). Given the improvements in medicine, science, and laws supporting individuals with disabilities, the need for AAC has increased. Laws such as The American with Disabilities Act (ADA) (PL-101-336, 1990) have made society aware of the rights of persons with disabilities, including those with communication impairments. About than 4 million people in the United States today have significant communication disabilities and cannot rely on natural speech to communicate daily needs (Beukelman and Mirenda 2013). These individuals are severely limited in their interactions with friends, family, and community members, and consequently the inability to communicate effectively impacts their social, educational, and vocational participation. Laws and policies protecting the rights of people with disabilities include those who have communication disorders as well. Advocacy groups such as the Communication Disabilities Access Canada (www.cdacanada.com) is an example of an organization that promotes and advocates for the rights of those who have speech and language disabilities, and the United States Society for Augmentative and Alternative Communication (USSAAC) (https://www.ussaac.org) states that it believes "everybody has the right to communication and advocates for access to communication in all environments for people who use or need AAC." According to the National Joint Committee for the Communicative Needs of Persons with Disabilities (NJC), communication is "a basic right of all human beings." It is the responsibility of professionals to provide the supports to those individuals with severe communication disabilities. All persons with a disability of any extent or severity have a basic right to communicate. These rights from the Communication Bill of Rights were put forth by the National Joint Committee for

Table 17.1 Communication Bill of Rights.

The Communication Bill of Rights (2016), which updated the original 1992 document, was developed by the Organizational Members of the National Joint Committee for the Communication Needs of Persons with Severe Disabilities (NJC). Members of the committee come from an interdisciplinary group. The updated Bill of Rights states that people with difficulty communicating due to a disability have the following 15 rights.

1. The right to interact socially, maintain social closeness, and build relationships
2. The right to request desired objects, actions, events, and people
3. The right to refuse or reject undesired objects, actions, events, or choices
4. The right to express personal preferences and feelings
5. The right to make choices from meaningful alternatives
6. The right to make comments and share opinions
7. The right to ask for and give information, including information about changes in routine and environment
8. The right to be informed about people and events in one's life
9. The right to access interventions and supports that improve communication
10. The right to have communication acts acknowledged and responded to even when the desired outcome cannot be realized
11. The right to have access to functioning AAC (augmentative and alternative communication) and other AT (assistive technology) services and devices at all times
12. The right to access environmental contexts, interactions, and opportunities that promote participation as full communication partners with other people, including peers
13. The right to be treated with dignity and addressed with respect and courtesy
14. The right to be addressed directly and not be spoken for or talked about in the third person while present
15. The right to have clear, meaningful, and culturally and linguistically appropriate communications.

Source: Brady et al. (2016).

the Communication Needs of Persons with Severe Disabilities (See Table 17.1).

> If you want to know what it is like to be unable to speak, there is a way. Go to a party and don't talk. Play mute. Use your hands if you wish but don't use paper and pencil. Paper and pencil are not always available for a mute person. Here is what you will find: people talking; talking behind, beside, around, over, under, through and even for you. But never with you. You are ignored until finally you feel like a piece of furniture.
>
> (Rick Creech, young man with CP, cited in Musslewhite and St. Louis 1988, p. 104)

Who needs AAC?

Persons who rely on AAC exhibit a wide range of disabilities across the life span, from the young student to the elderly man (Figure 17.2–17.4). Beukelman and Mirenda (2013) state: "There is no typical person who relies on AAC. They come from all age groups, socioeconomic groups, and ethnic and racial backgrounds" (p. 4). All people who use AAC, regardless of their disability (permanent or temporary), have one unifying characteristic: their communication needs are not achieved by speech alone. Individuals who are non-verbal or minimally verbal due to a congenital or acquired disorder depend on other modes of communication to participate in daily interactions with others. Individuals born with a disability, or a congenital disorder such as Down syndrome or cerebral palsy, may need access to AAC. Sarah, an eight-year-old elementary school student with cerebral palsy, utilizes AAC to interact with her classmates and teachers, who do not understand her unintelligible speech. She is understood by family members and close friends; however, to unfamiliar listeners she relies on a speech-generating device with pre-stored messages (e.g. "What are we doing today?") and core vocabulary to generate novel messages (e.g. "This weekend I watched my favorite movie!"). Or consider Ben, a student diagnosed with autism who attends school. He has only a few words to express himself and is frequently frustrated by his inability to communicate even his basic wants and needs. He also has difficulty understanding the spoken word. His speech-language pathologist (SLP) created a visual schedule to support his comprehension of the daily school routine, and to augment his lack of verbal speech, she provided him with a low-tech AAC device with important messages such as "I am all done," "I need a break," "I am thirsty," and "I am tired." Another example, of an AAC user is 62-year-old George, who enjoys attending social and community events; however, he cannot clearly articulate his personal thoughts and opinions as a result of a stroke. He wants to remain active in the community, therefore utilizes a speech- generating device and types his messages.

AAC assessment

Let's consider two clients:

- Jack, a kindergartner aged 5, is diagnosed with cerebral palsy. He is unable to speak, uses vocalizations to express emotion and effectively answers yes/no questions with eye blinks and head nods. He has limited control of his body, which includes significantly

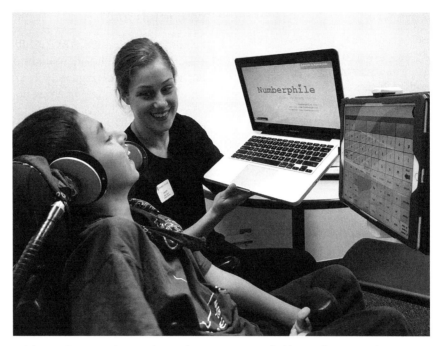

Figure 17.2 Student with CP using AAC. Picture taken and permission provided by Meghan Kennedy.

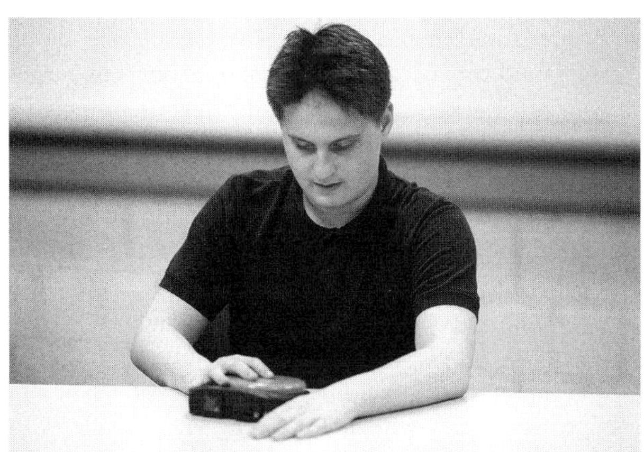

Figure 17.3 Student with autism using AAC.

impaired gross and fine motor skills. He uses a wheelchair for ambulation. Previous language testing by the SLP revealed his receptive language skills were age appropriate. His parents' primary goal is to help their son to communicate so he can successfully participate in school and be prepared academically.

- Stephen, a 55-year-old man diagnosed with amyotrophic lateral sclerosis (ALS), has owned and operated his own construction company for over 20 years. He is the breadwinner and is concerned about the welfare of his family and business. At this time, his speech is unaffected, but he and his wife want to prepare for the future. His wife is a positive support and wants to help her husband maintain his quality of life.

It is clear these individuals are candidates for an AAC assessment. Consider the following questions: How would you identify and implement a successful AAC system? What do you have to consider to ensure a successful AAC assessment? Who needs to be involved in the assessment process? What technology options will be presented? Do all the options need to be high-tech for the client to achieve their goals?

Unlike other speech and language assessments, the objective of an AAC assessment is not making a diagnosis, as the disorder or communication impairment has been acknowledged by previous evaluations (e.g. cognitive, language, or motor). The primary focus of an AAC evaluation is to systematically identify how the client can utilize a communication system to enhance and increase their communication skills, and improve their quality of life. The premise of an AAC evaluation is that all persons can communicate; there are no candidacy guidelines for utilizing an AAC system (Wasson et al. 1997). In 2004, the American-Speech- Language Hearing Association (ASHA) endorsed in a technical report that the Participation Model was a sound clinical framework for carrying out an AAC assessment: The report states: "The participation model emphasizes the importance of communication partners as a source for program development as well as potential sources of barriers to communication. Communication partners can facilitate the successful implementation of AAC by providing individuals with emotional, conversational, and technological support." The Participation Model as

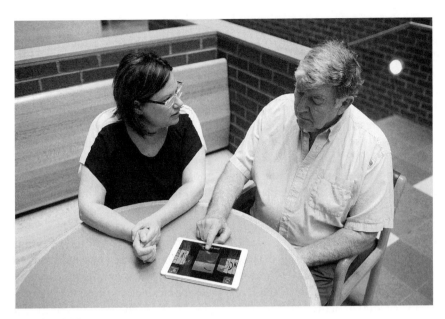

Figure 17.4 Older man using AAC.

described by Beukelman and Mirenda (2013) is a systematic approach, based on the functional involvement of persons without disabilities of the same chronological age. The evaluation encompasses gathering and synthesizing information to make an informed decision regarding the individual's communication needs. The foundation of the evaluation is providing an individual with the opportunity to participate and be an involved communicator. The assessment principles, as outlined in Beukelman and Mirenda (2013) include: (i) identify participation patterns and communication needs, (ii) assess the opportunities and barriers to utilize the AAC system, (iii) plan and implement interventions for today and tomorrow, and (iv) evaluate intervention effectiveness and participation (p. 109).

The team

The optimal AAC assessment framework will involve a *team*. As described in the Human-Tech Ladder, the team is a critical level of consideration impacting the success of human-tech interventions. A team may include parents, teachers, social workers, occupational therapists, and physical therapists, and most importantly the AAC candidate! The focus of an assessment should always begin with the client (Glennen and Decoste 1997; Hill and Corsi 2012). Focusing on the client first establishes a solid foundation for assessment and future intervention. The AAC process is considered a continuous assessment of the client's skills, future and present, focusing on the client's strengths and capabilities, rather than on his or her disability(ies). The team will establish a client profile by reviewing information about the individual, which may include a case history, past evaluations, identifying current AAC systems, including low- to high-tech, as well as the client's current performance and achievements (Hill and Corsi 2012). A vital principle in the assessment process is to include family or significant communication partners, such as teachers, friends, coworkers, and those who will be interacting with the candidate at school, at home, or in the community. Communication partners play a critical role in the success of the AAC user's ability to use a device (Light et al. 1985). The communication partner creates the opportunities for personal interactions, and simple changes in the communication partner's behavior can significantly alter how the AAC user communicates (Kent-Walsh and Rose-Lugo 2005; Kent-Walsh and McNaughton 2005). Effective communication partners are critical to the success of an individual using an AAC system. Research indicates that too often communication partners of individuals using AAC devices take the majority of conversational turns, provide fewer opportunities for communication, and ask predominantly yes-no questions. In order to communicate effectively with partners, the individuals must use their devices effectively to initiate interactions, respond frequently, and produce a wide range of communicative functions with the device (Light, Collier, and Parnes, cited in Kent-Walsh and Binger 2008).

Completing an ecological or environmental inventory (Beukelman and Mirenda 2013) will assist the evaluator in determining the communication needs of an individual by documenting his or her communication opportunities and interactions in a variety of real-world environments.

An ecological approach examines the individual's functioning in relationship to activities and environments in which he or she will or is expected to participate. Upon completion of those observations, the communication needs of the individual are reviewed and goals are identified in those environments where the AAC tools will be used. The rationale to examine communication contexts is that the AAC user needs to be a dynamic, involved communicator in activities and routines, not a passive participant. It is important that communication is implemented in motivational and interactive contexts, where language has meaning, consequences, and significance. What environment will the AAC tools and/or devices be used in? Who will be the communication partner(s)? How will the individual utilize the device, academically or vocationally? Is the disability acquired or congenital? What language needs to be available on the individual's device to help him or her return to work? Think about these questions as they apply to the case studies presented here. For example, Patrick was diagnosed with a traumatic brain injury (TBI), and was employed at the time of his motor vehicle accident, Testing reveals that he presents with an expressive language impairment, and can communicate at this time with only facial expressions and gestures. What AAC tool will help him return to work so he can communicate effectively with his coworkers? A toddler, Jaclyn, was diagnosed with cerebral palsy. She is a beginning communicator, how will she acquire language? "The average 18 month old child has been exposed to 4,380 hours of oral language at a rate of 8 hours/day from birth. A child who has a communication system and receives speech/language therapy two times per week for 20–30 minute sessions will reach this same amount of language exposure in 84 years" (Korsten n.d.).

Following observations of an individual in their natural environment, such as home, work, school, or in the community, it's important to establish a systematic framework for choosing which AAC system will have the most impact and be most appropriate in those daily environments. This is referred to as *feature matching*, a clinical decision based on a set of rules and relevant questions, rather than presumptions. Feature matching, a term we have heard in other chapters as well, is essential to an AAC assessment when determining an individual's strengths and capabilities relevant to the features of an AAC system (Glennen 1997). As defined by Shane and Costello (1994): "We submit that selecting the most appropriate AAC system (including hardware, software, and intervention strategies) is the result of a systematic process by which a person's strengths, abilities, and needs (current and future) are matched to available tools and strategies, a process often referred to as feature matching." The evaluator must be aware of the current technology, and think critically about making a clinical match that addresses the needs of the AAC candidate. How we chose to integrate a communication system into an individual's daily life will be essential to their success and ability to achieve communication competence. The team will review the AAC candidate's participation patterns, and information about vision, hearing, and motor and language skills, including seating and positioning, to provide the appropriate device or system match. If motor access is a concern, a number of factors need to be considered, such as how the communication system will be accessed, for example by *direct selection* (e.g. point or touch target directly from selection set) or *indirectly* via scanning (e.g. wait for a facilitator or electronic device to scan through desired items and then the item is chosen). Each individual presents with unique, separate needs, therefore each evaluator needs to review the AAC options (hardware and software) available and determine the best match or fit for their client. The client may utilize no-tech or *unaided* (e.g. gestures, sign language, eye gaze, facial expressions) communication strategies at home to those who are familiar with his or her speech pattern; however, other persons in the candidate's life who are unfamiliar may not understand the client's impaired speech production, therefore the individual may need to augment their communication by utilizing a more high-tech device. Dedicated devices, or speech-generating devices (SGDs), are specifically used for speech generation, and the hardware and software are solely dedicated for the purposes of communication. Please see Table 17.2 for a variety of AAC strategies and options.

Table 17.2 Augmentative and Alternative Communication Strategies and Options.

Aided means to represent an idea	Unaided means to represent an idea
Real objects	Gestures
Line drawings	Natural sign language (e.g. ASL, SEE)
Pictures (e.g. Picture Communication Symbols or PCS)	Fingerspelling or manual alphabets
Text-paper and pen	Eye gaze, eye blinks
Communication book/boards	Facial expressions
Electronic communication aids	Natural speech
Voice output communication aids (VOCAS)	Body movements
Speech-generating devices (SGDs)	Vocalizations

These electronic devices assist individuals who are unable use natural speech, and the communication system provides the communicator the opportunity have access to voice output during person-to-person exchanges. The technology relevant to SGD ranges from simple to complex, and can include low-/mid-tech and high-tech communication options. Please see Table 17.3 for a variety of AAC strategies and options.

The individual can select photos, pictures, letters, words, phrases, or sentences, alone or in combination, and have the information spoken aloud by the dedicated SGD to produce language via digitized speech (i.e. digitally recorded human voices) or synthesized speech (i.e. speech that sounds similar to the human voice but generated by a computer). The language on the SGD can be represented by text, symbols, or photographs, or a combination, as represented in Figures 17.5–17.7.

Devices considered in contrast to dedicated systems are non-dedicated devices, these are full operating computers that can run software programs and do more than generate language. Prime examples are the handheld devices or mobile technologies prevalent on the market today. Consumers have the availability of mobile devices and mobile applications (apps). Farral (2015) indicated: "These mobile technologies have had a huge impact on the field of Augmentative and Alternative Communication (AAC), causing major social change around the way in which individuals, families, and other services perceive AAC." Persons using a non-dedicated system can access the Internet and have access to email, research, reading, or use social media resources such as Twitter, Facebook, Pinterest, or blogs. McNaughton and Light (2013) recognize potential benefits of mobile technologies for the field of AAC, including "increased awareness and social acceptance of AAC in the mainstream." The evaluator needs to consider the skills and features to determine the appropriate communication system for the individual, so the AAC user can communicate with a variety of persons in a variety of environments. Consider a child at circle time or playing

Table 17.3 No-Tech to High-Tech Augmentative and Alternative Communication (AAC) Options.

No-tech	Low-tech	Mid-tech	High-tech
Does not involve technology or are non-electronic, e.g. gestures, facial expressions, or communication books or boards with messages represented via photographs, written words, or drawings.	Consists of communication books or boards with messages represented via photographs, written words, or drawings.	Utilizes technology that is relatively simple, such as simple battery-operated devices, and may include a voice output device such as the BIGmack (e.g. single switch device).	Consists of communication systems that are more advanced technology, such as dedicated speech-generating devices solely for the purposes of communication (i.e. Tobii DynaVox devices or PRC devices)

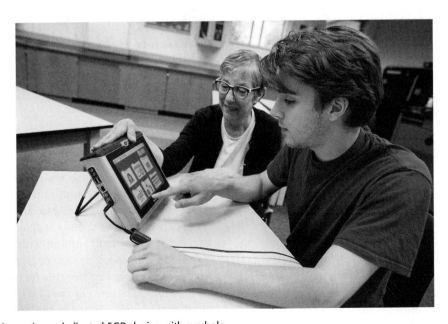

Figure 17.5 Student using a dedicated SGD device with symbols.

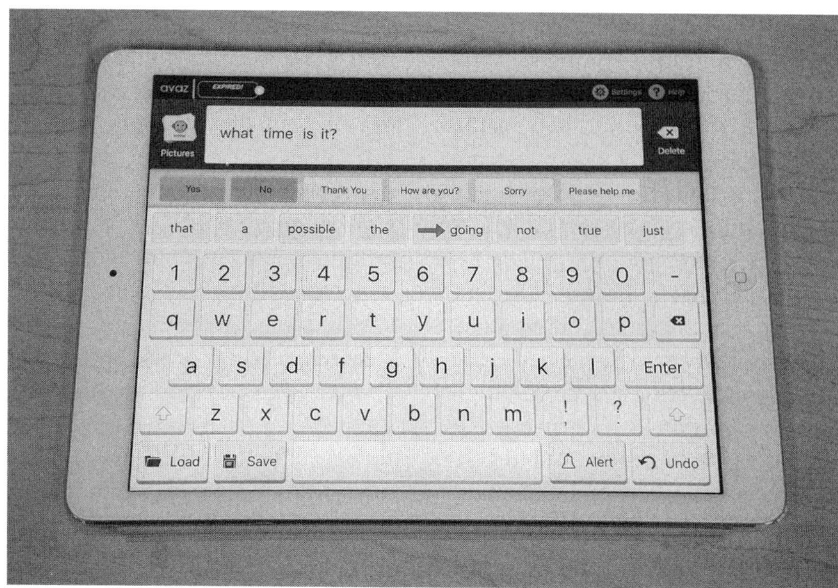

Figure 17.6 SGD device with letters and words.

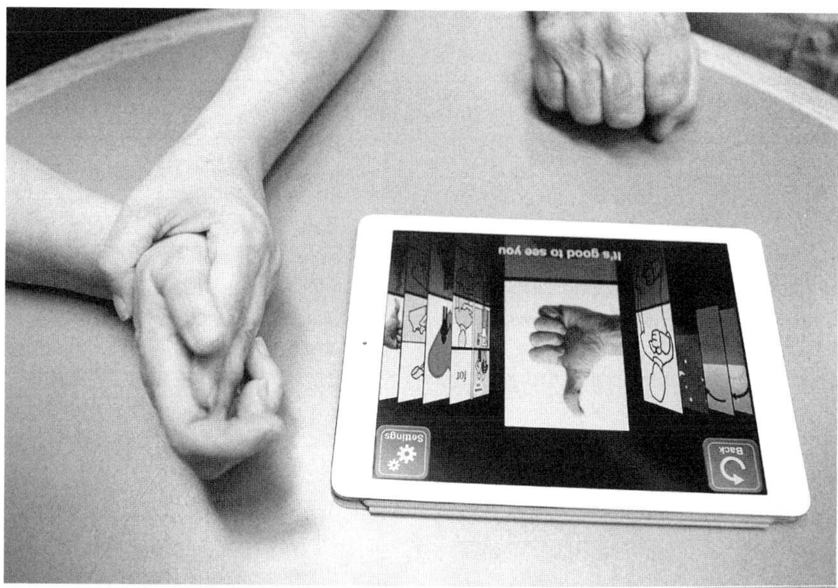

Figure 17.7 SGD device with photos and words.

with a peer. What strategies does she utilize to express an idea or thought? What natural gestures, vocalizations, or body language are used for expression? Rather than verbally requesting, does she reach for a toy? Does she push or pull another child to get their attention? Does the child lead you to what she wants? The child's ability to utilize a number of communicative tools and strategies clearly demonstrates the importance of multimodal communication (e.g. all the communication strategies an individual uses for expression). If the child has a dedicated SGD, but the device is not available, the child needs to rely on other communication methods. Teaching or encouraging gestural communication, or providing no-tech communication solutions, such as a picture board, can be valuable to an individual. Gestures, facial expressions, and body language are always available to the individual, without with having to rely on a communication book, board, or high-tech AAC device. An unaided symbol system that can be an effective communication strategy for person's with little or no functional speech is manual sign, the majority of which was designed for people with hearing impairments but which in recent years has been utilized for language development for improving comprehension, as well as expression (Beukelman and Mirenda 2005). If a child diagnosed with autism enters a preschool program, we have knowledge that capitalizing on visual strategies (Shane et al. 2009) is an effective intervention plan. Similar to a child who uses AAC, an adult needs to utilize multimodal communication strategies as well to participate in a social context. Language will be needed to participate in small talk, including messages that support greetings and story-telling, to be a successful conversational partner; if language is not accessible, the individual will be not be an effective conversational partner. A multimodal communication system is the key to successful expression (Fried-Oken 2008). Options for low-tech tools might be customized, such as communication books (small photo albums for pictures, symbols, words lists) or an SGD with multiples messages and information.

AAC intervention – psychosocial and physical levels of the human-tech ladder

Capitalizing on motivation and focusing on an individual's strengths and abilities, rather than on the individual's speech and language deficits, is an intervention approach that is recognized in the field of AAC. Communication by means of AAC is a complex process and can impose substantial motor, cognitive, sensory, and linguistic demands on the individual learning an AAC system (Thistle and Wilkinson 2013). Light (2003) noted that the motivation to communicate drives the individual's desire to participate in communication interactions. If motivation is low and communicative demands are high, the individual is likely to sacrifice communication opportunities and not participate (Clarke et al. 2001). Like other speech and language interventions, the primary instructor will be the SLP. The SLP will help support and create motivational communication opportunities for the client who utilizes AAC. Schnoll and Zimmerman (2001) noted that adults are engaged learners and are psychosocially motivated when they have choices, value what is being learned, enjoy the experience, and believe they will be successful. Team members, family, peers, coworkers, and community members play a significant role in assisting the individual utilizing a communication system. Research shows that without supportive communication partners, abandonment of a communication system is likely (Waller et al. 2005).

Some parents, caregivers, and communication partners may assume that providing AAC will impede speech development. However, a number of empirical studies actually report speech skills improve following AAC intervention (Beukelman and Mirenda 2005; Romski and Sevcik 1996). To improve speech and language skills it is important to remember that AAC is a multimodal communication system and should incorporate all communication strategies that an individual may utilize, including unaided (e.g. vocalizations, gestures, sign language) or aided communication strategies (e.g. communication books, boards, or SGDs). AAC interventions can play a significant role in communication and language development, including comprehension and expression. The most influential, valuable, and constant people in an individual's life are family members (Iovannone et al. 2003), and training family members and caregivers in how to access, implement, and program the AAC system is essential to the intervention process, to support continued use and reduce rejection of the communication system (Johnson et al. 2006).

Interventions implemented by trained parents are just as successful as clinician-implemented interventions (Law et al. 2004). Research indicates that communication partners significantly influence the success of individuals who use AAC, particularly beginning communicators. Communication partners frequently control interactions with communicators by: (i) asking a high frequency of closed-ended questions, (ii) taking the majority of conversational turns, (iii) providing few opportunities for children using AAC to initiate or respond in conversation, (iv) controlling the topic and direction of conversation, (v) frequently interrupting the utterances of children using AAC, and (vi) focusing on the AAC system during interactions (Light et al. 1994). Due to the communication partner's control of the communication interaction, children using AAC are often passive communicators who initiate fewer interactions, produce a limited number of communicative interactions, and respond infrequently. Professionals teaching an AAC system need to have the knowledge to train and support significant communication partners (Fishman 2011). It is imperative that clinicians implement communication partner interventions to maximize the AAC user's communicative participation in daily life activities and events. Communication partner or facilitator support is critical because many AAC users are not given the opportunity to socially communicate or participate in conversational exchanges with others. One reason for this may be that AAC devices are frequently programmed with basic wants and needs (Beukelman and Mirenda 2005). Requesting basic wants and needs is important for health, safety, and behavior regulation;

however, when observing daily communication interactions, we have much more to talk about! Psychosocial relevance is crucial for motivation when creating an intervention program if parents, caregivers, and the SLPs are to help an individual become a competent communicator (Rodgers and Brown 2005). An AAC system that only has requests programmed ("I am hungy!" or "I need to use the bathroom!") can become mundane, boring, and rote. Rather, enable the AAC communicator to share his or her weekend news or favorite movie. It is the interactions of the communication partners, the messages shared, that create communication interest and success; the AAC device alone does not make an individual an effective communicator (Beukelman and Mirenda 2005).

Individual psychosocial and physical factors must be considered when providing intervention with AAC systems. The AAC systems should be individualized and programmed to motivate the individual to embrace communication. When planning intervention strategies, the devices and AAC tools need to be individualized by customizing the layout, the symbols, and the access method (e.g. direct, indirect). A communication system may be represented by picture communication cards, books, or voice output technologies. One individual may utilize photographs to represent language; another may communicate with text-based symbols or chose to utilize a combination of symbols, photographs, and text. It is important to customize a device to avoid the AAC system being limited to requests frequently delegated to basic wants and needs ("I need a drink of water"). Communication should be interactive, conversational, and enjoyable, beyond basic requests. Consider Grace, a six-year-old girl with Down syndrome. Before beginning AAC treatment, it is essential to ask her educational team and parents questions such as "What does she love?" "What activities does she enjoy?" "Music?" "The park?" "Horses?" The interventionists want to create a psychosocially motivating, pleasant, and fun atmosphere for Grace to embrace the communication supports. Recognizing the importance of the psychosocial level of the Human-Tech Ladder is critical to implementing an AAC system in a motivational manner and is the first step to advance and promote communication. The individual needs to be a part of the communication process. Individuals with complex communication needs fit into Maslow's hierarchy of needs. They may get their basic needs met; however, communication goes beyond basic physiological and safety needs. An AAC user has psychosocial needs such as love and belonging, as well as the need to be respected by others to promote self-esteem, experience purpose, and reach self-actualization (e.g. to realize one's full potential). As interventionists we need to look beyond basic requests for food, drink, or the restroom. There are more interesting topics to talk about! When considering a general, everyday communicator, the breadth of a conversation transcends basic needs. Let's talk about our beach vacation or what we did over the weekend. How often do we talk about when we used the bathroom! Intervention should take into consideration creating a competent communicator. The skills required to use an AAC device may be different than verbal communicators; however, the purposes for communicating are the same for everyone. Light (1989) identified four main purposes for an AAC communicator that may be the same for you and your communication needs: (i) express wants and needs, (ii) establish and maintain social closeness, (iii) share information, and (iv) fulfill social etiquette routines.

The social utilization of an AAC device is critical for success. The focus of a successful AAC system and intervention is participation. An AAC system provides the user access to language via symbols, text, or both. Language is used to interact with others and maintain relationships. Timler et al. (2005) defined social communication as, "The intersection of language and social behaviors observed during peer interactions … that is, the verbal and nonverbal behaviors children display as they approach peers, maintain conversations, and resolve conflicts during peer interactions." The job of the AAC interventionist is to ensure that clients have access to the fullest possible range of communication modes and purposes, given each person's specific desires, needs, and abilities. Expression of *wants and needs* is a communicative function used to regulate the behavior of others to achieve a desired need or object. Messages programmed may include hunger, medical conditions (e.g. pain), or daily wants, needs, and activities. This can typically make programming messages or words on an AAC device predictable, useful, and relatively easy. Individuals with complex communication needs require AAC systems to support their participation and communication in a variety of settings, including work, school, and in the community (Collier et al. 2012). It is no longer enough for an AAC just to request food or an activity; individuals need access to communication to participate fully at school for learning, to establish friendships, and to collaborate with a colleague at work. The mother of eight-year-old Brian said it best: "There's more to life than cookies" (Light et al. 2002, p. 187). *Social closeness* refers to the communication necessary to establish, maintain, and develop personal relationships. Imagine not being able to tell someone you care about "I love you" or how difficult it would be for a child to bond with peers and develop friendships without the language needed (e.g. telling a joke to classmates or expressing sympathy to a friend). *Information transfer* or sharing encompasses more complicated communication interactions because it involves messages that are more complex in nature, and less predictable. Frequently, messages are novel and personal, typically covering a wide range of topics, for example, weekend news, asking and answering questions in school, or talking with friends about an upcoming event. Another purpose of communication, as described by Light (1988), is *social etiquette* or following certain social conventions such as saying "please" and "thank you." These phrases are predictable, which makes them easily programmable on a communication system.

How can these communication needs be accomplished? What tools need to be provided? The choice of communication systems that are developed and implemented should involve a team-driven approach, to maximize the use of the AAC system. As mentioned previously, communication partners are vital to the success of AAC intervention; naturalistic client- and family-centered approaches are recommended when introducing AAC systems (Romski and Sevcik 1996). Family and significant others should be included in all stages of the AAC program. (Bjorck-Akesson et al. 2000). If a child diagnosed with autism enters a preschool program, we have knowledge that capitalizing on visual strategies (Shane et al. 2009) is an effective intervention plan. When working with young children, for example, the philosophy is that AAC has an input and output to teach language. AAC tools can be utilized to stimulate language in a play environment during natural routines, and communication partners are essential to this learning process. Let's consider a two-year-old, a new language learner with minimal verbal speech, who loves books and is motivated to participate in literacy activities. As an interventionist we want to encourage both expressive communication and literacy development. An AAC solution might be to present a mid-tech tool such as a BIGmack (e.g. single message voice output) and utilize a repetitive line in a story (e.g. "Brown Bear, Brown Bear, what do you see?"). The child can participate in an enjoyable and motivational interaction with a voice by touching the BIGmack and repeating the line of the story!

Historically, AAC users face having to abandon their communication device due to the lack of social acceptability of the AAC system (Waller et al. 2005). Opportunities need to be provided for the AAC user to communicate and be accepted and responded to with positive, supportive interaction. The latest mobile technology and numerous apps provide individuals with the opportunity be socially accepted or be part of the "cool factor." Tablets, such as the iPad, and laptops are mainstream, popular, and acceptable SGDs in the community. For example, for a group of adult clients who utilized speech-generating software on their iPads in a restaurant setting, the wait staff was kind, patient, and accepted the clients' communication interactions when they ordered their meals, creating a positive communication interaction for these individuals. With the advances in technology of small, portable tablets such as the iPad, with its ease and social acceptability, we may hope to see a decrease in abandonment of devices. The growing familiarity of computers and tablets and the increasing number of people using them will hopefully encourage continued support of and use of an AAC system. Technology can be utilized as a means of communication for work, recreation, leisure, and study. For example, texting your teenage son the time you will pick him up from school, or emailing a colleague information about an important project, is using language for communication. The idea of technology connecting humans can be understood when considering the number of media currently in use, including Facebook, email, and texting. These communication exchanges, carried out with language but not speech, are very powerful. An AAC system provides access to communication, to language. If a child born with a congenital disorder such as cerebral palsy, autism spectrum disorder, or Rett syndrome will never speak, or an individual loses his or her ability to speak due to a TBI or cerebral vascular accident (CVA), they certainly are entitled to the same basic right to communicate and access language as a verbal individual. An in this modern age, technology is making this more possible, prevalent, and available.

> Full access to e-mail, cell phones, digital music, e-commerce, digital photo albums, and e-books, are all activities that require digital independence. These are fundamental communication in the twenty-first century and are necessary for full participation schools, the workplace the community at large. We must ensure that AAC technology … supports greater participation in today's Information society.
>
> (DeRuyter et al. 2007)

As stated previously, motivation and communication partner support are crucial when creating an intervention program if the team and SLP are to help a client become a competent communicator. The AT tools, that is the hardware and software, can change people's lives; however, the AAC device alone does not make an individual a competent communicator (Beukelman 1991). Light and colleagues (Light 1989; Light et al. 2003) identified four major areas of communication competency: linguistic, social, strategic, and operational. "Communication competency is about people. It is not about computer technology or AAC systems. Technology is just the tool, it is just the tool, it is the people and the interactions between them that must be our main focus" (Light 1997).

Linguistic competence refers to the understanding and expression of one's native language or having knowledge of the "code." For a verbal communicator, the linguistic code is simply speaking or writing to share information. For an AAC user, the code may be represented by photographs, pictures, words, signs, text, or a combination. This is referred to as the "symbol set" or the language display. For example, a child who is a beginning communicator will have less exposure to abstract language concepts; therefore, a concrete, contextual representation such as photographs code may be implemented. Photographs are transparent (e.g. a symbol recognizable in the absence of its referent). Like typical language learners, the AAC user needs to have frequent opportunities to use the communication symbols in a variety of contexts to understand the symbols' meaning and relevance. Family, friends, communication specialists, and other facilitators can play a major role in assisting those who rely on AAC to accomplish this challenging mission (Beukelman and Mirenda 2013). Ongoing opportunities in natural contexts for practicing expressive language can be provided by facilitators, helping the individual to learn the symbol or code of the system (Romski and Sevcik 1996). For example, an elementary school student may have a goal to communicate a variety of pre-stored messages (e.g. What's that? What's your name? Do you have any pets? or "What did you do this weekend?) during a conversational interaction with a peer. Gus Estrella, an AAC user, advises, "Dig in, get the support of both the school and the social services agencies, get the devices funded, and make us work our little tails off until we master enough language to become competent communicators and please remember pre-language does not mean 'no' language. It means there's a mind in this individual that needs to be developed" (Estrella 1997, p. 8). Operational competence, or "the technical skills needed to operate the AAC system accurately and efficiently" (Beukelman and Mirenda 2013, p. 12), is a critical skill for an AAC user to learn. Training will be required for the user to learn how to operate and maintain the device. Remember Stephen, the 55-year-old man with ALS? With the progression of his ALS, he will need to learn how to access a switch to operate his SGD. Operational competence is an important consideration when choosing a communication device, regardless of whether the system is a low-tech or high-tech system. Specifically, the needs are to update vocabulary, develop communication displays as needed, protect the device against damage and breakage, modify the system for future needs, and ensure day-to-day availability of the device (Beukelman 1991). New vocabulary may need to be added when the AAC user is learning a new topic at school, training for a new job, or sharing news from a recent event. Parents, family, teachers, or caregivers can benefit from training, as they may be responsible for programming and maintaining the device if the client is unable to do so independently.

Social competence is the skill at the heart of communication and vital to the human connection. Social competence includes initiating, maintaining, and terminating a conversation in a variety of communication environments, with a number of communication partners. The individual may need to communicate at school, at home, at church, at a party, or with his or her doctor. Research suggests that it is essential for AAC users to have a positive self-image, have an interest in communicating, be responsive, and put conversational partners at ease (Light 1988). "Augmentative and Alternative communication can provide a person with the ability to have and develop strong and rewarding relationships with others. Deny a person the ability to articulate intelligibly and that person is sentenced to live in social, intellectual and emotional isolation" (Prentice 2000, p. 213). The opportunities to practice social competence in natural contexts are essential for success, for both the facilitators and communicators. Communication is a dynamic and transactional process, in which conversational partners influence each other through the course of exchanges. Research suggests that optimum communication exchanges depend both on the communication skills of children who use AAC and on those of their communication partners; however, this is often overlooked (Kent-Walsh and Rosa-Lugo 2006). A goal for a high school student who utilizes a SGD might be to ask to play a game or to ask partner focus questions such as "How about you?" or "What's new?" to a peer to establish or maintain a friendship.

Strategic competence, or the ability to repair a communication breakdown, is a skill that can be demonstrated with both aided and unaided communication strategies; for example, a phrase like "please be patient with me while I type my message" can be programmed on the user's SGD, or the individual can use body language, gestures, and/or facial expressions that enhance or further clarify his or her message. For example, John, who has medical concerns and utilizes an SGD, will plan ahead for his visit to the physician. He will compose questions prior to his visit so he can contribute effectively to the conversation related to his medical needs.

Consider the case studies in Boxes 17.1–17.3 and the evidence in Box 17.4.

Summary

As we can see from this chapter, there are multiple levels of the Human-Tech Ladder which come into play in order to get communications systems in place for those who need them. Communication is a human right and

Box 17.1 Case study: Assessment and intervention – Stephen

We once again refer to Stephen, a 55-year-old man diagnosed with ALS who owns and operates his own construction company. He enjoys golf and social engagements with friends and family. He currently is able to speak; however, due to the progressive nature of his disease, Stephen will eventually lose his ability to use speech for communication and will need to rely on other modes of communication, including aided and unaided communication strategies. His SLP recommends that he participate in an AAC assessment with his family to determine his communication needs for today, tomorrow, and the future.

Stephen will need the support of caregivers and significant others for the AAC systems to be effective and successful in his daily life. The SLP will recommend an SGD that has the availability of direct selection, as well as scanning capabilities and eye gaze, to ensure that Stephen continues to have access when his motor skills fail and he can achieve operational competence. In addition, to ensure operational success, Stephen will need access to a symbol system that supports his language and literacy skills. Therefore, he will need access to a keyboard and word predication so he can generate novel thoughts, and not rely on others to determine his messages. In addition, to ensure access to letters on his device, his SLP will recommend voice banking (i.e. recording his speech for later use) so Stephen can put his own voice on his SGD in pre-stored messages, for example, using his own recorded voice to say "I love you" to his spouse.

Stephen will also need to have access to multiple communication supports in addition to an SGD, for strategic repairs, such as a communication board or low-tech alphabet board.

Box 17.2 Case study: Assessment and intervention – Jack

We once again refer to Jack, a boy diagnosed with cerebral palsy who is non-verbal; he is now seven years old. He utilizes unaided forms of communication, including eye gaze, vocalizations, gestures, head nods, and body language. However, he does have access to language for communication. His cognitive and communication skills have been evaluated and determined to be age appropriate. He has been receiving speech-language therapy services for most of his young life. At the age of 2.5 years he participated in an AAC assessment. To complete the assessment, his participation patterns and communication needs were assessed utilizing an ecological inventory. Two important environments were examined, including home and his preschool program. The major barrier encountered by Jack and his team during the assessment was access; Jack has limited control of his hands so direct selection would be a difficult; however, the opportunities for communication in a variety of environments, with a number of communication partners, were immense, and those who worked with Jack set high exceptions! The team and his parents knew that when he had access to language a window into his thinking and thoughts would become available.

The device chosen by the team at age 2.5 was the DynaVox V, with direct selection. This SGD provided language both with pictures and with text. The text-based representation of language was important because Jack was demonstrating some early literacy skills and was able to access messages on his SGD with the written word only presented. Jack demonstrated success with this system; he understood the "code," or language. He demonstrated age-appropriate social skills with low-tech (i.e. yes/no board) and high-tech systems (i.e. DynaVox V) by turn-taking with a peer, teacher, or parent during conversational exchanges. However, the major hurdle or challenge was access; he was able to use direct selection but with inconsistency due to his limited fine motor skills. Therefore, when he was five years old, switch scanning was tried with the DynaVox V and it was successful! With the changing technological opportunities (e.g. the presentation of tablet technology), at the age of seven Jack had access to an iPad with communication software and used two-switch scanning to operate the system. With the continued support of committed communication partners, Jack will achieve operational, linguistic, social, and strategic competence!

In addition to helping Jack master his communication skills, the SLP will be responsible for teaching and training parents and significant others the importance and value of being successful conversational partners. The SLP will ensure that Jack is being taught multimodal communication strategies, including unaided strategies such as eye blinks for "yes" and "no," as well as provide continued training of aided communication systems, including low-tech (i.e. vocabulary boards) and high-tech systems (i.e. eye gaze systems to interface with a computer), so that he can participate effectively in these communication interactions at school, at home, and in the community. Jack exhibits excellent potential to be a competent and successful AAC user with the assistance of a committed team, dedicated family, and continued assessment of new technologies.

Box 17.3 Case study: Assessment and intervention – Sarah

Again referring to Sarah, an 18-year-old young woman diagnosed with cerebral palsy, is attending college in the fall and has achieved the linguistic, social, operational, and strategic communication competence needed to make her journey and academic participation in college possible.

At the age of two Sarah participated in an AAC evaluation with the support of her parents, occupational therapist, and physical therapist. The SLP completed the evaluation and determined that Sarah was a candidate to utilize AT tools to support her lack of verbal output. Sarah at age two was unable to verbalize and was sincerely frustrated, as evidenced by her tantrums and screaming. It was evident Sarah needed alternative means of communication. It was recommended that Sarah utilize a multimodal communication system including sign language, picture communication books, gestures, facial expressions, and the true words that she could verbalize. At the age of 3.5, Sarah still was not developing age-appropriate speech and language. Therefore, a dedicated SGD was obtained so she had access to a voice output device, and most importantly access to language! Sarah was able to utilize direct selection to access the messages on the SGD, and when given partner support she was successful utilizing this AAC system to interact with her peers at preschool, at home with her family, and with teachers, therapists, and other community members.

Another important milestone Sarah achieved on her journey as an AAC communicator was access to literacy. As Sarah transitioned from preschool to kindergarten, she learned how to type and spell on an SGD keyboard and began the joy of literacy! She learned how to type to generate novel messages to effectively communicate in academic and social settings, in addition to communicating with pre-programmed messages. Sarah demonstrated operational, social, and linguistic competence with her SGD, and her ability to use sign language, gestures, and facial expressions supported her strategic competence. Sarah was able to repair a message with unaided communication strategies if her SGD did not have the necessary messages or was not available at the time of the conversational interaction.

Today Sarah is attending college and continues to use speech-generating software (an app) on her iPad dedicated to communication. She strives for self-advocacy and to be an active member of her community!

Box 17.4 Here's the evidence

Soto, G. and Clarke, M.T. (2017). Effects of a conversation-based intervention on the linguistic skills of children with motor speech disorders who use augmentative and alternative communication. *Journal of Speech, Language, and Hearing Research* 60(7): 1980–1998.

Key Words: communication-based intervention, children with motor speech disorders, augmentative and alternative communication (AAC)

Purpose: Young children who use AAC often experience significant language delays. The literature reports that there are positive effects of using verbal scaffolding procedures with conversation-based interventions on language development in children who are not AAC users. These scaffolding techniques allow children to hear language used in a meaningful ways, which helps to build more complex utterances from the child as they are able to contrast the response with their own. While evidence exists that these techniques work with children who have language delays, the techniques have not been studied with children who have motor speech disorders and use AAC. The purpose of this study is to investigate the effect of this scaffolding technique within a conversation-based intervention on the expressive vocabulary and grammatical skills of children in this group.

Sample/Setting: Eight children (three girls and five boys) ranging in age from 8 to 14 who used a high-tech speech-generating device (SGD) were recruited for this study.

Method: A multiple probe design across participants was used to investigate the use of a conversation-based intervention on the expressive vocabulary and grammatical skills of the participants. Baseline and post-intervention data were collected and analyzed using transcription and coding of video tapes of the sessions along with analyses of language samples within 60 minute observation periods. Analyses were done visually and statistically.

Findings: Data analyses indicated that all participants had a limited use of verbs, pronouns, bound morphemes, and spontaneous clauses during the baseline session. After the intervention sessions, all four linguistic measures increased and were generalized and maintained above intervention levels once the intervention had stopped.

Critical Thinking Questions:

1. Having read this research article, what do you understand to be the limitations of this research? Are there any limitations not stated?
2. What other findings did you take away from this article?
3. What implications does this article have for practice?

should be available to all people. As this chapter demonstrates, civil rights legislation which advanced the rights of people with disabilities (ADA 1990, Rehabilitation Act 1973) and legislation which provided funding to get AT into the hands of those who need it (Technology-Related Assistance for Individuals with Disabilities Act 1988) moved a human need into the realm of legislation and policy. Organizations where humans participate may have different rules regarding how people can access AAC, but these policies are in place, as demonstrated by the different case studies in the chapter. The importance of team involvement in implementing successful AAC is emphasized throughout the chapter. The psychosocial impact of communication and the technology and environmental intervention (TEI) options that support motivation to speak are also emphasized. For example, with devices such as tablets and apps that support communication becoming part of the everyday technology that all people use, the stigma of using these devices as AAC is decreased. The AAC user can now be as "cool" as anyone else who uses a tablet, instead of different. Of course, new policy issues arise from the use of everyday technology as AAC in the funding arena, but these issues are now being discussed and negotiated at the legislative/policy level of the Human-Tech Ladder and will no doubt influence how the societal needs of those who need communication TEI continue to be met. Finally, the chapter demonstrated the importance of matching TEI to a person's physical and cognitive level in order to successfully implement interventions to enable participation in communication. Individuals who require AAC need the assistance of dedicated, knowledgeable communication partners, and interventionists, as well as the tools and strategies that match their unique communication needs. The goal of AAC is for the communicator to be understood and validated as a person with thoughts, ideas, emotions, values, and opinions. Similar to a verbal individual, the AAC user desires to share information, express wants and needs, and establish social relationships. These AAC objectives can be accomplished if the individual has access to multimodal communication strategies, including aided and unaided communication tools represented by no-tech, low-tech, mid-tech, and high-tech solutions. As with Jack, Sarah, and Stephen, the ability to maintain social roles, be full, active participants in society, and be validated as communicators is the ultimate goal. Each individual has the opportunity to achieve linguistic, social, operational, and strategic competence with the support of knowledgeable interventionists, devoted team members, and dedicated communication partners.

References

American Speech-Language-Hearing Association (1982). Language. Retrieved from https://www.asha.org/policy/rp1982-00125/.

American Speech-Language-Hearing Association (2015). Augmentative and alternative communication (AAC). Retrieved from https://www.asha.org/public/speech/disorders/aac/.

Americans with Disabilities Act of 1990 (1990). Pub. L. No. 101-336, 104 Stat. 328.

Beukelman, D.R. (1991). Magic and cost of communicative competence. *Augmentative and Alternative Communication* 7 (1): 2–10.

Beukelman, D.R. and Mirenda, P. (2005). *Augmentative & Alternative Communication: Supporting Children & Adults with Complex Communication Needs.* Baltimore, MD: Paul H. Brooks.

Beukelman, D.R. and Mirenda, P. (2013). *Augmentative and Alternative Communication: Supporting Children and Adults with Complex Communication Needs*, 4e. Baltimore, MD: Paul H. Brooks.

Bjorck-Akesson, E., Granlund, M., Light, J.C. and McNaughton, D. (2000). Goal setting and problem solving with AAC users and families. Presentation at the Ninth International Conference of the International Society for Augmentative and Alternative Communication, Washington, DC.

Brady, N.C., Bruce, S., Goldman, A. et al. (2016). Communication services and supports for individuals with severe disabilities: guidance for assessment and intervention. *American Journal on Intellectual and Developmental Disabilities* 121 (2): 121–138.

Calculator, S.N. (2009). Augmentative and alternative communication (AAC) and inclusive education for students with the most severe disabilities. *International Journal of Inclusive Education* 13: 93–113.

Clarke, M., McConachie, H., Price, K., and Wood, P. (2001). Views of young people using augmentative and alternative communication systems. *International Journal of Language & Communication Disorders* 36: 107–115.

Collier, B., Blackstone, S., and Taylor, A. (2012). Communication access to businesses and organizations for people with complex communication needs. *Augmentative and Alternative Communication* 28 (4): 205–218.

Costello, J.M., Shane, H.C. and Caron, J. (2013). AAC, mobile devices and apps: growing pains with evidence based practice. Retreived from https://vantatenhove.com/files/papers/AACandApps/CostelloShaneCaron-WhitePaper.pdf.

DeRuyter, F., McNaughton, D., Caves, K. et al. (2007). Enhancing AAC connections with the world. *Augmentative and Alternative Communication* 23 (3): 258–270.

Estrella, G. (1997). The development of wisdom. The First Annual Edwin and Esther Prentke AAC Distinguished Lecture. Retrieved from https://minspeak.com/documents/prentkelecture/173-Estrella%201997.pdf.

Farral, J. (2015). Implementation of iPads for AAC in a specialist school. *Perspectives on Augmentative and Alternative Communication* 24 (2): 51–59.

Fishman, I. (2011). Guidelines for teaching speech-language pathologists about the AAC assessment process. *Perspectives on Augmentative and Alternative Communication* 20: 82–86. https://doi.org/10.1044/aac20.3.82.

Fried-Oken, M. (2008). Augmentative and alternative communication treatment for persons with primary progressive aphasia. *Perspectives on Augmentative and Alternative Communication* 17: 99–104.

Glennen, S.L. (1997). Augmentative and alternative communication. In: *The Handbook of Augmentative and Alternative Communication* (ed. S.L. Glennen and D.C. DeCoste). San Diego, CA: Singular Publishing Group.

Glennen, S.L. and DeCoste, D.C. (1997). *The Handbook of Augmentative and Alternative Communication.* San Diego, CA: Singular Publishing Group.

Hyatt, G.W. (2011). The iPad: a cool communicator on the go. *Perspectives on Augmentative and Alternative Communication* 20: 24–27. https://doi.org/10.1044/aac20.1.24.

Hanson, E., Beukelman, D.R., and Yorkston, K. (2013). Communication support through multimodal supplementation: a scoping review. *Augmentative and Alternative Communication* 29: 310–321.

Hill, K. and Corsi, V. (2012). The role speech-language pathologists in assistive technology assessments. In: *Assistive Technology assessment: A Handbook for Professionals in Disability, Rehabilitation and Health Professions* (ed. M.J. Scherer and S. Federici), 301–336. Boca Raton, FL: CRC Press.

Iovannone, R., Dunlap, G., Huber, H., and Kincaid, D. (2003). Effective educational practices for students with autism spectrum disorders. *Focus on Autism and Other Developmental Disabilitites* 18 (3): 150–165.

Johnson, J., Inglebret, E., Jones, C., and Ray, J. (2006). Perspectives of speech-language pathologists regarding success versus abandonment of AAC. *Augmentative and Alternative Communication* 22 (2): 85–99.

Kent-Walsh, J. and Binger, S. (2008). Tales from school trenches: AAC service-delivery and professional expertise. *Seminars in Speech and Language* 29 (2): 146–154.

Kent-Walsh, J. and McNaughton, D. (2005). Communication partner instruction in AAC: present practices and future directions. *Augmentative and Alternative Communication* 21 (3): 195–204.

Kent-Walsh, J. and Rosa-Lugo, L. (2006). Communication partner interventions for children who use AAC: storybook reading across culture and language. *The ASHA Leader* 11 (3): 6–7, 28–29.

King, T.W. (1999). *Assistive Technology: Essential Human Factors.* Boston, MA: Allyn & Bacon.

Korsten, J. (n.d.). Augmentative & alternative communication immersion. Retrieved from https://aacimmersion.weebly.com/the-proof.html.

Law, J., Garrett, Z., and Nye, C. (2004). The efficacy of treatment for children with developmental speech and language delay/disorder: a meta-analysis. *Journal of Speech, Language, and Hearing Research* 47: 924–943.

Light, J.C. (1988). Interaction involving individuals using augmentative and alternative communication systems: state of the art and future directions. *Augmentative and Alternative Communication* 4: 66–82.

Light, J.C. (1989). Toward a definition of communicative competence for individuals using augmentative and alternative communication systems. *Augmentative and Alternative Communication* 5: 1367–1144.

Light, J.C. (1997). Communication is the essence of human life: reflections on communication competence. *Augmentative and Alternative Communication* 13: 61–70.

Light, J.C. (2003). Shattering the silence: development of communicative competence by individuals who use AAC. In: *Communicative Competence for Individuals Who Use AAC: From Research to Effective Practice* (ed. J.C. Light, D.R. Beukelman and J. Reichle), 3–38. Baltimore, MD: Paul H. Brookes.

Light, J.C., Arnold, K.B., and Clark, E.A. (2003). *Finding a place in the "social circle of life." In: Communicative Competence for Individuals Who Use AAC: From Research to Effective Practice (ed. J.C. Light, D.R. Beukelman and J. Reichle)*, 361–397. Baltimore, MD: Paul H. Brookes.

Light, J.C., Collier, B., and Parnes, P. (1985). Communicative interaction between young nonspeaking physically disabled children and their primary caregivers: part I – discourse patterns. *Augmentative and Alternative Communication* 1: 74–83.

Light, J.C., Binger, C., and Kelford-Smith, A. (1994). Story reading interactions between preschoolers who use AAC and their mothers. *Augmentative and Alternative Communication* 10: 255–268.

Light, J.C. and McNaughton, D. (2012). Supporting the communication, language, and literacy development of children with complex communication needs: state of the science and future research priorities. *Assistive Technology* 24: 34–44.

Light, J.C. and McNaughton, D. (2015). Designing AAC research and intervention to improve outcomes for individuals with complex communication needs. *Augmentative and Alternative Communication* 31: 85–96.

Light, J.C., Parsons, A.R., and Drager, K.D.R. (2002). "There's more to life than cookies": developing interactions for social closeness with beginning communicators who require augmentative and alternative communication. In: *Exemplary Practices for Beginning Communicators: Implications for AAC* (ed. J. Reichle, D.R. Beukelman and J.C. Light), 187–218. Baltimore, MD: Paul H. Brookes.

McNaughton, D. and Light, J.C. (2013). The iPad™ and mobile technology revolution: benefits and challenges for individuals who require augmentative and alternative communication. *Augmentative and Alternative Communication* 29 (2): 107–116.

Mirenda, P. (2014). Revisiting the mosaic of supports required for including people with severe intellectual or developmental disabilities in their communities. *Augmentative and Alternative Communication* 30: 19–27.

Musselwhite, C.R. and St. Louis, K.W. (1988). *Communication Programming for Persons with Severe Handicaps.* Boston, MA: College-Hill.

Prentice, J. (2000). With communication anything is possible. In: *Speaking Up and Spelling It Out* (ed. M. Fried-Oken and H.A. Bersani), 208–214. Baltimore, MD: Paul H. Brookes.

Prizant, B. and Wetherby, A. (1989). Providing services to children with autism (ages 0–2 years) and their families. *Focus on Autism and Other Developmental Disabilities* 4 (2): 1–16.

Rehabilitation Act (1973). (29 U.S.C. § 701 et seq.).

Rodgers, N. and Brown, L. (2005). AAC: if you're not into it yet, you should be! *Perspectives on Augmentative and Alternative Communication* 14 (2): 2–5.

Romski, M.A. and Sevcik, R.A. (1996). *Breaking the Speech Barrier: Language Development Through Augmented Means.* Baltimore, MD: Paul H. Brookes.

Rummel-Hudson, R. (2011). A revolution at their fingertips. *Perspectives on Augmentative and Alternative Communication* 20 (1): 19–23.

Schnoll, R. and Zimmerman, B.J. (2001). Self-regulation training enhances dietary self-efficacy and dietary fiber consumption. *Journal of the American Dietetic Association* 101: 1006–1011.

Schunk, D. and Zimmerman, B.J. (2008). *Motivation and Self-Regulated Learning: Theory, Research, and Applications.* New York: Lawrence Erlbaum.

Shane, H.C. and Costello, J. (1994). Augmentative communication assessment and the feature matching process. Mini-seminar presented at the Annual Convention of the American Speech-Language-Hearing Association, New Orleans, LA (17–21 November).

Shane, H.C., O'Brien, M., and Sorce, J. (2009). Use of a visual graphic language system to support communication for persons on the autism spectrum. *Perspectives on Augmentative and Alternative Communication* 18: 130–136.

Staehely, J. (2000). Prologue: the communication dance. In: *Speaking Up and Spelling It Out* (ed. M. Fried-Oken and H.A. Bersani), 1–12. Baltimore, MD: Paul H. Brookes.

Teachman, G. and Gibson, B. (2014). "Communicative competence" in the field of augmentative and alternative communication: a review and critique. *International Journal of Language & Communication Disorders* 49 (1): 1–14.

Technology-Related Assistance for Individuals with Disabilities Act of 1988 (1988). (PL-100-407).

Thistle, J. and Wilkinson, K. (2013). Working memory demands of aided augmentative and alternative communication for individuals with developmental disabilities. *Augmentative and Alternative Communication* 29 (3): 235–245.

Timler, G., Olswang, L., and Coggins, T. (2005). "Do I know what I need to do?" A social communication intervention for children with complex clinical profiles. *Language, Speech, and Hearing Services in Schools* 36 (1): 73–85.

Vicente, K. (2006). *The Human Factor: Revolutionizing the Way We Live with Technology*. New York: Routledge, Taylor & Francis Group.

Waller, A., Balandin, S.A., O'Mara, D.A. and Judson, A.D. (2005). Training AAC users in user-centred design. Retrieved from https://www.researchgate.net/publication/250835931.

Wasson, C.A., Arvidson, H.H., and Lloyd, L.L. (1997). AAC assessment process. In: *Augmentative and Alternative Communication: A Handbook of Principles and Practices* (ed. L.L. Lloyd, D.R. Fuller and H.H. Arvidson), 169–198. Boston, MA: Allyn & Bacon.

Williams, B. (2000). More than an exception to the rule. In: *Speaking Up and Spelling It Out* (ed. M. Fried-Oken and H.A. Bersani), 245–254. Baltimore, MD: Paul H. Brookes.

18

Hearing loss and hearing-related factors: Technology and environmental interventions

Amy Rominger and Leisha R. Eiten

Outline

Assistive Technologies and Environmental Interventions in Healthcare: An Integrated Approach, First Edition.
Edited by Lynn Gitlow and Kathleen Flecky.

Companion website: www.wiley.com/go/gitlow/assitivetechnologies

Learning outcomes

After reading this chapter, you should be able to:

1. Define relevant terminology used to describe hearing loss and its associated difficulties.
2. Describe the impact of hearing loss in educational, vocational, or workplace and psychosocial domains.
3. Apply the Human-Tech Ladder (Vicente 2006) to hearing loss and hearing-related factors.
4. Delineate relevant tools and strategies for assessment of technology needs and environmental interventions for individuals with hearing loss.
5. Compare various technology options for specific listening environments, such as in the classroom, the workplace, the home, or for social settings.

Active learning prompts

Before you read this chapter:

1. Identify several strategies you could creatively apply when encountering a difficult listening environment, such as a setting with significant background noise or poor acoustics or an environment in which the speaker of interest is far away from you.
2. Complete a web search using the words "assistive technology" and "hearing loss." How many online catalogs note products for direct consumer (individual client or family member) purchase? How many products are in each available category? If you were a consumer looking to purchase a product for the first time, could you utilize the information provided by the catalog to understand and choose the item you need?
3. Investigate the range of assistive hearing technologies that are available at your academic institution for persons who experience hearing loss. What surprised you about your investigation?
4. Contact a local playhouse or movie theater and determine what hearing technologies are available to individuals who experience hearing loss or are impacted by hearing-related factors. What did you learn about these settings related to hearing concerns?

Key terms

Cochlear implant
Conductive hearing loss
Frequency modulation (FM) system
Hearing aid
Hearing impairment
Hearing threshold
Induction loop
Infrared system
Mixed hearing loss
Personal sound amplification products (PSAPs)
Sensorineural hearing loss
Telecoil
Vicente's Human-Tech Ladder model

Introduction

What is hearing? In some contexts, hearing is thought of as a sense that provides an awareness of sound (Hearing Loss Association of America n.d.). In more technical anatomy and physiology terms, hearing is the transfer of sound waves through the auditory system to the brain. In functional terms, hearing can be thought of as an avenue for connecting with others and with the outside world. This connection can be through speech and language; one example is a baby learning to understand and use speech. It could also be a thought-provoking, exciting lecture or understanding instructions and treatment plans from a doctor. Expressions of emotion or excitement and the enjoyment of music are also conveyed through sound. Hearing plays a critical role in connecting to the outside world. For people with hearing loss, assistive technology can be an excellent way to help re-establish links to the world around them. This chapter aims to introduce the impact of hearing loss and hearing-related factors and how to consider technology and environmental interventions (TEI) that may be helpful to an individual who has lost some, or all, of their auditory connections to their environment.

Definitions related to hearing loss

The terms hearing impairment, hearing disability, and hearing handicap are often used interchangeably; however, the World Health Organization's (WHO) International Classification of Function (ICF) specifies a distinction between each of these terms (World Health Organization 2001b). Impairment refers to the problems with a structure in the body or its function, specifically one that includes loss and a significant deviation from the norm for that structure. In the case of auditory function, hearing impairment or hearing loss is a deviation from normal hearing. Hearing impairment and hearing loss are interchangeable terms when referring to the loss or reduction of function of the auditory system. Even though the term hearing impairment is often used to describe auditory system dysfunction, referring to someone as a hearing impaired person should be avoided, as it deviates from person-first language that is recommended when referring to individuals with disabilities (Speech-Language & Hearing Association n.d.). For example, a patient or client is not referred to as a "hearing impaired patient," but instead as a "patient with hearing impairment" or a "patient with hearing loss."

Disability refers to the outcome of the combination of the structural impairment in the body (the hearing loss), how this impairment interacts with the person's physical and social environment, and his or her individual characteristics and qualities. This WHO resolution (World Health Organization 2001b) updates previous definitions of disability to include an individual's interaction with their environment when discussing their limitations in activity participation. The term hearing handicap has been used to refer to the obstacles imposed by society on those with hearing disabilities; however, the word "handicap" carries a stigma for many people and is not recommended for use following this new WHO resolution.

Prevalence of hearing loss

According to the WHO (2018), there are around 466 million people who have hearing loss and 34 million of them are children.

For the adult population included in these statistics (defined as older than 12 years of age), hearing loss is typically an acquired condition. Acquired means that the individual was not born with the loss, but rather it developed at some time after birth.

Some common causes of acquired hearing loss include ear infections, infectious diseases, use of drugs that are toxic to the ear (termed *ototoxic*), noise exposure, head trauma, and age-related hearing loss. Hearing loss is increasingly common in the aging population, with the presence of hearing loss increasing with every decade of aging and reported as affecting close to 63% of adults over the age of 70 (Lin et al. 2011). The marked prevalence of hearing loss in the aging population makes it one of the most common chronic health conditions in the United States (Mathers et al. 2008). The WHO estimates even higher hearing loss prevalence in countries without ready access to medical and surgical services, where otherwise-treatable causes of hearing loss are often untreated, resulting in permanent loss (WHO Estimates 2013).

Hearing loss is not just an adult or aging problem. It is estimated that approximately 1–6 newborns per 1000 are born with permanent hearing loss (Centers for Disease Control and Prevention 2010; Cunningham and Cox 2003; Harlor and Bower 2009). Congenital hearing loss is increasingly diagnosed early in infancy due to the implementation of universal newborn hearing screening (UNHS) and Early Hearing Diagnosis and Intervention (EHDI) programs in most states and provinces. Children can also acquire hearing loss in later childhood, which accounts for the overall increase in prevalence in childhood (Boulet et al. 2009; Centers for Disease Control and Prevention 1997; Niskar et al. 1998).

Descriptive characteristics of hearing loss

Degree

Permanent hearing loss can vary greatly in both degree and configuration or shape. When determining the degree of hearing loss, an audiologist will play a series of tones, finding the lowest level at which a person can detect those tones. Once the lowest level of detection or *hearing threshold* is determined, it is plotted on an audiogram using a specified set of symbols (Martin and Clark 2014). An audiogram is a standard graph that acts as a visual representation of an individual's hearing abilities for the range of tones tested. A typical audiogram graph and the symbols used to represent threshold are pictured in Figure 18.1. Frequency, or pitch, is displayed across the top of the graph in units called Hertz (Hz); intensity, or loudness, is displayed down the side of the graph in units called decibels Hearing Level (dB HL).

The range of frequencies that are typically tested and displayed on an audiogram represents the frequencies or tones that are most important for speech understanding (Katz 2014). Tones range from low-pitched bass sounds with lower numbered frequencies on the left side of the graph to high-pitched treble sounds with higher numbered frequencies to the right side of the graph. The range of intensity or loudness is from very quiet at the top of the graph with low dB numbers to very loud at the bottom of the graph with high dB numbers.

After an individual's hearing thresholds are determined, the thresholds are assigned a category for degree of hearing loss based on the decibel level of their responses. There is some variability between the American Speech-Language and Hearing Association (ASHA), the American Academy of Audiology (AAA), and other published studies in the categorization of degree of hearing loss (American Academy of Audiology n.d.; American Speech-Language and Hearing Association n.d.; Clark 1981). In general, *normal hearing* is a range of responses that are observed between −10 and 25 dB HL for adults and −10 and 15 dB HL for children, rather than the ability to respond to a single level of sound.

People with normal hearing threshold responses for all frequencies on the standard audiogram should be able to easily hear soft, average, and loud sounds in most listening situations, even in background noise. *Mild hearing loss,* which ranges from 26 to 40 dB HL, results in difficulty hearing soft sounds and causes increased difficulty understanding speech in noisy backgrounds. *Moderate hearing loss,* ranging from 41 to 55 dB HL and *moderately-severe hearing loss,* from 56 to 70 dB HL, result in an inability to hear soft sounds as well as increasing difficulty hearing moderately loud sound (Katz 2014; Kramer 2013).

People with untreated hearing loss of a moderate degree or worse can have considerable difficulty understanding speech in all listening situations, both in quiet

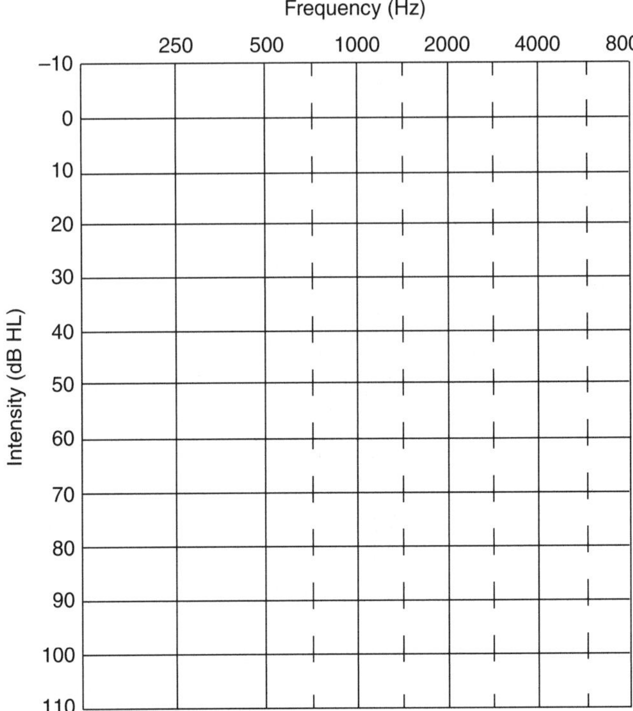

Symbol key	Right	Left
AC unmasked	○	X
AC masked	△	□
BC unmasked	<	>
BC masked	[	]
No response	↙	↘
Soundfleld	S	

Figure 18.1 Art of typical audiograph with symbols.

Table 18.1 Degrees of Hearing Loss and Their Impact on Understanding Speech.

Degree classification	Decibel range of hearing threshold	Impact on understanding speech
Normal hearing	−10–25 dB HL	• Will hear most, if not all, speech sounds
Mild hearing loss	26–40 dB HL	• Will do well in one-on-one conversations • May miss consonants • Will have increased difficulty for soft speech and in background noise
Moderate hearing loss	41–55 dB HL	• Will miss many speech sounds at normal conversational levels, even if face-to-face • Will have some difficulty using the telephone
Moderately-severe hearing loss	56–70 dB HL	• Will miss most speech sounds at normal conversational levels • Will have moderate difficulty using the telephone
Severe hearing loss	71–90 dB HL	• Will miss all normal conversational speech sounds • Will miss many loud speech sounds • Will likely need to rely on visual cues • Will have significant difficulty using the telephone
Profound hearing loss	91 + dB HL	• Cannot hear speech sounds, even if very loud, without amplification • May detect loud sounds as vibrations rather than auditory signals • May only hear extremely loud environmental sounds

Note. Adapted from the American Speech-Language and Hearing Association (2015) and the American Academy of Audiology (n.d.).

and in background noise. *Severe hearing loss,* which ranges from 71 to 90 dB HL, allows some loud sounds to remain audible, but communication without some type of amplification is difficult. *Profound hearing loss*, with hearing levels louder than 90 dB HL, may allow only extremely loud sounds to be audible. People with profound hearing loss may not be able to identify sounds or understand speech even if hearing aids are used (Katz 2014; Martin and Clark 2014). See Table 18.1 for more detailed effects of different degrees of hearing loss.

Configuration

The configuration of a hearing loss is the pattern of the loss across the frequencies (pitches) of sound that are important for understanding speech. Configuration of loss can be thought of as the shape of an individual's hearing levels when viewed on the audiogram, or more specifically, the degree of loss at each pitch. Common hearing loss configurations include *sloping* losses, *flat* losses, *rising* losses, *notched* losses, and *cookie-bite* losses. See Figure 18.2 for examples.

An individual with a sloping loss has better hearing for low-frequency sounds, such as vowels, and poorer hearing for high-frequency consonant sounds like "s" and "t." A flat configuration represents the same degree of hearing loss across all the important speech frequencies. A rising configuration, the opposite of a sloping configuration, indicates that the individual has poorer hearing for low frequencies, such as vowels, and better hearing for high frequencies, such as consonants. A notched hearing loss depicts a hearing loss that is only present at one frequency or very few neighboring frequencies. A "cookie bite" or U-shaped loss depicts better hearing ability for both very low and very high frequencies, with poorer hearing for middle speech frequencies (Katz 2014; Kramer 2013).

Another configuration characteristic, *symmetric* or *asymmetric*, can be used to compare the degree and shape of hearing loss from ear to ear. Describing hearing losses by using the configuration attribute allows one to quickly and efficiently determine which speech sounds a person may or may not hear. Many different degrees and configurations of hearing loss are possible, though children show a greater amount of variability in degree, configuration, and symmetry of their hearing losses than do adults (Pittman and Stelmachowicz 2003).

Type of hearing loss

In addition to describing degree and configuration, the type of hearing loss is also important in characterizing the loss. There are three primary types of hearing loss: *conductive* hearing loss, *sensorineural* hearing loss, and *mixed* hearing loss. The type of hearing loss is directly related to the part of the auditory anatomy that is dysfunctional. The auditory system is responsible for transferring sound waves from the environment all the way up to the brain for interpretation (Martin and Clark 2014). The peripheral auditory system can be divided into three distinct sections: the outer ear, the middle ear, and the inner ear (Figure 18.3).

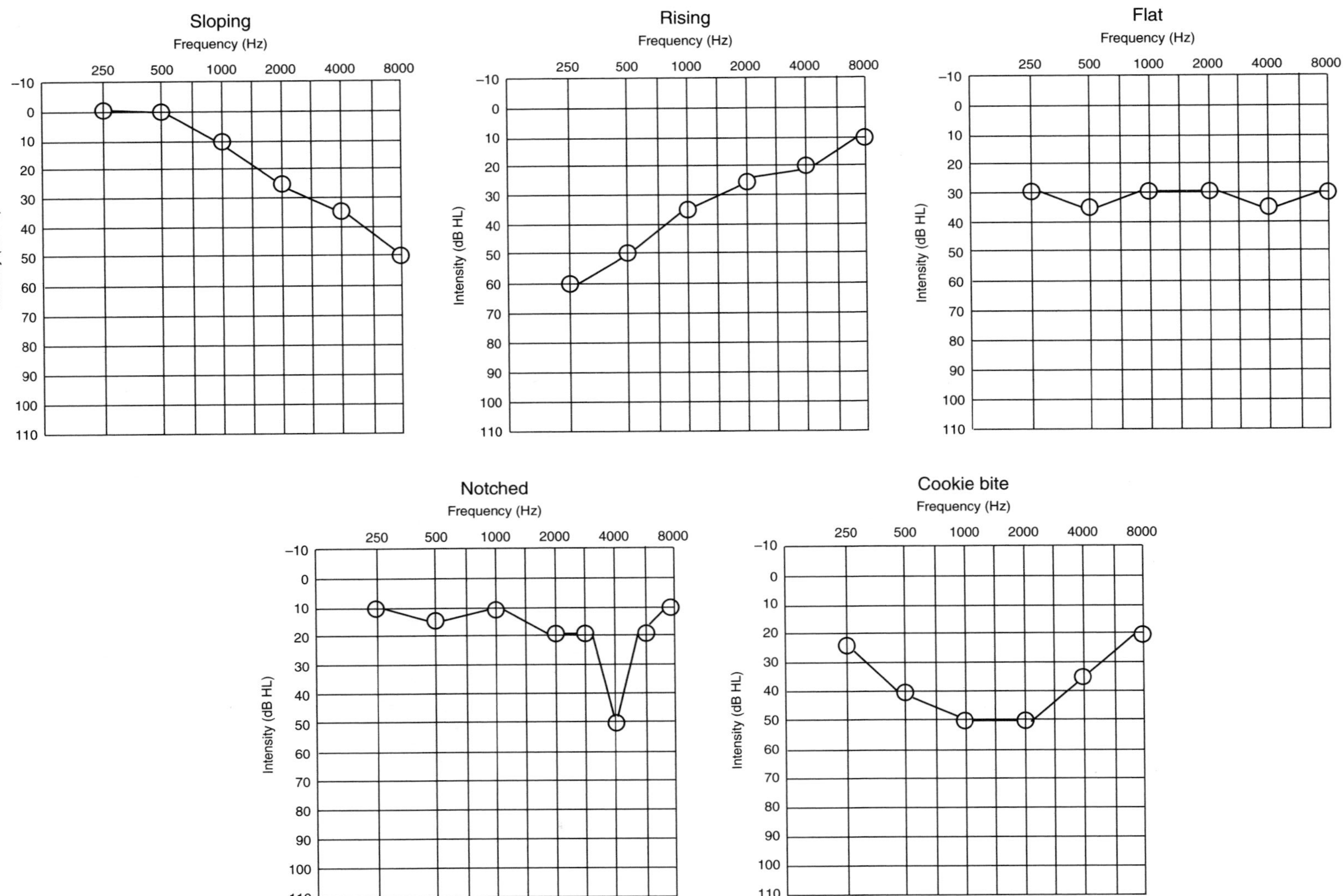

Figure 18.2 Configurations of hearing loss. Note

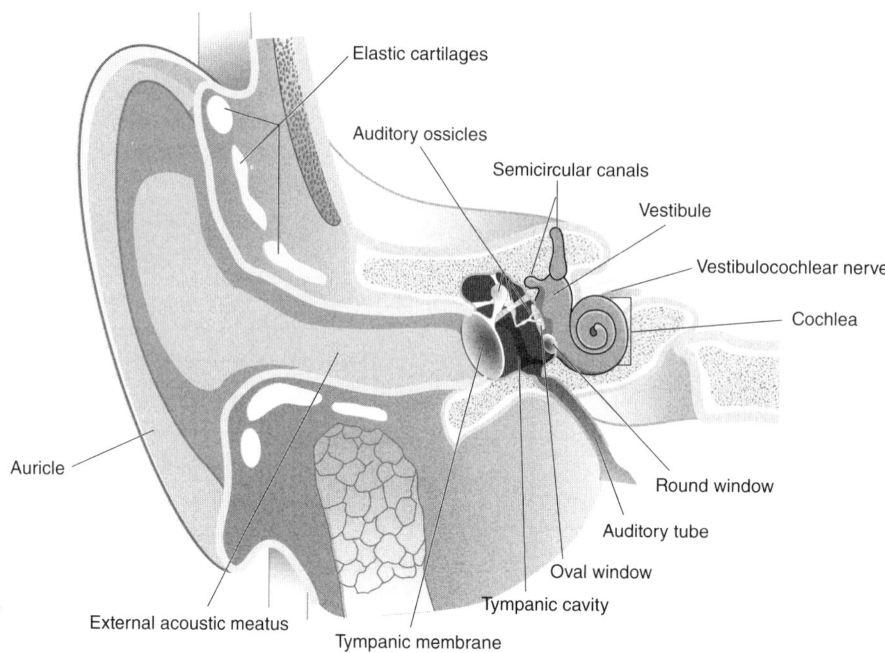

Figure 18.3 Anatomy of the ear.

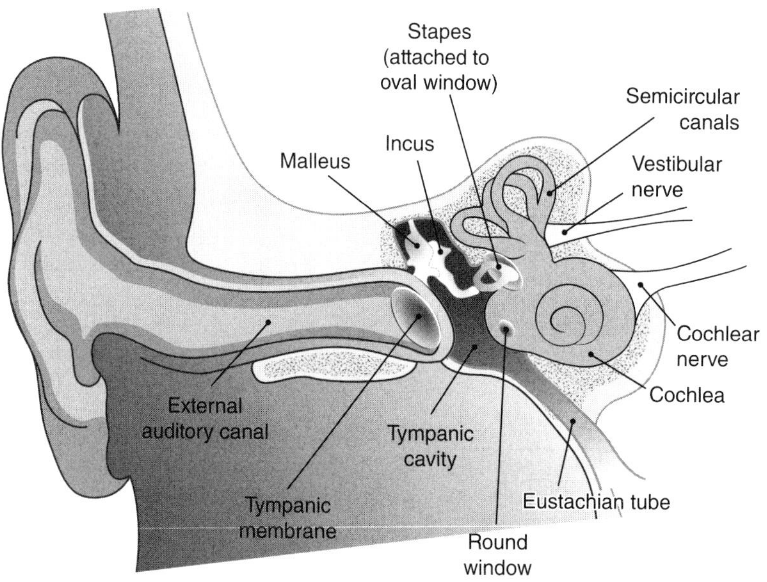

Figure 18.4 Artwork of close-up anatomy of tympanic membrane and cochlea. Source: Chittka and Brockmann (2005).

The outer ear is the portion of the auditory system that is responsible for collecting sound waves from the environment and transferring them down the ear canal to the tympanic membrane, also known as the eardrum (Seikel and King 2015). The tympanic membrane serves as the barrier between the outer ear and middle ear, and when the sound wave reaches it, the membrane is set into vibratory motion. The middle ear relies on three bones, known as ossicles, to transfer sound from the vibrating tympanic membrane to the inner ear (Seikel and King 2015). Because the ossicles are connected to the tympanic membrane, when the tympanic membrane is set into motion by sound, the chain of bones is also set into motion, further transferring sound along the auditory pathway until it reaches the opening to the inner ear. The cochlea is the spiral-shaped inner ear structure that transforms the sound into a signal that the brain can interpret (Seikel and King 2015). See Figure 18.4.

A conductive hearing loss occurs when there is some form of pathology in the outer and/or middle ear.

Common pathologies observed in these two sections of the auditory system include wax (cerumen) or foreign body blockage of the ear canal, deformities of the outer ear or middle ear, and fluid buildup resulting from ear infection (Katz 2014). Anything that causes a barrier to sound travel through the outer and/or middle ear will cause some degree of conductive hearing loss. Conductive hearing losses can often be treated with medicine or through surgery, which frequently results in a reversal of the hearing loss (Katz 2014).

A sensorineural hearing loss occurs when the pathology lies in the inner ear and/or the auditory nerve. A sensorineural hearing loss is typically due to damage to the hair cells in the cochlea and/or to auditory nerve fibers. Although there are many potential causes of this damage, some common causes are noise exposure, trauma, or the normal aging process (Katz 2014). Sensorineural hearing loss is almost always a permanent loss that cannot be reversed through medication or surgery. It is commonly treated with the use of amplification, such as hearing aids or cochlear implants (Katz 2014).

A mixed hearing loss results from a combination of a conductive hearing loss and a sensorineural hearing loss. In this instance there is some type of blockage of sound transfer through the outer and/or middle ear plus dysfunction of the inner ear and/or of the auditory nerve (Katz 2014). As discussed before, the sensorineural portion of the loss is typically not reversible; however, the conductive portion of the loss may be reversible through medical intervention if appropriate (Katz 2014; Seikel and King 2015).

Effects of hearing loss

The possible effects of hearing loss are significant and wide-ranging for infants, young children, and adults alike. These effects can present as speech and language delays, educational difficulties, social-emotional issues, vocational and workplace barriers, and interpersonal relationship problems. Numerous studies have evaluated children with hearing loss of varying degrees and have reported both short- and long-term effects on academic performance, speech and language development, and social-emotional development (Reyes 2008; Tye-Murray et al. 1995; Yoshinaga-Itano 2001; Yoshinaga-Itano and Sedey 1998). Hearing loss decreases the ability to hear speech and this decrease has a direct impact on the development of speech and language, since a child's speech and language output relates to what he or she hears (Tye-Murray 2008). According to Tye-Murray (2008), the overall ability to understand the speech of a child with hearing loss, also known as intelligibility, decreases as the degree of hearing loss increases. If a child is unable to hear specific speech sounds, then it is less likely that they will produce those speech sounds correctly.

Additionally, the intelligibility of speech in this population can also be influenced by how young the child was when their hearing loss was identified, how much speech therapy they have received, how soon after identification they were fit with appropriate amplification, and how consistently they have worn their amplification. Mitchell and Karchmer (2004) report that approximately 92% of infants with hearing loss are born to parents with normal hearing who use spoken language to communicate. If an infant cannot hear their parent's spoken language, early language input and learning can be dramatically affected. Not only can the ability to understand language be delayed, so can the ability to express language. Effects on expressive language are more significant in children without early identification of hearing loss or appropriate early intervention, including technology interventions (Moeller 2000; Yoshinaga-Itano 2001; Yoshinaga-Itano and Sedey 1998).

Educational

When there is difficulty communicating in the classroom, academic achievement has been shown to suffer, and children with hearing loss consistently fall short of the academic norms of their normal-hearing peers (Long et al. 1991; Md Daud et al. 2010; Stinson and Antia 1999). Difficulty communicating in the classroom can come from a number of sources, including the inability to keep up with the teacher's spoken message, an inability to hear speech in background noise, difficulty following the rapid speech of multiple talkers, and decreased access to the spoken academic content. Socially and emotionally, children can have difficulty developing relationships with their classmates due to their language problems, low self-esteem, or the one thing most children dread: being different from their peers. Identity issues may develop, specifically during adolescence and the teenage years. Loneliness and bullying have been reported as two of the top reasons why adolescents with hearing loss don't self-identify or admit to having a hearing loss (Kent 2003).

Psychosocial

For adults, many of the same issues arise regarding social-emotional stability. The impact of hearing loss on the ability to understand speech, whether it is within interpersonal communication or when gathering information in social situations, can lead to a withdrawal from those social settings. When it becomes difficult to

Box 18.1 Visual simulation

A visual simulation of what it might be like to listen to *The Pledge of Allegiance* with a moderate high-frequency hearing loss.

I ledge a legion oo uh lag uh uh Unied a uh Ameriuh, and oo uh Re ubli or whi ih and, one Na on under God, indivible, wih liberee and ju ih or all.

Missing speech sounds highlighted in gray:

I pledge allegiance to the Flag of the United States of America, and to the Republic for which it stands, one Nation under God, indivisible, with liberty and justice for all.

carry on a conversation at a party, understand dialogue in a movie, or understand the main points of a leader during a religious service, an individual with hearing loss may stop participating in those activities (see Box 18.1). This withdrawal and isolation has been shown to lead to a decrease in self-worth and an increase in depression (Arlinger 2003; Cacciatore et al. 1999; Chew and Yeak 2010; Veras and Mattos 2007). The National Council on the Aging (Seniors Research Group 1999) found that adults who did not wear appropriate amplification (e.g. hearing aids) were more prone to bouts of depression, were more anxious, had higher levels of paranoia, and had an overall decrease in quality of life. On the other hand, the authors also found that those older adults who used the appropriate technology to treat their hearing losses were more likely to participate in social activities and reported better quality of life, including improved relationships and mental health.

Vocational and workplace

As the aging population gets larger, more and more adults with hearing loss are expected to remain in the workplace. Vocational issues caused by hearing loss should not be overlooked. Difficulty hearing in meetings, especially when more than one person is talking, and struggling to keep up with or understand instructions can lead to more stress in the workplace (Jennings and Shaw 2008). Quality of life in adults with hearing loss is strongly related to whether their individual needs in their particular environments are being adequately addressed, specifically through appropriate technology.

The human-tech ladder, hearing loss, and hearing-related factors

The Human-Tech Ladder, as has been discussed in previous chapters, is a concept developed by Vicente (2006) to explain how technology can be designed and implemented for human use on a hierarchical scale of human factors.

When developing technological and environmental interventions for individuals with hearing loss, one must consider physical, psychological, team, organizational, and political factors (Vicente 2006). Hearing loss itself is a physical factor, with a number of resulting psychological factors to be considered. These are the two primary factors to consider when designing technological and environment interventions for this population, as they have the most direct impact on the individual. Many of the situations in which individuals with hearing loss experience difficulty can be mitigated through consideration of these two human factors. However, attention must be paid to the other three factors as they have an indirect impact on the assistive technology choices available.

Physical factors

The first level of consideration on Vicente's Human-Tech Ladder (2006) is the physical attributes of an individual. This includes their body's stature, size, dexterity, strengths, and weaknesses. When addressing hearing loss, the first thing to consider is the structure of the ear. Where is the pathology? Is the visible portion of the ear, the outer ear, intact? If the individual is given a listening device, how will it couple to the ear? There are some pathologies of the ear, such as microtia, an underdevelopment of the outer ear, which can make it difficult for the individual to use hearing aids or certain types of headphones (Katz 2014). In some cases where there is no outer ear structure present, double-sided wig tape, toupee tape, or a soft headband can be used to hold the device in place.

Even when hearing loss is the focus of intervention, other physical factors need to be taken into consideration. In the pediatric population it is not uncommon for a child to pull hearing aids or cochlear implants off their ears. Another frequent issue with young children is that their ears are small and the cartilage is not as rigid, so heavy devices can fall off. In these cases a low-technology loss-prevention device such as EarGear™, Safe-N-Sound™, or Oto/Critter Clips™ should be considered. A snug cap on the child's head is another simple solution that allows for a tight fit against the head so that the child does not pull off the listening devices.

Adults and older adults

For individuals on the other end of the age spectrum, some common physical difficulties with using hearing technology have to do with upper limb mobility, strength, dexterity, and sense of touch. Many hearing devices are small or have small controls, which makes care, maintenance, and manipulation of the devices challenging. A person with poor dexterity may not be able to grip a small battery for insertion into the device. This is especially true for small hearing aids, which require a battery change as often as once a week. A low-tech solution is to use a small tool with a magnet on the end to pick up the battery and help with insertion into the device or removal when it needs to be changed. With certain types of neuropathy or other loss of feeling in the fingers, it may be difficult to locate or manipulate the controls on the assistive devices. Some hearing aids can be ordered with modified control wheels with extra height. If this is not an option, it may be useful to use a hardened dot of glue or a thick sticker on specific controls that need identification through touch.

Persons with visual concerns

Visual limitations can pose challenges to the implementation of technology. A common question from new hearing aid users is, "How do I know which one goes on which ear?" Most hearing aids have a small colored indicator on the battery door that lets the user know in which ear they belong. For individuals with vision impairment, visual indicators may be difficult to detect, so the use of a larger colored sticker or a sticker with a designated texture can be placed on the body of the hearing aid based on the user's needs. Vision impairment can also pose a barrier to the use of captioning or text supplements while watching television or using the telephone.

Persons with disabilities: Deafness and blindness

Individuals with the dual disability of deafness and blindness present a particular challenge to all professionals involved, as visual supplements to assist with hearing loss and auditory supplements to assist with vision loss may not provide effective assistance for the individual to communicate with others or to be aware of the variety of sights and sounds around them. Individuals with this dual disability require careful team management to determine the degree of residual visual and hearing abilities and how to best supplement/substitute for each individual's needs. Some possible considerations are to find technologies that convert visual and auditory signals to touch/vibratory stimulation, or to use a combination of visual and/or auditory amplification, if possible.

Psychological factors

The second level on the Human-Tech Ladder relates to psychological factors (Vicente 2006). Some of the psychosocial consequences of hearing loss have been discussed earlier in this chapter, therefore the focus here will be on the psychological factors that need to be taken into consideration when choosing technology for an individual with hearing loss.

Young children

When an infant or a young child is first diagnosed with hearing loss it can come as a shock to their parents, especially if there is no history of childhood hearing loss in the family. In addition to experiencing the surprise, anger, and/or denial of the grieving process that can follow this diagnosis, parents receive a great deal of new and complex recommendations and treatment plans for their child. Parents of children with newly diagnosed hearing loss often report that they feel inundated with complex information (Russ et al. 2004).

The combination of intense emotions and the flood of new information about hearing loss, treatment options, communication options, education options, and technology options has led to parents feeling overwhelmed and confused (Fitzpatrick et al. 2008). Sass-Lehrer (2004) suggests following a model of intervention that focuses on self-empowerment and centers on the family. Written literature with simple information about the diagnosis and next steps can be helpful. It gives parents something to refer to later, when emotions are not as high and they are better able to process new information.

Additionally, information on connecting with parent support groups or with parents who have already navigated this diagnosis can be invaluable. While these suggestions do not strictly fit into the definition of technology, they certainly conform to Vicente's inclusion of non-hardware as technology (2006). Fostering education and a sense of understanding for parents can go a long way in ensuring proper selection, compliance, and appreciation of the hardware technology that may be used with their child.

Adolescents

For adolescents, and adults, one psychological factor to consider is the balance between finding technology that is appropriate for the person's audiologic needs and technology that the person is willing to use. The fear of negative feedback causes some individuals to reject any type of technology that is visible to others. Adolescents and teens may refuse to wear a device in the classroom because they do not want to stand out as different from their classmates. If a child's classroom teacher needs to wear a visible microphone to connect with hearing aid or cochlear implant technology, the child with hearing loss may feel that the microphone represents a visible beacon at the front of the classroom that highlights their disabilities.

This teen-aged population may be extremely concerned and self-conscious about what could be termed the "hearing aid effect." This effect happens when outside observers rate hearing aid wearers more negatively in categories such as intelligence, attractiveness, reliability, and personality, primarily based on having visible hearing aids (David and Werner 2016; Danhauer et al. 1980; Dengerink and Porter 1984; Mulac et al. 1983; Silverman and Klees 1989). The hearing aid effect can be caused not only by the onlooker's poor thoughts about individuals with hearing aids, but also by the projection of poor self-esteem and self-worth by the hearing aid user onto themselves (Doggett et al. 1998).

Some classroom teachers may have a negative reaction to wearing hearing assistance equipment such as a microphone. In the demanding and sometimes chaotic setting of classroom teaching, some teachers may feel that using and maintaining classroom hearing technology is too much to add to an ever-growing list of responsibilities. This can lead to the child with hearing loss feeling as if they are a burden or problem for the teacher. The best solution is to find technology hardware that meets the user's needs while also allowing them to feel comfortable using it. Vicente's broader definition of technology (2006) is useful in finding this balance; this includes counseling the child on their audiologic needs, educating the child and the teachers/educators working with the child, and coming up with a training schedule for everyone involved.

Adults

While adults may experience some of the same psychological factors as adolescents and teens, a slightly different perspective is needed. While an adolescent or teen is in the middle of developing their self-identity, an adult with later-developing hearing loss has already established their identity and self-concept as a hearing person. When an acquired hearing loss has an onset after the establishment of identity, a crisis can sometimes ensue. Johnson (2011) suggested that these individuals go through a grieving process because of detachment between the person they have always perceived themselves as being and their new reality.

The workplace can be an environment where this disconnect can have a heavy impact. The hearing aid effect may cause them to be worried about being seen as a poorer performer, or they may be worried they will lose their position to someone younger. When establishing a technological fit for these individuals, it is important to find devices that will fit in seamlessly with everyday tasks and needs. Interpersonal relationships can also be a realm where an adult may struggle with hearing loss as part of their identity. Spouses have reported feeling embarrassed, frustrated, angry, lonely, and annoyed when faced with an adult partner with hearing loss (Donaldson et al. 2004). To mitigate these issues, a person's important communication partners must be considered when choosing a technological intervention.

Team factors

Children

The primary team for implementing hearing assistance technology will change based on the population in question. A team rehabilitation approach is standard practice for preschool and school-aged children (Katz 2014). A child with hearing loss may have physicians, audiologists, speech-language pathologists, teachers of the hard-of-hearing, classroom teachers, and other allied health/rehabilitation professionals on their team along with their parents. Each professional brings a different perspective on how to overcome barriers to maximize access to information. Technological and environmental intervention is included in formalized educational planning and relies heavily on multidisciplinary team decisions. Under the Individuals with Disabilities Education Act (IDEA), which falls under the political human factors category, in order for children with hearing loss to have mandatory technological interventions in the educational setting, an individualized family service plan (IFSP) or individualized education plan (IEP) is necessary (IDEA Part B Regulations 2006; IDEA Part C Regulations 2011). The process for creating these documents requires a multidisciplinary team. For children with multiple sensory or system disorders or with limited physical ability to manipulate hearing assistance technology, the team may include more members. With so many moving parts to a team, detailed and accurate documentation and excellent communication is necessary.

Adults

For most adults whose only impairment is hearing loss, a technology team will likely be small (Katz 2014). It will mostly consist of the individual, their audiologist or hearing instrument dispenser, their spouse or other family members, and possibly an ear, nose, and throat (ENT) physician. Other rehabilitation professionals would not likely see a person whose only concern is hearing loss; however, primary healthcare providers are of critical importance in recognizing signs of developing hearing loss and in referring individuals for evaluation and consultation regarding hearing and communication concerns. When a person with hearing loss has multiple physical or cognitive concerns, a larger rehabilitation team is helpful in setting technology priorities and in reviewing the type of hearing assistant technology that would be most beneficial to the individual. Even though this is ideal, in reality it can be difficult to coordinate services with multiple professionals. Audiologists must often rely on family and friends to assist with technology decisions for an adult with multiple disabilities, and other rehabilitation professionals may be unaware of what hearing assistance technologies are available or how to use them.

Organizational and political factors

Regulation

Regulation for the licensing of audiologists and hearing instrument specialists is handled by the individual state where the professional practices. For audiologists, many states base their licensing requirements on the certification requirements of the ASHA, which provides accreditation to higher-education programs and outlines skills and knowledge necessary for clinical practice and certification (ASHA 2015). ASHA, as well as the AAA, provides practice recommendations and continuing education opportunities for all appropriately credentialed audiologists.

Federal law dictates who is legally entitled to hearing loss accommodations in the educational setting, in public places, and in the workplace. The IDEA guarantees services to children with qualifying disabilities. These services may include the provision of assistive hearing technology to ensure equal access to information for children from birth to 3 years under Part C and 3–21 years under Part B (IDEA Part B Regulations 2006; IDEA Part C Regulations 2011). For adults, the Americans with Disabilities Act (ADA) guarantees access to employment and public services for individuals with hearing loss (Americans with Disabilities Act 1990). The ADA prohibits employers from discriminating against qualified individuals with hearing loss for gaining employment and receiving fair compensation. Additionally, it requires employers to provide reasonable accommodations for these individuals, which could include technological or environmental interventions. It also guarantees equal access to public services, access to public buildings, and access to transportation, among other rights. Included in this provision is the specific mention of auxiliary aids to assist in gaining equal access.

Regulatory oversight for amplification and telecommunications is extensive. The Food and Drug Administration (FDA) (Regulatory Requirements for Hearing Aid Devices and Personal Sound Amplification Products 2009) has regulatory control over hearing aid technology. The FDA clearly defines hearing aids as devices for the use of treating hearing loss, while personal sound amplifying products (PSAPs) are for recreational use and are not intended to treat hearing loss (Regulatory Requirements for Hearing Aid Devices and Personal Sound Amplification Products 2009). It is critical to understand this distinction, so that when certain hearing assistance technology is recommended, the purpose and intended use is not misunderstood. Aside from the FDA, individual states have legislative control over the dispensing of hearing aids and assistive devices in their jurisdiction.

Legislation

The laws regarding which professionals are licensed to dispense hearing aids and assistive devices vary from state to state. The Federal Communications Commission (FCC) controls telecommunications technology. In 2010, regulations were updated to increase the access of individuals with disabilities to modern communications (21st Century Communications and Video Accessibility Act 2010). This act allows individuals with hearing loss access to telephone and video services, including Voice over Internet Protocol (VoIP) service, non-interconnected VoIP, electronic messaging services, and interoperable video messaging services. Additionally, this act regulates how many and which devices must have hearing aid compatibility, allowing for greater access to telephone services for individuals with hearing loss.

Selecting assistive technology for hearing loss

The broad goal of TEI for people with hearing loss is to restore or improve communication access in order to establish or maintain social and emotional connections. Those connections happen with significant others, family members, and friends, as well as within the larger community in which a person lives and works. In addition to enabling social communication, appropriate technology should be available to promote safety and independence in a person's living situation. TEI intervention can also be applied in a narrow way by choosing a specific technology that addresses only the environments or situations that the individual finds problematical (Katz 2014; Kramer 2013).

Professionals who develop intervention recommendations need to think beyond the typical assumptions of what technology is and embrace the broad view of technology given by Vicente (2006): technology is both physical and non-physical and is any tool that can help humans reach their goals. In terms of working with individuals with hearing loss, it is especially important to consider "softer" elements, such as environmental manipulation and adjustments to interpersonal communication, in addition to the more typical hardware technologies. The assessment tools discussed in this section will address ways to gather information on the activity limitations and participation restrictions imposed by hearing loss. It is important to remember how these limitations and restrictions interact with Vicente's Human-Tech Ladder (2006).

Awareness of activity limitations and participation

There is no universally accepted, standard measure to determine the activity limitations and participation restrictions imposed by hearing loss. Since activity limitations are the disadvantages that a hearing loss inflicts on a person's daily communicative functions, the amount of difficulty that a person experiences will be highly individualized. Hearing loss is often referred to as a "hidden" limitation since it is not always immediately apparent to others. Some individuals may compensate well for their loss, but others may be in denial about the effects of their hearing loss on their daily functions. It may be difficult to determine the effects of a hearing loss when other cognitive or communicative impairments are also present. Recent research has linked hearing loss with declines in memory and thinking skills in adults over the age of 70 years (Lin 2012). Based on the evidence from Lin's research (2012), hearing handicap can disguise itself within cognitive decline and may be a significant contributor in that decline. It can also be a hidden factor behind social isolation and depression in adults (Seniors Research Group 1999).

Assessment tools

When assessing hearing-related difficulties, an unstructured interview can often be used to gather pertinent information about daily communication function. The individual may be able to pinpoint their most significant sources of frustrations and identify their goals in this informal manner. If prompting is needed in order to determine if hearing difficulties exist, a screening questionnaire can be used. Short questionnaires like the 10-item National Institute on Deafness and other Communication Disorders (NIDCD) survey (NIDCD 2015), allow social workers, allied health professionals, physicians, family members, or the individual to determine if hearing difficulty exists and if further investigation is needed. One advantage of this type of tool is that it is quick, free, and easy to administer. However, it does have limitations in that more in-depth information may be desired. An interview technique called *motivational interviewing* (Clark 2010) can also be used to intentionally motivate a client or patient to recognize their difficulties and to identify possible solutions.

Various structured scales and screening tools are available for use when more detailed information is needed. The WHO International Classification of Functioning Checklist (2001a) includes a number of hearing and communication functions in its review of a person's activity limitations and participation restrictions. The ICF Checklist is a general overview of activity and participation; therefore, a tool that focuses on hearing-specific difficulties may be more suitable. The Hearing Handicap Inventory for the Elderly (HHIE) (Ventry and Weinstein 1982), the Hearing Handicap Inventory for Adults (HHIA) (Newman et al. 1990), and the Client Oriented Scale of Improvement (COSI) (Dillon et al. 1997) are some of the hearing-specific instruments available for use in the clinical setting. These screening tools have been primarily developed for adults and ask the individual, or their frequent communication partners, to judge the degree of difficulty they experience in a variety of communication situations. The COSI asks the person with the hearing loss to identify their top five specific listening needs, offering the added benefit of allowing the individual to have more direct participation in their own intervention. Depending on the instrument used, it may also provide a rating of disability or a recommendation for further testing when indicated.

Listening and hearing inventories have been developed for young infants and school-aged children as well. Pediatric inventories primarily rely on parent and teacher report of the child's listening behaviors and speech and language development. The Parents' Evaluation of Aural/Oral Performance of Children (PEACH) (Ching and Hill 2007), the Early Listening Function (ELF) (Anderson 2002), and the Infant-Toddler Meaningful Auditory Integration Scale (IT-MAIS) (Zimmerman-Phillips et al. 2000) are a few assessments available for infants and toddlers with hearing loss. The Children's Home Inventory of Listening Difficulties (CHILD) (Anderson and Smaldino 2000), the Listening Inventory for Education (LIFE) (Anderson and Smaldino 1998), and the Teachers' Evaluation of Aural/Oral Performance of Children (TEACH) (Ching et al. 2007) are some tools used to assess school-aged children. Some inventories for older school-aged children, such as the LIFE and the CHILD, have a child interview component as well. Pediatric-based inventories and scales indicate listening situations

Table 18.2 Select Tools for Assessing Hearing Difficulties and Needs in the Pediatric Population.

Name of assessment	Description	Reference
Infants and toddlers (Birth–3 years)		
Developmental Index of Audition and Listening (DIAL)	Checklist of auditory milestones and listening needs	Palmer and Mormer (1999)
Functional Auditory Performance Indicators (FAPI)	Hierarchical list of auditory skills that helps to determine what a child can and can't do auditorily	Stredler-Brown and Johnson (2004)
Infant-toddler: Meaningful Auditory Integration Scale (IT-MAIS)	Parents report, through an interview with the clinician, their child's spontaneous responses to sound	Zimmerman-Phillips et al. (2000)
Parents' Evaluation of Aural/Oral Performance of Children (PEACH)	Parents evaluate the effectiveness for amplification in children Note: can also be used for school-aged children	Ching and Hill (2005)
Early Listening Function (ELF)	Evaluates the distances at which a child can detect auditory stimuli	Anderson (2002)
School-aged children (3–21 years)		
Auditory Behavior in Everyday Life (ABEL)	Evaluates everyday auditory behaviors, such as auditory awareness and conversational skills	Purdy et al. (2002)
Child's Home Inventory of Listening Difficulties (CHILD)	Parents rate their child's auditory behavior in the home	Anderson and Smaldino (2000)
Teachers' Evaluation of Aural/Oral Performance of Children (TEACH)	Teachers evaluate the effectiveness for amplification in children	Ching et al. (2005)
Screening Instrument for Targeting Educational Risk (SIFTER)	Teacher assesses whether a child is at risk for academic failure Note: there is also a preschool version available for children three to five years	Anderson (1989)

Table 18.3 Select Tools for Assessing Hearing Difficulties and Needs in the Adult Population.

Name of assessment	Description	Reference
Adults (21+ years)		
Hearing Handicap Inventory for Adults (HHIA) and Hearing Handicap Inventory for the Elderly (HHIE)	Measures the social and emotional consequences of hearing loss Note: the purpose of each questionnaire is similar, however, they are adjusted for their respective age groups	Newman et al. (1990) Ventry and Weinstein (1983).
Client-Oriented Scale of Improvement (COSI)	Questionnaire documenting the individual's hearing goals, needs, and improvements.	Dillon et al. (1997)
Communication Profile for the Hearing Impaired (CPHI)	Evaluates communication performance, communication strategies, environment, and personal adjustment	Demorest and Erdman (1987)
Abbreviated Profile of Hearing Aid Benefit (APHAB)	Documents outcomes of hearing aid fitting	Cox and Alexander (1995)

and environments where the infant or child responds reliably to sound and where they do not, but do not rate disability. All can be used as a starting point to determine if hearing technology intervention is needed, if it will be accepted by the person with hearing loss, and what environments may most need technology intervention (Tables 18.2 and 18.3).

Hearing assistance technologies

People with mild to moderately-severe degrees of hearing loss will most often use hearing aids as a primary amplification technology to assist with auditory/verbal communication. Those with severe degrees of hearing loss may access auditory/verbal communication with either hearing aids or cochlear implants as their primary hearing intervention. People with severe to profound degrees of hearing loss may choose to access auditory/verbal communication with cochlear implant technology or may use manual/visual communication methods such as sign language without any hearing interventions. It is important to remember that the effect of hearing loss on communication function varies greatly between individuals even when similar degrees of hearing loss exist (Gelfand 2009; Roeser et al. 2007).

Hearing aids and cochlear implant technologies

For people with hearing loss who rely on auditory/verbal communication, assistance technology is focused on amplification devices, assistive equipment, and communication strategies. Hearing aids and/or cochlear implants are the primary technology typically used for individuals with permanent hearing loss. Hearing aids allow for personalized amplification of sound based upon an individual's degree and configuration of hearing loss. It is not a one-size-fits-all situation. Specialized and individualized fitting protocols ensure that a person with hearing loss is getting enough sound amplification for frequencies where they have hearing loss, while at the same time limiting the output so that sounds levels are not over-amplified or damaging (Musiek et al. 2011; Pensak and Choo 2015).

Hearing aids

The use of hearing aids to treat hearing loss has been shown to improve quality of life, including decreased depression, better communication with family and friends, better relationships, better perceived physical health, and more emotional stability (Arlinger 2003; Chisolm et al. 2007; Seniors Research Group 1999). Hearing aids, no matter what their style or size, use miniaturized microphones, digital processors, and miniaturized speakers (often called receivers), and are powered by small batteries to amplify sounds acoustically (Figure 18.5). Current hearing aid developments include increasingly sophisticated digital sound processing, including extended frequency bandwidth, loudness compression, noise reduction, and feedback suppression. Digital circuitry now allows wireless communication between a pair of hearing aids using methods similar to cell phone signals, resulting in more seamless performance (Dillon 2012).

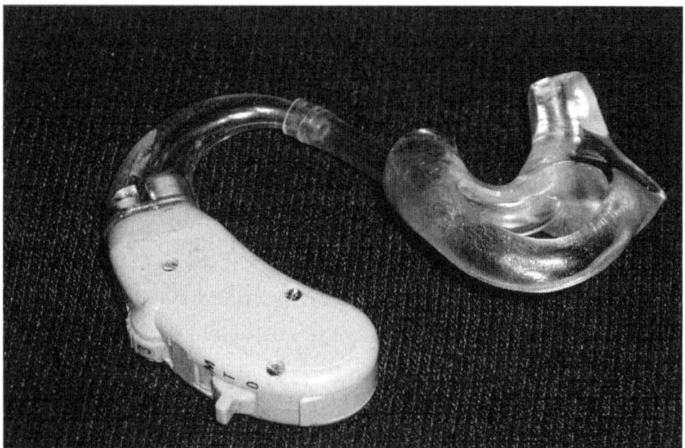

Figure 18.5 Picture of a Hearing aid. Source: Photo taken by Udo Schröter – Own work, CC BY-SA 3.0, https://commons.wikimedia.org/w/index.php?curid=181643

Cochlear implants

For individuals with sensorineural hearing loss who cannot receive benefit from hearing aids, typically those with severe to profound hearing loss who have poor speech understanding abilities, cochlear implants can be an amplification option that does not depend on acoustic amplification (Figure 18.6). Cochlear implants use miniaturized microphones, digital processors, and external transmitters, powered by small batteries, to connect with magnetic receivers and electrodes implanted in the skull and inner ear (cochlea) (Watzman and Roland 2014). The external parts of the cochlear implant process sound and send electrical signals to the internal electrodes in the cochlea in order to stimulate the hearing nerve directly. Cochlear implants can be implanted on one or both ears. Cochlear implant candidacy and funding for cochlear implants is highly regulated (Devices@FDA 2015), and decisions about bilateral versus unilateral implantation will depend on many factors such as communication performance, listening needs, and physical and emotional health. Some unilateral cochlear implant users continue to wear a hearing aid on their non-implanted ear and function "bimodally"; that is, with both electrical and acoustic input (Dillon 2012; Watzman and Roland 2014)

Hearing aid and cochlear implant technology is constantly being updated. With digitization, device software and processing strategies can be upgraded and implemented quickly. A great deal of attention is also being applied to improving the water- and dust-resistance of hearing aid and cochlear implant housing to allow better function in real-life environments that expose devices to dust, dirt, and moisture. (Taylor and Mueller 2011; Watzman and Roland 2014). No matter how sophisticated the digitization becomes, it is important to remember that the most critical sounds that these devices amplify or process are speech sounds. Music and environmental sounds are important for listening enjoyment and environmental awareness, but communication is a critical function of daily living and is a top priority. It is beyond the scope of this chapter to review all the possible processing options available in modern hearing

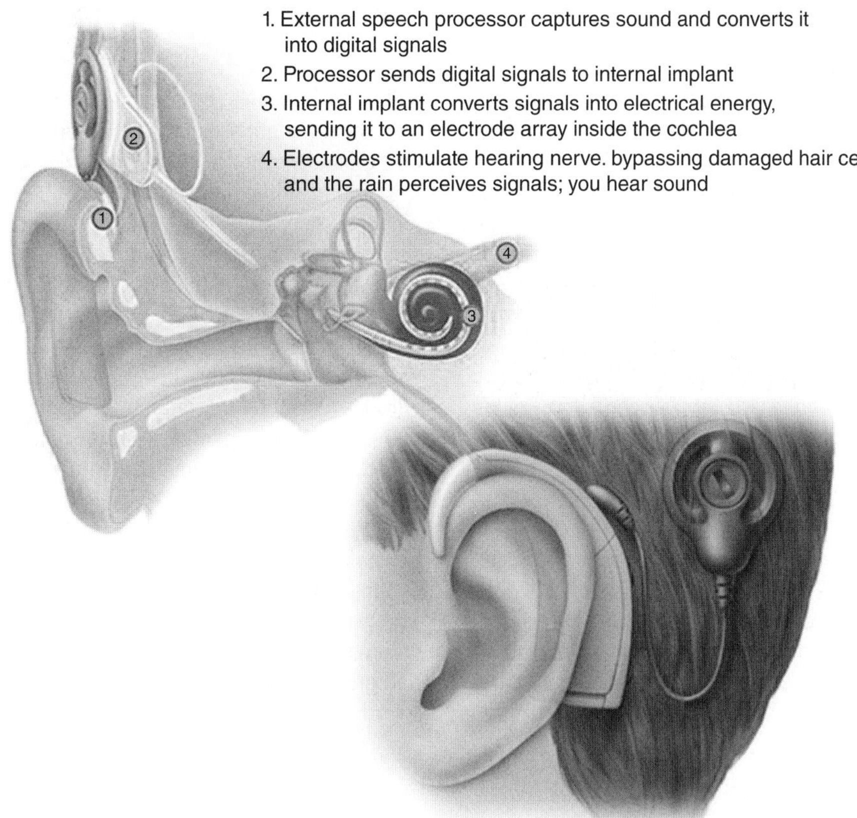

1. External speech processor captures sound and converts it into digital signals
2. Processor sends digital signals to internal implant
3. Internal implant converts signals into electrical energy, sending it to an electrode array inside the cochlea
4. Electrodes stimulate hearing nerve. bypassing damaged hair cells, and the rain perceives signals; you hear sound
1
2
3
4

Figure 18.6 Photo of cochlear implant. Source: https://commons.wikimedia.org/wiki/File:Cochlear-implant.jpg. Public Domain.

aids and cochlear implants. See the Additional Learning Resources section of this chapter to learn more about this topic.

Although one of the goals of this text is to find low-tech environmental interventions when possible, the amplification of speech and other sounds is highly technical. Today's hearing aids and cochlear implants are sophisticated digital devices and require expertise and skill in selecting, programming, evaluating, and monitoring.

Moreover, hearing aid and cochlear implant technology itself is highly sophisticated, yet the operation of the technology should be as simple as possible for the individual user (Taylor and Mueller 2011; Katz 2014). The most sophisticated and expensive device can be a poor technology intervention if the user cannot operate its controls, if they cannot get it in or out of their ears, or if it has not been fitted properly based on available best-practice guidelines. An expensive hearing aid that gets left in the drawer is a completely ineffective technology intervention; therefore, a great deal of the hearing aid and cochlear implant selection and fitting process involves working with an individual and their family to determine a multitude of individualized factors. Some primary factors to consider are provided in Box 18.2.

Box 18.2 Guiding questions for hearing assistive technology

- Will the technology be a single or multiple-use technology? In other words, does the technology provide benefit for only one situation or environment, or can it be used for multiple environments?
- How will the technology connect with the user's hearing aids or cochlear implants?
- Does the user need additional hardware or technology that must be worn and manipulated to access the signal?
- If the technology will connect with hearing aids or cochlear implants, will those devices need to be reprogrammed or adjusted to accept the additional input?
- What are the overall costs of the system and availability of funding sources?

Additionally, there should be ongoing monitoring of benefit and patient outcomes with the amplification technology to ensure that it was a good fit for the individual's needs and lifestyle. Technology interventions should be closely tied to the individual's needs, and not solely based on the hearing loss diagnosis. Two people

Box 18.3 Case study 1

The individual: John is a 76-year-old widower who lives independently in his own home by himself. He has been diagnosed with a moderate high-frequency sensorineural hearing loss in both ears. A majority of his day is spent watching television and reading the newspaper or books. He has a daughter who lives out of state with her family: a spouse and two young children. In order to catch up with each other, they speak on the phone a few times per week. John occasionally gets together with two of his friends for coffee and lunch at a small diner in town.

The hearing difficulties: Upon a visit to his audiologist, prior to getting hearing aids, John reports that he spends most of his days in quiet environments, but occasionally he will go to social outings in environments with a minimal amount of background noise. Even though he turns the volume up on the television he still has some difficulty following the dialogue, especially for programs that have characters with foreign accents. He does pretty well hearing on the telephone, but occasionally has difficulty hearing his grandchildren during their weekly phone calls.

The technology interventions: It is recommended, based on his individual needs and difficulties, that John obtain hearing aids with mid-level technology for both ears. His hearing aids should contain digital technology that addresses some background noise. He should consider getting a telecoil in the hearing aids in addition to using an in-line amplifier or an amplified telephone, to address the difficulties he has while speaking with his grandchildren on the telephone. For television viewing he could try using closed captioning, or he could obtain an infrared system made especially for TV viewing that includes a receiver with a neckloop that is compatible with the telecoil in his hearing aids. It is unlikely that he will need to obtain additional technology to deal with the minimal noise he experiences at the diner. In this situation he should employ some environmental modifications, such as sitting in a corner booth away from the counter and grill, with his back toward the room, and his hearing aids in the program for "noise."

Summary of technology: Hearing aids with noise reduction and telecoil, telephone amplifier, closed captioning or TV infrared system, use of good communication strategies while in background noise.

Box 18.4 Case study 2

The individual: Sue is a 42-year-old woman who lives with her husband. She has been diagnosed with a moderate high-frequency sensorineural hearing loss in both ears (note: the same diagnosis as Case Study 1). Sue is a CEO of a major corporation. A majority of her day is spent in conference rooms, on the telephone, or at lunch meetings in restaurants. In her free time, she loves to go to the local theater and she attends religious services once a week.

The hearing difficulties: Upon a visit to her audiologist, prior to getting hearing aids, Sue reports that she has significant difficulty hearing her dining partners during lunch meetings at noisy restaurants. She also has a hard time following the fast-moving conversation around the conference table at her office. She does okay on the telephone; however, on occasion she will have difficulty following along with what the caller is saying. She is fearful that these misunderstandings on the telephone will cost her future clients. She has some difficulty hearing certain dialogue at the theater, and she often needs her husband to translate what is said during religious services.

The technology interventions: It is recommended, based on her individual needs and difficulties, that Sue obtain hearing aids with high-end technology for both ears. Her hearing aids should contain digital technology that aggressively handles high levels of background noise. She should consider getting a telecoil in the hearing aids. While an amplified telephone may help her on the phone, due to her high levels of worry regarding this situation she may want to consider obtaining a captioned telephone, which her state provides for free to individuals with hearing loss. Another option would be to obtain hearing aids that have streaming technology available. This will allow her direct input to the hearing aids from both the landline telephone and a mobile phone. The local theater and her place of worship both have induction loop systems in place already, so she can access amplified sound through the telecoil in her hearing aids. Additionally, she should try to sit as close to the speaker as possible. Since two of the three difficult environments she encounters have induction loop systems, she should consider having the conference room at her office looped as well. This would allow her to tap into an amplified signal without purchasing any additional personal equipment. She should request restaurant meetings during the mid-afternoon rather than at the lunch hour, as there will be less background noise. She should try to sit near a wall, with her back facing the room and her hearing aids in their most aggressive noise-reduction program. She should make sure to always face the individual speaking to her. If these solutions do not work, she should consider a smaller and quieter restaurant or she should invite her dining partners back to her office where she can take advantage of the loop system.

Summary of technology: Hearing aids with aggressive noise reduction and telecoil, captioned telephone, induction loop systems, use of good communication strategies while in background noise.

with the same hearing loss can have completely different intervention needs based on their lifestyle and daily environments. These differences are illustrated in Box 18.3 Case Study 1 and Box 18.4 Case Study 2.

When amplification alone is not enough

Even though hearing aids and/or cochlear implant devices are most often the primary TEI for people with hearing loss who depend on auditory/verbal communication, they are not the end point in terms of hearing assistance. Hearing aids and cochlear implants are designed to provide *optimum* amplification for listening within a 1–2 m range in relatively quiet listening backgrounds. Background noise, distance from a sound source, and reverberation (echo) can all impact the ability to receive a clear, audible signal (Gelfand 2009; Roeser et al. 2007). These distorting effects on sound occur for everyone, even those with normal hearing. Anyone who has tried to have a conversation across a large table in a noisy bar or restaurant has experienced the deleterious impact of distance, background noise, and reverberation.

The impacts of these three sound characteristics on listening are even greater for people with hearing loss (Crandell 1993; Finitzo-Hieber and Tillman 1978; Helfer and Wilber 1990; Nábělek 1988). Even with sophisticated digital noise reduction processing, amplification systems cannot completely remove background noise without also reducing the audibility of speech. The level of background noise in comparison to the level of the signal of interest (often speech) is referred to as the signal-to-noise ratio (SNR) (Pensak and Choo 2015). If a talker is more than 2 m from the listener with hearing loss, the sound level of the talker's speech drops dramatically and a hearing aid or cochlear implant microphone is not able to completely compensate for the reduced input level. At a 2 m listening distance the SNR decreases, making it more difficult to hear a softer speech signal against a noisy background (Dillon 2012). Supplementary hearing assistance technology may be needed to improve audibility and speech clarity in those listening situations where hearing aids or cochlear implants alone are not enough for clear hearing and understanding, or when the SNR decreases so much that it is challenging to hear speech over background noise (Taylor and Mueller 2011: Watzman and Roland 2014).

In order to enable a person to fully participate in different communication environments in their daily social interactions and in their community, the use of hearing assistance technologies in addition to hearing aids or cochlear implants should be considered. This will require evaluation of the successes and struggles the person encounters with listening and communicating in daily listening environments, such as in social groups, telephone conversation, entertainment activities (e.g. plays, music events, movies, and television), and in places of worship. The type of additional hearing assistance technology that is chosen will be guided by a number of factors, as noted in Box 18.5.

The main advantage of hearing assistance technologies related to hearing aids and cochlear implants is that they provide a more direct connection between a sound source and the listener without distance and background noise degrading the signal. For example, instead of trying to listen to a TV show from across the room with other sounds interfering, the sounds from the television can be routed directly into the hearing aids or cochlear implant as if the person was listening with the TV speaker in his or her ears. This is referred to as remote microphone technology. Remote microphone systems can couple to or connect with hearing aids and cochlear implant systems in a variety of ways and offer a significantly improved SNR (Pensak and Choo 2015).

Box 18.5 Here's the evidence

Kent, B. and Smith, S. (2006). They only see it when the sun shines in my ears: exploring perceptions of adolescent hearing aid users. *Journal of Deaf Studies and Deaf Education*, 11(4): 461–476.

Key Words: adolescent hearing aid users, stigma, psychosocial support

Purpose: To explore the experiences and perceptions of hearing aid use by adolescents with hearing loss.

Sample/Setting: Sample of mainstream-educated adolescents who are fitted with hearing aids. Interviews took place in the school setting.

Method: Narrative design with interviews.

Findings: Adolescent hearing aid users report that a sense of "normality" is the biggest factor in whether they wear their hearing aids or not on a regular basis. Positive self-identity was tied to social relationships with peers and interactions with hearing adolescents. Those who had positive relationships with their peers, or who felt that having a hearing loss was "normal," were more likely to have a confident sense of self and to wear hearing aids. On the other hand, those who felt different from their peers reported a desire for belonging and tended not to wear hearing aids as consistently.

Critical thinking questions:

1. What are your thoughts on the design of this study? What elements make it a strong piece of evidence, and what elements could be changed to make it stronger? Are there any limitations?
2. How does the sample and/or setting of this study translate to the population and/or setting in which you practice or will be practicing?
3. How could this study contribute to the design of other future studies?

Frequency modulation (FM) systems

One assistive technology option is a frequency modulation (FM) system. FM systems use the same technology that radio stations use, and they operate on frequencies specifically reserved for assistive devices. Some newer systems use digital transmission similar to cell phone transmission rather than radio transmission and are referred to as digitally modulated (DM) systems (Valente et al. 2007). FM or DM systems can be used in any situation where high background noise levels and distance from the talker or sound source is likely to affect the individual's ability to hear and understand. With these systems, the speaker talks into a microphone, which passes the sound to a transmitter. The transmitter wirelessly sends the speech signal to a miniature receiver that can be attached to a hearing aid or cochlear implant. The receiver can also work through a wireless streamer or telecoil neckloop (see information about streaming technology, telecoils, and neckloops below). This type of remote microphone system allows the signal of interest, often speech, to be received directly in the hearing aid or cochlear implant, rather than relying on the microphones of the hearing aid or cochlear implant to pick up the sound signal from across the room (Dillon 2012).

FM/DM systems are frequently used in educational settings due to their ability to connect simultaneously to many different hearing aid and cochlear implant models as well as to classroom audio distribution systems with loudspeakers. This is especially helpful if there are multiple children using the technology. FM/DM transmitters can be adapted to connect with large- and small-area public address (PA) systems, computers, televisions, and telephones. While these systems can be useful for the reasons given above, there are some limitations to consider. FM systems can be prone to interference from other FM signals (Valente et al. 2007).

Additionally, each classroom or building uses its own frequency channel to send the radio signal; therefore, the user must switch channels when changing locations, making it cumbersome for users who may struggle with technology. DM systems have overcome many of the interference and channel problems that FM systems have experienced. FM and DM systems require separate receiver equipment to be attached to the hearing aid or cochlear implant (Taylor and Mueller 2011). This addition can be undesirable for some people who do not want another piece of equipment to purchase or maintain.

Infrared systems

Infrared systems use light transmitters called emitters to wirelessly transmit signals that are just outside of human sight range. These light signals are similar to those used in remote controls for electronics. An infrared system is similar to an FM or DM system in that a microphone picks up sound and sends it wirelessly from a transmitter to a receiver that the person with hearing loss uses (Valente et al. 2007). The difference from an FM system lies in the method of wireless transmission. Due to the size of the infrared receiver, infrared systems are most often used with PSAPs such as TV amplifiers, and with audio distribution systems that connect to loudspeakers in meeting rooms and classrooms (Kramer 2013). Infrared systems are usually less expensive than FM systems, making them an excellent option for personal use in the home and in small group situations. Just like any assistive device, there are limitations to infrared use. Infrared systems require a line-of-sight connection between the transmitter and receiver because of the light transmission; therefore, any situation where objects may interfere with the light beam may not be appropriate for this type of technology. If an infrared system is desired in a large area, multiple units may need to be used. Similar to FM systems, infrared systems require a special receiver to be connected to a hearing aid or cochlear implant (Valente et al. 2007).

Telecoils and induction loop systems

Telecoils and induction loops are hearing assistance technologies that have been available for many years but are experiencing a resurgence in use across the United States. Telecoils are small metal coils that are built into many hearing aids and cochlear implants. The coil picks up and amplifies electromagnetic signals coming from personal neckloops, small- or large-area induction loops, and telephones (Dillon 2012). Small- and large-area induction loops are special loops of wire that can be put in homes and public places. The sound from the talker is transmitted through this induction loop wire and can be heard directly in an individual's hearing aid or cochlear implant via the telecoil when the listener is in or near the induction loop (See Figure 18.7).

An advantage to this system is that no additional receiver, streamer, or equipment is required beyond an active, accessible telecoil program in the hearing aid or cochlear implant. Induction loop systems can be connected to PA systems, televisions, and computers (Valente et al. 2007). There is no limit to how many users can receive the information from the induction loop, as long as they are within receiving range of the loop and have an active telecoil available. Aside from permanently installed induction loops, this technology can also be used to connect users to other types of systems without having a device-specific receiver. Personal induction neckloops are dedicated individual systems that can

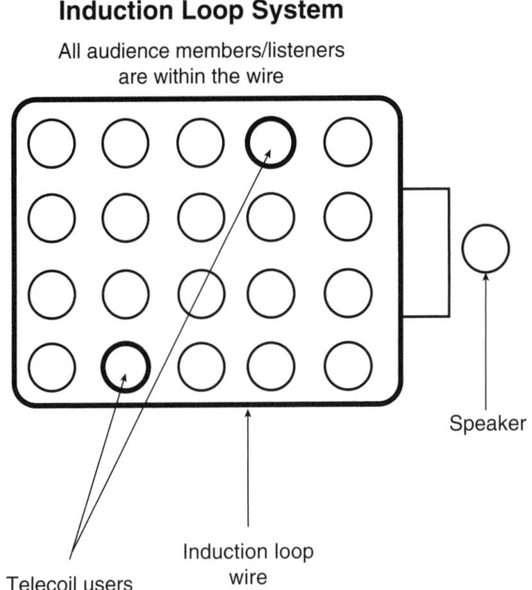

Figure 18.7 Schematic of an induction loop system.

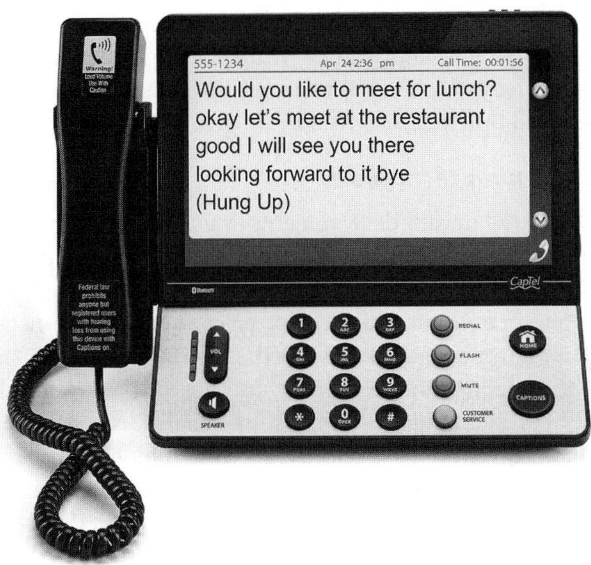
555-1234
Apr 24 2:36 pm
Call Time: 00:01:56
Would you like to meet for lunch?
okay let's meet at the restaurant
good I will see you there
looking forward to it bye
(Hung Up)
CapTel

Figure 18.8 Captioned telephone CapTel 2400i phone.
Source: Courtesy of Ultratec.

receive FM, Bluetooth, or infrared signals and send those signals to a hearing aid or Cochlear Implant's telecoil using a small loop worn around the neck (Taylor and Mueller 2011). There are many positives to using an induction loop system. However, in order to benefit from this technology a user must have an active telecoil, which is not automatically included in all hearing aids. Additionally, even though there has been considerable growth in the number of loop systems available, limited access in public places in the United States still exists.

Telephones

The telecoil of a hearing aid also helps users make better connections with telephones. Under the Hearing Aid Compatibility Act of 1988 (HAC Act) the FCC has the responsibility for ensuring that all landline telephones manufactured in the United States or imported for use in the United States after 1988 are hearing aid compatible. Additionally, all "essential" telephones must also be hearing aid compatible under the HAC Act (Hearing Aid Compatibility for Wireline Telephones n.d.). Essential telephones are defined by the FCC as "coin-operated telephones, telephones provided for emergency use and other telephones frequently needed for use by persons using hearing aids" (Hearing Aid Compatibility Act 1988). Essential phones might include workplace phones, phones in confined settings like hospitals and nursing homes, and phones in hotel and motel rooms that are available to the public or those that are frequently used by hearing aid users.

With the increase in wireless telephone use, the FCC updated the HAC Act to include regulations for digital wireless telephone (mobile phone) compatibility with hearing aids. There are two methods through which a phone can be considered compatible with hearing aids. The first is through a radio-frequency (RF) rating. This rating, called the M-rating, determines how much interference is likely between the telephone and the hearing aid. In order to be considered compatible, a wireless telephone must have a rating of M3 or higher. The other method through which compatibility can be determined is by rating the strength of the electromagnetic signal while the hearing aid is in telecoil mode. This T-rating must be at a T3 level or higher for a phone to be considered as compliant (Hearing Aid Compatibility for Wireline and Wireless Telephones 2015). Many wireless service providers have multiple phone models available that are hearing aid compatible. A user seeking this type of compatibility may even have the option of trying out a phone's compatibility in the service center or store prior to purchase.

Another telephone option to consider is a caption telephone. Caption telephone systems use relay or caption operators with fast, high-quality voice-recognition technology to quickly display captions of what the caller says on a large, easy-to-read built-in screen (Figure 18.8). Captioning allows users to read what's being said during the conversation, while the user talks normally into the telephone (Valente et al. 2007). Most caption phones also provide an amplified volume control, allowing users to listen and read simultaneously. Currently available caption phone systems require a high-speed internet connection for the captioning function. Some systems may require a telephone landline, but others allow for both landline and cell phone connections (Valente et al.

2007). As a provision of the ADA, the FCC has established a fund to give individuals with hearing loss access to captioned telephone service at no cost, if they are referred by a qualified healthcare provider.

Streaming technology

One of the newest developments available in hearing aid connectivity is wireless "streaming." Using digital signals similar to cell phone signals, hearing aids with built-in wireless communication can be programmed to connect to an intermediate device called a streamer (Katz 2014). The streamer can then communicate with a variety of devices including cell phones, personal music devices, landline telephones, televisions, and remote personal microphones, often using Bluetooth transmission. With wireless streaming, a variety of different inputs can be heard directly in a person's hearing aid(s) instead of relying on the microphone to pick up faraway or hard-to-hear signals. Each model of streamer works exclusively with a manufacturer's specific hearing aid model and is programmed to transmit to only one or two sets of hearing aids (Kramer 2013). Streamers should be ordered through an audiologist or hearing aid dispenser to ensure proper compatibility and programming.

Assistive technology for persons not using amplification

Personal amplifiers

Personal amplifiers or "listeners" may be helpful for some people, but most of these devices have a limited range of amplification available and are not designed to compensate for hearing losses that are beyond the mild hearing loss range. The FDA refers to these devices as PSAPs. They cannot be defined as hearing aids, and they are not intended as a substitute for hearing aids (Regulatory Requirements for Hearing Aid Devices and Personal Sound Amplification Products 2009). They can be used for close one-on-one communication and are often used for TV listening. PSAP systems can be wireless, using a microphone and transmitter that are wirelessly connected to a receiver and amplifier using infrared or radio signals (Katz 2014). The system could also be hard-wired, with the microphone directly connected to an amplifier. PSAPs work in much the same way as the technologies discussed for those with hearing loss; however, they are not coupled with hearing aid or cochlear implant technology (Kramer 2013). The person using a PSAP uses headphones or earbuds connected to the amplifier/receiver and has some amount of volume control for listening. Tablet and smartphone applications are also available to convert the mobile device into a personal amplifier using the system's built-in microphone along with headphones or external speakers. A volume control wheel or switch often controls the PSAP's amplification of the incoming signal. Wireless receivers with headphones that are connected to PA systems in theaters, museums, and places of worship also fit into the PSAP category. As with other personal amplifiers, they are not designed for assisting with hearing losses that are more than a mild loss and are not considered a hearing aid by FDA rules (Regulatory Requirements for Hearing Aid Devices and Personal Sound Amplification Products 2009).

Amplified telephones are frequently used by people who do not wear hearing aids. FCC rules (HAC Act 1988) require that wireline telephones manufactured after 1989 have some amount of volume control adjustment available. High-volume telephones are also available that allow additional power beyond the HAC Act minimum standards. Telephones that allow high volume levels can accommodate individuals with mild to moderate hearing losses whether or not they use hearing aids (Dillon 2012). People who do not wear hearing aids can only take advantage of the extra volume provided and not the available telecoil/electromagnetic technology. Caption telephones (see above) with adjustable volume controls would also be an appropriate technology choice for people who do not wear hearing aids but who need assistance with hearing and understanding on the phone (Katz 2014). Table 18.4 summarizes technology solutions for hearing difficulties in a variety of settings.

Alerting and alarm systems

Alerting and alarm systems are often a neglected consideration, but are critical for independent living and safety. A major focus when choosing alerts and alarms is making sure that the individual will be able to be alerted even when they are not wearing personal amplification (Pensak and Choo 2015). This means exploring whether the person would be best alerted by an amplified, vibratory, or visual type of signal. Technology can be chosen to address each individual alerting need independently, or a more extensive alerting system can be installed that connects multiple signal inputs into one receiver (Valente et al. 2007). An alerting system that is installed in the home can have smoke and carbon dioxide alarms, as well as doorbell transmitters that are directly wired into the home's electrical system. These can be connected to a wireless wristwatch or pager receiver that provides distinctive vibrotactile signal patterns for each type of alarm. Visual alerts and bed/pillow shakers can also be connected into the system (Katz 2014).

Table 18.4 Select Suggestions for Addressing Hearing Difficulties in Various Settings.

Difficult listening situation	Soft technology solutions	Hard technology solutions
Classroom	• Preferential seating in the front and center of the classroom • Tennis balls on the bottom of chairs and desks • Carpeting, cork tiles, felt, or soft fabrics on hard surfaces	• FM system • Captioning for films and videos
Restaurant	• Avoid sitting near the noisiest spots (bar area, near the kitchen, etc.) • Avoid busy times when there is more noise • If wearing hearing aids with directional capabilities, sit with back toward the background noise • If not wearing hearing aids, sit with back toward wall • Opt for a booth over a table if possible	• Personal FM system • If wearing hearing aids, ensure they are on the "noise" setting • PSAP, such as a one-on-one communicator
Party or crowded area	• Stay near the edges of the room, where there is less surrounding noise • Face communication partners to make use of facial cues • Use good communication strategies	• If wearing hearing aids, ensure they are on the "noise" or "crowd" setting • FM system • PSAP, such as a one-on-one communicator
Watching television		• Infrared system • Loop system • Closed captioning • Streaming technology
At a play or movie	• Preferential seating in the front and center or near a loudspeaker	• Infrared system (if available) • Loop system (if available)
Telephone		• Telecoil • In-line amplifier • Amplified telephone • Acoustic-to-magnetic adaptor • Captioned telephone • Streaming technology

There are a variety of alerting needs that should be considered. These include: alarm clocks, doorbells, knocks on the door, ringing telephones, fire alarms, carbon monoxide alarms, baby/child monitors, timers for appliances such as the stove and oven, computer prompts, and pagers (Valente et al. 2007). There are many alerting and alarm products available, and a wide range of prices and product quality can be found. There are many assistive technology websites online, most of which can be found with a brief Internet search. Examining the different online catalogs can be helpful to provide further education on what current products are available. Even though acquiring a device online can be quick, easy, and inexpensive, a hands-on demonstration of equipment should be considered prior to purchase. These demonstrations can help the user evaluate the effectiveness and ease-of-use of different alerting options. Technology demonstration centers are available in many locations to show how assistive equipment is used and how each type of alerting system operates. Some audiology and hearing aid dispensing centers also have the technology available for demonstration. Hearing loss support groups such as the Hearing Loss Association of America (HLAA) can be an excellent source of information about different alerting and signaling options and implementation (Hearing Loss Association of America n.d.).

TEI and the deaf population

Within the Deaf Community, Deafness is not considered a handicap or disability but a matter of pride and a cultural choice. For culturally Deaf individuals, communication emphasis is on manual or visual language (American Sign Language [ASL] in the United States) with technology that supports visual communication (Holcomb 2012). Technology interventions are available to assist with communication between Deaf individuals and hearing/speaking individuals who do not use manual communication (Kramer 2013). Sign Language interpreting and captioning services provide communication access in a variety of important public settings such as physicians' offices, hospitals, government buildings, organized meetings, educational settings, and in public entertainment venues such as movie theaters and playhouses.

Technology priorities will vary with the individual, but in general, text and visual supplements are needed to provide communication access in a variety of environments and to provide connections with different forms of media, including telephones and television (Gelfand 2009). Visual supplements such as captioning can be provided in multiple ways. Communication access real-time translation (CART) is a method of live captioning, which can be used in many settings, including schools and the workplace. CART utilizes a stenograph-type device and CART stenographer to quickly type the speech message and convert it to text (Kramer 2013). Another option for face-to-face communication and interpreting real-time speech is to use speech-to-text translation software, such as Dragon, Apple's Siri, or those available through numerous smartphone and tablet applications. This does not require an intermediate person to do the typing translation; however, the technology is not as accurate at converting the spoken message to text as a CART system. Closed captioning is another visual representation of spoken language that can be helpful while watching television or movies.

Teletypewriters (TTYs) and Telecommunication devices for the deaf (TDDs) are dedicated systems that are used to provide text communication for the telephone. TTYs look similar to a typewriter and serve to send written text messages back and forth over phone lines. TDDs are essentially the same as TTYs, but smaller and more portable (Kramer 2013). Telephone relay services are available to provide telephone communications between someone using a text telephone device and another person who does not have a telephone with text capabilities. With continued developments in cell phone communications and data streaming, text communication has become the norm for everyone, not just for people with hearing loss or deafness. Many of the previously dedicated telecommunication assistance services have been incorporated into conventional smartphone and computer tablet technologies and have made telecommunications significantly easier to access for individuals who are Deaf or Hard of Hearing (Katz 2014). With many different real-time video communication applications such as Skype available, manual/visual telephone conversations can take place between individuals who are Deaf without using text telephone devices or an intermediate translator.

Hearing service dogs may be appropriate for some individuals. Hearing dogs are trained to alert people to household sounds that need to be identified for everyday safety and independence (Shafer 2005). They are trained to make physical contact and lead their person to the source of the sound. They also can provide general sound and environmental awareness in public. By providing sound awareness and companionship, they provide increased freedom and independence for individuals who are deaf (Shafer 2005). Several hearing service dog training programs are available in the United States, for example, Assistance Dogs International and Dogs for the Deaf.

Environmental modifications and communication strategies

As previously mentioned, distance from the speaker, reverberation, and background noise make understanding speech difficult for everyone, but especially for individuals with hearing loss (Crandell 1993; Finitzo-Hieber and Tillman 1978; Helfer and Wilber 1990; Nábělek 1988). One of the ways to reduce these barriers to speech understanding is by implementing environmental modifications. Environmental modifications could be considered soft technology, since there is no direct hardware-based assistive device being manipulated.

For the pediatric population, one of the most difficult listening environments is in the classroom. There are multiple sources of reverberation due to the presence of many hard surfaces: desk tops, floors, chalkboards or whiteboards, and windows (Smaldino and Flexer 2012). Additionally, there are multiple sources of background noise in the classroom, including noise from children moving around, scraping tables and chairs, talking, and heating, ventilation, and air conditioning (HVAC) units as well as noise from outside of the classroom (Crandell et al. 2004). Reverberation in combination with background noise can significantly interfere with the teacher's speech signal. In many instances, the teacher moves around the classroom while teaching, creating a changing distance between them and the student with hearing loss (Crandell et al. 2004).

One environmental modification is to decrease the distance between the teacher and the student. This is often referred to as "preferential seating," meaning the child is seated as close to the teacher as possible, in the front row and with their best hearing ear centered toward the teacher (Smaldino and Flexer 2012). An attempt should be made to soften hard surfaces in a classroom. This could involve the use of felt or cork on the walls, window treatments on windows, carpeting on areas of the floor, and cut tennis balls attached to the legs of chairs and desks. Staggering desks instead of lining them up in linear rows can help as well. The child with hearing loss should sit as far away from HVAC units as possible. The teacher should encourage the use of some type of object that can be passed among students to indicate when they can speak, to prevent multiple students speaking at once. It can also be helpful for the child to receive new vocabulary words or outlines of new lessons prior to the class period (Crandell et al. 2004).

For children and adults alike, it is important to reduce background noise as much as possible. This means reducing or removing other sounds sources such as television or music while having a conversation. If at a party or event, the individual with hearing loss should try moving to the edges of the room, or moving an important conversation to a quiet room or hallway (Smaldino and Flexer 2012).

The person with the hearing loss should learn what strategies work best for them to understand speech and how to self-advocate and inform others of the ideal way to verbally communicate with them (Kramer 2013). One communication strategy to consider is the use of clear speech. Clear speech is a term used to describe slightly slower, strong (but not too loud), well-articulated (but not overly articulated) speech. The individual with hearing loss may need to request that a speaker look directly at them while speaking in order to receive a more direct speech signal and to take advantage of facial cues. They may also need to ask for clarification, repetition, or rephrasing if a spoken message is missed (Katz 2014). Requesting that a family member not try to communicate from another room or when his or her back is turned can be difficult, as long-standing communication habits are difficult to change. When attending lectures, movies, plays, or religious services, preferential seating close to the primary talker or loudspeakers can improve the ease of listening and the clarity of sound. Preparations prior to the event by reading plot summaries and lecture overviews and learning new terms and vocabulary can be helpful. This allows the individual with hearing loss to focus more on the larger message rather than struggling with individual words or concepts.

Summary

The number of individuals with a diagnosed hearing loss is surprisingly large and continues to increase. With hearing loss remaining near the top of the list of most common chronic conditions in older adults, the need for TEI is apparent. Unidentified and untreated hearing loss can result in speech and language, academic, vocational, social, and interpersonal relationship issues. While hearing aids and cochlear implants are the primary technology of choice for treating hearing loss, they are not always enough to keep an individual connected with the outside world. A range of technologies are available to improve access to speech and environmental sounds in situations where hearing aids and cochlear implants are not worn or when they do not provide enough help for the individual's specific listening needs.

Technological intervention for hearing loss falls along a continuum from counseling about proper communication strategies and low-technology environmental modifications to highly sophisticated hardware and digital processing. Formal and informal assessment is necessary to determine proper interventions on an individual basis. With various causes, types, degrees, and configurations of hearing loss and their intricate interactions with Vicente's Human-Tech Ladder, an individualized technological intervention plan is imperative.

References

21st Century Communications and Video Accessibility Act (2010). Pub. L. 111-260 C.F.R.

American Academy of Audiology (AAA) (n.d.). Hearing & hearing loss. Retrieved from http://www.howsyourhearing.org/hearingloss.html.

American Speech-Language and Hearing Association (ASHA) (2015). Degree of hearing loss. Retrieved from http://www.asha.org/public/hearing/degree-of-hearing-loss.

Americans with Disabilities Act (ADA) (1990). Pub. L. No. 101-336, 104 Stat. 328 C.F.R.

Anderson, K.L. (1989). *SIFTER: Screening Instrument for Targeting Educational Risk in Children Identified by Hearing Screening or Who Have Known Hearing Loss: User's Manual*. Danville, IL: Interstate Printers & Publishers.

Anderson, K.L. (2002). ELF – Early Listening Function. Retrieved from https://successforkidswithhearingloss.com/wp-content/uploads/2011/08/ELF-Oticon-version.pdf.

Anderson, K.L. and Smaldino, J.J. (1998). *Listening Inventory For Education (LIFE)*. Tampa, FL: Educational Audiology Association.

Anderson, K.L. and Smaldino, J.J. (2000). Children's Home Inventory for Listening Difficulties (CHILD). Retrieved from https://wyominginstructionalnetwork.com/wp-content/uploads/2018/05/C.H.I.L.D-Children%E2%80%99s-Home-Inventory-Listening-Difficulties.pdf.

Arlinger, S. (2003). Negative consequences of uncorrected hearing loss – a review. *International Journal of Audiology* 42 (Suppl 2): 2S17–2S20.

Boulet, S.L., Boyle, C.A., and Schieve, L.A. (2009). Health care use and health and functional impact of developmental disabilities among US children, 1997–2005. *Archives of Pediatrics & Adolescent Medicine* 163 (1): 19–26.

Cacciatore, F., Napoli, C., Abete, P. et al. (1999). Quality of life determinants and hearing function in an elderly population: Osservatorio Geriatrico Campano Study Group. *Gerontology* 45 (6): 323–328.

Centers for Disease Control and Prevention (1997). Serious hearing impairment among children aged 3–10 years – Atlanta, Georgia, 1991–1993. *MMWR. Morbidity and Mortality Weekly Report* 46 (45): 1073–1076.

Centers for Disease Control and Prevention (2010). Identifying infants with hearing loss – United States, 1999–2007. *MMWR. Morbidity and Mortality Weekly Report* 59 (8): 220–223.

Centers for Disease Control and Prevention (n.d.). Communicating with and about people with disabilities. Retrieved from https://www.cdc.gov/ncbddd/disabilityandhealth/pdf/disabilityposter_photos.pdf.

Chew, H.S. and Yeak, S. (2010). Quality of life in patients with untreated age-related hearing loss. *Journal of Laryngology and Otology* 124 (8): 835–841. https://doi.org/10.1017/S0022215110000757.

Ching, T. and Hill, M. (2007). The Parents' Evaluation of Aural/Oral Performance of Children (PEACH) scale: normative data. *Journal of the American Academy of Audiology* 18 (3): 220–235.

Ching, T., Hill, M. and Psarros, C. (2005). Teacher's Evaluation of Aural/Oral Performance of Children (TEACH). Retrieved from https://www.outcomes.nal.gov.au/teach.

Chisolm, T.H., Johnson, C.E., Danhauer, J.L. et al. (2007). A systematic review of health-related quality of life and hearing aids: final report of the American Academy of Audiology Task Force on the Health-Related Quality of Life Benefits of Amplification in Adults. *Journal of the American Academy of Audiology* 18 (2): 151–183.

Chittka, L. and Brockmann, L. (2005). Perception space – the final frontier. *PLoS Biology* 3 (4): e137. https://doi.org/10.1371/journal.pbio.0030137.

Clark, J.G. (1981). Uses and abuses of hearing loss classification. *ASHA* 23 (7): 493–500.

Clark, J.G. (2010). The geometry of patient motivation: circles, lines and boxes. *Audiology Today* 22 (4): 32–40.

Cox, R.M. and Alexander, G.C. (1995). The abbreviated profile of hearing aid benefit. *Ear and Hearing* 16 (2): 176–186.

Crandell, C.C. (1993). Speech recognition in noise by children with minimal degrees of sensorineural hearing loss. *Ear and Hearing* 14 (3): 210–216.

Crandell, C.C., Kreisman, B.M., Smaldino, J.J., and Kreisman, N.V. (2004). Room acoustics intervention efficacy measures. *Seminars in Hearing* 25 (2): 201–206.

Cunningham, M. and Cox, E.O. (2003). Hearing assessment in infants and children: recommendations beyond neonatal screening. *Pediatrics* 111 (2): 436–440.

Danhauer, J.L., Blood, G.W., Blood, I.M., and Gomez, N. (1980). Professional and lay observers' impressions of preschoolers wearing hearing aids. *Journal of Speech and Hearing Disorders* 45 (3): 415–422.

David, D. and Werner, P. (2016). Stigma regarding hearing loss and hearing aids: a scoping review. *Stigma and Health* 1 (2): 59–71.

Demorest, M.E. and Erdman, S.A. (1987). Development of the communication profile for the hearing impaired. *Journal of Speech and Hearing Disorders* 52 (2): 129–143.

Dengerink, J.E. and Porter, J.B. (1984). Children's attitudes toward peers wearing hearing aids. *Language, Speech, and Hearing Services in Schools* 15 (3): 205–209.

Devices@FDA (2015). Retrieved from http://www.accessdata.fda.gov/scripts/cdrh/devicesatfda/index.cfm?sia=1.

Dillon, H. (2012). *Hearing Aids*, 2e. New York: Thieme Medical.

Dillon, H., James, A., and Ginis, J. (1997). Client Oriented Scale of Improvement (COSI) and its relationship to several other measures of benefit and satisfaction provided by hearing aids. *Journal of the American Academy of Audiology* 8 (1): 27–43.

Doggett, S., Stein, R.L., and Gans, D. (1998). Hearing aid effect in older females. *Journal of the American Academy of Audiology* 9 (5): 361–366.

Donaldson, N., Worrall, L., and Hickson, L. (2004). Older people with hearing impairment: a literature review of the spouse's perspective. *Australian and New Zealand Journal of Audiology* 26 (1): 30–39.

Finitzo-Hieber, T. and Tillman, T.W. (1978). Room acoustics effects on monosyllabic word discrimination ability for normal and hearing-impaired children. *Journal of Speech, Language, and Hearing Research* 21 (3): 440–458.

Fitzpatrick, E., Angus, D., Durieux-Smith, A. et al. (2008). Parents' needs following identification of childhood hearing loss. *American Journal of Audiology* 17 (1): 38–49.

Gelfand, S. (2009). *Essentials of Audiology*, 3e. New York: Thieme Medical.

Harlor, A.D.B. and Bower, C. (2009). Hearing assessment in infants and children: recommendations beyond neonatal screening. *Pediatrics* 124 (4): 1252–1263.

Hearing Aid Compatibility Act of 1988 (1988). (H.R.2213). Retrieved from https://www.congress.gov/bill/100th-congress/house-bill/2213.

Hearing Aid Compatibility for Wireline Telephones (n.d.). Retrieved from http://www.fcc.gov/guides/hearing-aid-compatibility-wireline-telephones.

Hearing Loss Association of America (n.d.). Retrieved from http://www.hearingloss.org.

Helfer, K.S. and Wilber, L.A. (1990). Hearing loss, aging, and speech perception in reverberation and noise. *Journal of Speech, Language, and Hearing Research* 33 (1): 149–155.

Holcomb, T.K. (2012). *Introduction to American Deaf Culture*. Oxford: Oxford University Press.

IDEA Part B Regulations (2006). 34 CFR § 300 and §301 C.F.R.

IDEA Part C Regulations (2011). 34 CFR § 303 C.F.R.

Jennings, M.B. and Shaw, L. (2008). Impact of hearing loss in the workplace: raising questions about partnerships with professionals. *Work* 30 (3): 289–295.

Johnson, C.E. (2011). *Introduction to Auditory Rehabilitation: A Contemporary Issues Approach*. Boston, MA: Pearson Education.

Katz, J. (2014). *Handbook of Clinical Audiology*, 7e. Philadelphia, PA: Lippincott Williams & Wilkins.

Kent, B. (2003). Identity issues for hard-of-hearing adolescents aged 11, 13, and 15 in mainstream setting. *Journal of Deaf Studies and Deaf Education* 8 (3): 315–324.

Kramer, S. (2013). *Audiology: Science to Practice*, 2e. San Diego, CA: Plural Publishing.

Lin, F.R. (2012). Hearing loss in older adults: who's listening? *Journal of the American Medical Association* 307 (11): 1147–1148.

Lin, F.R., Niparko, J.K., and Ferrucci, L. (2011). Hearing loss prevalence in the United States. *Archives of Internal Medicine* 171 (20): 1851–1853.

Long, G., Stinson, M.S., and Braeges, J. (1991). Students' perceptions of communication ease and engagement: how they relate to academic success. *American Annals of the Deaf* 136 (5): 414–421.

Martin, F.N. and Clark, J.G. (2014). *Introduction to Audiology*, 12e. Boston, MA: Pearson.

Mathers, C., Fat, D.M., and Boerma, J. (2008). *The Global Burden of Disease: 2004 Update*. Geneva, Switzerland: World Health Organization.

Md Daud, K., Noor, R., Sidek, D.S., and Mohamad, A. (2010). The effect of mild hearing loss on academic performance in primary school children. *International Journal of Pediatric Otorhinolaryngology* 74 (1): 67–70.

Mitchell, R.E. and Karchmer, M.A. (2004). Chasing the mythical ten percent: parental hearing status of deaf and hard of hearing students in the United States. *Sign Language Studies* 4 (2): 138–163.

Moeller, M.P. (2000). Early intervention and language development in children who are deaf and hard of hearing. *Pediatrics* 106 (3): e43.

Mulac, A., Danhauer, J., and Johnson, C. (1983). Young adults' and peers' attitudes towards elderly hearing aid wearers. *Australian Journal of Audiology* 5: 57–62.

Musiek, F.E., Baran, J.A., Shinn, J.B., and Jones, R.O. (2011). *Disorders of the Auditory System*, 1e. San Diego, CA: Plural Publishing.

Nábělek, A.K. (1988). Identification of vowels in quiet, noise, and reverberation: relationships with age and hearing loss. *Journal of the Acoustical Society of America* 84 (2): 476–484.

National Institute on Deafness and other Communication Disorders (2015). Do you need a hearing test? Retrieved from https://www.nidcd.nih.gov/health/do-you-need-hearing-test.

Newman, C.W., Weinstein, B.E., Jacobson, G.P., and Hug, G.A. (1990). The Hearing Handicap Inventory for Adults: psychometric adequacy and audiometric correlates. *Ear and Hearing* 11 (6): 430–433.

Niskar, A.S., Kieszak, S.M., Holmes, A. et al. (1998). Prevalence of hearing loss among children 6 to 19 years of age: the Third National Health and Nutrition Examination Survey. *Journal of the American Medical Association* 279 (14): 1071–1075.

Palmer, C.V. and Mormer, E. (1999). Goals and expectations of the hearing aid fitting. *Trends in Amplification* 4 (2): 61–71.

Pensak, M.L. and Choo, D.L. (2015). *Clinical Otology*, 4e. New York: Thieme Medical.

Pittman, A. and Stelmachowicz, P. (2003). Hearing loss in children and adults: audiometric configuration, asymmetry, and progression. *Ear and Hearing* 24 (3): 198–205.

Purdy, S.C., Farrington, D.R., Moran, C.A. et al. (2002). A parental questionnaire to evaluate children's Auditory Behavior in Everyday Life (ABEL). *American Journal of Audiology* 11 (2): 72–82.

Regulatory Requirements for Hearing Aid Devices and Personal Sound Amplification Products(2009). Food and Drug Administration 21 CFR 874.3300.

Reyes, R. (2008). Early intervention for hearing impairment: appropriate, accessible and affordable. *Annuals of Academic Medicine Singapore* 37 (12 Suppl): 55–52.

Roeser, R.J., Valente, M., and Hosford-Dunn, H. (2007). *Audiology Diagnosis*, 2e. New York: Thieme Medical.

Russ, S., Kuo, A., Poulakis, Z. et al. (2004). Qualitative analysis of parents' experience with early detection of hearing loss. *Archives of Disease in Childhood* 89 (4): 353–358.

Sass-Lehrer, M. (2004). Early detection of hearing loss: maintaining a family-centered perspective. *Seminars in Hearing* 25 (4): 295–307.

Seikel, J. and King, D.W. (2015). *Anatomy and Physiology for Speech, Language and Hearing*, 5e. Clifton, NY: Cengage Learning.

Seniors Research Group (1999). *The Consequences of Untreated Hearing Loss in Older Persons*. Washington, DC: The National Council on the Aging.

Shafer, D. (2005). A tail of hearing service: service dogs can fill gaps for people with hearing loss. *ASHA Leader* 10 (3): 4–20.

Silverman, F.H. and Klees, J. (1989). Adolescents' attitudes toward peers who wear visible hearing aids. *Journal of Communication Disorders* 22 (2): 147–150.

Smaldino, J.J. and Flexer, C. (eds.) (2012). *Handbook of Acoustic Accessibility: Best Practices for Listening, Learning, and Literacy in the Classroom*. Stuttgart, Germany: Thieme Medical.

Stinson, M. and Antia, S. (1999). Considerations in educating deaf and hard-of-hearing students in inclusive settings. *Journal of Deaf Studies and Deaf Education* 4 (3): 163–175.

Stredler-Brown, A. and Johnson, C.D. (2004). Functional auditory performance indicators. Retrieved from https://www.phonakpro.com/content/dam/phonakpro/gc_hq/en/resources/counseling_tools/documents/child_hearing_assessment_functional_auditory_performance_indicators_fapi_2017.pdf.

Taylor, B. and Mueller, H.G. (2011). *Fitting and Dispensing Hearing Aids*, 2e. San Diego, CA: Plural Publishing.

Tye-Murray, N. (2008). *Foundations of Aural Rehabilitation: Children, Adults, and Their Family Members*. Clifton, NY: Cengage Learning.

Tye-Murray, N., Spencer, L., and Woodworth, G.G. (1995). Acquisition of speech by children who have prolonged cochlear implant experience. *Journal of Speech, Language, and Hearing Research* 38 (2): 327–337.

Valente, M., Hosford-Dunn, H., and Roeser, R.J. (2007). *Audiology Treatment*, 2e. New York: Thieme Medical.

Ventry, I.M. and Weinstein, B.E. (1982). The hearing handicap inventory for the elderly: a new tool. *Ear and Hearing* 3 (3): 128–134.

Ventry, I.M. and Weinstein, B.E. (1983). Identification of elderly people with hearing problems. *ASHA* 25 (7): 37–42.

Veras, R.P. and Mattos, L.C. (2007). Audiology and aging: literature review and current horizons. *Revista Brasileira de Otorrinolaringologia* 73 (1): 128–134.

Vicente, K.J. (2006). *The Human Factor: Revolutionizing the Way People Live with Technology*. New York: Routledge, Taylor & Francis Group.

Watzman, S.B. and Roland, T. (2014). *Cochlear Implants*, 3e. New York: Thieme Medical.

WHO Estimates (2013). Retrieved from http://www.who.int/pbd/deafness/estimates/en/.

World Health Organization (2001a). *ICF Checklist*. Geneva, Switzerland: World Health Organization.

World Health Organization (2001b). International Classification of Functioning, Disability and Health. Geneva, Switzerland: World Health Organization. Retrieved from https://www.who.int/classifications/icf/en/.

World Health Organization (2018). Deafness and hearing loss fact sheet. Retrieved from http://www.who.int/mediacentre/factsheets/fs300/en/.

Yoshinaga-Itano, C. (2001). The social-emotional ramifications of universal newborn hearing screening, early identification and intervention of children who are deaf or hard of hearing. *Sound Foundations Through Early Amplification: Proceedings of the Second International Pediatric Audiology Amplification Conference*. Chicago, IL.

Yoshinaga-Itano, C. and Sedey, A.L. (1998). Language of early- and later-identified children with hearing loss. *Pediatrics* 102 (5): 1161–1171.

Zimmerman-Phillips, S., Robbins, A., and Osberger, M.J. (2000). Assessing cochlear implant benefit in very young children. *The Annals of Otology, Rhinology & Laryngology. Supplement* 185: 42–43.

Additional resources

Consumer guide to hearing aid features and technology options: http://www.consumerreports.org/cro/hearing-aids/buying-guide.htm

American Speech-Language and Hearing Association: www.asha.org

American Academy of Audiology: www.audiology.org

19

Technology and environmental intervention for visual impairment

Stacy Smallfield

Outline

Assistive Technologies and Environmental Interventions in Healthcare: An Integrated Approach, First Edition.
Edited by Lynn Gitlow and Kathleen Flecky.

Companion website: www.wiley.com/go/gitlow/assitivetechnologies

Learning outcomes

After reading this chapter, you should be able to:

1. Compare and contrast the terms blindness, legal blindness, and low vision.
2. Describe common eye diseases that result in visual impairment.
3. Apply the Human-Tech Ladder (Vicente 2006) to individuals with visual impairment.
4. Describe strategies to assess the AT needs of individuals with visual impairment.
5. Identify potential technology and environmental interventions for individuals with visual impairment.

Active learning prompts

Before you read this chapter:

1. Consider all of the activities included in your daily routine. You may find it helpful to record your activities in a journal. Reflect on which activities require the use of vision. What type of vision (e.g. near, far, central, peripheral) do they require?
2. Compare and contrast the terms blindness, legal blindness, and low vision using at least two different sources.
3. Learn about common visual impairments using the interactive website http://webaim.org/simulations/lowvision or the computer tablet application VisionSim.
4. Interview a friend about his or her daily activities. You may find Questions 6 through 9 found in Box 19.1 helpful as a way to guide your interview. Consider how many of the tasks require reading in order to complete.
5. Consider the technology devices you use every day, such as a smartphone, television, computer, or tablet computer. Describe the role that the visual system plays in operating these devices.
6. Locate the built-in accessibility features on your personal computer. Become familiar with how to adjust each of the settings. Note which accessibility features are particularly helpful for an individual with visual impairment.

Key terms

Bioptic telescopes
Electronic magnification
Legal blindness
Low vision
Optical magnification
Prisms
Scotomas

Box 19.1 Select interview questions when completing an assessment for AT for visual impairment

1. Describe your previous history with seeking professional assistance for your visual impairment.
2. Do you have other medical conditions in addition to your visual impairment that influence how you perform everyday activities?
3. (Provide a picture or a scene to look at.) Describe what you see.
4. Describe your social support system. Do you live with family members or other care providers? Do you have family and friends nearby?
5. Describe your home.
6. Describe what a typical day is like for you. Are you employed? What hobbies or leisure interests do you enjoy?
7. Which of the activities that you perform in a typical day are most important to you? Which do you have to do? Want to do? Need to do?
8. Do you like to read? What type of reading do you do on a regular basis? (i.e. newspaper, mail, books, financial statements, recipes, electronic communication)
9. Do you drive? What other methods of community mobility have you used?
10. What types of equipment or strategies do you use now to assist you? How did these come about?
11. Describe your history of falling.

Technology and environmental intervention (TEI) for visual impairment

The visual system is our most far-reaching sensory system (Moore, as cited in Titcomb et al. 1997). We are able to avoid oncoming cars, hit a fastball, perceive a friend's emotions, post a picture to Instagram, and knit a scarf all because of the intricate functioning of the visual system. Many of the tasks that we do in a day – apply makeup, acquire the news, make a purchase, travel to school, prepare a meal, play a game, send a text – we do with the help of our vision. As you reflect upon the activities that comprise your daily routine (refer to the first Active Learning Prompt above), you quickly realize that you use your vision for almost every component of every task in which you participate. So, you can easily see how vision loss can have a profound impact on daily life. TEIs ranging from no-tech to high-tech can be very instrumental in assisting individuals with vision loss perform everyday activities. The purpose of this chapter is to discuss the role of assistive technology (AT) in enhancing occupational performance for those with visual impairment.

Definitions of visual impairment

Vision loss of varying degrees affects over 285 million people worldwide, including 39 million with complete blindness and 246 million with partial vision loss despite the use of corrective lenses (World Health Organization [WHO] 2010). Because older adults are at higher risk for developing many of the eye-related conditions that lead to vision loss (Stuen and Faye 2003; WHO 2018), researchers project the prevalence of blindness and low vision to increase dramatically over the next 20 years as the population ages (Varma et al. 2016). In the United States specifically, experts predict that the number of people with vision loss will double by the year 2050 (Varma et al. 2016).

There are several terms that are used to describe visual impairment, including blindness, legal blindness, and low vision, and there is some overlap between these terms, as you may have found while you completed the second Active Learning Prompt at the beginning of the chapter. While some individuals experience blindness, or a complete loss of vision, many others experience limited vision loss in which some usable vision remains. This limited vision loss is often referred to as *low vision*, and includes the range of vision between normal vision and blindness (Lighthouse International n.d.-c). Low vision is more common than complete blindness (Congdon et al. 2004; WHO 2010) and can be further

Table 19.1 Classification of Vision Loss.

Range of vision loss	Description of vision loss	Range of visual acuity
(Near-) normal vision	Normal acuity Near normal acuity	20/12–20/25 20/32–20/63
Low vision	Moderate visual impairment Severe visual impairment Profound visual impairment	20/80–20/160 20/200–20/400 20/500–20/1000
(Near-) blindness	Blindness	Less than 20/1000–no light perception

Source: Adapted from International Council of Ophthalmology (2002).

classified as moderate, severe, or profound (International Council of Ophthalmology 2002). *Legal blindness* is the point at which a person with vision loss becomes eligible for state and federal services and benefits; specifically, a person with a visual acuity of 20/200 or worse in the better eye or a visual field restriction equal to 20° or greater in the better eye is legally blind (Lighthouse International n.d.-a). Therefore, someone who has low vision may also be legally blind if his or her remaining best-corrected vision is 20/200 or worse. However, it is important to note that not all people who are legally blind experience complete blindness. Refer to Table 19.1 for the Snellen (US) equivalents of each of these classifications of vision loss. Many TEI are available to maximize and supplement remaining vision so that individuals with vision loss can participate in occupations of choice to the fullest extent.

Select eye conditions that lead to visual impairment

There are several eye-related diseases that lead to vision loss, and as previously stated, older adults are most at risk for developing these conditions (Stuen and Faye 2003; WHO 2018). These include cataract, age-related macular degeneration (ARMD), diabetic retinopathy, glaucoma, and hemianopia. While some of these conditions are treatable, several of them are not curable and thus lead to irreparable vision loss. This makes TEIs for people with visual impairment even more critical. Each of these conditions will be discussed briefly, and you can refer to the third Active Learning Prompt to locate online resources and applications that demonstrate what a person living which each of these conditions may experience.

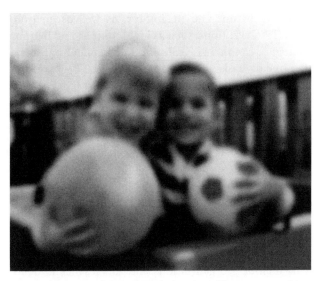

Figure 19.1 A scene as it might be viewed by a person with cataract. Source: National Eye Institute, National Institutes of Health (NEI/NIH).

Cataract

Simply stated, cataract is the clouding of the lens of the eye (National Eye Institute [NEI] 2015a). This decreases the amount of light that is able to pass through the lens and results in blurry, cloudy vision (Stuen and Faye 2003; NEI 2015a). Additionally, colors may appear less vibrant, glare may become problematic, and night vision may become more difficult (NEI 2015a). Refer to Figure 19.1 for a scene as it might be viewed by a person with a cataract. Cataracts can be removed through surgery and replaced with a lens implant. However, because many people worldwide cannot afford cataract surgery or are not surgical candidates due to other medical conditions, it is the leading cause of blindness worldwide (WHO 2010).

Age-related macular degeneration

ARMD is the most common cause of vision loss in the US older adult population (NEI 2018). Named for the macula, or the central portion of the visual field responsible for the sharpest vision, ARMD occurs when the macula deteriorates because of either fatty deposits (drusen), which is dry ARMD, or leaky blood vessels under the retina, which is wet ARMD. This deterioration results in blind spots called *scotomas* that are scattered throughout the central portion of vision, and limit the ability to read, write, drive, recognize faces, engage in hand crafts, and perform other activities that require central vision. Refer to Figure 19.2 for a scene as it may be viewed by a person with ARMD. In dry ARMD the deterioration is limited to the macula and complete blindness does not occur. Peripheral vision is spared and

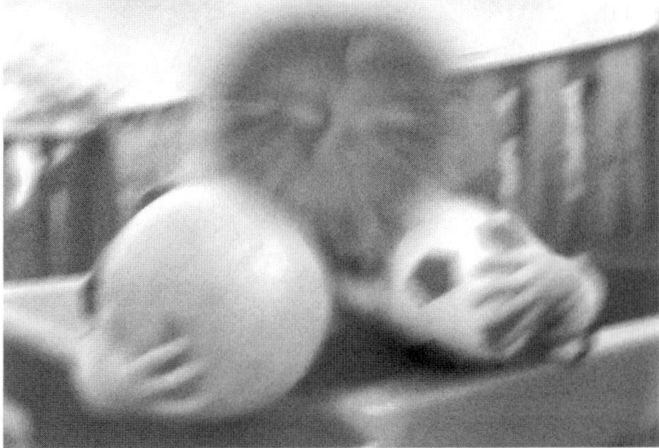

Figure 19.2 A scene as it might be viewed by a person with age-related macular degeneration. Source: National Eye Institute, National Institutes of Health (NEI/NIH).

can be used to replace central vision; however, visual acuity in the periphery is not as clear, thus, many TEIs including electronic and optical magnification are useful to those with ARMD in order to maximize this remaining vision. Wet ARMD can lead to blindness if left untreated or if it causes retinal detachment. A small number of individuals with wet ARMD qualify for laser surgery or medicinal injections to stop the progression of the disease, but there is no cure for ARMD (NEI 2018).

Diabetic retinopathy

Diabetic retinopathy occurs as the result of a longstanding history with diabetes (NEI 2015b). Similar to ARMD, diabetic retinopathy produces scotomas in the visual field because of leaking blood vessels in the retina (NEI 2015b). However, unlike ARMD, diabetic retinopathy is not limited to the macula. You may have observed this difference when you completed the third Active Learning Prompt. Both central and peripheral vision may be affected by diabetic retinopathy, which can eventually lead to complete blindness. In fact, diabetic retinopathy is the leading cause of blindness in adults living in the United States (NEI 2015b). Researchers have found that blood sugar, blood pressure, and cholesterol regulation can assist in slowing the development and progression of diabetic retinopathy (NEI 2015b). In severe stages of the disease, laser surgery intervention may be useful in shrinking the leaking blood vessels (NEI 2015b).

Glaucoma

Glaucoma occurs when there is an abnormal amount of pressure on the optic nerve in the eye (NEI 2015c). This abnormal pressure squeezing the optic nerve produces peripheral vision loss that is often referred to as tunnel vision. Refer to Figure 19.3 for a scene as it might be

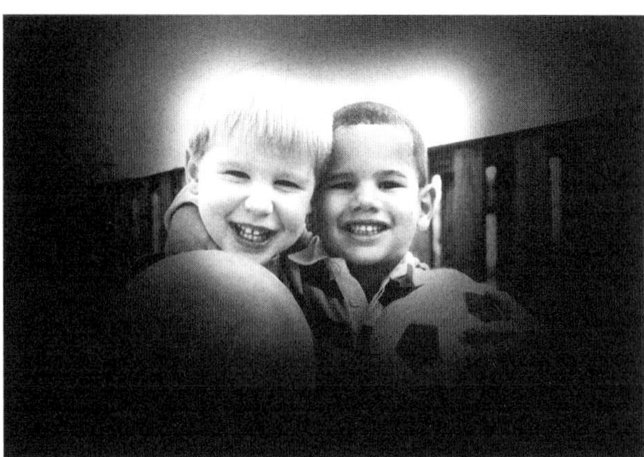

Figure 19.3 A scene as it might be viewed by a person with glaucoma. Source: National Eye Institute, National Institutes of Health (NEI/NIH).

viewed by a person with glaucoma. As you recall in the third Active Learning Prompt, vision loss with glaucoma progresses from the outer visual field in toward the central field, similar to looking through a tunnel. This is a much different pattern of vision loss compared to the scotomas that occur as the result of ARMD or diabetic retinopathy, and results in a limited ability to identify movement or objects in the surrounding environment. Because early glaucoma is not painful and does not have symptoms, most people do not receive medical attention for it until a significant amount of vision has been lost; it can progress to the central vision and eventually lead to complete blindness (NEI 2015c). The pressure in the eye can be controlled through medication, typically in the form of eye drops, or through surgical intervention (NEI 2015c).

Hemianopia

Lastly, hemianopia (also called hemianopsia) is the result of pathways in the brain that carry visual information becoming damaged, usually as the result of stroke, brain injury, or tumor (Lighthouse International n.d.-b). The result is damage to half of the visual field. When damage occurs to the same side of both visual fields, it is further defined as homonymous hemianopia, whereas when damage occurs to opposite visual fields it is called heteronymous hemianopia (Lighthouse International n.d.-b). Functionally, individuals experiencing hemianopia often bump into or ignore objects and people on the side of the affected visual field; therefore, mobility is impaired. When the damage occurs on the left side, individuals also have difficulty reading because the beginning of each line is difficult to detect. The damage may resolve somewhat over time, but once again TEIs can be useful for this population. AT, including prisms and magnifiers, as well as environmental interventions, such as high-contrast and lighting strategies, can increase safe and independent participation in daily tasks.

Application of the human-tech ladder to individuals with visual impairment

As introduced in Chapter 1, Vicente's (2006) Human-Tech Ladder is one way of organizing our thoughts about the fit between the person, the environment, and the technology we use.

There are five rungs to Vicente's (2006) Human-Tech Ladder which progressively move from the physical and psychological attributes of the person outward to the team members, organizations, and policies that influence the development, prescription, funding, and access to technology (Vicente 2006). Together, each rung of the Human-Tech Ladder can be applied to the way we conceptualize the interaction between a person with a visual impairment, their environment, and the technology they use.

Physical

The first rung or lowest level of the Human-Tech Ladder is the physical attributes of the person, such as body shape and size, joint motion, strength, balance, coordination, and others that may influence the design and use of a particular piece of technology (Vicente 2006). These physical attributes should influence both the hard and the soft aspects of technology, such as the size, shape, or type of material that is being developed and being considered for a particular user (Vicente 2006). For example, technology with highly contrasting colors (i.e. black and white) would be a better match to a person with visual impairment as compared to one that has low contrast. Similarly, technology with enlarged print size (i.e. a minimum of 18-point font) would be more valuable than one that did not have enlarged print.

While impairment of the visual system is of primary attention when considering the physical attributes, people with visual impairment may also have other chronic conditions that affect their physical functioning and thus the match to the physical attributes of a piece of technology. We know that 80% of older adults aged 65 and older manage at least one chronic condition and those aged 75 and older manage at least three chronic conditions (Triple Tree 2011). This means that many older adults living with vision loss also manage other conditions such as arthritis, hearing limitations, cardiorespiratory diseases, and others that impair their ability to participate in their daily occupations. Not only do they have to find ways to perform everyday tasks with an impaired visual system, but these impairments of other body structures that may limit normal joint motion, strength, activity tolerance, coordination, balance, and more also affect their performance and so should be considered.

For example, an older adult with glaucoma may also have a history of arthritis in her hands which limits her joint range of motion, strength, and coordination. This person may have a difficult time dispensing eye drops as a treatment for her glaucoma because of the combination of vision loss and limited hand function. Similarly, an older adult with diabetes may have additional impairments in tactile sensation and ambulation due to peripheral neuropathy. This person may have a difficult time with meal preparation tasks because of the combination of vision and tactile sensation impairment. Choosing technology with the appropriate physical attributes that accommodate individual-specific needs is an important consideration at this first rung of the Human-Tech Ladder.

Psychological

The second rung of the Human-Tech Ladder continues to focus on the individual, but rather than the physical attributes of the person, the emphasis at this step is the fit between the individual's psychological status and the technology (Vicente 2006). According to Vicente (2006), psychological factors include mental functioning, such as memory capacity, understanding cause/effect relationships, and the ability to cognitively understand how to use the technology. A piece of technology may be appropriate for a person from a physical standpoint, but if it is not simple and intuitive, the likelihood that it will get used to the fullest extent is not very good. This is especially true for those with visual impairment because without the assistance of full vision, a person with visual impairment relies much more on cognitive strategies to manage their daily activities. Technology that has tolerance for error is going to be more suitable for those with visual impairment. Credit card kiosks that accept a card swipe without preference for which way the card is facing would be an example of technology that has tolerance for error for a person with a visual impairment. Keys that are functional from either direction or vending machines that accept dollar bills from either end would be other examples of this.

People with visual impairment rely heavily on their cognition in order to be successful in carrying out their daily activities. They often rely heavily on their memory as a substitution for their vision to locate common items they use throughout the day and often use common objects as TEI. Basic TEI such as placing a rubber band around a bottle to distinguish shampoo from conditioner or using a safety pin system to color-code and organize clothing (for example, pin one safety pin to all black colored pants, two safety pins to all navy blue colored pants, etc.) are simple but effective AT strategies that people with visual impairment can use if there is a match between the psychological attributes of the person and the technology (hardware and software).

Individuals with vision loss may also have difficulty adjusting to vision loss. This type of psychosocial concern also needs to be considered when assessing and planning TEI for this population. For example, the individual who has not yet accepted his or her vision loss and is still hoping for a cure may not be ready to accept technology as a strategy for maximizing functional performance. Similarly, depression or anxiety may be present in individuals coping with vision loss. These psychosocial factors can have a significant influence on the type of TEI, if any, that is integrated into his or her daily routine.

Team

The third rung of the Human-Tech Ladder includes the team members involved in the development, provision, and training of the technology (Vicente 2006). Any team requires adequate communication and coordination to achieve the goals of the team. It is no different when providing clients with TEI. There are many professionals with valuable expertise to add to the effectiveness of a comprehensive AT plan of care. All of these viewpoints must be integrated into one comprehensive plan in order to achieve the most effective outcome for the client.

There are a number of interprofessional team members who may be involved in the provision of technology to individuals with visual impairment, in addition to the person with visual impairment and his or her family members or caregivers. As a team they are responsible for the assessment, equipment provision, and training in the use of all TEIs that are part of the plan of care. Each member has a unique set of roles and responsibilities. Eye care professionals, such as those from the fields of ophthalmology and optometry, are critical for completing a formal and thorough eye exam. In addition to the exam, they would be responsible for the prescription of any medication, corrective lenses, or optical devices. Occupational therapy practitioners, vision rehabilitation therapists, and certified low vision therapists may be involved in the training in the use of optical or electronic devices as well as other non-optical intervention strategies and environmental modifications for the performance of daily activities, educational activities, work tasks, and leisure interests (Academy for Certification of Vision Rehabilitation & Education Professionals [ACVREP] n.d.-a, n.d.-c; Kaldenberg and Smallfield 2013). Occupational therapists also contribute knowledge about the interaction between the skills of the person, the occupations he or she chooses to perform, and the environment(s) in which the occupations are performed to the interprofessional team (American Occupational Therapy Association 2014). Orientation and mobility specialists train individuals with vision loss or complete blindness how to navigate their home and community surroundings. This includes training in the use of a long cane as well as in the use of public transportation and other mobility options for those with visual impairment (ACVREP n.d.-b). Finally, rehabilitation counselors provide employment-related counseling to those with vision loss or blindness.

Organizational

The organizational level is the fourth rung of Vicente's (2006) Human-Tech Ladder. There are several organizational structures that may be considered when applying Vicente's (2006) Human-Tech Ladder to people with visual impairment and they typically can be classified in one of two systems, namely the blindness system and the medical system. In the United States, several organizations, including schools, state vocational services, other community-based programs, and the Veteran's Administration medical system, historically have comprised the blindness system. Optometrists, orientation and mobility specialists, low vision therapists, and rehabilitation teachers commonly work in these organizations. These organizations provide comprehensive services to people who are blind and visually impaired and since these organizations operate on state and federal funding, a certain level of service is provided to those who qualify for services at no additional cost to the client.

The organizations that comprise the blindness system can be contrasted to the traditional medical or healthcare delivery system in the United States. Organizations within the healthcare system, such as medical clinics and hospitals, did not emphasize treatment for people who are blind and visually impaired until 1990, when there was a change in reimbursement so that medical providers, including occupational therapists, could receive reimbursement for providing services to clients with vision loss (Warren 1995). Therefore, individuals with visual loss had increased access to care because occupational therapy practitioners, who commonly work in the medical system rather than the blindness system, were then able to provide services and receive medical insurance reimbursement for the services they provide. Furthermore, the Balanced Budget Refinement Act of 1999 (Pub. L. 106-113) included legislation that allowed doctors of optometry to meet the supervision requirements for Medicare beneficiaries (American Optometric Association Federal Relations Committee 1999).

Political

Finally, policy and political considerations comprise the fifth and top rung of the Human-Tech Ladder (Vicente 2006). This includes not only policies that influence the provision of hard and soft AT but also public opinion, social values, and cultural norms. The development and provision of AT services and equipment are greatly influenced by existing laws, regulations, and sociocultural norms and cannot be overlooked when considering all options for TEIs for people with visual impairment.

As you may have noticed in the earlier discussion on organizational influences on the development and provision of AT services and equipment, policy has had a significant influence. The change in policy that took effect in 1990, which stated that visual impairment is recognized as a physical impairment under federal guidelines, influenced the type of healthcare professionals who can provide services and training to individuals with vision loss. The addition of occupational therapy practitioners as recognized service providers who can receive reimbursement for their services contrasts with previously recognized providers of services to the blind and visually impaired through the blindness system.

Furthermore, policy or lack thereof can greatly influence access to technology. Specifically, unlike for intervention such as prescription medications, people with vision loss can purchase optical and electronic magnification and many other TEIs off the shelf. However, this ease of access in obtaining the technology comes at the price of receiving little to no training in how to use the technology appropriately. This in turn can result in abandonment of the technology because the user does not know how to use it correctly or to its fullest capacity. Additionally, there are many regulations and licensure laws governing the training and education level of the professionals who do prescribe client-centered technology and the proper training in the use of such devices.

In addition to policy changes, this macro level of the Human-Tech Ladder also considers the social and cultural considerations of AT and how this technology is perceived by the general public. For example, some individuals with visual impairment may try to hide their vision loss from others. Therefore, they may not want to use specially designed AT such as a long cane, talking watches, or optical magnifiers when they are out in public. However, they may be more willing to use technology that blends in with that used by the general public, such as a tablet computer with applications specific to visual impairment, or a talking navigation device that is sold commercially. Social perceptions of disability may be a significant driving factor in the selection and use of AT.

Considerations in assessment for AT for visual impairment

Prior to providing any technology or environmental intervention for individuals with vision loss, an assessment of the current fit between individual skills, the environment, and the tasks they desire to perform should be completed. Any current technology and strategies that are being used should be included in that assessment. A thorough understanding of the current status of the individual along with the supports and barriers he or she may have in performing occupations of choice informs the selection and recommendation of new or additional TEI.

Theoretical models of practice

Assessment and intervention when working with people with vision loss should be guided by a theoretical model. Theories, models of practice, and frames of reference serve as ways to explain a given phenomenon. Applied to AT and vision loss, the purpose of a theory, model of practice, or frame of reference would be to view performance of daily occupations through a given lens and then explain why a particular intervention strategy would be expected to produce a higher level of independence in those daily tasks.

There are several theories, models of practice, and frames of reference that may be applicable when considering appropriate AT for people with vision loss. The purpose of this chapter is not to provide a comprehensive listing of all of the possible theories that could be applied, or a detailed description of all of them, but rather to provide a sampling of theories that may be appropriate and a description of how they can be applied when considering an assessment of the appropriateness of AT for vision loss.

Potential theoretical approaches that may be useful when working with individuals with vision loss may include the Transtheoretical Model of Health Behavior Change (Prochaska and Velicer 1997), the Person-Environment-Occupation Model of Occupational Performance (Law et al. 1996), Ecology of Human Performance, (Dunn et al. 1994), or the Rehabilitative (compensatory) frame of reference (Seidel 2003). While the Transtheoretical Model of Health Behavior Change is a model frequently used when addressing public health issues, it is useful to apply when working with individuals with visual impairment because it provides a framework in which to consider an individual's readiness to make adaptations or changes in their health status (Prochaska and Velicer 1997). If an individual has not yet come to terms with permanent visual loss, there is a decreased likelihood that recommended TEIs will be implemented into a daily routine. According to the Transtheoretical Model of Health Behavior Change, targeting education and intervention recommendations based upon an individual's readiness to accept the information will prove to be most effective (Prochaska and Velicer 1997).

The Person-Environment-Occupation-Model of Occupational Performance (Law et al. 1996) and the Ecology of Human Performance model (Dunn et al. 1994) are models of practice developed by occupational therapists that emphasize the influence of the environment on the performance of daily activity. According to these models, the individual cannot be separated from the environment in which they perform daily life tasks, and so the environment needs to be considered along with an individual's skills and abilities when selecting appropriate TEIs. For example, an older adult with ARMD likes to read the morning paper. Gathering information about the setting in which this activity is performed (i.e. at the kitchen table, or in the recliner chair in the living room) is critical so that appropriate recommendations can be made. In this case, the lighting for each setting may be drastically different from the other, and so intervention strategies can be tailored to meet the individual's needs when characteristics of the environment are known.

Finally, the Rehabilitative or compensatory frame of reference (Seidel 2003) is also useful when considering the assessment for AT needs for an individual with visual impairment. A compensatory approach acknowledges that restoration of function is not always achievable (Seidel 2003), and thus performance in daily tasks can be enhanced through technology or other adaptive strategies. This frame of reference can be combined with other theoretical approaches in order to meet all aspects of a client's plan of care. Further information about each of these select theoretical approaches and their application to AT assessment and intervention can be found in Table 19.2.

After one or more theoretical approaches with which to guide the assessment and intervention planning process are selected, an AT assessment should include a thorough history of both the client's health and their performance of daily activities. First, understanding the client's medical condition is important as this influences

Table 19.2 Select Theoretical Models for Assessment and Intervention for Visual Impairment.

Theoretical approach	Description	Application to technology and environmental adaptation for visual impairment
Stages of Change/ Transtheoretical Model of Health Behavior Change (Prochaska and Velicer 1997)	• Provides a structure for determining the readiness of an individual to make changes in behaviors. • Progresses from no awareness that a change is needed through the process of adopting and maintaining a behavior change.	• This model is useful for determining if an individual with vision loss is ready to be introduced to technology and environmental interventions to support performance of daily activities. • The level of education and intervention provided to an individual with vision loss will vary depending upon their readiness to make changes.
Person-Environment-Occupation Model of Occupational Performance (Law et al. 1996)	• Divides the components of daily occupation into qualities of the person, environmental contributors, and attributes of the occupation itself. • Useful for evaluating how a client performs an occupation in a specific environment in order to identify appropriate intervention strategies.	• Intervention strategies to improve performance of daily tasks can be targeted at the person, the environment, or the occupation. For example: ∘ Person: Instruction in scanning techniques or scotoma awareness ∘ Environment: Reducing clutter, increasing contrast and illumination ∘ Occupation: Modify check writing to automatic bill pay; adapt stovetop cooking to microwave meals for increased safety.
Ecology of Human Performance (Dunn et al. 1994)	• Emphasizes the interwoven relationship between a person and the environment. • Identifies a variety of intervention approaches that can target the individual, the environment, or both.	• The alter intervention strategy targets the environment by placing the individual with visual impairment in a setting that maximizes his or her functional abilities. • The adapt intervention strategy emphasizes the use of strategies or technology to maximize the individual's occupational performance in context.
Rehabilitative/Compensatory Frame of Reference (Seidel 2003)	• Recognizes the benefit of assistive devices and compensatory methods when independence cannot otherwise be restored. • Assistive technology, therapeutic adaptations, and environmental modifications can be suitable intervention strategies to compensate for physical and cognitive impairments.	• A person can maximize remaining vision through the use of electrical and optical magnification, learning to use a preferred retinal locus, increasing lighting with their environment, and other compensatory strategies.

the selection of TEIs. The nature of the medical condition will lead to functional limitations. For example, one would anticipate that a client with diabetic retinopathy may also have additional complications from diabetes mellitus including peripheral neuropathy, which may produce sensation changes. A diagnosis of diabetes mellitus also indicates that the client is managing a chronic condition and will have medication management and lifestyle modification needs as a result. On the other hand, a diagnosis of cataract for an older adult who is a good surgical candidate to have the cataract removed means that the client has much different needs that should be taken into account. Knowing the history of the presenting diagnosis as well as the client's past medical history is critical to the overall assessment for AT needs. The medical history may be gathered through an interview with the client and/or care providers or it may also be gathered through a review of the client's medical record, or both.

Client profile

In addition to having a thorough understanding of a client's medical condition, it is also important to gather information about the types of activities or occupations in which the client participates. In the *Occupational Therapy Practice Framework* (American Occupational Therapy Association 2014) this is termed the "occupational profile." Like the information gathered in the medical history, information about the types of activities that are meaningful to a client with visual impairment will greatly influence the TEIs that are considered during intervention planning. In the fourth Active Learning

Prompt you completed an interview of someone you know to determine what activities he or she participates in on a daily basis. Compare how many of these were the same or different than the ones that you perform. Likewise, two clients with the same diagnosis will have very different AT needs based on the activities they perform on a regular basis. For example, a librarian who enjoys staying current in literature will use different TEIs than a chef who wants to be able to participate in food preparation activities. Gathering information about a client's vocation, hobbies, interests, daily tasks and routines, and obligatory occupations allows the therapist to collaborate with the client to develop a truly meaningful intervention plan and makes the assessment for AT client-centered. Additionally, gathering information regarding social, financial, physical, temporal, personal, cultural, and virtual contexts is critical as these factors will also influence the selection of TEIs. Refer to Box 19.1 for additional interview questions related to a client's medical and occupational history that may be useful during an assessment for technology needs when working with individuals with visual impairment.

One formal assessment tool that is useful for gathering information about an individual's occupational performance history is the Canadian Occupational Performance Measure (COPM; Law et al. 2005). The COPM is a semi-structure interview in which the client describes the activities they need or want to do. The client then prioritizes the activities so that intervention can be focused on the ones that are of most importance to them. During the assessment, the client rates his or her ability to perform and satisfaction with of each of the prioritized activities on a scale of 1–10, with 1 being poor performance and low satisfaction and 10 being good performance and high satisfaction. The COPM is then re-administered at the end of intervention to determine the level of change in performance and satisfaction. Rebovich and Zevoda (2013) discuss the clinical utility of the COPM in assessing older adults with vision loss and conclude that it is a valuable tool in promoting collaboration between the client and the therapist as it promotes individualized, client-centered care. Because it is a standardized tool, it is also useful for reporting functional outcomes among this client population.

Performance in context

Another useful standardized assessment of function for individuals with visual impairment is the Self-Report Assessment of Functional Visual Performance Profile (SRAFVP; Mennemen et al. 2012). The SRAFVP consists of 22 tasks on which the client with vision loss rates their performance as either unable (1), difficult (2), or independent (3) and 16 additional tasks in which the client's performance is observed and rated by the AT practitioner using the same three-level scoring system. Sample self-report items include reading, meal preparation, financial management, shopping, and writing, while sample performance items include reading the time on a watch, climbing stairs, dialing a telephone, and managing medication. Ideally, the assessment should be completed in the client's natural home environment using any assistive devices as they normally do. The SRAFVP can be used to gather both baseline and re-assessment data that can be used in reporting functional outcomes and measuring changes in function as the result of occupational therapy intervention, including TEIs (Mennemen et al. 2012).

Observation of actual performance in priority activities is a critical step of the assessment process. Observation of task performance provides the opportunity to identify where the breakdown in task performance occurs. While the SRAFVP does include performance items (Mennemen et al. 2012), additional observation of task performance of occupations not included in the SRAFVP may be indicated depending upon the client's priorities for intervention. Equally important to developing a good understanding of the client occupations is a clear understanding of the environment in which meaningful occupations are performed. Observation of task performance in the natural environment in which it occurs is ideal. This enhances the intervention planning as TEIs can be tailored to the specific environment in which the activity occurs. For example, observing a client with visual impairment reading the newspaper in their armchair where they routinely read the newspaper, rather than observing them in an outpatient clinic setting, provides a richer observation experience which can in turn lead to more tailored intervention.

One aspect of the environment that is especially important to assess for a client with visual impairment is the level of illumination in the locations where priority tasks are performed. Lighting has a significant influence on task performance among this population (Figueiro 2001) and therefore should be thoroughly addressed in both assessment and intervention. Obtaining objective data regarding lighting levels using a commercially available light meter can be useful as a guide for intervention planning. While observation of occupation in context is not always feasible, it provides valuable information and should be implemented when practical.

Personal skills and abilities

Finally, assessment for AT when working with clients with visual impairment should also include a detailed assessment of their visual skills and other personal skills and abilities. This might include but is not limited to testing visual skills such as acuity, contrast sensitivity, visual field, and oculomotor control, scanning, and visual cognitive tasks. Many of these can be tested informally; however, the author recommends using standardized assessment such as the Brain Injury Visual Assessment Battery for Adults (biVABA) (Warren 1998), which contains the testing instructions and equipment for a thorough functional visual assessment.

Additional standardized assessments are available with which to assess reading, which is often significantly influence by vision loss. Two common assessments of reading skills include the MNRead Acuity Charts (Mansfield et al. 1994) and the Pepper Visual Skills for Reading Test (VSRT), also known as the Pepper Test (Watson et al. 1995). The MNRead measures both acuity level and reading speed and assists the therapist in identifying the smallest type size at which a person can read at his or her maximum speed (Mansfield et al. 1994). The MNRead charts have demonstrated reliability (Subramanian and Pardhan 2006; Patel et al. 2011). Similarly, the Pepper Test assesses reading accuracy and speed (Watson et al. 1995) and is a reliable and valid assessment of reading for individuals with visual impairment (Baldasare et al. 1986; Watson et al. 1990, 1995).

Beyond specific visual skills, it is important to consider a client's broader skills and abilities as they relate to the performance of daily activities. Since many people with visual impairment are older adults, other health conditions may cause limitations in other factors such as muscle strength and range of motion, balance and coordination, sensation, and cognition. These other limitations can directly influence TEI recommendations. For example, a person with visual impairment as the result of a traumatic brain injury who also has cognitive impairments may not be able to use a complex software program that contains text-to-speech functions. Other less cognitively complex TEIs may be more suitable for this client. Psychosocial factors such as isolation, depression, and anxiety should also be accounted for in a comprehensive AT assessment as these will all influence the type and amount of TEI recommended. Refer to Table 19.3 for a select list of standardized assessment tools that may be useful when conducting an assessment for AT needs for an individual with visual impairment.

Select TEI strategies for visual impairment

Once a thorough assessment for AT has been completed, the information gleaned from it can be used to develop intervention options. When considering TEIs for visual

Table 19.3 Select standardized assessment tools for visual impairment.

Assessment	Reference	Items assessed
Canadian Occupational Performance Measure (COPM)	Law, M., Baptiste, S., Carswell, A. et al. (2005). *Canadian Occupational Performance Measure Manual*, 4e. Ottawa, Canada: CAOT Publications.	• The top occupational performance issues are identified and rated according to: ∘ perceived performance ∘ satisfaction with performance
Self-Report Assessment of Functional Visual Performance Profile (SRAFVP)	Mennemen, T.A., Warren, M., and Yuen, H.K. (2012). Preliminary validation of vision-dependent activities of daily living instrument on adults with homonymous hemianopsia. *American Journal of Occupational Therapy*, 66(4): 478–482.	Performance of daily tasks: • 22 self-report items • 16 performance-based items
Brain Injury Visual Assessment Battery for Adults (biVABA)	Warren, M. (1998). *Brain Injury Visual Assessment Battery for Adults*. Lenexa, KS: visABILITIES Rehab Services.	Components of visual function including: ∘ Acuity ∘ Visual field ∘ Oculomotor control ∘ Contrast sensitivity ∘ Visual attention ∘ Visual scanning
MNRead Acuity Charts	Mansfield, J.S., Legge, G.E., Luebker, A., and Cunningham, K. (1994). *MNRead Acuity Charts: Continuous-Text Reading-Acuity Charts for Normal and Low Vision*. Long Island City, NY: Lighthouse Low Vision Products.	• Reading acuity • Reading speed
Pepper Visual Skills for Reading Test (VSRT)	Watson, G. R., Whittaker, S., and Steciw, M. (1995). *The Pepper Visual Skills for Reading Test*, 2 e. Lilburn, GA: Bear Consultants.	• Reading accuracy • Reading speed

impairment, it is important to remember that a comprehensive intervention plan will include multiple TEIs and will likely include multiple options for each of the priority tasks identified in the assessment process. Identifying multiple intervention options for each priority task will provide an opportunity for collaboration with the client to discuss each of the potential solutions, trial them, and select the most appropriate one(s).

It should be noted that living with vision loss is living with a chronic illness. Therefore, in addition to the selection and implementation of appropriate TEI, clients need to be trained to solve challenges that come up in the future. A comprehensive intervention plan for clients with visual impairment should also include training in the problem-solving strategies needed to be successful in the future. These problem-solving strategies can be considered as part of the soft technology that goes along with hard technology. Strong research evidence supports the use of a problem-solving approach with individuals with visual impairment (Berger et al. 2013).

The remainder of this chapter will focus on describing a wide variety of potential TEIs for people with visual impairment. Because visual impairment significantly affects one's ability to read, and reading is a critical part of many daily tasks, potential TEIs for reading will be discussed first. This will be followed by TEIs that can be useful when considering general activities of daily living. Finally, since technology use in the form of smartphones, tablet computers, and computers in general is increasingly becoming the societal norm, specific information regarding soft technology that can be applied to these devices will be discussed.

AT for reading and viewing

There are many types of assistive devices that can enhance an individual's ability to perform tasks involving reading. There are many types of reading that people perform throughout the day; these include near reading for either brief or extended periods of time as well as distance reading or viewing for either brief or extended periods of time. Think back to Active Learning Prompt 4, in which you were asked to complete the interview of a friend to gain information about their daily activities. How many of these activities include a reading component? Now think about just the activities that require reading. Is the reading at a near distance (such as reading a text message on a smartphone) or a far distance (such as reading a street sign while driving in the car)? Does your friend perform those activities for only a few seconds (looking at a price tag) or for hours at a time (watching a movie in the theater)? The kind of activity will influence the type of AT that is most appropriate for that task.

Optical magnification

Optical magnification is one type of AT that can be used to increase the ability of an individual with visual impairment to complete reading and viewing tasks. Optical magnifiers are non-electronic devices that magnify, or enlarge, an image that is presented through a glass lens. The lens of an optical magnifier is similar to the lenses in a pair of glasses; however, the lenses are of higher power, and therefore often heavier than typically found in eyeglasses, although these types of lenses can be mounted in eyeglasses as well. The strength of the magnification determines the size of the lens; the stronger the magnifier the smaller the usable view of the lens. Therefore, it is important to remember that stronger magnification is not necessarily better. There are many types of optical magnifiers, including handheld magnifiers, stand magnifiers, spectacle magnifiers, and telescopes. Each will be discussed briefly, including a discussion of the tasks in which each may be appropriate.

As the name implies, individuals with visual impairment hold a handheld magnifier in their hand. Handheld magnifiers are meant to be used for reading tasks within a close distance, such as reading restaurant menus, price tags, and medication or food labels. They are portable and most efficient when used for brief reading tasks. Handheld magnifiers come with or without illumination which can aid in reading (see discussion of illumination below) and in a variety of powers.

While handheld magnifiers are best for brief reading tasks, stand-based magnification is used for more extended reading and viewing of material at a close distance. Stand magnifiers are placed on a table or other surface when in use and are guided along the reading material with the hand. Reading the mail or other written correspondence, the newspaper or a magazine, or financial statements are select reading tasks for which stand magnifiers are appropriate. Similar to handheld magnification, stand magnifiers are available either with or without built-in illumination. The lighting source can vary; for example, incandescent, light-emitting diode, or halogen bulbs may be used. Clients should be allowed the opportunity to trial several different lighting sources to determine which type is most suitable and least straining on their eyes. Illuminated magnification needs to have a power source, and both battery-operated and electricity-powered options are available. Battery-operated devices are more portable but come with the added cost and task of maintaining charged batteries. Electrical-powered lit magnification is less portable but does not have the added maintenance of batteries.

Spectacle magnifiers appear similar to regular eyeglasses; however, the lenses are of higher power, and thus heavier. The advantage to spectacle magnification is that it provides a hands-free option of viewing close material for an extended period of time. Spectacle magnification is appropriate for tasks such as sewing and woodworking in which two hands are often used to perform the task over a period of time. The power of the lens dictates the distance at which the material must be held (or focal distance) in order to maintain an image that is in focus. The higher the power, the shorter the working distance. It is often difficult for people to maintain this reduced focal distance.

Telescopes are the final type of optical magnification that will be discussed here. While we often think of using long telescopes for viewing objects such as the stars at a distance, shorter, more practical telescopes are available for use by individuals with visual impairment to perform daily occupations that require either near or far reading and viewing. Telescopes can either be handheld or mounted onto the top portion of eyeglasses. Handheld telescopes are used monocularly for brief spotting tasks such as reading street signs, whereas mounted telescopes can be either monocular or binocular, and are often used for activities such as driving, watching movies in the theater, or performing hobby or craft activities. When a telescope is mounted onto eyeglasses, the individual with visual impairment can use his or her regular prescription lenses for typical viewing and then tip his or her head down in order to view through the bioptic for a magnified view of select images. Monocular telescopes require the user to manually focus the image; some *bioptic telescopes* are available with autofocus technology. Most bioptic telescopes used for driving are fixed focused at infinity and are not focusable because the tasks that are completed with theses telescopes often do not allow for the time to focus (Brilliant 1999). More information about selecting the most appropriate optical magnification device for near and far visual activities can be seen in Table 19.4.

While many devices can be ordered without a prescription, often higher-powered magnifiers must be ordered by an eye care or rehabilitation practitioner. It is also important to note that the soft technology of teaching and training in the use of the device can be critical to proper and long-term use. Fok et al. (2011) reported that an individual with vision loss uses on average 6.1 AT devices and approximately 16% of these are abandoned. Contributing factors to abandonment may be the amount of training received in the proper use of the device in order to integrate it into daily habits and routines.

Electronic magnification

Electronic (video) *magnification* is an alternative to optical magnification and can be used when optical magnification is insufficient or for prolonged reading. Rather than viewing print or other objects through a high-powered lens to

Table 19.4 Select Optical Magnification Devices for Reading and Viewing.

Device	Type of reading	Select reading tasks
Handheld magnification	Brief reading of material at a close distance	• Medication labels • Food labels • Restaurant menus • Price tags
Stand-based magnification	Protracted reading of material at a close distance	• Written correspondence • Newspaper • Magazines • Financial statements
Spectacle magnification	Hands-free protracted reading or viewing of material at a close distance	• Newspaper • Magazines • Books • Hobby or craft activities
Handheld telescopes	Brief viewing of items at medium or far distances	• Street signage • Aisle signage • Bus number • Field enhancement (if used in reverse)
Bioptic telescopes	Hands-free, extended viewing of material at far distances	• Road signs while driving • Television viewing • Computer use • Hobby or craft activities

enlarge the image, electronic magnification functions much like a video camera in that when the camera focuses on print material or another item of interest it is projected onto a larger viewing screen such as a monitor, a television, or a built-in screen on the device itself.

Electronic magnification is also commonly referred to as closed-circuit television (CCTV) because early models consisted of a moveable table, a camera, and a television screen in a closed system. The print material is placed on the moveable base; the area that is under the camera is projected onto the screen. However, now there are many types of portable and even head-mounted models of electronic magnification available in addition to stand-based models. Refer to Figure 19.4 for an example of stand-based electronic magnification. An individual with visual impairment can also access electronic magnification as an application on a tablet computer. Refer to Table 19.5 for a select listing of electronic magnification applications that can be downloaded to a table computer or smartphone for use.

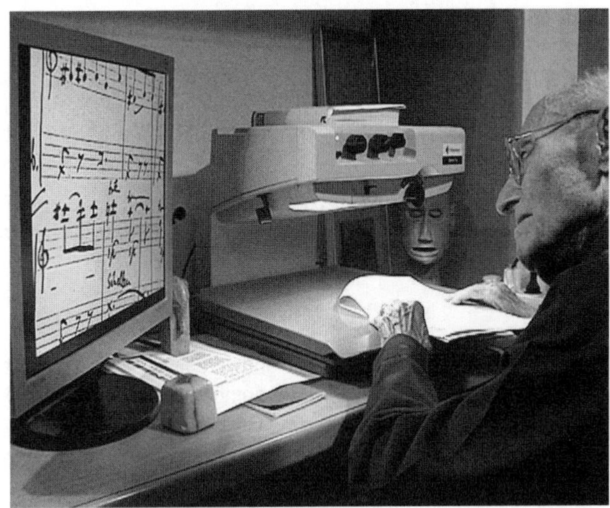

Figure 19.4 Electronic magnification. Source: Photo: Etan Tal. Licensed under CC0.

Table 19.5 Tablet Computer Applications for Visual Impairment.

Topic	Description	Select mobile computer applications
Magnification	• Increases size, spacing, and contrast for reading • Each application has different features, including light, optical character recognition, and contrast adjustments	• Vision assist (iOS) • Magnifier (TiAu) (iOS) • Easy Reader Pro (iOS) • iCanSee (iOS) • Magnifying Glass With Light (iOS) • ZoomReader (iOS) • Magnificent Magnifier (Android) • Magnify (Android) • EyeSight (iOS) • Lumin (iOS) • Zoomcontacts (iOS)
Audio books	• Provides a library of audio books • Adjustable font size and contrast • Access to your local library's eBooks	• Learning Ally Audio (iOS) • Read2Go (iOS) • OverDrive Media Console (iOS, Android) • DaisyWorm (iOS)
Memory aids	• Full voiceover accessibility support • Custom sounds	• Alarmed~Reminders + Timers (iOS) • RxmindMe Prescription/Medicine Reminder and Pill Tracker (iOS)
Navigation aids	• Talking map • Voiceover capabilities • Pedestrian navigation	• Navigon North America (iOS) • Ariadne GPS (iOS) • MotionX GPS Drive (iOS) • AroundMe (iOS, Android) • BlindSquare (iOS) • Navigon North America (iOS) • Ariadne GPS (iOS) • MotionX GPS Drive (iOS) • AroundMe (iOS, Android) • BlindSquare (iOS)

(*Continued*)

Table 19.5 (*Continued*)

Topic	Description	Select mobile computer applications
Money identification	• Recognizes and speaks many forms of currency	• LookTel Money Reader (iOS) • EyeNote (iOS)
Color identification	• Speaks names of colors • Useful for dressing and other tasks requiring color identification	• GreenGar Studios' Color Identifier (iOS) • Color ID Free (iOS, Android) • Color Visor (iOS) • AidColors (iOS) • ColoredEye (iOS)
Object identification	• Recognizes and verbally describes objects • Accesses shopping information by scanning bar codes • Uses sighted workers to identify objects • Records audio messages that can be accessed by scanning paper labels • Scans logos to access talking menus	• TalkingTag (iOS, Android) • VizWiz (iOS) • oMoby (iOS, Android) • Digit Eyes (iOS) • All Access Talking Menus & More (iOS) • AudioLabels (iOS) • TapTapSee (iOS)
Text-to-speech	• Multiple voices in multiple languages • Reads PDFs out loud • Reads emails, responds to voice commands • Reads web pages	• Voice Dream Reader (iOS) • vBookz PDF Voice Reader (iOS, Android) • Talkler-Email for your Ears (iOS) • SayText (iOS) • Web Reader (iOS, Android) • Voice Brief (iOS)
Speech-to-text	• Voice recognition software • Dictates to social media platforms	• Dragon Dictation (iOS) • Dragon Mobile Assistant (Android) • Vlingo (iOS, Android) • AccessNote (iOS)
Word prediction	• Customizable word prediction • Text-to-speech option	• Type-O HD –Writing is for Everybody (iOS) • Fleksy-Happy typing (iOS, Android)
Braille	• Type on touch screen using Braille	• BrailleTouch (Android, iOS) • BraillePad Pro (iOS)
Other daily living aids	• Clock, calculators, phone • Record lists • Reads newspapers, local and national • Internet browsing	• Big Clock HD (iOS) • Talking Clock Widgets (Android) • Talking Clock for iOS (iOS) • Chime (iOS, Android) • Talking Calculator (iOS, Android) • List Recorder (iOS) • NoSquint (iOS) • AutoRingtone Pro Talking CallerID Ringtones (iOS) • BigBrowser (iOS) • Earl (iOS)

Advantages of electronic magnification include the ability to adjust the power of magnification easily as needed, and many models provide full color images in addition to black and white images. Reverse polarity, or the ability to change the foreground and background to the opposite color, is also an option on many models. Electronic magnification can be used for viewing in addition to reading tasks; refer to Box 19.2 for select viewing tasks for which electronic magnification can be used.

Evidence for optical and electronic magnification

Smallfield et al. (2013) conducted a systematic review of the literature that included a review of research about the effectiveness of optical and electronic magnification for improving the performance of reading tasks for older adults with low vision. They found limited evidence supports the use of AT devices (both optical and electronic magnification) compared to no device (Smallfield et al. 2013).

Box 19.2 Beyond reading: Uses for electronic magnification

- Cutting and painting fingernails
- Selecting jewelry
- Looking at photos
- Looking at bugs on leaves
- Checking for spots on clothing
- Coloring
- Knitting
- Distinguishing medications
- Hand crafts

However, when comparing optical magnification to electronic magnification, moderate evidence supports the use of stand-based electronic magnification for improving reading speed and duration (Smallfield et al. 2013). Goodrich and Kirby (2001) found that handheld electronic magnification is more favorable than optical magnification for reading tasks, while Culham et al. (2004) determined that head-mounted electronic magnification is less favorable as compared to optical magnification. In short, stronger evidence supports the use of electronic magnification, specifically stand-based systems, rather than optical magnification. However, because a variety of factors influence device selection, including financial resources, the specific activity performed, and the environment in which the task is performed (see earlier discussion on the Human-Tech Ladder for others), both optical and electronic magnification are valuable AT options to improve reading performance in clients with visual impairment. Refer to Box 19.3 for more a more in-depth study of the current research base regarding interventions to support the occupation of reading for older adults with low vision.

Prisms

In addition to optical and electronic magnification to enhance the performance of reading and viewing tasks, for individuals specifically with peripheral field deficits due to hemianopia, prisms are a useful way of expanding the field of view. *Prisms* work by bending light toward the base of the prism (Hemianopia.org n.d.); the degree of bend increases as the diopters of a prism increase (1 prism diopter roughly increases field awareness by 0.5 of a degree) (Hemianopia.org n.d.). Therefore, the field of view that is cut off by the hemianopia can be expanded by placing the base of the prism toward the side of the peripheral field deficit. Prisms can be ground into eyeglasses or placed on eyeglasses using an adhesive prism, called a Fresnel prism (Hemianopia.org n.d.).

Box 19.3 Here's the evidence

Smallfield, S., Clem, K., and Myers, A. (2013). Occupational therapy interventions to improve the reading ability of older adults with low vision: a systematic review. *American Journal of Occupational Therapy* 67: 288–295. doi:10.5014/ajot.2013.004929.

Key Words: evidence-based practice, occupational therapy, reading, self-help devices, low vision

Purpose: To gather the current evidence to support the use of optical, non-optical, and electronic magnification devices to support the occupation of reading for the performance of daily activities.

Sample: 32 peer-reviewed journal articles.

Method: Systematic review.

Findings: There is moderate evidence to support both electronic magnification and illumination to enhance reading. Limited evidence supports optical magnification.

Critical Thinking Questions:

1. Why do you think there such limited research on the benefits of optical magnification for the performance of reading tasks?
2. If you designed a study to examine the benefits of using an assistive device for reading, what would you want to know? How would you design the study?
3. Having read this article, what additional research do you think is needed in addition to that already discussed in the study?

Because prisms are a type of optical lens, they should be prescribed by an eye care professional. Bowers et al. (2008) found that 20 of 43 participants with homonymous hemianopia who were fitted with 40 diopter press-on prisms were still using them one year later and that the participants reported the prisms to be useful in functional mobility and avoiding obstacles.

Absorptive filters

Absorptive filter glasses are those that absorb unwanted light. They are available in many tints and are useful for enhancing contrast and reducing glare (Eschenbach Optik n.d.). Absorptive filter eyewear is particularly used for outdoor use to enhance the ability to distinguish foreground from background or for identifying potential obstacles. For example, absorptive filters can enhance the ability to distinguish concrete steps or curbs or view the walking path on a sunny day after freshly fallen snow.

Non-optical devices for reading and viewing

In addition to optical and electronic magnification strategies to enhance reading performance for those with visual impairment, there are several non-optical strategies that should also be considered. While not often considered as AT, when using a broad definition of AT that includes environmental intervention, large print can be considered in this category. Specifically, while electronic and optical magnification are methods of enlarging small print to make it more readable, presenting reading material in large print is another potential solution to the challenge. Moderate evidence supports a minimum of a 14–16 point font size to improve the readability of print (Russell-Minda et al. 2007).

Many novels and other literature are available in large print; the reader is referred to the public library system, which often carries a selection of materials in large print. It is also possible to obtain many pieces of literature electronically on computers, tablet computers, and dedicated electronic reading devices which function as electronic magnification as previously described, including the ability to enlarge the print to the desired size. Depending upon the type of reading task, copy machines and computers can be additional methods of enlarging print material to the needed or desired size. Finally, a simple, black, bold marker may be a useful piece of AT when an individual with visual impairment has to read his or her own handwriting. Larger, darker print achieved by this type of marker may be easier to read than that from a delicate fine point pen.

Illumination and contrast for reading and viewing

Finally, lighting and contrast are essential considerations when discussing TEI for individuals with visual impairment. While at first blush colored filters, or overlays that can be placed over reading material in order to enhance the contrast between the background and the written material, may seem to be an effective TEI for enhancing reading activities, Eperjesi et al. (2004) determined that colored overlays do not enhance reading speed for older adults with low vision. Black text on a white background, or vice versa, provides the highest contrast. However, there is moderate research evidence to support illumination as a TEI for improving reading performance (Smallfield et al. 2013). Lighting levels, especially in the home environment, are often well below recommended levels for reading for those with visual impairment. Bowers et al. (2001) and Eldred (1992) have determined that ideal illumination levels range between 1000 and 7000 lx, while most homes are typically at 50 lx.

A relatively easy way to improve reading performance is to introduce mechanisms for increasing the amount of lighting in areas of the home in which reading occurs. For example, adding a task lamp by the recliner chair where the newspaper is read or adding under-cabinet lighting in the kitchen where meal preparation is typically performed can make a measurable difference in reading performance for an individual with visual impairment. Researchers have also determined that, specific to individuals with ARMD, there is no single type of lighting (halogen, incandescent, florescent, etc.) that is most effective (Eperjesi et al. 2007; Haymes and Lee 2006). Therefore, it is important to be client-centered when discussing lighting options with clients to ensure that a light source that does not produce glare or eye strain is selected. Figueiro (2001) has developed a practical guide that can be used by clients and family members to enhance lighting within the home environment.

AT for daily activities

In addition to specific tasks that require reading performance, there are many other daily activities that may be enhanced by TEIs. Beyond enlargement of print material, an individual with visual impairment can use his or her other senses, such as the senses of hearing and tactile sensation, to maximize performance of daily routines. A basic search on the Internet or in a low vision product catalog will reveal several potential solutions. A sample of TEIs that maximize tactile sensation, hearing, or a combination of both will be described here. Additionally, general environmental interventions that are helpful to those with visual impairment will be shared.

Sensory substitution strategies

When the sense of vision becomes impaired, other senses can be used to gain the same or similar information for task completion. Tactile sensation, audition (the sense of hearing), and vibratory sense are commonly used by individuals with visual impairment to maximize performance of daily tasks. For example, templates and signature guides are tactile strategies to assist in writing in a straight line. They are typically available in a dark color so as also to increase contrast with white paper to maximize use of residual vision. Refer to Figures 19.5 and 19.6 for examples of templates for writing checks and letters, respectively. Folding items such as paper currency in a certain manner to distinguish one from another is another example.

Rubber bands are a simple tactile strategy in order to distinguish similar items from each other. One or multiple bands can be placed around soup cans, shampoo or conditioner bottles, or other types of like containers. Rubber bands are available in a variety of thicknesses

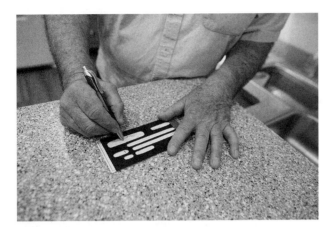

Figure 19.5 A guide for writing checks.

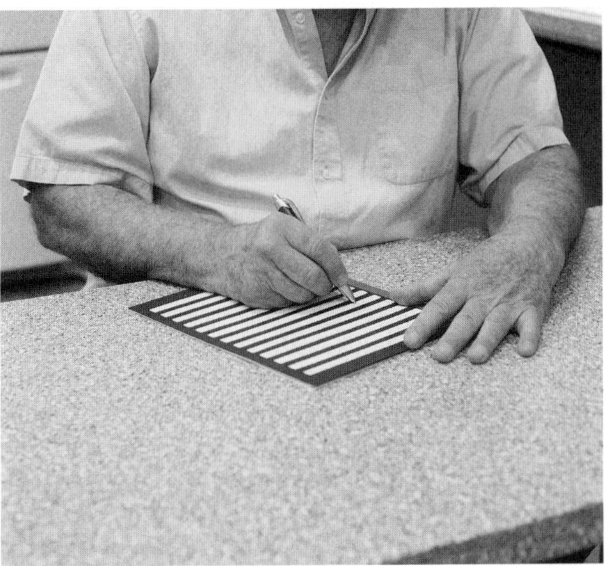

Figure 19.6 A guide for writing letters.

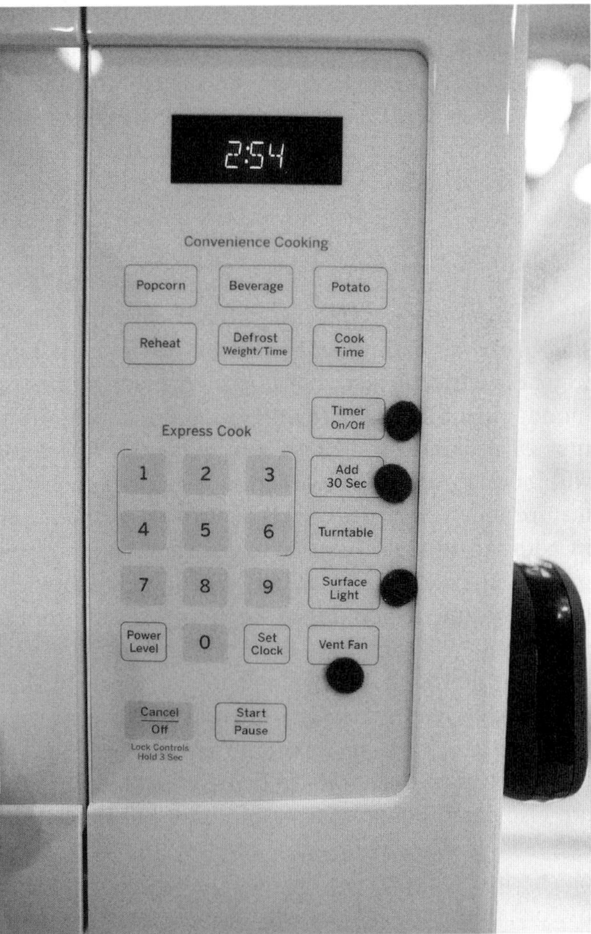

Figure 19.7 Raised dial markings on a household appliance.

and colors in order to provide further options. Similarly, safety pins can be used in a similar manner on clothing in order to distinguish colors that are similar to each other. A coding system can be developed in which the most commonly worn color receives no pins, the next color receives one pin, and so forth. The pins can be laundered and left on the piece of clothing permanently.

Raised dots are another way of providing tactile sensation as a way to gain information that is typically obtained by sight. Raised indicators, such as those already included on a keyboard to identify where hands placement should be on the home row, can be used as appliance markings, remote control cues, or on other items in which distinction between controls is needed. Raised dots can be homemade with fingernail polish or puff paint or they can be purchased commercially with a sticky back that can be applied to most surfaces. Refer to Figure 19.7 for an example of raised markings on a dial. It is important to note that when determining the ideal location for raised dots a temporary solution should be used before the intervention is made permanent so that changes can be made if necessary. Raised dots are available in bright contrasting colors so that the individual with visual impairment can use his or her remaining vision to see the raised marking; however, transparent raised markings are also available if the client desires the adaptation to be less evident to others.

A white cane is commonly used by individuals with visual impairment to assist with safe and independent functional mobility. The white cane can be viewed as an extension of tactile sensation and is a means of identifying objects, steps, or curbs in the path of travel, prior to coming into contact with them. While some individuals with visual impairment may not wish to identify as having a visual impairment by using a white cane for functional mobility, a white cane can alert others to the visual impairment, which can ease potential awkward encounters. There are several models of white canes available, ranging from the traditional long cane, to a folding white cane. There are hi-tech versions of the white cane available or being developed, such as those in which the cane itself is replaced with an ultrasonic light ray (Whittington 2013) or those with a built-in global positioning system (Young 2011). There are also shoes available that replace the white cane with vibration alerts (Coxworth 2011) and soon there may be eyeglasses built with cameras that will replace the white cane (Cockerton 2012).

The sense of hearing can also be used to gain information that is typically gathered through vision. There are several talking devices, such as talking watches, alarm clocks, color identifiers, tape measures, money identifiers, thermometers, and more. Most movies available on digital versatile disc (DVD) come with a descriptive video service that includes a voiceover feature which describes what is happening on the screen in addition to what the characters are saying and the other sounds of the movie. This version of the movie is typically found by looking in the special features of the main menu.

In addition to movies, many books are available in a text-to-speech format. The National Library Services provides free books on tape to those who are blind or visually impaired (Library of Congress n.d.), but there are also many other sources of audio books that are commercially available. These can be purchased online or checked out through the local library. They can be listened to through computers, tablet computers, smartphone applications, dedicated electronic reading devices, and DVD players, depending upon how the talking book was purchased.

Finally, in addition to talking devices, movies, and books, other technology can but used to provide an auditory signal rather than actual speech in order to alert an individual with visual impairment. For example, a boil alert is a simple metal disc that can be placed in a pot of water to be boiled. Once the water begins to boil the boil alert rattles, indicated that the water is indeed boiling. Similarly, a liquid level indicator can be placed on the rim of a cup to alert the user when to stop pouring liquid into the cup. Once the sensors (located on the inside of the cup) on the liquid level indicator detect the liquid, the device provides an auditory cue so that the pourer stops filling the cup.

Evidence for sensory substitution strategies

Researchers have not studied the use of sensory substitution strategies as a stand-alone intervention as extensively as optical and electronic magnification devices (Kaldenberg and Smallfield 2013). Sensory substitution strategies may be included as part of multicomponent intervention that includes other strategies such as magnification, but this is not clear in the current research literature. Therefore, while these types of TEIs are used extensively with individuals with visual impairment, more research needs to be conducted to determine the effectiveness of these technologies.

Environmental interventions

In addition to technology ranging from rubber bands to talking books, environmental modifications are an important component of the interventions provided to maximize the daily performance of individuals with visual impairment. These include organizational strategies and maximizing contrast between foreground and background.

Individuals with visual impairment may find it useful to organize their living environment. This allows them to use their memory to assist in locating items throughout their home. Consistently storing items in the same location allows the individual with visual impairment the ability to locate them easily without the need to visually search, thus enhancing overall function. A common example of this is having a small shelf or hook at the entry of the home on which to place keys upon entry. This allows the individual to easily locate the keys the next time he or she leaves the home. The same concept can be applied to utensils and food storage in the kitchen, clothing items in the closet and dresser drawers, toiletry items in the bathroom, and more. Reinforcement of this concept among others who live in the home is crucial to the success of organizational strategies.

Similar to consistent organization of items within the home, keeping the home environment free of clutter is also a useful strategy with visual impairment. Eliminating unneeded items from the living space reduces visual clutter, allowing an individual with visual impairment easier access to necessary items, and increases safety during functional mobility in the space. For example, rather than storing old newspapers or magazines, it may be useful to remove them so that they do not distract and make it more difficult to find the most recent issue.

The use of high contrast throughout the home is another environmental intervention that may be considered for those with visual impairment. Contrast enables an individual with vision loss to more easily distinguish between an item of interest and the background. For example, a dark wall color in the bathroom makes the white bathroom fixtures more easily noticeable. A white cutting board makes dark colored vegetables easier to identify. This same concept applies to solids and patterns. Replacing patterns in the living environment such as placemats, wallpaper, or carpeting with that of a solid color is another method of decreasing visual clutter which has the potential to increase the ease of performing daily living tasks. Boxes 19.4 through 19.7 provide additional TEI ideas for the performance of daily activities in the kitchen, bathroom, outdoor spaces, and with clothing management, respectively.

Evidence for organizational and contrast strategies

Similar to sensory substitution strategies, there is insufficient evidence to support the use of organizational strategies for older adults with low vision (Kaldenberg and Smallfield 2013). Therefore, this is an area in need of further research, because currently there is not enough literature to either support or refute this intervention approach. However, there is limited evidence to support the use of contrast strategies (Eperjesi et al. 2004) as an environmental intervention, but further research in this area is needed.

AT for computer access

Finally, because computers and other portable computerized devices are almost ubiquitous in today's society, it is worthwhile to discuss specific technologies that may be useful for an individual with visual impairment when

Box 19.5 Select visual TEIs in the bathroom

- High contrast can be helpful to distinguish foreground from background
    - Dark colored walls with white bathroom fixtures
    - Dark colored towels on white bathroom fixtures
    - Add contrast between tub/shower surround and any tub/shower chair
- Solid color towels are preferable over patterned ones to reduce visual clutter
- Grab bars around toilet and shower areas as a physical and tactile assist with functional mobility in these areas
- Drawer organizers can decrease clutter so that toiletry items can be easily located
- A rubber band can be placed around the conditioner bottle to distinguish it from the shampoo bottle
- A wall-mounted dispenser with clearly labeled sections can be used for shampoos, soaps, and conditioners; the contents of each section can be memorized
- Task lighting should be used
    - Lit mirror for makeup application (this can come with or without magnification)
    - Night lights for walking to the bathroom at night
    - Adequate lighting throughout the sink, toilet, and shower areas

Box 19.4 Select visual TEIs in the kitchen

- Different shaped plastic containers can assist in distinguishing food items. Further identify items by using tape to craft upper case letters on the top of container (e.g. V = vegetable soup)
    - Spaghetti sauce = square containers
    - Soup = round containers
- Use a barcode labeling system
    - Record a short message that is matched to a barcode, the message is played when the barcode is scanned
- Shapes and identifying features of canned products can be used to identify contents
    - Pull tops, rounded bottom edges
    - Sound of different food products when shaken
- Organize food products on different shelves
- Funnels of various sizes can be used when pouring liquids
- A cookie sheet can catch crumbs when wiping off countertops and tables
- Stemless wine glasses are useful for avoiding mishaps
- Oven mitts that cover the entire arm can increase safety over the stove or in the oven
- High-contrast placemats and cutting boards can be helpful to distinguish foreground from background
    - A solid dark placemat underneath a white plate
    - White mug for dark coffee
    - White cutting board for slicing dark colored vegetables
- Drawer organizers can decrease clutter so that utensils can be easily located
- Clean out leftovers from the refrigerator on a regular basis to avoid eating spoiled foods
- Rubber bands can be placed around food cans to aid in distinguishing one from another
- Large print labels made from laminated index cards can be attached to food items and then reused as a grocery list when the item needs to be purchased again
- Task lighting should be used in food preparation areas
    - Mounted under cabinets
    - Recessed lighting overhead placed in key locations
    - Task lamp
- High-contrast electrical tape and a bold permanent marker, nail polish, or raised dots can be used to simplify the microwave keypad, stovetop dials, and other kitchen control by highlighting only the most commonly used buttons
- An auditory or vibratory liquid level indicator can be used when filling glasses to avoid overflow
- A boil alert can be used in the bottom of a pot to provide an auditory cue that water is boiling and to prevent the water from boiling over
- Solid color towels, placemats, and napkins are preferable over patterned ones to decrease visual clutter

Box 19.6 Select visual TEIs for outdoor enjoyment

- High-contrast landscaping such as light flowers in front of dark green bushes provides easier enjoyment of the outdoors
- Scented plants can assist in identifying them
- A color identifier can be used to discover the color of flowers
- Landscape lighting or rope lighting can light paths or highlight destinations
- A rope trail is useful for walks, hiking, or as a path from one building to the next
- A radio can be used to assist with navigation back to the shore when swimming
- Global positioning systems with auditory directions can assist with navigation

Box 19.7 Select visual TEIs for clothing management

- Single-use detergent can be used to avoid pouring liquids or powders
- Clothes pins can be used as a tactile marking to distinguish similar colored items from each other. Pins can be placed on the inside of the tag. For example:
  - Black = no pin
  - Navy blue = 1 pin
  - Brown = 2 pins
- Sock clips can be used to join socks together after wearing so as to avoid the need to match socks after laundering
- No-wrinkle shirts and pants reduce the need to iron
- Outfits can be hung up together to avoid having to match shirt to pants

accessing computers. Refer to Active Learning Prompt 5 and consider for a moment how many computerized devices you use in a day. Now consider how you use your vision to assist in operating them. We use a visual display on a computer, tablet computer, or smartphone to consume information; we use our vision to see the keyboard or other input device to ensure that we are accurately telling the computer what we would like it to do. You can easily see how visual impairment makes accessing computerized technology more difficult. The purpose of this section of the chapter is to discuss hard and soft technologies that are designed to allow an individual with visual impairment increased access to computers and portable computerized technology.

Built-in accessibility features

Most computer operating systems now come with several accessibility features. In Active Learning Prompt 6 you located these features in the control panel and practiced adjusting the features which are particularly helpful for individuals with visual impairment. Two of these features include a text-to-speech function, which reads the text from the screen out loud, and a magnification function, which enlarges the images on the screen. The size and color of the mouse pointer on the screen can also typically be adjusted to best meet the user's needs, and the computer display can be set up in high contrast.

Adaptive computer technologies

In addition to the already existing accessibility features available in most computer operating systems, software packages can be added to maximize independence in computer use for those with visual impairment. Some of these include ZoomText Screen Magnifier/Reader by Ai Squared, Manchester Center, VT; JAWS Screen Reading Software by Freedom Scientific, St. Petersburg, FL; and Dragon NaturallySpeaking by Nuance Communications, Burlington, MA. While these software programs are available for purchase, there are free screen readers available through the Internet as well. NonVisual Desktop Access (NVDA; NV Access n.d.) is a free screen reader that can be used with a Microsoft Windows operating system. In addition to software applications, large keyboards with high contrast and other hardware is also available. It is important to note that Fok et al. (2011) found that adaptive computer technologies such as specialized software programs, as opposed to more normative devices such as large television screens and computer monitors, were among the most common AT devices that were abandoned by participants in their research.

Tablet computer applications

Finally, in addition to the software and hardware available for traditional desktop and laptop computers, there are a growing number of software applications available for tablet computer users who have visual impairment. These applications range from magnification applications to color identifiers, currency identifiers, talking calculators, and more. Refer to Table 19.5 for a select listing of applications which may be useful for those with visual impairment.

Summary

In sum, the number of individuals with visual impairment in the United States is expected to increase significantly due to the aging of the population. Diagnoses such as ARMD, diabetic retinopathy, glaucoma, cataract, and hemianopia are common in the older adult population and can have a profound effect on visual function. Because vision loss associated with these diagnoses is uncorrectable (except in the case of cataract removal),

TEIs can play a critical role in maximizing performance of daily occupations for those with vision loss.

The selection of TEI for an individual with visual impairment should be based upon a thorough assessment of personal skills and abilities, the desired occupations, and the environment in which those occupations are performed. AT selections should be made based upon the specific occupation(s) that the client needs or wants to perform. Therefore, the intervention plan for each client will be very unique as the therapist collaborates with the client to identify the TEI that will be the best fit for the client when taking all factors of the Human-Tech Ladder into account. It is important to remember that a comprehensive intervention plan for a client with visual impairment will include multiple pieces of technology and environmental strategies.

There is a wide range of potential TEIs that can be useful for those with visual impairment. Many daily occupations involve a reading component. Therefore, TEIs that enhance reading and viewing are typically prescribed for those with vision loss. While electronic magnification is particularly useful for improving reading performance, optical magnification is also a common option to assist in the performance of occupations that involve reading. For those with peripheral field deficits, prisms may be a useful way to expand the field of view and improve functional mobility both in the home and in the community.

Along with magnification and other optical aids to support the reading necessary for daily occupations, there are a number of other TEIs that can support individuals with visual impairment. There are many commercially available talking devices that substitute the typical visual display with auditory output. Similarly, many TEIs use tactile sensation to augment reduced visual skills. Environmental strategies such as adequate illumination, high contrast, decreased clutter, and increased organization all serve as additional ways of maximizing independence in the performance of daily occupations. Finally, there are a growing number of computer applications available to make accessing computers and other mobile computerized devices even more possible than it has been in the past.

While several TEIs were discussed in this chapter, it is impossible to cover them all due to the number of devices available and the number of new devices and applications that have come on the market even since this chapter was written. Because each client's environment is so unique, the potential intervention options are truly endless. It is important to note that the soft technology, or the training associated with all of these devices, is critical to their success and decreases the risk that the device will be abandoned. In fact, the true success of any piece of AT or environmental adaptation comes when the client integrates it into his or her daily routine so that it is no longer considered a piece of technology, but rather, a way of life.

Acknowledgments

The author would like to acknowledge Betsy Haag and Gayl Yarnell for their contributions to the content in the tables and boxes in this chapter.

References

Academy for Certification of Vision Rehabilitation & Education Professionals (n.d.-a). Certified low vision therapist scope of practice. Retrieved from https://www.acvrep.org/certifications/clvt-scope.

Academy for Certification of Vision Rehabilitation & Education Professionals (n.d.-b). Certified orientation and mobility specialist scope of practice. Retrieved from https://www.acvrep.org/certifications/coms-scope.

Academy for Certification of Vision Rehabilitation & Education Professionals (n.d.-c). Certified vision rehabilitation therapist scope of practice. Retrieved from https://www.acvrep.org/certifications/cvrt-scope.

American Occupational Therapy Association (2014). Occupational therapy practice framework: Domain and process. *American Journal of Occupational Therapy* 68 (Suppl. 1): S1–S48. http://dx.doi.org/10.5014/ajot.2014.682006.

American Optometric Association Federal Relations Committee (1999). *Bulletin 26: Low Vision Services Under Medicare*. Washington, DC: Author.

Baldasare, J., Watson, G., Whittaker, S., and Miller-Shaffer, H. (1986). The development and evaluation of a reading test for low vision individuals with macular loss. *Journal of Visual Impairment and Blindness* 80: 785–789.

Berger, S., McAteer, J., Schreier, K., and Kaldenberg, J. (2013). Occupational therapy interventions to improve leisure and social participation for older adults with low visions: a systematic review. *American Journal of Occupational Therapy* 67: 303–311. https://doi.org/10.5014/ajot.2013.005447.

Bowers, A.R., Meek, C., and Stewart, N. (2001). Illumination and reading performance in age-related macular degeneration. *Clinical and Experimental Optometry* 84: 139–147. 10.111/j.1444-0938.2001.tb04957.x.

Bowers, A.R., Keeney, K., and Peli, E. (2008). Community-based trial of a peripheral prism visual field expansion device for hemianopia. *Archives of Ophthalmology* 126 (5): 657–664.

Brilliant, R. (1999). Driving with a bioptic telescope: concepts and techniques. Retrieved from https://ocutech.com/driving-with-a-bioptic-telescope-concepts-and-techniques/.

Cockerton, P. (2012). Guide glasses for the blind: new hi-tech specs could replace white canes and dogs. *Mirror* (22 November). Retrieved from www.mirror.co.uk/news/technology-science/science/hi-tech-specs-developed-by-oxford-university-1450827.

Congdon, N., O'Colmain, B., Klaver, C.C. et al. (2004). Causes and prevalence of visual impairment among adults in the United States. *Archives of Ophthalmology* 122: 477–485. https://doi.org/10.1001/archopht.122.4.477.

Coxworth, B. (2011). Haptic shoe could replace the white cane. *New Atlas* (17 October). Retrieved from http://www.gizmag.com/le-chal-haptic-shoe-for-blind/20186.

Culham, L.E., Chabra, A., and Rubin, F.S. (2004). Clinical performance of electronic, head-mounted, low-vision devices. *Ophthalmic and Physiological Optics* 24: 281–290.

Dunn, W., Brown, C., and McGuigan, A. (1994). The Ecology of Human Performance: a framework for considering the effect of context. *American Journal of Occupational Therapy* 48: 595–607.

Eldred, K.B. (1992). Optimal illumination for reading in patients with age-related maculopathy. *Optometry and Vision Science* 69: 46–50. https://doi.org/10.1097/00006324-199201000-00007.

Eperjesi, F., Fowler, C.W., and Evans, B.J. (2004). The effects of coloured light filter overlays on reading rates in age-related macular degeneration. *Acta Ophthalmologica Scandinavica* 82: 695–700. https://doi.org/10.1111/j.1600-0420.2004.00371.x.

Eperjesi, F., Maiz-Fernandez, C., and Bartlett, H.E. (2007). Reading performance with various lamps in age-related macular degeneration. *Ophthalmic and Physiological Optics* 27: 93–99.

Eschenbach Optik (n.d.). Absorptive filters and protective eyewear. Retrieved from https://www.eschenbach.com/products/absorptive-filters.asp.

Figueiro, M.G. (2001). *Lighting the Way: A Key to Independence*. Troy, NY: Lighting Research Center.

Fok, D., Polgar, J., Shaw, L., and Jutai, J. (2011). Low vision assistive technology device usage and importance in daily occupations. *Work* 39: 37–58.

Goodrich, G.L. and Kirby, J. (2001). A comparison of patient reading performance and preference: optical devices, handheld CCTV (Innoventions Magni-Cam), or stand-mounted CCTV (Optelec Clearview or TSI Genie). *Optometry* 72: 519–528.

Haymes, S.A. and Lee, J. (2006). Effects of task lighting on visual function in age-related macular degeneration. *Ophthalmic and Physiological Optics* 26: 169–179. https://doi.org/10.1111/j.1475-1313.2006.00367.x.

Hemianopia.org (n.d.). How prisms work. Retrieved from http://www.hemianopia.org/index_files/Howprismswork.htm.

International Council of Ophthalmology (2002). Visual standards: aspects and ranges of vision loss with emphasis on population surveys. Retrieved from http://www.icoph.org/downloads/visualstandardsreport.pdf.

Kaldenberg, J. and Smallfield, S. (2013). *Occupational Therapy Practice Guidelines for Older Adults with Low Vision*. Bethesda, MD: AOTA Press.

Law, M., Cooper, B., Strong, S. et al. (1996). The Person-Environment-Occupation Model: a transactive approach to occupational performance. *Canadian Journal of Occupational Therapy* 63: 9–23.

Law, M., Baptiste, S., Carswell, A. et al. (2005). *Canadian Occupational Performance Measure Manual*, 4e. Ottawa, Canada: CAOT Publications.

Library of Congress (n.d.). That all may read…: National Library Service for the Blind and Physically Handicapped (NLS). Retrieved from https://www.loc.gov/programs/national-library-service-for-the-blind-and-physically-handicapped/about-this-service/.

Lighthouse International (n.d.-a). Social Security Administration: definition of legal blindness. Retrieved from http://li129-107.members.linode.com/about-low-vision-blindness/definition-legal-blindness/.

Lighthouse International (n.d.-b).What is hemianopia? Retrieved from http://li129-107.members.linode.com/about-low-vision-blindness/vision-disorders/hemianopia/.

Lighthouse International (n.d.-c).What is low vision? Retrieved from http://li129-107.members.linode.com/about-low-vision-blindness/all-about-low-vision/.

Mansfield, J.S., Legge, G.E., Luebker, A., and Cunningham, K. (1994). *MNRead Acuity Charts: Continuous-Text Reading-Acuity Charts for Normal and Low Vision*. Long Island City, NY: Lighthouse Low Vision Products.

Mennemen, T.A., Warren, M., and Yuen, H.K. (2012). Preliminary validation of a vision-dependent activities of daily living instrument on adults with homonymous hemianopsia. *American Journal of Occupational Therapy* 66: 478–482.

National Eye Institute (2018). Facts about age-related macular degeneration. Retrieved from http://www.nei.nih.gov/health/maculardegen/armd_facts.asp.

National Eye Institute (2015a). Facts about cataract. Retrieved from http://www.nei.nih.gov/health/cataract/cataract_facts.asp.

National Eye Institute (2015b). Facts about diabetic eye disease. Retrieved from http://www.nei.nih.gov/health/diabetic/retinopathy.asp.

National Eye Institute (2015c). Facts about glaucoma. Retrieved from http://www.nei.nih.gov/health/glaucoma/glaucoma_facts.asp.

NV Access (n.d.). About NVDA. Retrieved from https://www.nvaccess.org/about-nvda/.

Patel, P.J., Chen, F.K., Da Cruz, L. et al. (2011). Test-retest variability of reading performance metrics using MNREAD in patients with age-related macular degeneration. *Investigative Ophthalmology and Visual Science* 52: 3854–3859. https://doi.org/10.1167/iovs.10-6601.

Prochaska, J.O. and Velicer, W.F. (1997). The Transtheoretical Model of Health Behavior Change. *American Journal of Health Promotion* 12 (1): 38–48. https://doi.org/10.4278/0890-1171-12.1.38.

Rebovich, A. and Zevoda, E. (2013). Clinical utility of the COPM in assessing older adults with vision loss. *Gerontology Special Interest Section Quarterly* 36 (3): 1–4.

Russell-Minda, E., Jutai, J.W., Strong, G. et al. (2007). The legibility of typefaces for readers with low vision: a research review. *Journal of Visual Impairment and Blindness* 101: 402–415.

Seidel, A. (2003). Rehabilitative frame of reference. In: *Willard & Spackman's Occupational Therapy*, 10e (ed. E.B. Crepeau, E.S. Cohn and B.A. Boyt Schell), 238–240. Philadelphia, PA: Lippincott Williams, & Wilkins.

Smallfield, S., Clem, K., and Myers, A. (2013). Occupational therapy interventions to improve the reading ability of older adults with low vision: a systematic review. *American Journal of Occupational Therapy* 67: 288–295. https://doi.org/10.5014/ajot.2013.004929.

Stuen, C. and Faye, E. (2003). Vision loss: normal and not normal changes among older adults. *Generations* 27: 8–14.

Subramanian, A. and Pardhan, S. (2006). The repeatability of MNREAD Acuity Charts and variability at different test distances. *Optometry and Vision Science* 83: 572–576. https://doi.org/10.1097/01.opx.0000232225.00311.53.

Titcomb, R.E., Okoye, R., and Schiff, S. (1997). Introduction to the dynamic process of vision. In: *Functional Visual Behavior: A Therapist's Guide to Evaluation and Treatment Options* (ed. M. Gentile), 3–54. Bethesda, MD: American Occupational Therapy Association.

Triple Tree (2011). Innovation & the health care needs of seniors. Retrieved from https://www.triple-tree.com/strategic-insights/2011/october/innovation-the-health-care-needs-of-seniors/.

Varma, R., Vajaranant, T., Burkemper, B. et al. (2016). Visual impairment and blindness in adults in the United States: demographic and geographic variations from 2015 to 2050. *JAMA Ophthalmology* 134 (7): 802–809.

Vicente, K. (2006). *The Human Factor: Revolutionizing the Way People Live with Technology*. New York: Routledge, Taylor & Francis Group.

Warren, M. (1995). Nationally speaking: including occupational therapy in low vision rehabilitation. *American Journal of Occupational Therapy* 49: 857–860.

Warren, M. (1998). *Brain Injury Visual Assessment Battery for Adults*. Lenexa, KS: visABILITIES Rehab Services.

Watson, G., Baldasare, J., and Whittaker, S. (1990). Validity and clinical uses of the Pepper Visual Skills for Reading Test. *Journal of Visual Impairment and Blindness* 84: 119–123.

Watson, G.R., Whittaker, S., and Steciw, M. (1995). *The Pepper Visual Skills for Reading Test*, 2e. Lilburn, GA: Bear Consultants.

World Health Organization (2010). Visual impairment and blindness 2010. Retrieved from http://www.who.int/blindness/data_maps/VIFACTSHEETGLODAT2010full.pdf.

World Health Organization (2018). Blindness and vision impairment. Retrieved from https://www.who.int/news-room/fact-sheets/detail/blindness-and-visual-impairment.

Yanko Design. (2013). Eyestick: blind stick with eyes. Retrieved from https://www.yankodesign.com/?s=eyestick.

Young, M. (2011). Xun Ye's Origin GPS helps the visually impaired get to their destination. Trend Hunter (28 June) Retrieved from https://www.trendhunter.com/trends/origin-gps.

Additional resources

Kaldenberg, J. and Smallfield, S. (2013). *Occupational Therapy Practice Guidelines for Older Adults with Low Vision*. Bethesda, MD: AOTA Press.

Berger, S. (ed.) (2013). Special issue on effectiveness of occupational therapy interventions for older adults with low vision. *American Journal of Occupational Therapy* 67 (3): 263–265.

20

Technology and environmental interventions to promote community mobility

David Joseph Feathers

Outline

Learning outcomes

After reading this chapter, you should be able to:

1. Outline the human–environment interactions that are present for community participation.
2. Describe the Skills, Rules, and Knowledge (SRK) framework (Rasmussen 1983) within the context of technology and environmental interventions.
3. Understand the barriers faced by diverse individuals as they move around the community through a research study on community accessibility.
4. Address barriers to community mobility through inclusive ergonomic design.

Active learning prompts

Before you read this chapter:

1. Look up definitions of:
   a. Ergonomic design; Skills, Rules, and Knowledge (SRK) framework; inclusive design;
   b. Accessible transportation.
2. Investigate some paratransit options in your area.

Assistive Technologies and Environmental Interventions in Healthcare: An Integrated Approach, First Edition.
Edited by Lynn Gitlow and Kathleen Flecky.

Companion website: www.wiley.com/go/gitlow/assitivetechnologies

Key terms

Community mobility
Skills, Rules, and Knowledge (SRK) framework
Community accessibility
Micro-environmental interactions
Meso-environmental interactions
Macro-environmental interactions
Inclusive ergonomic design

Introduction

The World Health Organization (WHO) International Classification of Functioning, Disability and Health (ICF) model, discussed in Chapter 2 of this book, offers a systems view of disability: it is ever-present, it exists in a continuum throughout one's life, and it can be mitigated or reduced by appropriate technology and environmental design interventions. In the United States, there are millions of adults who face one or more substantial physical barriers to getting around in their community. As a result, many persons who face mobility barriers either curtail the frequency and duration of trips outside their home, maintaining a routine that includes only the essentials. Some individuals remain in the home and utilize delivery services, which can bring them food, clothing, entertainment, and so forth. Others depend on caregivers for support, and connectivity to the community is a shared experience for the individual and caregiver(s).

This chapter outlines inclusive ergonomic design approaches and gives examples using community-based case study research data to assess and address physical mobility issues in community-dwelling adults. It will attempt to link human factors systems thinking, accessible and inclusive design, and human performance requirements germane to mobility and accessibility issues within the community. There are four parts to this chapter: Part I, entitled "Accessibility and the Human–Environment Interactions of Community Participation," discusses the range of scales of accessibility, from small things like features of a door, to large things such as a downtown area of a city. Part II, entitled "Inclusive Designing and the SRK Model," discusses Rasmussen's Skills, Rules, and Knowledge (SRK) model as it applies to physical access and accessibility within and around the community. Part III, "Profiles from the Community," showcases three individuals and offers some context to community-based issues. Finally, Part IV, "Evidenced-based Design and Research for Community Participation," discusses current research and future directions of research and design for community-based mobility. Community involvement is a complex topic and this chapter only addresses a small fraction of all considerations for accessibility and inclusive design. Throughout the chapter you will see different levels of Vicente's (2006) Human-Tech Ladder represented, which addresses this complexity. For example, in the first part, "Political" and "Social" considerations that influence community participation are presented.

Part I: Accessibility and the human–environment interactions of community participation

An accessible community can create new opportunities for social inclusion, address healthcare disparities, promote well-being, and provide equal opportunities for attaining employment, remaining employed, and advancing in a career. The human–environment interactions of community participation should include multiple considerations, such as:

- accessible transportation modalities
- accessible domestic environments
- destination facilities that support access.

Additionally, there must be ways to address how to aggregate accessibility for each domain, coordinating all domains to support individual assessment and decisions, which enable planning routes, engaging in public events, and participating in the community. Accessibility must address all aspects of this human–environment interaction to ensure basic levels of inclusive community participation.

Transportation

Accessibility research has investigated and provided an evidence base for designs of the built environment and products we use every day (e.g. Steinfeld et al. 1979). This evidence base informs accessible design of many important features of human–environment interactions. For example, Title II of the Americans with Disabilities Act (ADA) establishes accessibility standards for vehicles used for public transportation, and calls for alternative means of transportation (e.g. paratransit) to supplement fixed transportation routes if the existing system cannot be made accessible (Americans with Disabilities Act 1990). These alternative means of transportation should be comparable to the existing route system, and many local transportation agencies have made their existing system accessible (NCD 2005) or have grown their paratransit systems to accommodate an ever-growing population of riders (NCD 2007). Despite a growing

Box 20.1 Here's the evidence

Layton, N. (2012). Barriers and facilitators to community mobility for assistive technology users. *Rehabilitation Research and Practice*. 2012 (Art No.: 454195). Retrieved from https://www.hindawi.com/journals/rerp/2012/454195.

Key Words: assistive technology (AT), environmental interventions, community mobility, disability

Purpose: To investigate the impact of AT solutions used to engage in community mobility upon the lives of adults with a disability.

Sample/Setting: A sample 100 users of assistive technology devices, from the population of those 18 years and over with disabilities in Victoria, Australia. They were recruited using advertisements and snowball sampling methods.

Method: Survey.

Findings: While participants use a variety of AT, environmental interventions, and personal care, a range of barriers and enablers to community mobility were identified. These include access to AT devices, environmental interventions, public transport, and inclusive community environments. Substantial levels of unmet need result in limited personal mobility and community participation.

Critical Thinking Questions:

1. After reading this research article, what do you understand to be the limitations of this research? Are there any limitations not stated?
2. If you were to replicate this study using a different method or design, what designs would you use to increase the rigor and why?
3. Based on the findings of this study, what additional research is needed that is not addressed in the discussion section?

number of accessible transportation systems, many barriers to community participation, employment, enjoyment, independence, and interdependence still exist (Box 20.1).

According to the National Council on Disability report (2007), a lack of accessible and affordable transportation is a major barrier to employment for many people with disabilities (NCD 2007). The ADA addresses issues of discrimination and accessibility in public transit, and these are an important part of the picture but not the complete picture; connecting the nodes (connecting location to location) is key: "elimination of these barriers will enhance the labor pool available to employers and increase employment opportunities for people with disabilities" (NCD 2007, p. 45).

Community access

Designing for community access and participation presents challenges on many scales. Three scales of community interaction are outlined below, and each represents unique opportunities for technology and environmental design interventions. Micro-environmental interactions are those involving specific human–object interactions (e.g. opening a door with a doorknob versus a handle); meso-environmental interactions involve human and near-environment interactions (e.g. moving across a room to operate a light switch); and macro-environmental interactions constitute larger, aggregated, and more complex interactions (e.g. getting across a downtown area to meet a friend at a coffee shop) (e.g. Saarinen 1976).

Each level (micro, meso, and macro) can receive design attention, but it is difficult to prioritize interventions, allocate limited resources effectively, and determine the impact of interventions across scale. Iterative technology and environmental design improvements should be led by evidence, and existing models can assist in this process. These levels (micro, meso, and macro) will be discussed in relationship to inclusive design and community participation in the upcoming sections.

For most individuals in the United States, the personal car is the primary means to access community resources and employment. This means of transportation has a strong cultural identity and preference, despite alternative transportation infrastructure being available. The personal car is an example of a micro-environmental interaction, and many available options can be considered in order to make this environment accessible. In the United States, the National Highway Traffic Safety Administration (NHTSA) is the federal entity with "the authority to regulate the manufacture of automotive adaptive equipment and modified vehicles used by persons with disabilities" (NHTSA n.d.). Berkowitz et al. (1998) reported the average cost of personal vehicle modification was \$6497 (>\$9500 in 2014 dollars), which is cost prohibitive for many people, but costs may be covered or partially subsidized by insurance programs, rehabilitation services, federal programs, and foundations. For persons who cannot afford these costs, a reliable and accessible transportation structure must be utilized, which may be an affront to an individual's strong cultural leaning toward the independence provided by personal automobile transportation.

Part II: Inclusive designing and the SRK model

Rasmussen's SRK framework was created to understand human decision-making performance and information processing within complex human–machine systems (Rasmussen 1983). It can be applied to situations where an individual or a group of individuals need to perform daily tasks that involve a series of decisions and actions, such as getting to work using public transportation. It can be applied to almost any circumstance where decision-making behaviors can be evaluated, and can prove to be a powerful systematic framework to evaluate and compare existing designs and new designs. The work of Kim Vicente (whose road map was used to structure this book), along with that of Rasmussen, has evaluated human performance, error, and support of design solutions for interface designs of complex systems, such as nuclear power plant operations, where information needs to be timely, appropriately salient, and robust against misinterpretation (e.g. Vicente and Rasmussen 1992). Recently, the SRK framework has been used to guide evidence-based improvements for inclusive design of products (e.g. McAdams and Kostovich 2011). In this context, inclusive design considers the individual's capacities as they perform tasks, such as traveling from one part of the community to another.

In this chapter, the SRK framework is considered within the context of inclusive design. Three case studies from a research study provide unique examples of community mobility, getting to the grocery store. These case studies exemplify how the framework can systematically describe how individuals use the existing transportation system. Themes from these case studies are presented to showcase opportunities for improvements in technology designs, environmental designs, how individuals use these designs, and how to organize and present information needed for wayfinding and other supports for community interaction.

The SRK framework can be applied on all three scales of community interaction: micro-environmental, meso-environmental, and macro-environmental. Figure 20.1 is an outline of the framework, where each box on the left-hand side represents a decision, and each box on the right-hand side represents a discrete and actionable step toward executing a human response. It starts with the human receiving information (input). If there is a direct connection between what the individual thinks she or he is receiving and what she or he needs to do, then a response is executed. An example of a direct connection can be getting to work without having to read a map or ask for directions. If there is not a direct connection, then the individual will need to refer to rules (e.g. a map)

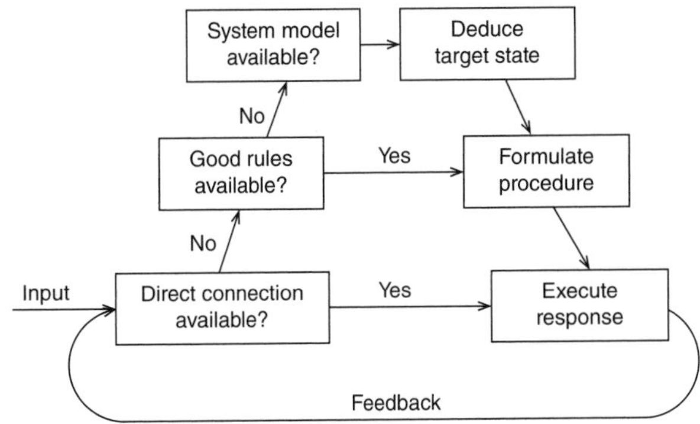

Figure 20.1 The Skills, Rules, and Knowledge (SRK) framework, with decision variables, and feedback loop.

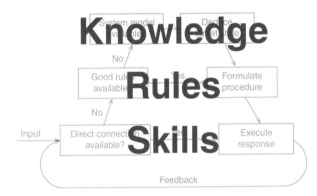

Figure 20.2 The Skills, rules, and knowledge (SRK) "levels."

or seek an understanding of a system model (e.g. ask for directions). If a person does not have a direct connection, or any good rules, or does not know how to create a system model, they may risk committing an inappropriate action or error. In the case of community mobility, errors may be wrong turns, getting lost, or perhaps boarding the wrong bus. These errors will likely cause delays and frustration, and may make the individual vulnerable in a variety of ways.

The SRK model allows for an understanding of what a person knows, how they behave in relationship to design interventions, and how they may react to unique or novel situations. For designers, an ideal design should promote skills-based actions, support the operator if rules are needed, and provide a systems model that ultimately leads to timely and appropriate responses. Figure 20.2 is an overlay of SRK "levels" atop a grayed-out Figure 20.1.

If the individual is operating at a skills-based level for a specific task, their actions are quick, seemingly automatic, and do not require additional information. However, if there are no direct connections apparent, then rules must be communicated and interpreted, and a procedure must be formulated to execute a response. If there are no good rules, or if the rules are not readily

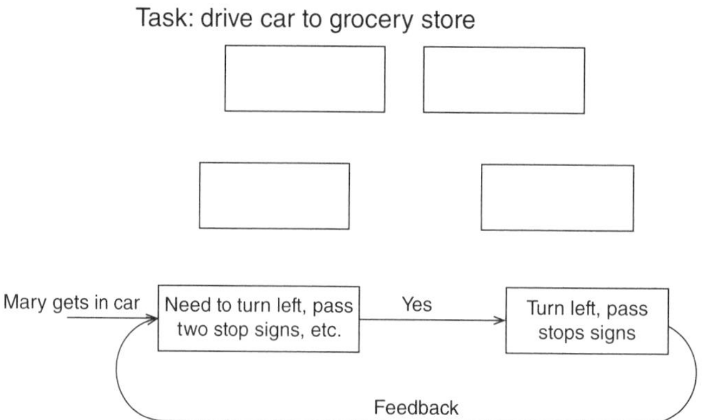

Figure 20.3 Skills-based behavior: Getting to the grocery store that Mary is familiar with.

interpreted as actionable, an operator must try to understand the system, deduce a target state, formulate a procedure, and ultimately execute a response. Feedback is given to the operator, which may help to establish rules, ultimately leading to a direct connection to facilitate a timely response. Many examples of this framework have been given, from power plant operators, to using a power window in a car (e.g. Vicente and Rasmussen 1988; Blackler et al. 2003; Gaunet and Briffault 2005). This framework is robust and can allow for analysis of micro-scale tasks, such as using a can opener, to macro-scale interactions, such as using a paratransit system. The SRK framework is flexible enough to allow for analysis of multiple individuals and can track improvements in performance by assessing whether an individual is operating at a "rules-based" level at the beginning and masters the task to operate at a "skills-based" level after a period of time. Since the framework has a feedback loop, it can serve to analyze processes from those with a few steps to those with many steps.

A macro-environmental example of the SRK framework within the context of community mobility is presented next, and demonstrates how this framework can offer guidance to human decision-making performance and facilitate a framework for supportive designs. Mary is familiar with where her local grocery store is in her town. If she were to use a car from her home, she would have to turn left, make a right after two stop signs, travel 2 miles, then turn left at the forth traffic light into the store parking lot. She is operating on a *skills-based* level (see Figure 20.3). There are direct connections available and salient cues within the environment prompt her timely responses. These actions are quick, and seem to happen without thought or effort. However, this was not always the case, as she needed to learn this way before she moved to town.

Additional information was once needed to develop her skills-based behavior; rules and a systems model were given to her in a variety of ways so that she could get to the skills-based level. When she first moved to town, she was told that the grocery store was down the hill and at the southern edge of town. This helped her build a system model of where this store is in relationship to her workplace and her home. This also provided some general rules, e.g. "if you are going to the grocery store, you need to make a left out of the driveway. Then make a right after two stop signs …" This helped her to establish further rules and refine her system model so that she could get to the store, not efficiently in the beginning, but successfully. As she learned more about the town, and where the grocery store is in relationship with other stores, parks, and other features, her system model and rules about where the store is within the context of the town was also expanding and becoming more robust.

When visitors ask her where the grocery store is, she offers rules in the form of directions, usually with the help of a map, since she has forgotten the name of each road she needs to drive on, although she travels it regularly! (See Figure 20.4.) She will also offer basic information to help build a system model (down the hill, southern edge of town), as described in Figure 20.5. They will likely get to the grocery store, but perhaps not as efficiently as someone who is experienced. Depending on the quality and robustness of the rules and system model, the visitors can be adaptable if there is a road closure, or some other disruption preventing them from getting to the store. If she offered only skills-based or rules-based directions (make left after two stop signs, etc.) they would not have the flexibility to adapt to changing conditions and it would be difficult to retrieve any errors (say, miscounted number of stop signs). For this example, while it is desirable to operate on a skills-based level, it can lead to inflexibility or errors if there are disruptions (e.g. time pressure, missed or misinterpreted cues, road closures representing a change in the system).

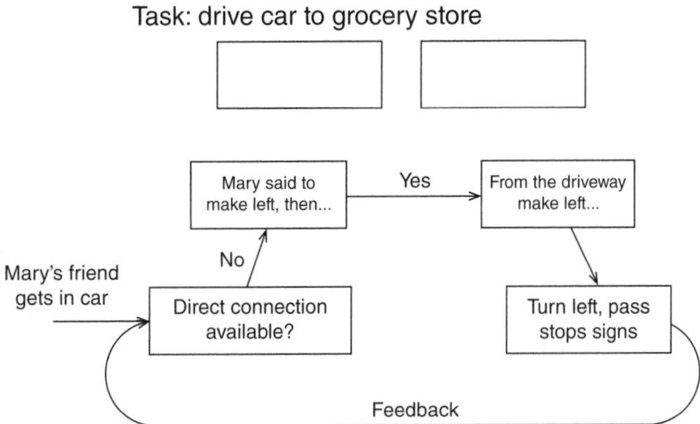

Figure 20.4 Rules-based behavior: Mary's friend is going to the grocery store following turn-by-turn directions from Mary.

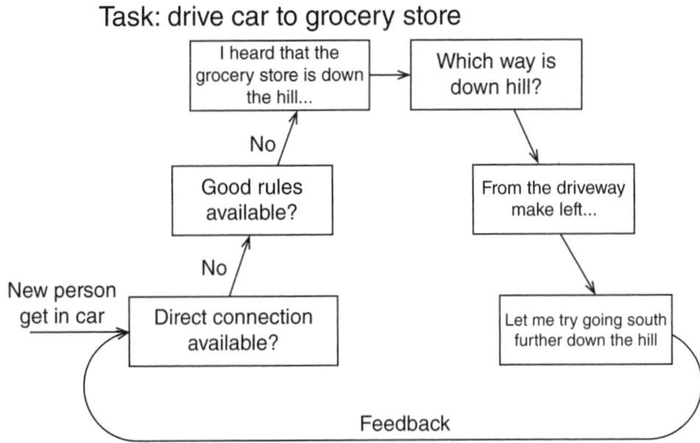

Figure 20.5 Knowledge-based behavior: getting to the grocery store for a new person to the area.

Individuals performing *simple* tasks should be operating at a skills-based level. They should not have to be looking for rules or attempting to construct a systems model in order to understand how to perform a task. For increasingly complex and novel situations, or for tasks that require additional resources, rules can and should be made available to allow for procedures to be followed. Once the procedure is established, appropriate responses can be executed. Eventually, skills-based behavior is fostered, rules can be recalled easily if a method of communicating these is designed well, and knowledge base can be reinforced through experience. These are all important attributes for successful performance and should be part of any designed system that intends to promote community mobility (see Toolbox).

Part III: Profiles from the community

Three case studies involving bus and paratransit use are presented below. These case studies were a part of a research project on universal design and accessible transportation conducted at Cornell University for a local transportation network. Selected individual responses are highlighted below, each represents a unique set of considerations, which are evaluated using the SRK framework. Solutions and ideas for each individual are presented, but constitute only one way to solve each respective issue; more appropriate and elegant solutions may be instituted. These cases highlight the systematic use of the SRK framework to design for greater community mobility. See Boxes 20.2–20.4.

Creating solutions through SRK assessment

Eddy is a tech-savvy person, and creating accessible solutions to address his goals in greater community involvement can have many options. Using the SRK framework, designs can be tested out as he uses a website (for example). As he talks though what are positive and negative features of one or more accessible transportation websites, a researcher can get a sense of how he requests information to be presented, and how to create new or search for existing websites or mobile applications that deliver the information that suits his needs. Designers and researchers can add the needs of other riders who will have varied needs such as high-contrast options or supplemental auditory displays for persons requiring visual or auditory support.

Creating solutions through SRK assessment

Sam is an expert at transportation systems, and her knowledge is needed to inform new, innovative design solutions (see Box 20.3). The SRK model can be used to guide solutions, test prospective design interventions, and allow consumers to compare competing designs. One of Sam's complaints concerned wait times for pickup and drop-off. The SRK framework can be used to assess gaps in understanding between route demands and passenger delivery, which is important for managers of these transportation networks as they gauge improvements. For example, new design solutions based on SRK analysis, such as a mobile device application that informs the

Box 20.2 Community mobility case study 1: Using technology to develop a mental map of accessible transportation

Eddy is a manual wheelchair user who has to get to work using accessible public transportation. When he first moved to town, he relied on paratransit to pick him up from his home, drive him to work, and return him home at night. He considered paratransit to be stigmatizing and was tired of waiting for over an hour to be either picked up or dropped off. He desired to use public transportation, which offered a regular schedule, and overheard a conversation at work about how the new bus system in his town had 100% accessible buses. He asked his coworkers if they knew where the buses ran, which was his first attempt to establish a systems model, building his "knowledge" level to then deduce target state by understanding what rules are available, formulate a procedure, and then execute a response. On his lunch break, he attempted to look up the route map posted on the transit system website (see Figure 20.6). He has used public transportation route maps before when he used to live in another city, and considers himself knowledgeable in map reading and way-finding using maps. He preferred first looking at the entire transit system map to assess area coverage, and to build a systems model based on route complexity, number of stops from his house to work, whether or not there are multiple bus routes connecting home to work, which could increase flexibility of pickup and drop-off times, and more. By performing these steps, Eddy is continuing to establish a knowledge base

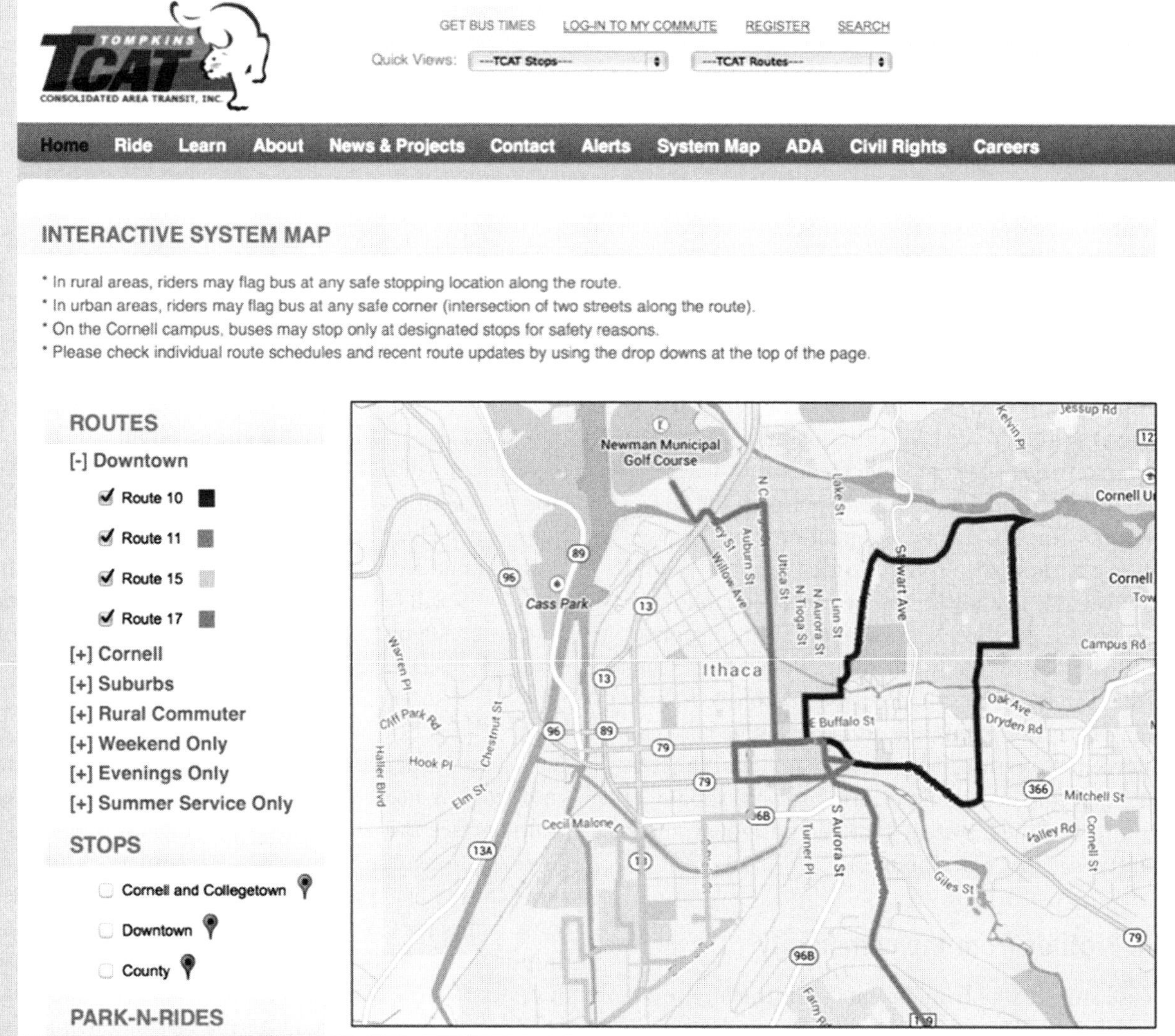

Figure 20.6 Overview map of transportation in Eddy's town to help build a systems model. Source: http://www.tcatbus.com/pages/system.

and making some assumptions regarding rules (e.g. multiple routes on major roads increase redundancy and therefore frequency of potential bus pickups).

Eddy builds his understanding of the system using the transit system map because this is his preferred mode of learning. The bus transportation website shows many potential solutions, there are many different ways to access the transit system information, and it is this type of flexibility that is central to inclusive environments and ergonomic design. Bus route maps can show all routes in the system, or selected routes, based on menu options. Other methods are also available: drop-down menus (showing all stops on a route) and fill-in boxes in which users can type an origin and destination. For visitors, some prefer not to build a systems model by looking at the route map; rather, they will prefer to fill in their origin and destination (skills-based level), which is available in the "Quick Views" sections located at the top of the web page. This reduces the cognitive load, but increases inflexibility, as it offers no additional information. Eddy, however, can use the fill-in boxes if he needs to go somewhere new, and he can do this with confidence as he has been developing a well-formed systems model to offer him flexibility if an unexpected event disrupts his journey.

Box 20.3 Community mobility case study 2: Developing a robust systems model of accessible transportation

Sam has been using paratransit for over 30 years and has been around to see the program grow and services improve over time. In relationship to the SRK model, she has a well-formed knowledge base and knows many rules of the paratransit system, which can give her abilities to adapt and respond to unique or novel situations. Sam has cerebral palsy, uses a power wheelchair, and is ADA eligible, meaning she can ride accessible transportation at a reduced rate or free (depending on the route), and make expedited route requests. She uses the transportation system regularly for most of the year: every day during the winter and twice a week during the summer. In the winter, Sam depends on paratransit for transportation from her home to work, and during warmer months she uses her power chair to travel the same 10 blocks.

If Sam were to use the regular bus system instead of the paratransit system, she would need to travel multiple blocks to the nearest bus stop, board a mainstream accessible bus, and travel nearly an entire bus route to eventually be dropped off at a central plaza, which is about two blocks from her office. While this option is a possibility, the process is time-consuming and difficult, and paratransit's vehicles are an excellent alternative for Sam.

While Sam does note possible improvements that paratransit might consider, she emphasizes the success of the program, especially when compared to other cities throughout the state. Sam notes that in many other cities, conversations about paratransit are not aimed at improving a system, but instead defending its existence. Sam explains that because the county she lives in has such a good paratransit infrastructure, community members are able to go beyond defending its existence, and aim to advance conversations about system-level issues such as travel and safety training, customer service training, eligibility requirements, and demand management.

Sam's complaints about paratransit focus on scheduling. As an ADA eligible person, she has the advantage of a 24-hour ride request, as opposed to the normal paratransit minimum of two business days' advance notice. However, she is subject to paratransit's policy allowing for an hour pickup window before a rider's scheduled appointment. This means that a rider with a 10 a.m. appointment can be picked up at 9 a.m., quickly driven to her destination, and forced to wait a lengthy period of time until the appointment is scheduled to begin. Beyond the obvious inconvenience that this causes, the policy can often inhibit the rider's ability to participate in certain activities. For instance, if Sam schedules a physical therapy (PT) appointment at 7:40 a.m., paratransit could schedule her pickup for 6:40 a.m. and drop her at her destination before the PT center is open. Sam can either wait outside until the facility opens, or deal with the complexity of rearranging her schedule to avoid early-morning PT. She cites this inconvenience, as well as wait times and general delays, as problems within the paratransit system. She would like to look at how paratransit "does its business," and decide whether the system could be run more efficiently.

consumer that the vehicle is three minutes away on Main Street, may begin to address some concerns and begin to create a more inclusive design solution, with improvements and innovations based on consumer needs.

Creating solutions through SRK assessment

Fran, and perhaps other rural residents, has difficulty communicating her transportation needs effectively because she tends to use more than one transportation network during a single trip (see Box 20.4). Each transportation network may function well independently, but when they need to be integrated, timely scheduling may not be a reality. This macro-scale issue can be considered within the SRK framework, as multiple agencies can work together to address node-to-node connections based on consumer preferences and ridership demands. To begin this analysis, a list of existing networks with timetables needs to be gathered. Then scenarios can be developed that test ridership demands, reliability/timeliness of routes during peak hours, challenging weather

Box 20.4 Community mobility case study 3: Rural accessibility

Fran, aged 34, is a resident of a neighboring community outside the county where she works, and travels nearly 20 miles to work every day. Her county is largely rural farmland and does not have a paratransit system. Because the bus serves only the county, Fran's journey to work has three sections. First, her mother drives her to the nearest town within her work county, where she catches a mainstream accessible bus to a downtown station. From there, paratransit picks her up and takes her directly to her job about 20 blocks away.

Fran has cerebral palsy and uses a power wheelchair. She explains that while the mainstream bus provides her with an indispensable service (she would not be able to get to work without it), relying on the bus system can be tricky during winter months. The "kneeling" mechanism that regular busses are equipped with cannot operate when the outside temperature drops below a certain point, and in such cases, Fran is unable to reach the third leg of her journey and is forced to stay home from work. Like many others, she also cites the one-hour pickup window as problematic.

conditions, etc. These scenarios can be analyzed using the SRK framework, ensuring that the transportation systems are readily understood and performance is equivalent for novice as well as expert consumers.

Part IV: Evidenced-based design and research for community participation: Current and future needs

Physical access to the community has improved through building practices, and new accessibility research has impacted federal, state, and local building codes. In the upcoming years, demographic shifts (e.g. aging population), as outlined in Jones and Sanford (1996) and Kaye et al. (2000), will impact the need for accessible built environments, therefore impacting community access and participation. Research needs exist on all three levels of environmental interaction, macro, meso, and micro.

Accessibility guidelines for macro-environmental considerations of public transportation services and an ever-growing research evidence base have investigated individual behaviors, human performance, and space needs for a variety of contexts, for example, accessible buses (D'Souza et al. 2010) and accessible taxis (Petzäll 1995). The Americans with Disabilities Act Accessibility Guidelines (ADAAG) for Transportation Vehicles (US Access Board 1998) addresses accessible facilities and transportation systems. The Accessible Public Transportation Rehabilitation Engineering Research Center, a cooperative research, development, and dissemination effort between the State University of New York at Buffalo and Carnegie Mellon University, has provided numerous studies on accessible and universally designed transportation systems (IDeA Center 2014). Research addressing consumer needs for system-wide concerns can be performed in a variety of ways, from focus groups to crowd-sourcing ridership issues.

New mobility device technologies and trends may influence accessibility and access guidelines (Cooper et al. 2008). Wheelchairs, for example, are getting larger in both length and width, and new guidelines must reflect these changes in order to accommodate physical accessibility to support community involvement (Paquet and Feathers 2004; Steinfeld et al. 2010).

Additional considerations

There are promising initiatives, which serve to promote flexible and cost-effective options supporting commuting needs, telecommuting, and flexible schedules, that can be instituted to assist persons with disabilities to acquire, maintain, and advance in employment opportunities. Cultural concerns were raised during the interviews collected, and represent another important layer of consideration for community access and participation. Two examples are outlined below.

Michelle is a person with a visual impairment and uses paratransit approximately twice per day for work-related travel. Michelle became ADA certified for reduced transit fares two years ago and has since used the paratransit system regularly for travel during the workday. She recognizes the quality of the paratransit system in the county but feels that a notable shortcoming lies in the lack of "sensitivity training" given to bus and paratransit drivers. She explains that while drivers are well trained in wheelchair and mobility assistance, few are familiar with cognitive and developmental disabilities or related needs, and as such will inadvertently act in disrespectful or insensitive ways. She does not blame the drivers for this but instead the system administration for failing to provide adequate training regarding the competence of persons with cognitive and developmental disabilities. The SRK framework can be used to assess scenarios where misunderstandings may exist and errors may be committed. For example, if a driver is not aware of how to instruct a rider with a cognitive disability that his stop is coming up, the SRK can be used to assess some possible intervening designs, such as a flashing light to indicate that the passenger's stop is approaching, or a symbol that may be more instructive. Ideally, the use and interpretation of this new design should be on a *skills-based* level. It may take several design interventions and trials to get this to work quickly and easily for both the driver and the passenger.

Gregory, aged 42, has cerebral palsy and uses the system to travel from his job to home after work on weekdays as a subscription paratransit rider. He's driven to work each morning by a friend who works similar hours. He says that paratransit simply makes it easier to do his job, and notes that "without the ADA, [he doesn't] know where he would be." Like Michelle, he is pleased with the paratransit system but notes his dissatisfaction with a lack of driver training in regards to treatment of persons with cognitive and developmental disabilities. He says through halted speech that "intellectually and cognitively [he is] fine ... and pretty self-sufficient," and that he is often offered assistance when it is not needed. Although Gregory also attributes the issue to a lack of training and not to individual drivers, he feels that the staff should understand the abilities of passengers, and respect their independence when appropriate.

The WHO ICF model reframes disability and places it within a continuum, on which all persons experience and can be addressed by appropriate design interventions. Millions of adults face one or more substantial physical barriers to getting around in their community. The case studies outlined in this chapter give a snapshot of personal stories concerning community mobility. This chapter paired these case studies with a particular inclusive ergonomic design approach, the SRK framework, to assess and address physical mobility issues in community-dwelling adults. Using a systematic approach to solving transportation-related problems is critical to find successful solutions. The SRK framework is an approach that assists in understanding how users interact with a system and assessing interventions in complex human–environment interactions. This framework has been shown to provide evidence-based solutions for increasing community participation through improved design on micro, meso, and macro levels.

Acknowledgments

The author expresses deep gratitude to the individuals volunteering their stories for the case study research project, and for the students in Universal Design class for transcribing components of the interviews.

References

Americans with Disabilities Act of 1990 (1990). Pub. L. No. 101–336, 104 Stat. 328.

Berkowitz, M., O'Leary, P.K., Kruse, D.L., and Harvey, C. (1998). *Spinal Cord Injury: An Analysis of Medical and Social Costs.* New York: Demos.

Blackler, A., Popovic, V., and Mahar, D. (2003). The nature of intuitive use of products: an experimental approach. *Design Studies* 24 (6): 491–506.

Clarkson, P.J., Waller, S.D., and Cardoso, C. (2015). Approaches to estimating user exclusion. *Applied Ergonomics* 46: 304–310. https://doi.org/10.1016/j.apergo.2013.03.001.

Coleman, R. (2002). *Living Longer: The New Context for Design.* Design Council Policy Papers series. London: Design Council.

Cooper, R.A., Cooper, R., and Boninger, M.L. (2008). Trends and issues in wheelchair technologies. *Assistive Technology* 20 (2): 61–72.

D'Souza, C., Steinfeld, E., Paquet, V., and Feathers, D. (2010). Space requirements for wheeled mobility devices in public transportation: analysis of clear floor space requirements. *Transportation Research Record: Journal of the Transportation Research Board* 2145 (1): 66–71.

Gaunet, F. and Briffault, X. (2005). Exploring the functional specifications of a localized wayfinding verbal aid for blind pedestrians: simple and structured urban areas. *Human-Computer Interaction* 20: 267–314.

Jones, M. and Sanford, J. (1996). People with mobility impairments in the United States today and in 2010. *Assistive Technology* 8 (1): 43–53.

Kaye, H.S., Kang, T., and LaPlante, M.P. (2000). *Mobility Device User in the United States – Disability Status Report (14).* Washington, DC: US Department of Education, National Institute on Disability and Rehabilitation Research.

Keates, S. (2007). *Designing for Accessibility. A Business Guide to Countering Design Exclusion.* Mahwah, NJ: Lawrence Erlbaum.

McAdams, D. and Kostovich, V. (2011). A framework and representation for universal product design. *International Journal of Design* 5 (1): 29–42.

National Council on Disability (NCD) (2005). *The Current State of Transportation for People with Disabilities in the United States.* Washington, DC: National Council on Disability.

National Council on Disability (NCD) (2007). *Empowerment for Americans with Disabilities: Breaking Barriers to Careers and Full Employment.* Washington, DC: National Council on Disability.

National Highway Traffic Safety Administration (n.d.). Driving safety: disabled drivers and passengers. Retrieved from http://www.nhtsa.gov.edgesuite-staging.net/Driving-Safety.

Nugent, T. (1961). The design of buildings to permit their use by the physically handicapped. National Academy of Sciences, National Research Council: NAS-NRC-910.

Paquet, V. and Feathers, D. (2004). An anthropometric study of manual and power wheelchair users. *International Journal of Industrial Ergonomics* 33 (3): 191–204.

Petzäll, J. (1995). The design of entrances of taxis for elderly and disabled passengers: an experimental study. *Applied Ergonomics* 26 (5): 343–352.

Rasmussen, J. (1983). Skills, rules, knowledge; signals, signs, and symbols, and other distinctions in human performance models. *IEEE Transactions on Systems, Man and Cybernetics* 13: 257–266.

Saarinen, T.F. (1976). *Environmental Planning: Perception and Behavior.* Boston, MA: Houghton Mifflin.

Steinfeld, E., Maisel, J., Feathers, D., and D'Souza, C. (2010). Anthropometry and standards for wheeled mobility: an international comparison. *Assistive Technology* 22 (1): 51–67.

Steinfeld, E., Schroeder, S., and Bishop, M. (1979). *Accessible Housing for People with Walking and Reaching Limitations*. Washington, DC: US Department of Housing and Urban Development.

US Access Board and Department of Transportation (1998). ADA Accessibility Guidelines for Transportation Vehicles. Federal Register (36 CFR Part 1192).

Vicente, K. (2006). *The Human Factor: Revolutionizing the Way People Live with Technology*. New York: Routledge, Taylor & Francis Group.

Vicente, K. and Rasmussen, J. (1988). On applying the Skills, Rules, and Knowledge framework to interface design. *Proceedings of the Human Factors and Ergonomics Society Annual Meeting* 32 (5): 254–258.

Vicente, K.J. and Rasmussen, J. (1992). Ecological interface design: theoretical foundations. *IEEE Transactions on Systems, Man, and Cybernetics* 22 (4): 589–606.

Toolbox: Resources

Accessibility within the home:

Chapter 10 discussed private environments and accessibility within the home (meso-environmental concerns). Since the majority of private residences do not have to be designed under the ADA, there may be resistance to adopting accessibility features or planning ahead to future accessibility projects. Concrete change (https://visitability.org/about-concrete-change/) has advocated for accessible features in the home. Their visitability initiative outlines three features:

- "At least one zero-step entrance approached by an accessible route on a firm surface no steeper than 1:12, proceeding from a driveway or public sidewalk.
- Wide passage doors.
- At least a half bath/powder room on the main floor." (http://www.udeworld.com/visbooklet/visitibilitybooklet.pdf)

Barrier-free research and inclusive design:

Micro-environmental accessibility has been subject to many research studies in the past several decades, which include for example, barrier-free research by Dr. T. Nugent (e.g. Nugent 1960), universal design research by Dr. E. Steinfeld (e.g. Steinfeld et al. 1979, 2010), and inclusive design research by Professors Clarkson, Coleman, and Keates (Clarkson et al. 2015; Coleman 2002; Keates 2007). Public spaces and features within spaces, such as doorways, elevators, and counter-top heights, should be designed following the ADAAG at a minimum (US Access Board 1998).

There are numerous federally sponsored research projects and centers that consider evidence-based accessibility and human-centered design strategies, please see the list below.

- Rehabilitation Engineering Research Center on Accessible Public Transportation: www.rercapt.org
- Rehabilitation Engineering Research Center on Universal Design and the Built Environment: http://idea.ap.buffalo.edu/home/index.asp
- Center for Inclusive Design and Environmental Access: http://idea.ap.buffalo.edu/home/index.asp

Federal sources for grants and information on accessible transportation and community access are provided below:

- United States Access Board: http://www.access-board.gov
- United States Department of Transportation: https://www.transit.dot.gov/regulations-and-guidance/environmental-programs/livable-sustainable-communities/livability-grant
- United States Department of Education: National Institute on Disability and Rehabilitation Research (NIDRR): https://www.ed.gov/category/program/national-institute-disability-and-rehabilitation-research

21

Leisure: Technology and environmental interventions

Nathan "Ben" Herz

Outline

Assistive Technologies and Environmental Interventions in Healthcare: An Integrated Approach, First Edition.
Edited by Lynn Gitlow and Kathleen Flecky.

Companion website: www.wiley.com/go/gitlow/assitivetechnologies

Learning outcomes

After reading this chapter, you should be able to:

1. Describe the importance of a variety of leisure and recreational activities to meaningful life participation and quality of life.
2. Apply the Human-Tech Ladder (Vicente 2006) to engagement in leisure within a range of technology and environmental interventions (TEI).
3. Describe relevant strategies in assessment and evaluation of leisure and TEI.
4. Identify the role of TEI in addressing the leisure interests of persons who experience physical, mental, or social disabilities.
5. Explain the role of new technologies, e.g. digital media, virtual reality, and gaming, in terms of TEI for leisure and recreational pursuits.

Active learning prompts

Before you read this chapter:

1. Reflect on your own definition of leisure in your life.
2. Describe how your participation in leisure activities impacts you and your life. How might your life change if you could not engage in these activities?
3. Using the Internet, research your favorite leisure activity to see what adaptations and assistive technologies are available to aid in an individual's participation.
4. Analyze the current trends in leisure with the impact of the new technology and digital alternatives to leisure pursuits (i.e. iPad impact on children's playing, Internet gaming).

Key terms

Digital media
Gaming
Leisure
Play
Recreation
Sports
Technology and environmental interventions (TEI)
Vicente (2006) Human-Tech Ladder
Virtual reality

Leisure defined

In this chapter, students will learn about a variety of technology and environmental interventions (TEI) related to leisure. They will learn when and how to implement technology interventions on a low- to high-technology continuum for individuals who want to participate in leisure activities. The application of technology to leisure activities encompasses a multitude of variables that affect successful participation. If student answers to the first active learning prompt, regarding what leisure means, were summarized, there would be many personal answers offered to define leisure. Some would define leisure as quiet time and relaxation and others would define it as active and stimulating. Leisure can be viewed as, "freedom from the demands of work or duty" or "time free from the demands of work or duty, when one can rest, enjoy hobbies or sports, etc." (Dictionary.com n.d.) The Occupational Therapy Practice Framework: Domain and Process (OTPF) defines leisure as "a non-obligatory activity that is intrinsically motivated and engaged in during discretionary time, that is, time not committed to obligatory occupations such as work, self-care, or sleep" (American Occupational Therapy Association 2014, p. S21). These activities play a significant role in an individual's life routines and have an important impact on health and quality of life (Vaughn 2010). While there are many definitions of leisure, common aspects of these definitions include that it is freely chosen, may be for pleasure, is actively engaging, may be anything which is motivating, and is free from obligation (Hurd and Anderson 2011). In addition to being defined personally and culturally, the meaning of leisure changes throughout the life span.

Leisure as part of a meaningful life

Leisure allows us to develop the necessary skills for life in our younger years. We learn rules and establish interactions with others, as well as begin, continue, and maintain friendships through the leisure activities we engage in as a child. A person who has an injury or illness may

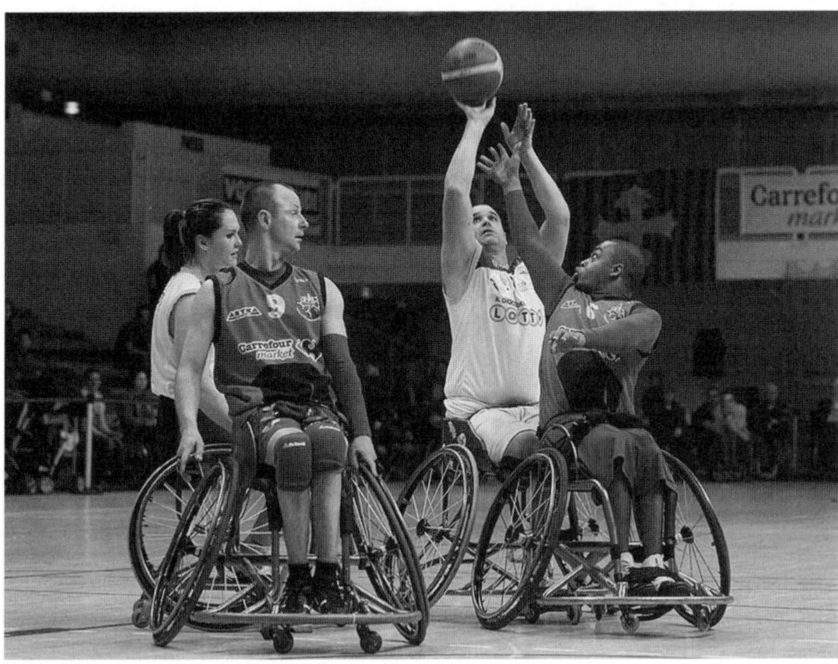

Figure 21.1 Photo of a wheelchair basketball game. Source: https://commons.wikimedia.org/wiki/File:Euroleague_-_LE_Roma_vs_Toulouse_IC-27.jpg. Licensed under CC BY SA 3.0.

choose to withdraw and not participate in leisure. That may be due to the inability to participate or to factors that contribute to a lack of confidence, fear, or in some cases depression or a lack of knowledge about alternative ways to engage in leisure pursuits (Figure 21.1) (Rimmer et al. 2004).

An individual can have a balanced lifestyle and participate in activities of daily living, work, and leisure. If an individual does not participate in all of the activities that he/she perceives as being important then there can be a decline in health in all aspects of the individual, including physical, emotional, cognitive, and social aspects. During our working life, leisure is a release for many people that allows them to escape the pressures of daily life and participate in something meaningful and robust that they value. As we age and head into retirement, leisure activity has been shown to increase cognitive and physical function and decrease the negative impacts of aging (Leitner and Leitner 2012).

Leisure activities can be viewed as a way to promote healthy endeavors through planning and participation, for example while one individual works out or goes for a run, another may consider other leisure activities that promote health as leisure such as cooking or other athletics. It is important that every assistive technology practitioner recognizes that every individual is different and has various activities that are meaningful to him/her.

Hamilton-Smith (1985) states, when discussing leisure, "I am talking about human experience, characterized by intrinsic motivation and/or satisfaction; by a subjective sense of freedom to choose and of freedom from constraint; and by the understanding that it is accepted by our own reference group as being leisure" (p. 15). Mee et al. (2004) observed that doing something purposeful is directly associated with the meaning of one's day and that engagement in activities that are personally meaningful to an individual contributes to a sense of purpose for that person. Indeed, having things to do that are meaningful fills life with purpose.

Leisure activities across the life span

As we examine the meaningfulness of leisure we need to understand that it has various meanings and influences across the life span. The influences vary from skill development to social interaction, as well as factoring into an individual's quality of life. Individuals choose leisure activities based on experience and success. Children who are athletic and play sports may continue to pursue those leisure pursuits, whereas those who do not enjoy those activities may choose more intellectual pursuits. These choices permeate into the later years and influence participation as an individual ages.

Children utilize play as a means to accomplish skill development and learning. Play is essential to development because it contributes to the cognitive, physical, social, and emotional well-being of children

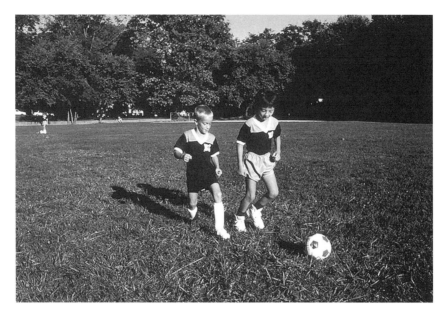

Figure 21.2 Photo of young children playing ball game. Source: Courtesy of National Cancer Institute.

and youth (Ginsburg 2007). "Mary Reilly recognized the complexity of play which she described as a 'cobweb' through which children learn mastery of their environment and gain the skills and competency in adulthood" (Vaughn 2010, p. 138). Play may have a leisure feel, while allowing a child to experience the world through adherence to rules, socialization, and interests. It is here that children establish many of their personality traits and characteristics. Play is actually the child's work and is seen as a normal everyday occurrence (Figure 21.2).

As children age into adolescents, there are various differences associated with both gender and socioeconomic leisure pursuits. For example, Livingston (2019) states that boys spend more time than girls in leisure pursuits. Additionally, some evidence exists stating that lower childhood socioeconomic status can result in lower engagement in leisure time physical activity as one ages (Elhakeem et al. 2015).

The wide range of options available in the field of leisure nowadays enables young adolescents to enjoy a great diversity of leisure experiences. The alternatives that are available range from social gathering to motion pictures, video gaming, and organized activities, allowing for a huge array of activities to choose from.

If we look at development through the theoretical perspective of Erikson (1959), the developmental goals for young adults are moving toward being independent from their parents and establishing themselves in the world of work. Their leisure interests may revolve around the work environment and family, as well as sports, group activities, exercise, outdoor activities, and dating, to name a few (Krishnagari and Southam 2006). A market analysis revealed that the young adult demographic, with more leisure time and fewer familial responsibilities, who are often opinion leaders and trendsetters, determine the success or failure of new leisure options. Young adults include more singles and are more ethnically diverse than older generations (Mintel n.d.).

In middle adulthood we must recognize the impact of leisure as a means to maintain friendships and that it also revolves around family in such a way as to meet Erickson's theory of generativity versus stagnation. In this case then individuals may take pleasure in increasing a younger individual's skills and talents as a way of leaving a legacy behind. Examples include being a coach or mentor. Leisure is related to aspects of life such as work, family, home life, community participation, and friendship (Krishnagari and Southam 2006).

The older adult has an increase in free time associated with the winding down of career expectations and family requirements. Associated roles may be a grandparent, parent, and/or retiree. Erikson's last stage is ego integrity versus despair and is described as the time in which life is reviewed for completeness and satisfaction. If activity levels are not maintained then there may be a deterioration of skills, strength, coordination, and endurance. There are some aspects of individual experiences which are associated with normal changes due to aging, such as decreases in hearing, vision, and sensory abilities. Specific examples of leisure activities that older adults engage in are dining out with friends, travel, card games, walking, swimming, and exercise (Krishnagari and Southam 2006).

The human-tech ladder

As presented in Chapter 1 in this text, the Human-Tech Ladder (Vicente 2006) is a framework that provides a means of considering the numerous factors that promote technology integration within human life. The framework proposes that there are a variety of contextual factors that need to be addressed when providing technology resources to humans. These factors may influence the design and implementation of that technology and include physical, psychological, team, organizational, and political variables.

As with any implementation of technology, the Human-Tech Ladder is based on a human or societal need. To demonstrate how the Human-Tech Ladder can be applied to leisure-based technology, we will focus on leisure that concentrates on physical activity, given its visibility as a societal need. Of course, there are many other types of leisure pursuits and we will refer to some of them later in the chapter.

Political

Starting at the top of the ladder, or the political rung of the ladder, we consider political factors, which may influence leisure. In recent years much national attention had been focused on increasing a person's physical activity. For example, one of the goals of Healthy People 2020 is to enhance health, fitness, and quality of life through daily physical activity. This includes all people and is especially important for people with disabilities who are at risk of being sedentary and inactive (Healthy People 2020 n.d.-b). Associated with this goal, in turn, federal initiatives are funded that support increasing physical activity. For example, one federal initiative associated with this goal is the Let's Move campaign promoted by First Lady Michele Obama, which encourages families to promote physical activity and healthy eating in their children's lives (Let's Move n.d.). These initiatives in turn trickle down to influence funding for programs that support this agenda.

Another example of a health project is The Healthy Steps program funded by the National Center for Chronic Disease Prevention and Health Promotion's Division of Adolescent and School Health developed by the New York State Department of Education in 2006 to combat childhood obesity a societally recognized need (Department of Health and Human Services, National Center for Chronic Disease Prevention and Health Promotion, Division of Adolescent and School Health 2009).

Moreover, a focus on increasing wellness through leisure at the federal level, influencing programming and funding, is the Veterans Administration Adaptive Sports Program. This program provides funding and programming to keep veterans with disabilities engaged in physical activities (US Department of Veterans Affairs n.d.). The program promotes keeping disabled veterans healthier by engaging them in leisure activities, in this case sports. Finally, the National Center on Health, Physical Activity and Disability (NCHPAD) was developed in 1999 through funds from the Centers for Disease Control and Prevention (CDC) to ensure that the needs of people with disabilities were promoted at the national level as well (American Association of Health and Disability n.d.). The use of adaptive technology and environmental intervention is critical to both initiatives. These examples illustrate how societal needs can provide support and funding for programs that focus on solving human problems, in this case the need for humans to engage in physical activity (see Box 21.1).

Organizational

At the next level of the Human-Tech Ladder we consider *organizational factors*. If we follow the societal need focusing on keeping people healthy and fit through physical activity, we can see how this might play out at the variety of organizations where leisure activities take place. In the workplace, for example, many employers have instituted evidence-based programs that are designed to promote wellness (Healthy People 2020 n.d.-a). These programs engage people in non-work-related activities, which promote participation in physical leisure activities that are shown to increase health and decrease the cost of work-related injuries. Given that the Americans with Disabilities Act protects the right of people with disabilities in workplace environments, these employees must be included in these initiatives as well. A variety of programs in residential facilities for elders might be focused on engaging residents in gardening activities. Gardening has been shown to be a leisure activity that promotes wellness using a multimodal approach in this population (Wang and MacMillan 2013). Finally, in school-based settings, children with disabilities must be included in physical activity programs along with their non-disabled peers (Columna et al. 2010).

Teams

The next rung on the Human-Tech Ladder is the *team*. In all of the instances we describe above, a variety of team members, including the client, rehabilitation therapists, educators, employers, and athletic trainers, are among those who may be involved in using technology to engage people with disabilities in wellness and physical activity programming. The CDC has a resource

Box 21.1 Here's the evidence

Caddick, N. and Smith, B. (2014). The impact of sport and physical activity on the well-being of combat veterans: a systematic review. *Psychology of Sport and Exercise* 15: 9–18.

Key Words: sports, physical activity, combat veterans, well-being, rehabilitation, post-traumatic stress disorder (PTSD)

Purpose: Analyze the current evidence of the influences of sports and physical activity on the well-being of combat veterans.

Sample/Setting: Research studies were examined that relate to combat veterans and veterans who have experienced injury, illness, or disability.

Method: Systematic review.

Findings: The authors found positive influences of physical activity and sports on the motivation and well-being of combat veterans who engaged in these activities; however, results of these studies should be interpreted with caution.

Critical Thinking Questions:

1. How does the sample and/or setting of this study translate to the population and/or setting in which you practice or will be practicing?
2. What do the findings of this review suggest about the potential for physical activity and sports activities for long-term rehabilitation?
3. How could this study contribute to the design of other future studies?

Box 21.2 I created the renegade all-terrain wheelchair

As a wheelchair user who loves the Maine outdoors, I struggled pushing my wheelchair down paths and tote roads to get to my favorite spots. There were many times I couldn't get to where I wanted and would have to turn back.

Even after a light snow, when deer hunting is at its best, I would be stuck in the house because of my inability to push the snow-filled wheels. While fishing or just going off-road, soft terrain would all but make it impossible for me to enjoy the outdoors.

Now, after developing the Renegade All-Terrain Wheelchair, I can wheel off-road and through soft terrain or several inches of fluffy snow with relative ease. My hands never touch muddy or wet wheels, keeping them warm and dry.

Renegade Wheelchairs. Retrieved from http://www.alphaonenow.org/userfiles/Renegade_mediakit_10_23_2012.pdf.

that provides information about how physicians and other healthcare providers can promote physical activities with their clients who have disabilities (Centers for Disease Control and Prevention 2018). School-based physical activity programs must also include students with disabilities, and it is likely that therapists, student peers, and paraprofessionals work together to make this happen (Heyne et al. 2012). All of these organizationally based programs include TEI within them.

Psychosocial

At the next level of the Human-Tech Ladder we consider the *psychosocial* factors which impact leisure engagement. There is much evidence from the literature that engagement in leisure promotes health and well-being for people across the life span, including those who have disabilities (Van Asselt et al. 2015). Additionally, lack of ability to engage in leisure pursuits may negatively impact health and wellness. The story of the development of the Renegade Wheelchair demonstrates the psychosocial value of engaging in leisure activities and the influence this value may have on technology development. John Rackely, an avid hunter and Maine outdoorsman, sustained a spinal cord injury while jumping on his daughter's trampoline. After his injury, he wanted to return to the woods. This passion spurred him to develop the Renegade Wheelchair. Box 21.2 tells his story in his own words (Rackley n.d.).

Physical

The needs at the bottom of the Human-Tech Ladder concern the physical characteristics which must be considered when matching a person with a leisure technology. There needs to be an understanding of the numerous physical capabilities of the individual as each one can affect one's level of participation in some way. For example, if we have a client with a C6 spinal cord injury who wants to shoot a firearm, the design of the technology must be matched to that individual's physical capabilities. The firearm needs to be mounted (at a height to sight the target) and may need to be adapted for execution of the trigger mechanism. The mount must be strong enough to receive the recoil from the firearm without causing injury or harm to the participant.

In summary, Vicente (2006) states, "If the human factor is taken into account, a tight fit between person and design can be achieved and the technology is more likely to fulfill its intended purpose" (p. 54). As we look at all the factors, it is evident that they can affect each other and influence clients' overall success in leisure pursuits. The rest of the chapter provides information regarding how to evaluate an individual's leisure needs along with a variety of low- to high-tech adaptations that are available to enable participation in leisure pursuits.

Assessment and evaluation of leisure

As stated above, the impact of leisure activities on an individual and their life is important for maintenance of health and wellness. The evaluation process is one that can occur in many different ways. While there are structured evaluations associated with leisure activities which will be described further, you may also take the unstructured route. As an example, in a clinic for people who have amyotrophic lateral sclerosis, the occupational therapists (OTs), physical therapists (PTs), and nurses participate in a structured evaluation; however, part of the process may include unstructured parts. In order to look at the whole person we must not forget to evaluate and gain knowledge about their interactions and participation.

Leisure elicits a different type of motivation and reason for participation. It can make an unmotivated client participate. As a therapist engages with clients, there is a need to develop a style/story, so that you may successfully gain the relevant information you need to complete a comprehensive evaluation. Review Chapter 2 of this text for more information on the theory-based evaluation and clinical reasoning process. Many times the interview process includes interview questions such as: (i) What do you do for fun? (ii) What do you like to do besides work or school?

For a more formal assessment tool, professionals in a clinic setting could utilize the Occupational Performance History Interview (OPHI), developed by Kielhofner in 1988 (Kielhofner and Henry 1988). The OPHI is a structured interview that can guide a professional to address a client's individual participation in life activities. The interview is based on the Model of Human Occupation (MOHO) originally introduced in 1985, by Kielhofner. Elements of the OPHI include: (i) organization of daily living routines, (ii) life roles, (iii) interests, values, and goals, (iv) perceptions of ability and responsibility, and (v) environmental influences (Kielhofner and Henry 1988). When assessing interests, values, and goals, we examine the area of leisure and specifically address the value of them in the individual's life.

There are other structured evaluations found in the area of leisure that pertain to the healthcare environment. Many are a part of various evaluations that include leisure but are not specifically focused on it. These include but are not limited to: the Canadian Occupational Performance Measure (COPM), Occupational Circumstances Assessment Interview Rating Scale (OCAIRS), Occupational Questionnaire (OQ), Bayer Activities of Daily Living Scale (B-ADL), Functional Rating Scale (FRS), and Kohlman Evaluation of Living Skills (KELS) (Asher 2014). These all have areas associated with the evaluation of leisure activities and participation. There are other assessment tools available that evaluate the social participation and activities of individuals but do not necessarily assess leisure specifically, looking more at the areas of specific daily living skills in the home as well as the community.

Quality of life measures

Other relevant tools included would be ones that assess an individual's quality of life. The Quality of Life Scale (QOLS) was originally a 15-item instrument that measured five conceptual domains of quality of life: material and physical well-being, relationships with other people, social, community, and civic activities, personal development and fulfillment, and recreation (Burckhardt and Anderson 2003). Other quality-of-life evaluations are available such as the SF-36 Health Survey (SF-36), Quality of Life Index (QL Index), and the Quality of Life Inventory (QOLI) (Asher 2014). All of these evaluations take into account the level of participation and abilities of an individual in relation to satisfaction with roles and activity levels.

Leisure-specific assessments

There are specific leisure assessments available, including the Leisure Assessment Inventory (LAI), which measures the leisure behavior of adults through its four components: (i) the Leisure Activity Participation Index (LAP), (ii) the Leisure Preference Index (L-PREF), (iii) the Leisure Interest Index (L-INT), and (iv) the Leisure Constraints Index (L-CON). The purpose of the LAI is to help professionals and caregivers use leisure to facilitate: development of leisure skills, maintenance and promotion of physical fitness and health, development of friendships, creation of residential environments that foster social networks, facilitation of community inclusion, preparation for retirement, and empowerment of individuals to live self-determined lifestyles (Hawkins et al. 1997).

Moreover, The Leisure Motivation Scale measures an individual's motivation for participating in leisure activities. The four primary motivators identified by research are: (i) intellectual (ii) social, (iii) competence-mastery, and (iv) stimulus-avoidance as the individual parts of the evaluation. It is useful for establishing the components of leisure activities that motivate the individual to participate (Beard and Ragheb 1983).

The relationship of leisure to injury and illness

If an individual has an injury or illness, the lack of participation in leisure activities takes its toll in many different ways, regardless of age. As we discussed briefly, leisure has an impact on each area of development. In an article by Caldwell (2005), a review of the literature provided information on how leisure can contribute to the physical, social, emotional, and cognitive health of an individual through prevention, coping, and transcendence, allowing for participants to also maintain their quality of life. As healthcare professionals, we need to address specific areas in which we participate in life and how they are affected by injury or illness, such as activities of daily living, instrumental activities of daily living, rest and sleep, education, work, leisure, and social participation. Research indicates that leisure is an integral and important part of our lives, as both an occupation and an avocation, for life satisfaction as well as contributing to a good quality of life (Vaughn 2010).

If an individual cannot participate in leisure and it is something they value, then there can be detrimental ramifications. The loss of the leisure role may contribute to decreased social participation, learning, self-esteem, and self-worth, and may increase depression. Research indicates that the perception of leisure satisfaction is the most significant predictor of life satisfaction. It is also related to development, well-being, and coping. Research has also shown that individuals who suffer from an illness or injury can disengage from pursuits that are purely for enjoyment and focus on activities of daily living and work (Krishnagari and Southam 2006).

In healthcare, it is vital that we address the whole person and integrate our treatment into a well-rounded and balanced life. We all need to examine the nature of dysfunction and the factors that contribute to it. As we provide intervention and education, we must look at the means necessary to improve the participation of the individual in all aspects of their life, including leisure, which can be the focus of treatment due to the intrinsic motivation it holds for individuals.

Role of TEI in participation

In order to promote participation in meaningful leisure activities, TEIs have the ability to use a full range of no-/low-tech to high-tech options, which can enable individuals to participate in an activity and be successful. According to Campbell and colleagues (2008), "when promoting participation, the focus of intervention shifts from skill-building to using strategies that ensure maximal participation as quickly as possible. Adaptation interventions include use of both low- and high-technology AT devices that allow children (individuals) to participate in the absence of being able to perform skills required in the activity or routine" (p. 97). Moreover, using the example mentioned earlier, adding a firearm mount to a power wheelchair for a client with a C6 spinal cord injury can allow them to participate once again in a hunt. Associated with the mount is devising a way for the trigger mechanism to fire; this can be done through the use of the individual's elbow and wrist movement, so when they engages the target, participation and success are possible. Having the ability to be a part of something valued and meaningful, that was thought to have been lost, is powerful and motiving. Little changes can make a difference in your client's life satisfaction and leisure pursuits (Vaughn 2010).

General leisure activities TEI strategies

In terms of general leisure activities, there are pieces of technology ranging from simple to complex that can be utilized to promote participation in board games, card games, paper games, and other tabletop games, as well as painting and drawing. In order to allow individuals to participate, there are specific aspects to consider. Knowing the different aspects of activities relating to print size, contrast, color, manipulation patterns, objects and movements, cognitive aspects (such as rules, sequences, and problem-solving), and gross movements is important to determine interventions and adaptations. Examples of simple assistive technology and adaptations might be built-up handles, straps, card holders/supports, and book stands.

Organized sports

Organized sports programs in the United States offer a variety of ways for all individuals to participate. Specific organizations provide adaptive ways to play as well as well-defined rules for the activities. Organized sports programs have created specific opportunities for individuals with an injury or illness to participate. Sports and recreation programs offer the opportunity to achieve success in a very short time period, allowing the participant to use this success to build self-confidence and focus on possibilities instead of dwelling on what can no longer be done. The ability to participate in a sport, such as cycling, skiing, and sailing, provides the opportunity to reunite with family and friends in a shared activity. The availability of programming in the United States is extraordinary. A sample of options includes, but is certainly not limited to, baseball, basketball, water skiing, sailing, scuba diving, canoeing, kayaking, tennis, cycling, golf, equestrianism, rock climbing, hunting, and fishing (See Box 21.3).

As mentioned before, participation in sports as children can be an important influence on development.

Box 21.3 Organized sports for the disabled

Name	Website
Disabled Sports USA	https://www.disabledsportsusa.org/about/
Miracle League	http://www.miracleleague.com
National Sports Center for the Disabled	http://www.nscd.org
Wheelchair and Ambulatory Sports USA	http://www.wasusa.org
The Lakeshore Foundation	http://www.lakeshore.org
Ability Plus	http://www.abilityplus.org
Office of National Veterans Sports Programs & Special Events	http://www.va.gov/adaptivesports

While not everyone does participate, statistics from the CDC show that a mother's participation in sports increases her child's likelihood to participate by 22%, while a father's participation increases his child's likelihood to try sports by 11% (Brown 2015). In a 2012 study by the Physical Activity Council, it was found that there are 206.7 million "active" Americans age six and older. Recognizing that there are varied levels of activity, the authors of the article estimate that 33% of Americans age six and older are active to a healthy level (or 94.8 million individuals) (http://physicalactivitycouncil.com). It is therefore a possibility that individuals we see in practice have already participated in sports and would make that a part of their rehabilitation. The opportunity to participate in sports has physical, psychological, and social benefits for the participants. Disabled veterans of all ages and abilities report better health, new friendships, and a better quality of life when participating in adaptive sports (Hawkins et al. 2011).

Examples of TEI for specific sports

Golf

Golf is a sport that can be accessed through both adaptive means and activity modification. In the area of specific adaptive equipment there can be modified carts (single ride) that allow you to sit supported as you swing the club (Figure 21.3). Other adaptations include the making of custom clubs and also gloves that will allow you to grasp the club without having the grip strength usually required. There are GPS systems available for determining distance, so that the visually impaired golfer can choose the correct club. When it comes to putting, the visually impaired individual may use a sound monitor placed at the hole for direction and distance. Simple modifications can be a built-up handle, the modified golf glove, and extensions for ball recovery as well as placement on the tee. A specific list can be found at the Disabled Sports USA website for adaptive equipment at https://www.disabledsportsusa.org/sports/adaptive-equipment/golf-equipment/.

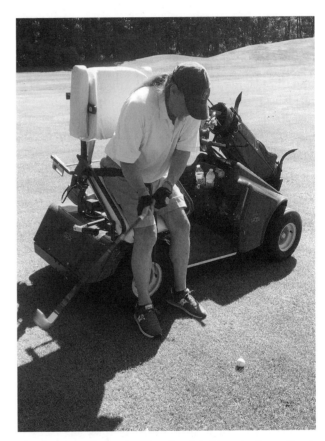

Figure 21.3 Photo of golfer using Solorider adaptive golf cart on the golf course (Sleeping Giant). Source: Used with permission of the Sports Association, Gaylord Hospital.

Hunting

Hunting may be another valued leisure pursuit that people with disabilities find challenging. The combination of being outdoors (terrain, weather, and the elements) and the skills necessary to participate may limit one's motivation to participate. The complexity involved in someone with specific needs going hunting stems from the integrated movements that are necessary to complete the activity. There are many components involved in the hunting process: one needs to stabilize the equipment, be able to visualize/focus on the target, and then pull the trigger (using fine motor coordination). So when an evaluation takes place for this activity, healthcare providers must also look at the integrated movements for the individual to be successful. Whether the equipment is a bow, crossbow, or firearm, there are many assistive technology adaptations available, from mounts for the equipment to specific items of sighting apparatus and modified trigger units, including but not limited to sip and puff switches.

For example, a support for rifles such as the Be Adaptive Model HQ100 can be found at the website http://beadaptive.com. Modified trigger pull mechanisms using a bite method, such as the Model BT100, can also be found at the Be Adaptive website. An example of a sighting option is the iScope, which attaches to most rifle scopes with four padded set screws. The device allows you to see a full screen view of what the sighting scope sees. Being able to see an image full screen without trying to look through the scope allows for comfortable, accurate shooting, particularly if you have mobility or vision problems.

Another relevant website to explore would be www.buckmasters.com, which offers a variety of adaptive shooting applications and can be a useful resource. You can also use an iPhone or an iPod touch. The iScope can be found at https://iscope.com/. There is a full range of no-tech to high-tech options available, from one that can be created from problem-solving and critical reasoning with materials found in the hobby shop and/or home to those available from the above-mentioned resources.

Outdoor mobility and TEI strategies

When looking at mobility, the TEI practitioner must consider the terrain and environment associated with the activity. Power wheelchairs may allow the freedom to move to and fro. Simple modifications include changing tires to wider ones and cambering the wheels. Many different wheelchairs have replaceable wheels that are more appropriate for the off-road environment, such as Fatso 24″ Off-Road Wheels or Wheelchair Off Road Rear Wheels 24″ found at Sportaid at http://www.sportaid.com/wheelchair-tires-tubes-parts/wheelchair-tires/all-terrain-wheelchair-tires. While these tires can be pricy, many are reasonable and will assist individuals with the mobility necessary to move within the desired terrain and environment successfully.

Another option for outdoor mobility would be the use of hand bikes. While many may not be designed for off-road work, they certainly can take the place of a two-wheel bike and offer the same experience. There are many to choose from and various styles, from leisure-type riding to racing options. One place to look for examples of hand bikes is at http://disabledgear.com/pages/handbikes – they have various manufacturers listed and links to websites for those interested in riding and competing on bikes.

Specific sports: Swimming

Swimming is a common activity everyone can participate in with simple modifications. Simple no-tech adaptations include floats, noodles, and rafts. Other items are floatation vests, head supports, and pool lift chairs. Many aquatic programs utilize universal design principles and use infinity (walk-in type) pools for ease of entrance and exit for those who have physical disabilities. The infinity pool avoids the expense of having a ramp or lift installed. Pool lifts are also common and use hydraulics to raise and lower a person into the pool. An example of this type of lift can be found at https://www.spectrumproducts.com/product-category/ada-pool-lifts-assisted-access/. These lifts are usually mounted on the side of the pool. If a pool has a ramp or walk-in design, individuals may use a chair made of PVC (similar to a shower chair) to roll in and out of the pool. If an individual chooses to swim at the beach and uses a wheelchair, mobility issues could arise from the width of the tires on the wheelchair and whether they are able to get across the sand. Once in the water, you can utilize the various flotation devices noted earlier.

Specific sports: Horseback riding

Specific resources for riding can be found at the Professional Association of Therapeutic Horsemanship International (PATH Intl.), formerly the North American Riding for the Handicapped Association (NARHA). The association tagline is "Ensuring excellence and changing lives through equine-assisted activities and therapies" (https://www.facebook.com/pathintl/). The PATH group governs and serves as a resource for the activities that encompass equine-assisted activities and therapies (EAAT). EAAT also includes therapeutic carriage driving, interactive vaulting (which is similar to gymnastics on horseback), and equine-facilitated learning/mental health (this activity uses the horse as a partner in cognitive and behavioral therapy, usually with the participation of a licensed therapist). EAAT also includes

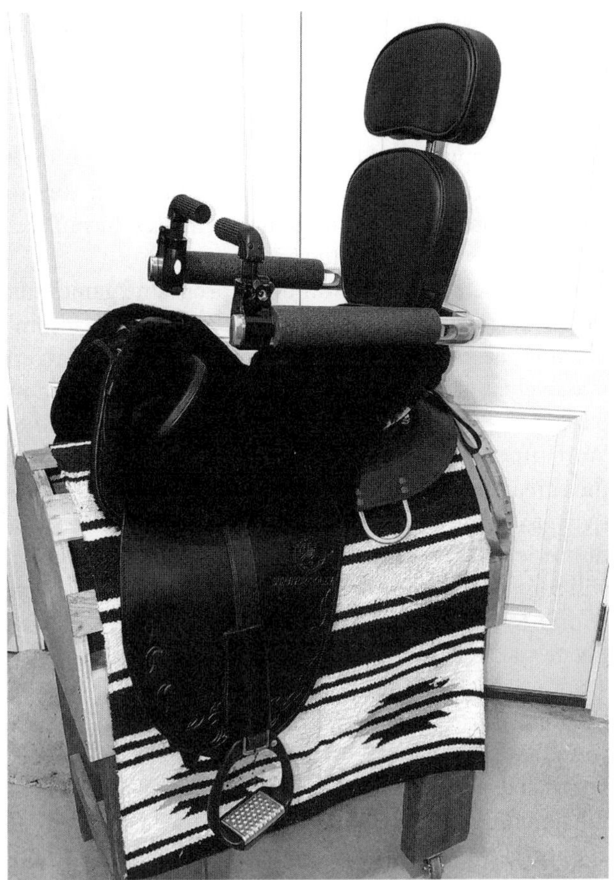

Figure 21.4 The independence saddle. Source: Permission to use photo provided by Independent Strides.

ground work, exercises that are done with the horse on the ground, and stable management. Details of the various programs as well as PATH certification and accreditation of centers and individuals are available on the PATH website (http://www.pathintl.org).

Horseback riding has many therapeutic benefits and has a rich history of participation. Individuals who use wheelchairs and those that have difficulties with mounting a horse (able-bodied as well) can use a mounting ramp, which includes a platform to bring themselves high enough to get on the horse. There are various assists that allow for an individual to participate in riding, such as a two-rider pad, modified saddles (i.e. extra strapping and pads), harness and gait belt combination, various other bolsters and pads, and padded gait belts (Figure 21.4). Many of these items can be found at www.freedomrider.com.

Digital media and TEI strategies

Three major electronic gaming system platforms, as well as PC and Mac computer gaming, are continually growing. Digital gaming has become a market that facilitates many leisure pursuits. Specific gaming platforms can enhance experiences and promote leisure activities that provide simulation and enable participation. The differences in platforms and computers allow for different levels (based on the platform/operating system) of participation and adaptations/modifications. The computer has become a common household item and one that the whole family uses for work, information gathering, education, and leisure. Barriers to participation for people with a variety of disabilities are associated with the digital age. Cognitive, motor, visual, and hearing impairments can compromise individuals' ability to participate in virtual games and environments. The impact of digital media gaming on leisure activities is significant. In a white paper collaboration between The AbleGamers Foundation and 7-128 Software (Robinson and Walker 2010), it was found that 25% of individuals over 50 play digital media (video) games, and in 2007 the US Census revealed that 61% of American households had computers. A survey conducted by a consulting firm found that overall videogame console ownership in American households increased from 44% in 2006 to 58% in 2009 (Robinson and Walker 2010). As the population ages, the likelihood of having a disability which may interfere with one's ability to play video games increases, as illustrated in Box 21.4.

Box 21.4 Survey results

5- to 15-year-olds – 7.2% males and 4.3% females report at least one disability

16- to 64-year-olds – 19.6% males and 17.6% females report at least one disability

65 and older – 40.4% males and 43.0% females report at least one disability

Drawing from cultural anthropology and gerontology, Reid and Hirji (2004) proposed explanations of how virtual reality (VR) gaming provides an enabling environment for clients with disabilities. Given the flexibility of many VR/gaming technologies, the virtual environment may be manipulated, controlled, and fine-tuned to accommodate existing abilities and functional limitations of the person that may eventually result in a satisfactory engagement. Many VR/gaming applications can be modified in order to successfully control the environment and improve an individual's level of participation. The feeling of accomplishment derived from being able to successfully participate and complete an activity to one's satisfaction is intrinsically rewarding and thus therapeutically beneficial. Many VR applications are set in a game format. Games set in a VR format allow the user to set goals, receive instant feedback, reinforce positive or efficient behaviors and, depending on the technology, automatically chart their progress (Bondoc et al. 2012).

Activities that are part of the VR/gaming genre may be used to restore, remediate, or develop a variety of client factors and performance skills, including range of motion, coordination, postural control, attention and concentration, motivation, self-confidence, and socialization. These attributes may be essential for client participation and engagement in meaningful activities (Bondoc et al. 2012). Thus using VR as an assistive technology to assist a client in regaining function and participation skills is gaining in popularity (Wickham n.d.).

Accessibility

Enabling access to digital media has been discussed in other chapters, for example Chapter 20. However, a brief overview will be presented here as well. Individuals can access a computer in many ways to address communication issues and environmental controls and to participate in video and online gaming. There are speech recognition programs that allow you to talk into a microphone and give directions for action, such as Dragon NaturallySpeaking (Nuance 2013). Microsoft also has voice recognition built into its operating system (Microsoft 2016) Touch screen access is another way to gain accessibility to computers, as are various switches and eye gaze technologies. Coupled with these interfaces, a reader program allows an individual to hear what is being done and be aware of the various ways in which an activity is taking place.

Accessibility is the key to participation in this area. As complex as it is, there are a few things that could make digital programs/gaming accessible for many out there, and there are four areas in which the ability to modify could increase participation and accessibility for individuals with disabilities. Modification of speed control, text-to-speech, color contrast, and programmable keys would allow most individuals with disabilities to participate in digital programs/gaming.

The ability to control the speed of the action can assist those with a decreased reaction time, allowing for completion of actions that may be otherwise missed. Text-to-speech allows for the activity to have instructions or actions communicated to the participant while participating. It changes the written words/directions from text on the screen to spoken words.

Color contrast issues can affect the individual who has visual problems, and modifying color contrast creates a way for a player to successfully participate along with those who have no visual issues. Programmable keys provide an alternative to using a mouse or full keyboard. There are other interfaces such as controllers that can be used for one-handed implementation for individuals with amputations or those with strokes who cannot utilize bilateral movements. Programming one key to access various aspects of the game eliminates the number of keystrokes that define the action.

While there are many different programs/games out there, few manufacturers have been proactive in accomplishing these changes. As an example, one of the largest massively multiplayer online games (MMO) changed its parameters to include some of these changes. World of Warcraft, added a way to move buttons to anywhere on the screen for easy access and allowed for mouse sensitivity to be adjusted for character movement through numeric ratings: the higher the number, the faster it will move. In the area of contrast/color, the developers' efforts to delineate between specific items have given greater accessibility to those with visual difficulties. They utilize symbols and other forms of identification to assist those with color issues to participate and be successful. Finally, the game has text-based warnings, but the hearing-impaired can play and understand what is happening as the action occurs with the text-to-speech application. The game can be played successfully without sound (AbleGamers 2010).

The AbleGamers Foundation is an organization that supports and assists individuals, both client and developer, with implementing accessibility in the digital age. The AbleGamers Foundation is dedicated to bringing greater accessibility in the digital entertainment space so that people with disabilities can gain a greater quality of life and develop a rich social life that gaming can bring (AbleGamers Foundation n.d.). The group has been involved in development of many forms of accessibility as it relates to digital media. They have developed the Adroit Switchblade controller in collaboration with Evil Controllers, and it can be found at the following website: https://ablegamers.org/xbox-adaptive-controller-the-evolution-of-accessibility/. The controller is one of a kind, allows for programmable keys and thumb sticks, and is affordable (Figure 21.5).

Gaming systems

Recent developments by the three major video gaming systems (Wii, Playstation, and Xbox One/Kinect) have changed the interface for participants. Gaming was once defined by controller use and now it is accessible with or without controllers (Xbox One/Kinect). Both the Wii and Sony Move utilize the remotes (accelerometers with

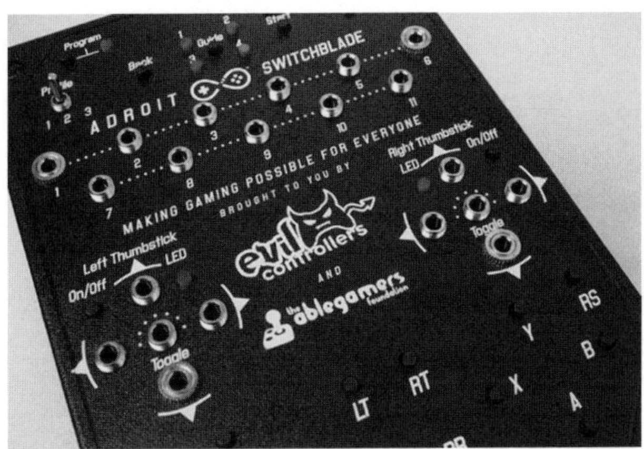

Figure 21.5 Adroit switchblade. Source: Used with permission of www.Evilcontrollers.com.

buttons) using Bluetooth technology, with the difference being that the Move uses camera technology whereas the Wii does not. The Xbox One/Kinect utilizes camera technology as well as a grid system that maps the playing area, immersing the participant in the game using the individual as a controller (physical cues, usually hands). The Move and Kinect systems work collaboratively with their respective hardware, the Xbox 360 and the PlayStation 3/4.

The major feature of the Wii console continues to be its wireless controller, the Wiimote, which may be used as a pointing device and can read motion and rotation on three planes. The controller comes with an accessory, the nunchuk, which provides additional controls for specific games that require two hands, boxing for example. The controller also contains sound and vibration to provide specific feedback to the gamer for specific actions that take place while participating, such as setting the hook in a fishing game. In this instance the feedback is that the vibration on the Wiimote occurs when the fish hits the hook, reminding the gamer to pull back to hook the fish on the line. The Wiimote can also be used to turn the console on and off. The Wii itself does not have the higher-resolution graphics found in the Sony and Xbox systems.

The Sony Move began in the form of the EyeToy, the company's earlier endeavor in the use of camera technology which was unique at the time. The Move, with the improved graphics and utilization of camera, accelerometers, and a gyroscope, gives feedback similar to that given by the Wii, but provides more opportunities. The Move creates a better interface between the player and system than the Wii, accomplishing this due to its wireless capabilities and camera technology. It does, however, come with a higher price tag. The graphics surpass those of the two other gaming systems, while it remains similar to the Wii in how the feedback and performance are implemented by responding to actual physical movement of the player.

The Xbox One/Kinect utilizes camera technology with a grid system that maps the playing area and immerses the participant in the game. The difference between the Kinect and the two other systems is that the participant is the controller. Once the system maps the playing area and identifies the player's, they become the interface. Along with the camera, the Xbox One/Kinect also uses gestures to begin the game and control it. Microsoft has introduced the Kinect for Windows, which allows for the sensor to be connected to a PC and gives flexibility to the system by not requiring the hardware of the console. The software development kit (SDK) is available. Changes associated with this new SDK most notably include the seated skeletal tracking now available. This tracking facilitates users who are sitting down, which is a feature that was missing from the earlier Kinect models, decreasing their flexibility. This is also now available in the newly introduced Xbox One. This mode focuses on tracking 10 joints of the upper body (head, shoulders, arms). Also added are new language settings to allow for regional language differences such as Australian English (Microsoft 2012).

The three commercial gaming platforms have the ability to now have a level playing field in terms of adaptation. The Kinect is no longer limited to having to use all four extremities to be successful. The Kinect, Wii, and Move are able to be activated in a seated posture without compromising the gaming experience. Many off-label modifications are also available. Options allow changing the controllers to single-switch designs and alternative positioning; for example, Wii bowling allows the Wiimote to be mounted on a hat, with a head/neck motion used to complete the bowling action and a single switch to release the ball.

Many of the off-the-shelf games allow individuals to participate in a modified position for success. In many cases those individuals that need the modifications prefer to utilize the off-the-shelf games as opposed to games specifically designed for people with disabilities. They want to play what everyone else does. It is for that reason it is important for healthcare providers to be creative in how they approach these modification challenges. The clients who we work with do not wish to be recognized for their limitation, but rather their ability to participate in games the same way as everyone else does. It is our responsibility to return them to their specific areas of interest and leisure for their self-esteem, emotional well-being, and recovery. Assistive technology allows them to participate in things that may have been thought gone forever. See Box 21.5.

Box 21.5 Case study

Jamie is a 24-year-old who was in an all-terrain vehicle (ATV) accident resulting in a C6-7 quadriplegia. He was riding out in a field and drove over a small sinkhole that threw him over the ATV landing on his head. Jamie was evacuated by emergency medical services to a regional trauma center where he was found to have a C6-7 incomplete fracture. Jamie is a college student who is a senior in biology and scheduled to graduate at the end of this final semester. He was on vacation in Colorado prior to beginning the semester. He lives in New York City and before the accident used primarily public transportation and his bike to get around. Jamie had worked for a bike delivery service to assist with his bills. Jamie is an outdoorsman and enjoys all of the related activities, including camping, hiking, shooting (not hunting), fishing, climbing, and mountain biking, and can be found in the mountains any chance he gets. In the city he enjoys the theater, concerts, going out with friends, and visiting new places.

Jamie has one younger sister who is 17 and parents who are divorced. Jamie lives with a roommate in a two-bedroom apartment in the city on the sixth floor of a building about six blocks from the school. His mother lives an hour from the city and is remarried and his father lives in Colorado where he was vacationing when the accident happened.

Medical course

Jamie was taken to surgery where his fracture was stabilized utilizing Harrington Rod fixation and he was put in a halo. Following surgery he was put into the intensive care unit for two days for observation and then moved to the orthopedic/neuro floor. While there he was able to use his non-dominant left upper extremity (UE) shoulder, elbow, wrist, and some finger flexion and extension musculature movements. On his right dominant side he demonstrates shoulder motion, elbow flexion, but not extension, and active wrist extension, which permits tenodesis, opposition of thumb to index finger, and some finger flexion.

He was moved to the acute care floor and therapists started working on gross movements and simple functional activities. Jamie was transferred from acute care to an inpatient rehabilitation facility where he spent four months recuperating and learning how to care for himself. He was extremely motivated and supported by his family. Jamie currently has a manual wheelchair and is independent in activities of daily living. He is able to drive independently with hand controls and independently able to transfer in and out of his car. He is preparing to complete his final semester in college and is living back in the city in the sixth floor apartment with his roommate. Jamie has worked hard get where he is and has done well with his rehabilitation. To his credit, he has displayed no signs of depression or anger.

Jamie is now ready to explore outdoor leisure opportunities and has been referred to you for assistance with adaptation and assistive technology to help with participation in successful leisure activities. He is open to any suggestions that will get him back to the outdoors and also biking (Figures 21.6 and 21.7).

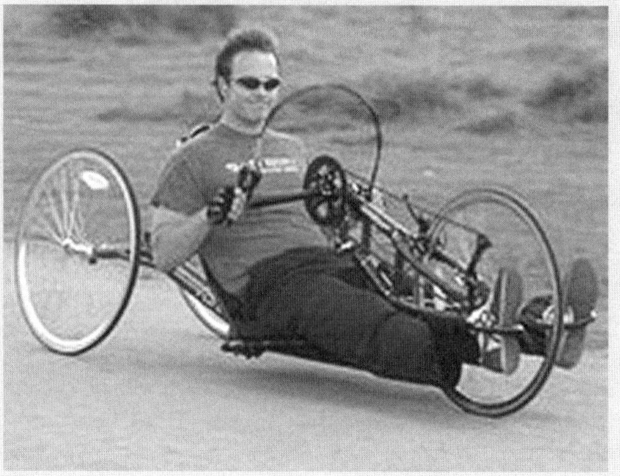

Figure 21.6 Handbike example. Source: David Hawgood (https://commons.wikimedia.org/wiki/File:Handcycle_in_Richmond_Park_-_geograph.org.uk_-_1315077.jpg). Licensed under CC BY SA 4.0.

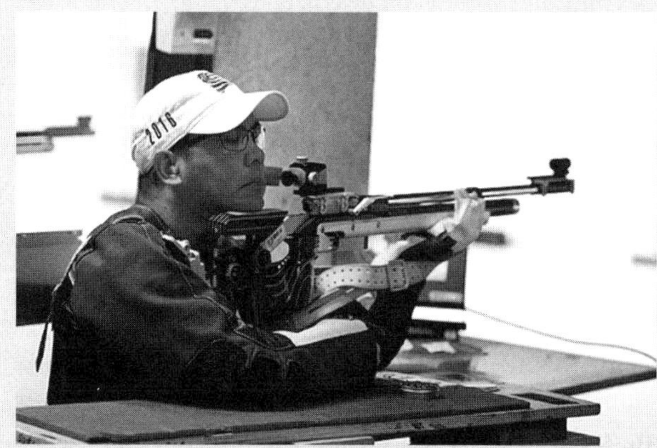

Figure 21.7 Adaptive target shooting. Source: Used with permission from www.NCHPAD.org.

Case study questions

1. What would you suggest for Jamie to begin exploring the area of leisure?
   Answer: Currently, there are a variety of activities he could do and in going to the mountains he would need some sort of off-road wheelchair. You can go a few different ways: large tires, three-wheeled hand bikes, or a power-based chair (although, if the battery dies then so does the ability to ambulate). A manual off-road wheelchair would probably be the best choice, and Jamie would want to work on conditioning and strengthening for the rigors of the

off-road environment. Alternatives could also be an off-road four-wheeled bike or, for level surfaces, a hand bike.

2. If Jamie wanted to target shoot, what recommendations would you make?
Answer: Jamie could employ a rest on his lap or wheelchair. Physically, he could shoot a rifle with little to no modification except for the stabilization of the right upper extremity, hence the recommendation for a rest. The weight of the firearm would also be factor to consider with regard to the necessity of the rest. Pulling a trigger should be accomplished with his left hand, so he may need to switch his opposition to establish his left as his dominant side. Alamo Four Star makes a tripod mount that could easily be used in any situation for hunting or target shooting.
3. Based on what you know about Jamie, are there any other suggestions that you could make regarding his leisure pursuits? Are there other ways Jamie can participate?
Answer: As mentioned earlier, he could begin to compete in off-road racing utilizing an off-road bike. He would also have the ability to use hand bikes, competitively or otherwise. The same is true of shooting as a sport; he can either participate for fun or as a competitor. Jamie's quality of life does not need to be compromised due to his injury. As he gains experience, he can also move to refereeing/judging in the various activities as well as participating. Jamie could also test equipment as well as write about his experiences in the outdoors. So there are various alternatives that could make it possible for him to participate in desired leisure activities.

Summary

Healthcare providers are responsible for an individual's healing, rehabilitation, and participation in leisure activities. The chapter illustrated various adaptations and interventions that enable those individuals who have an injury, illness, or disability to participate in a variety of leisure activities. As has been outlined in this chapter, leisure is such an important part of the human experience, for development, social interactions, learning, motivation, happiness, and success, to name just some of the issues addressed. By looking at the development of an individual across their life span, we can demonstrate the importance of leisure activities in a person's participation in and quality of life.

The chapter provides various assistive device references, which range from simple to complex. Many individuals choose to participate in leisure activities and it is the job healthcare providers to respect and support these choices. Leisure is a way in which we as individuals can express ourselves and who we are.

References

AbleGamers (2010). Disabled gamers' guide to the World of Warcraft. Retrieved from https://accessible.games/accessible-player-experiences/.

American Association of Health and Disability (n.d.). National Center on Health, Physical Activity and Disability (NCHPAD). Retrieved from www.aahd.us.

American Occupational Therapy Association (2014). Occupational therapy practice framework: domain and process. *American Journal of Occupational Therapy* 68: S1–S48.

Asher, I.E. (ed.) (2014). *Occupational Therapy Assessment Tools: An Annotated Index*, 4e. Bethesda, MY: AOTA Press.

Beard, J.G. and Ragheb, M.G. (1983). Measuring leisure motivation. *Journal of Leisure Research* 15 (3): 219–228. https://doi.org/10.1080/00222216.1983.11969557.

Bondoc, S., Powers, C., Herz, N., and Hermann, V. (2012). Virtual reality based rehabilitation. *OT Practice* 15: CE1–CE8.

Brown, Y.J. (2015). Disabled baseball programs. Retrieved from https://connectwithkids.com/tipsheet2015/2002/74_may29/baseball.html.

Burckhardt, C. and Anderson, K. (2003). The Quality of Life Scale (QUOLS): reliability, validity, and utilization. *Health and Quality of Life Outcomes* 1: 60. https://doi.org/10.1186/1477-7525-1-60.

Caldwell, L. (2005). Leisure and health: why is leisure therapeutic? *British Journal of Guidience and Counseling* 33: 7–26.

Campbell, P.M., Milbourne, S., and Wilcox, J. (2008). Adaptation interventions to promote participation in natural settings. *Infants and Young Children* 21 (2): 96–106.

Centers for Disease Control and Prevention (2018). Increasing physical activity among adults with disabilities. Retrieved from http://www.cdc.gov/ncbddd/disabilityandhealth/pa.html.

Columna, L., Davis, T., Lieberman, L., and Lytle, R. (2010). Determining the most appropriate physical education placement for students with disabilities. *Journal of Physical Education, Recreation & Dance (JOPERD)* 81 (7): 30–37.

Department of Health and Human Services, National Center for Chronic Disease Prevention and Health Promotion, Division of Adolescent and School Health (2009). Stepping up to promote healthy youth. Retrieved from http://www.cdc.gov/healthyyouth/stories/pdf/2009/success_09_ny.pdf.

Dictionary.com (n.d.). Leisure. Retrieved from https://www.dictionary.com/browse/at--leisure.

AbleGamers Foundation (n.d.). About AbleGamers. Retrieved from https://ablegamers.org/about-ablegamers/.

Elhakeem, A., Cooper, R., Bann, D., and Hardy, R. (2015). Childhood socioeconomic position and adult leisure-time physical activity: a systematic review. *International Journal of Behavioral Nutrition and Physical Activity* 12 (92): 10.1186/s12966-015-0250-0.

Erikson, E. (1959). *Psychological Issues*. New York: International Universities Press.

Ginsburg, K. (2007). The importance of play in promoting healthy child development and maintaining strong parent-child bonds. *Pediatrics* 119 (1): 182–191.

Hamilton-Smith, E. (1985). Can the arts really be leisure? *World Leisure & Recreation* 27 (4): 15–19. https://doi.org/10.1080/10261133.1985.10558892.

Hawkins, B.A., Ardovino, P., Rogers, N.B. et al. (1997). *Leisure Assessment Inventory*. Retrieved from https://www.idyllarbor.com/agora.cgi?p_id=A183&xm=on.

Hawkins, B.L., Cory, A.L., and Crowe, B.M. (2011). Effects of participation in a Paralympic military sports camp on injured service members: implications for therapeutic recreation. *Therapeutic Recreation Journal* 45 (4): 309–325.

Healthy People 2020 (n.d.-a). Evidence-based resource summary.

Healthy People 2020 (n.d.-b). Nutrition, physical activity, and obesity. Retrieved from: http://www.healthypeople.gov/2020/leading-health-indicators/2020-lhi-topics/Nutrition-Physical-Activity-and-Obesity.

Heyne, L., Wilkins, V., and Anderson, L. (2012). Social inclusion in the lunchroom and on the playground at school. *Social Advocacy and Systems Change Journal* 3: 54–68.

Hurd, A.R. and Anderson, D.M. (2011). *The Park and Recreation Professional's Handbook*. Champaign, IL: Human Kinetics.

Kielhofner, G. and Henry, A. (1988). Development and investigation of the Occupational Performance History Interview. *American Journal of Occupational Therapy* 42 (8): 489–498.

Krishnagari, S. and Southam, M. (2006). Leisure occupations. In: *Predretti's Occupational Therapy: Practice Skills for Physical Dysfunction*, 7e (ed. H.M. Pendleton and W. Schultz-Krohn), 412–426. St. Louis, MO: Elsevier.

Leitner, M. and Leitner, S.F. (2012). *Leisure in Later Life*, 4e. Urbana, IL: Sagamore.

Let's Move (n.d.). Get active. Retrieved from https://letsmove.obamawhitehouse.archives.gov/active-schools.

Livingston, G. (2019). The way U.S. teens spend their time is changing, but differences between boys and girls persist. Pew Research Center (20 February). Retrieved from https://pewrsr.ch/2GQ44jn.

Mee, J., Sumsion, T., and Craik, C. (2004). Mental health clients confirm the value of occupation in building competence and self-identity. *British Journal of Occupational Therapy* 67 (5): 225–233. https://doi.org/10.1177/030802260406700506.

Microsoft (2012). Kinect for Windows. Retrieved from https://support.xbox.com/en-US/xbox-on-windows/accessories/kinect-for-windows-setup.

Microsoft (2016). Windows Speech Recognition. Retrieved from https://support.microsoft.com/en-us/help/14213/windows-how-to-use-speech-recognition.

Mintel (n.d.). Young adult leisure trends. Retrieved from https://store.mintel.com/search#stq=Young+adult+leisure+trends&stp=1.

Nuance (2013). Dragon NaturallySpeaking. Retrieved from https://shop.nuance.com/store/nuanceus/custom/pbpage.resp-dragon-home-bf-2013-digital.

Rackley, J.W. (n.d.). Renegade Wheelchairs. Retrieved from http://www.alphaonenow.org/userfiles/Renegade_mediakit_10_23_2012.pdf.

Reid, D. and Hirji, T. (2004). The influence of a virtual reality leisure intervention program on the motivation of older adult stroke survivors: a pilot study. *Physical & Occupational Therapy in Geriatrics* 21 (4): 1–19.

Rimmer, J.H., Riley, B., Wang, E. et al. (2004). Physical activity participation among persons with disabilities: barriers and facilitators. *American Journal of Preventive Medicine* 26 (5): 419–425.

Robinson, E. and Walker, S. (2010). *Gaming on a Collision Course*. Harpers Ferry, WV: AbleGamers Foundation and 7–128 Software.

US Department of Veterans Affairs (n.d.). VA adaptive sports programs. Retrieved from https://www.blogs.va.gov/nvspse/.

Van Asselt, D., Buchanan, A., and Peterson, S. (2015). Enablers and barriers of social inclusion for young adults with intellectual disability: a multidimensional view. *Journal of Intellectual and Developmental Disability* 40 (1): 37–48. https://doi.org/10.3109/13668250.2014.994170.

Vaughn, L. (2010). Evaluation of play and leisure. In: *Occupational Therapy Essentials for Clinical Competence* (ed. K. Sladyk, K. Jacobs and N. MacRae), 135–150. Thorofare, NJ: Slack Inc.

Vicente, K. (2006). *The Human Factor: Revolutionizing the Way We Live with Technology*. New York: Routledge, Taylor & Francis Group.

Wang, D. and MacMillan, T. (2013). The benefits of gardening for older adults: a systematic review of the literature. *Activities, Adaptation & Aging* 37 (2): 153–181. https://doi.org/10.1080/01924788.2013.784942.

Wickham, J. (n.d.). VR and occupational therapy. Retrieved from http://www.jaclynwickham.com/itpthesis.

22

Physical factors focused on activities of daily living (ADLs) and electronic aids to daily living (EADLs)

Lynn Gitlow

Outline

Assistive Technologies and Environmental Interventions in Healthcare: An Integrated Approach, First Edition.
Edited by Lynn Gitlow and Kathleen Flecky.

Companion website: www.wiley.com/go/gitlow/assitivetechnologies

Learning outcomes

After reading this chapter, you should be able to:

1. Define activities of daily living (ADLs).
2. Describe Vicente's Human-Tech Ladder factors which impact the use of technology and environmental intervention (TEI) for ADLs.
3. List several assessment tools which, when used as part of a systematic evaluation, can be used to identify ADL difficulties.
4. List a variety of TEI for use by those with physical difficulties completing ADLs.
5. Provide a case study demonstrating the use of TEI for increasing independent function in ADLs.
6. List a variety of electronic aids to daily living (EADLs) available for those with physical access issues.

Active learning prompts

Before you read this chapter:

1. Describe your morning routine. Write down everything that you do for an hour after you wake up, noting how many times you make decisions, use your hands, and use creative ways to solve problems. What would happen if you could not use one of your hands to participate in your morning routine? What if you forgot what to do every day when you woke up? How would this impact the rest of your day?
2. Try to do your morning routine without bending your knees. How would this impact your ability to get in and out of bed? Use the bathroom and bathe?
3. Try to do your morning routine without the use of your hands? How would this impact your ability to get in and out of bed? Get around and in and out of your house?
4. Think of how your morning routine changes when you have houseguests or when you go away? How does that make you feel?

Key terms

Activities of daily living (ADLs).
Electronic aids to daily living (EADLs)
International Classification of Functioning, Disability and Health (ICF)
Self-care
ADL assessment tools

Introduction

It is reported that people spend two-thirds of their lives at home or engaged in activities of daily living (ADLs) (Module 9: Assistive technology to enhance independent living n.d.). "Most tasks of daily life are routine, requiring little thought or planning – things like bathing and dressing, brushing teeth, eating at the table, getting to work, meeting with friends, going to the theater. These are the daily activities that occupy most of our time and there are many of them" (Norman 1990, p.124).

Cynkin and Robinson (1990) describe these daily activities as those which make up the patterns of our lives. They undergird everything else that we do so that when our ADLs are disrupted this impacts everything else that we do in a day.

In this chapter we will discuss technology and environmental interventions (TEIs) that can be used to enable people to engage in everyday activities. Many of the options have been discussed in other chapters as well, such as the chapter on wheeled mobility and other mobility devices (Chapter 15), the chapter on cognitive interventions (Chapter 13), and more. But because ADLs are so important, this chapter will discuss options for enabling participation in these everyday tasks, particularly focusing on options for those who have physical problems.

Before starting to describe some of the devices that are categorized in this area, it is useful to return to our definitions of TEI. Remember that there is a full range of TEI options, from no-tech to high-tech, and we will give examples of a full range of ADL-related technologies in this chapter. For many of the options that we present here, once we write about them they may become obsolete, and they certainly may be by the time that you are reading this chapter, thus the author would like to emphasize the importance of the process of matching a person to a technology rather than forcing a technology to fit a person because we think it is cool or it's the latest new thing. Please refer to Chapter 2 and the case of Jake as an example of what happens when a technology and environmental intervention practitioner (TEIp) tries to force a technology to fit a person rather than starting out with a systematic evaluation. There will always be a cool new technology that will be available, but without doing a systematic theoretically guided evaluation that matches a person to TEI that is useful to them, no matter how exciting the technology may appear, it may not be useful without this evaluation. So please review Chapter 2 and remember to match the person to the technology that is right for them.

Human-tech ladder

Policy and legislation

The World Health Organization (WHO) and World Bank (2011) state that over 1 billion people report needing one or more assistive devices. Additionally, their World Report on Disability (2011) states that only 1 in 10 people have access to the assistive technology (AT) that they need. Certainly, the issue of access to AT is on international and national health policy agendas. While research exists supporting that users of AT require less caregiver support (Agree and Freedman 2003; Hoenig et al. 2003) and have decreased reported disability as a result of using AT (Spillman 2004), barriers to obtaining it are continually reported (WHO 2015).

When one investigates the types of assistive devices that people use to increase their participation in ADLs, it is difficult to find comprehensive statistics on their use. We suspect this goes back to the problems with understanding what AT really means and being able to investigate the need and use of all the devices that exist under this umbrella term of AT/TEI for ADL. Much of the data collected on AT use focuses on use of devices for mobility, hearing, and vision, and on prosthetic devices, thus data on the use of devices to improve performance in the area of ADL is difficult to find. It may be that mobility, hearing, and vision devices are needed for individuals to increase their independence in ADL, but studies are not designed in a way to elucidate these nuances. Research reporting AT use among those over 65 supports its efficacy in increasing one's ability to engage in ADLs. For example, a classic study on TEI for keeping elders functional Mann et al. (1999) revealed that AT and environmental modifications in participants' homes could slow their age-related decline, decrease caregiver costs, and decrease institutionalization.

The World Report on Disability recommends, "Increase access to assistive technology that is appropriate, sustainable, affordable, and accessible," given the barriers it identifies to both rehabilitation services and access to assistive technologies (WHO and World Bank 2011, p. 123). This report makes a variety of recommendations regarding how governments should proceed in addressing these access problems. Recommendations include reforming laws, policies, and delivery systems. In addition to recommendations regarding access to AT, this report also highlights the importance of promoting enabling environments to increase participation of people with disabilities in society. As previously mentioned, in the current and future landscape of health and wellness, and supported by our conceptual practice models, one cannot separate AT and the environment, thus our use of the term of TEI. The World Report on Disability recommends "creating a culture of accessibility" through effective law enforcement and regulations as well as enforcement of these regulations (WHO and World Bank 2011, p 193).

HealthyPeople 2020 also has an objective related to increasing access to TEI in order to "Reduce the proportion of people with disabilities who report barriers to obtaining the assistive devices, service animals, technology services, and accessible technologies that they need" (HealthyPeople.gov 2016). However, this objective has been archived at the time of this writing due to lack of supporting data. A paucity of supporting data has been identified throughout the text as an issue in the area of justifying TEI initiatives. The lack of research and outcomes data is a critical barrier to getting people the TEI that they need, along with a host of other factors.

Funding issues always are barriers to getting people the AT that they need, and this issue is more explicitly discussed in Chapter 4. Suffice it to say that getting AT and mainstream technologies into the hands of the people who need it to increase their participation in ADL remains a barrier that needs to be addresses at the policy and legislation level of the Human-Tech Ladder (WHO 2015).

Equally as important is lack of awareness of what exists to help people increase their independence in ADL. The WHO recognizes this problem and calls for policy development to overcome this issue through a variety of measures, including increasing practitioners who can provide TEI services to those who need them and adequate provision of devices to those in need (World Health Organization 2017).

All of these issues are among those that have policies implications. We cannot emphasize here strongly enough how important demonstrating the outcomes of TEI interventions is for advancing understanding and support of the need for these interventions at a policy and legislative level.

Definitions

There are many definitions of ADLs and we will mention several definitions and categorization schemes here to hone in on what we will cover in this chapter. The Medical Dictionary for Health Professions and Nursing defines ADLs as "Everyday routines generally involving functional mobility and personal care, such as bathing, dressing, toileting, and meal preparation (activities of daily living)" (Farlex Partner Medical Dictionary 2012). The Occupational Therapy Practice Framework, which guides the scope and practice of occupational therapy (OT) practitioners, defines ADLs as "activities oriented towards taking care of one's own body" (AOTA 2014, p. S16). These activities include (i) bathing and showering; (ii) toileting and toilet hygiene; (iii) dressing; (iv) swallowing and eating; (v) feeding; (vi) functional mobility; (vii) personal device care, and (viii) sexual activity (AOTA 2014).

According to the Abledata website, technology products for ADLs include those which assist a person in:

> Bathing, Carrying, Child Care, Clothing, Dispenser Aids, Dressing, Drinking, Feeding, Grooming/Hygiene, Handle Padding, Health Care, Holding, Reaching, Time, Smoking, Toileting, Transfer.
>
> (Abledata.com n.d.)

As you can see, there are many areas identified under the umbrella of TEI for ADL. Moreover, many devices that we might consider in other categories can improve one's ability in the use of ADL as well, such as mobility devices, devices for vision, and hearing and cognitive aids. Since those have been discussed in other chapters, we will try to focus on ones that have not yet been discussed elsewhere in the book. For the purposes of this book, we shall present information on TEI as presented in the ADL section of the International Classification of Functioning, Disability and Health (ICF) Browser (n.d.). This includes, "TEI for SELF CARE d510 Washing oneself (bathing, drying, washing hands, etc.) d520 Caring for body parts (brushing teeth, shaving, grooming, etc.) d530 Toileting d540 Dressing d550 Eating d560 Drinking d570 Looking after one's health" (ICF Browser n.d.).

While most of the chapter will focus on TEI for ADLs, the end of the chapter will conclude with electronic aids to daily living (EADLs). These devices, once called environmental control units (ECUs), provide alternative access to electronic devices in the home that are routinely used, such as light switches, TV controls, bed controls, and door openers (Oddo 2010). We add them to this chapter because those who have ADL difficulties resulting from body structure and function problems are likely to need assistance with these objects in their environments as well. Based on our conceptual practice models, we must consider the environment when evaluating a person for TEI intervention (Erikson et al. 2004). Please see Chapter 2 for a more in-depth discussion of conceptual practice models.

Organizational level

There has been much attention given in other chapters to the influence that organizational setting has on the provision of TEI. Funding and focus on what equipment is considered as relevant is certainly dictated by organizational purpose, and we refer you to the chapters that discuss these issues in more detail (Chapters 4, 6, 7, and 8). However, we would like to emphasize one issue here that needs to be considered by all TEIp, and that is the issue of providing ethical practice guided by professional standards for practice.

According to the code of ethics of the Rehabilitation Engineering and Assistive Technology Society of North America (RESNA), it is the clinician's responsibility, among other things, to "Hold paramount the welfare of persons served professionally" and "Inform and educate the public on rehabilitation/assistive technology and its applications" (RESNA n.d.-a).

Additionally, the Standards of Practice state "Individuals shall inform the consumer about all device options and funding mechanisms available regardless of finances, in the development of recommendations for assistive technology strategies" (RESNA n.d.-b).

Organizational pressures may try to influence the TEIp to be cost conscious and encourage them to minimize TEI recommendations. Likewise, a practitioner who knows that a client has limited income or access to funds may hesitate to recommend costly TEI to that client. The caveat here is to make the recommendation based on a theoretically systematically guided evaluation supported by best practice regardless of organizational pressures or what you think a client might be able to afford. In most cases, people find the support that they need to get the TEI that they feel will increase their participation in everyday activities. The key, of course, is that the client believes that the AT will make a difference for him or her (Wielandt et al. 2006).

While finances are barriers to getting AT and this has often been cited in the literature, the TEIp is still encouraged to discuss the best options and alternatives to these options with their clients regardless of pressures that may be exerted from organizational influences. As reported in the literature, the most frequent source of payment for AT is the client himself or herself

(Carlson et al. 2002). For more detailed information on funding in different environments, please refer to the information in Chapter 4 on funding.

Team considerations

As mentioned in Chapters 9 and 10, the provision of TEI is a team sport. Regardless of where the client is (home, school, etc.), when decisions are made to recommend TEI for increasing participation in ADL a number of practitioners may be involved. For example, in a home setting the nurse may be the first person to see the client and home and recognize that the person has TEI-related needs. The nurse may then recommend that the OT or physical therapist (PT) come in and assess the client's need for AT. The physician may then need to document the medical necessity for the recommendations (Federici et al. 2012). Similarly, in a school setting the students may need AT to assist with eating lunch or putting on gym clothes, and those involved in these activities may all be involved in the TEI recommendations and service necessary to evaluate and train students in their use (QIAT Leadership Team 2015).

Psychological level

ADLs are very culturally embedded activities, as are the tools used to carry out these activities (Chang et al. 2006). The reader is referred to chapter on psychosocial influences of TEI decisions (Chapter 11) for a reminder of the importance of this level of consideration. An excellent example of how culture influences everyday ADLs is an article describing the making of tea by Deborah Hannam (1997) entitled "More than a cup of tea: meaning construction in an everyday occupation." Making sure to understand the meaning of ADLs when doing your evaluation is critical to matching a person to TEI that will be successful for that person. Using both quantitative and qualitative assessments can be helpful in getting a full picture of this meaning (Ahluwalia et al. 2010; Scherer 2005). Positive psychological outcomes have been reported in the literature from users who have increased their independence and competence in performing ADLs. For example, in a study conducted by Kumar and Phillips (2013), participants reported increased independence and confidence in self-feeding after using a mobile arm support. Negative psychosocial effects were reported as well in this same study, including that clients felt as though the equipment signaled that they had disabilities. It is important to remember to consider that the psychosocial impact of TEI use on a user can be both positive and negative, and these factors have an impact on whether or not the client will use the recommended TEI (Scherer 2005).

All of the cognitive considerations discussed in the chapter on cognition (Chapter 13) must be considered as well when recommending a TEI for increasing participation in ADLs. See Box 22.1 for a case study.

Box 22.1 Case study: Miguel

Miguel is a six-year-old boy who has cerebral palsy. The author met him while working in Ecuador with members of the Community Inclusion Through Technology, International (CITTI) project team (http://www.cittiproject.org). While observing Miguel at school, members of the project team noticed that he was not able to hold a utensil and feed himself. We fabricated a low-tech tool to enable him to do this task. The team provided Miguel with the adaptation and tried to show him how to use it, but he would have none of it. He constantly threw the adaptation on the floor. One day when the team came to work they noticed that Miguel was eating lunch and that his father was feeding him. After a discussion with his family and in-country team, our team found out that the family came every day to feed their son. This was a part of their family ritual time and Miguel feeding himself independently was not something that he or the family was interested in doing. They wanted Miguel to be able to communicate and increase his independence in walking. The CITTI project team learned a valuable lesson from this case. As we have mentioned over and over in this book, first find out what the client and caregivers want to do with TEI and then proceed from that point. Do not try to impose a technology on a client.

Physical level

There are many reasons that people use TEI to participate in ADLs. In 2014, the National Center for Health Statistics (CDC) (2016) reported that over 70 million non-institutionalized persons in the United States have "at least one basic action difficulty." As mentioned above, definitions are difficult to compare and understand in this area, and what the causes for these difficulties are remains undefined; however, there is a high incidence of people needing help with basic ADLs. The predicted global increase in chronic health conditions such as diabetes, cardiovascular disease, cancer, and mental health disorders (WHO and World Bank 2011) will inevitably impact the number of people who will have difficulty in carrying out ADLs. Please see Box 22.2 for a study which investigates the impact of using technology assistance to carry out ADLs. These chronic illnesses and other related causes of disability might be accompanied by body structure and function problems such as decreased strength, decreased range of motion (ROM),

Box 22.2 Here's the evidence

Hoenig, H., Taylor, D.H., and Sloan, F.A. (2003). Does assistive technology substitute for personal assistance among the disabled elderly? *American Journal of Public Health* 93(2): 330–337.

Key Words: technological assistance, personal assistance, ADL limitations

Purpose: To investigate if the use of technology assistance used by elders with limitations in ADLs is associated with fewer hours of assistance provided by other personal assistants.

Sample/Setting: Sample consisted of 2683 people who had one or more ADL limitations drawn from respondents to the 1994 National Long-Term Care Survey.

Method: Survey design.

Findings: For those with ADL limitations there was a consistent relationship between assistive technology and personal assistance indicating fewer hours of help when technological assistance was used.

Critical Thinking Questions:

1. After reading this research article, what do you understand to be the limitations of this research? Are there any limitations not stated?
2. If you were to replicate this study using a different method or design, what designs would you use to increase the rigor and why?
3. Based on the findings of this study, what additional research is needed that is not addressed in the discussion section?

decreased endurance, and fine motor complications. For example, weakness, low endurance and fatigue, limited ROM, lack of coordination and poor dexterity, loss of use of one side of the body or one upper extremity, lower-extremity amputation with prosthesis, limited vision, decreased sensation and pain including low back pain, and bariatrics are reasons that have been presented by Radomski and Trombly (2014) to discuss ADL solutions for clients. Other texts include paraplegia and quadriplegia/ tetraplegia in this groups of diagnoses (Pendleton McHugh and Schultz-Krohn 2013) when discussing TEI solutions for those who have ADL limitations. Literature has described the use of technology for ADLs to increase independence for those with scleroderma and leprosy, among other diagnoses (Maia et al. 2016; Sandqvist et al. 2004). Additionally, many diagnosis-related websites will catalog products that can be useful to help with everyday living. For example, the Arthritis Foundation (n.d.) has an Ease of Use section devoted to describing products that are easy for those who have arthritis symptoms such as pain and weakness or other physical limitations to use to increase or maintain their independence in everyday life activities. Similarly, the National MS Society (n.d.) has a section of its website devoted to describing tools that will enable you to continue to the everyday things of life. More of these resources will be listed in the Toolbox at the end of the chapter.

For the purposes of this text, we will describe TEI for ADLs using the ICF activities categories, presenting examples of TEI solutions along the continuum of possibilities that exist. These include Self-care: Washing oneself (bathing, drying, washing hands, etc.); Caring for body parts (brushing teeth, shaving, grooming, etc.); Toileting; Dressing; Eating; Drinking; and Looking after one's health (ICF Browser n.d.). Additionally, we will include some information on electronic aids to daily living (EADL), which provide access to the environment in the home as well. Again, the reason that this information is included in this chapter is that our conceptual practice models tell us to consider the person within their environment, and it is likely that those with body structure and function problems are likely to need environmental interventions as well.

Evaluation and assessment tools

Once you have chosen your conceptual practice model to guide your evaluation and have identified the clients' barriers to ADL performance, a variety of assessment tools can be used to further assess these barriers. Numerous resources are available for the clinician to use when looking at assessment tools to use when working with someone who has ADL problems. One is the Rehabilitation Measures Database available online at http://www.rehabmeasures.org/default.aspx. Using the search function to search for ADL brings up information and references to a number of assessment tools that can be useful for identifying a client's ADL needs.

The following list of assessment tools were listed at this Functional Assessment Tool website (http://docplayer.net/4799216-International-encyclopedia-of-rehabilitation.html).

Some of the assessment tools are listed below in Table 22.1.

The WHO Disability Assessment Schedule 2.0 has a section which looks at Self-care – hygiene, dressing, eating & staying alone – and is available online at http://www.who.int/classifications/icf/whodasii/en.

Table 22.1 ADL Assessment Tools.

ADLs	Barthel Index (Mahoney and Barthel 1965) FIM™ Instrument (Guide for the Uniform Data Set for Medical Rehabilitation 1997) Katz Index (Katz et al. 1963) LIFEware℠ System (Baker et al. 1997)

There are numerous standardized assessment tools that can be used to identify an individual's ADL status, and more references will be listed in the Toolbox at the end of the chapter.

TEI for ADLs

This next section of the chapter will discuss TEI for options for the activities identified above as ADL according to the ICF. Table 22.2 lists the ICF breakdown of the activities of washing oneself and caring for body parts.

Bathing and washing

Numerous no-tech to high-tech options are available to enable a person to increase either participation in bathing and washing or caring for their body parts. One may wash oneself in a variety of settings, including in the sink, in a shower, in a bath, in a pond, etc., depending on one's context, and as we mentioned above, culture as well as context will greatly impact how one participates in the ADLs. We will present the material in this section of the chapter using a case study (Box 22.3). The case study is presented first, followed by a full range of options from no-tech to high-tech that one can consider to increase participation in these activities. Then we will describe the solutions that were used in the case study. Feel free to use this case study to challenge yourselves to come up with answers before seeing what happened.

Table 22.2 From the ICF Self-Care Chapter.

d510 Washing oneself
d5100 Washing body parts
d5101 Washing whole body
d5102 Drying oneself
d5108 Washing oneself, other specified
d5109 Washing oneself, unspecified
d520 Caring for body parts
d5200 Caring for skin
d5201 Caring for teeth
d5202 Caring for hair
d5203 Caring for fingernails
d5204 Caring for toenails
d5208 Caring for body parts, other specified
d5209 Caring for body parts, unspecified

Source: http://apps.who.int/classifications/icfbrowser with permission of the WHO.

Box 22.3 Case study: Lauren

Lauren is an 87-year-old obese woman with multiple chronic disabilities, including obesity and arthritis, which results in pain and decreased joint ROM and decreased strength. She is seen at an outpatient clinic where she states that she is most interested in improving her balance and overall strength to be able to engage in activities at home, such as feeding her cat and getting her coal to heat her house. She uses a walker or two canes for mobility.

She lives alone but will not allow therapists to come to her house for a home evaluation to assess the tasks she is asking for help with: feeding the cat and doing the coal. She states that she is independent in all self-care tasks and has no problems with feeding and cooking. After several visits to the clinic, seeing a variety of providers, a team conference reveals that several providers, including massage, OT, and the physician, have noticed that Lauren has a persistent body odor which leads them to wonder about her ability to carry out self-care tasks. They ask the OT to investigate more in depth what is going on with Lauren in the area of self-care. The therapist explains the situation to Lauren, and she agrees to participate in a more thorough assessment of her self-care abilities.

After completing relevant sections of the Klein Bell Activities of Daily Living Scale, (Klein and Bell 1982), a standardized ADL assessment focusing on self-care, the OT finds out that Lauren does have some issues with self-care tasks. Most importantly, the OT finds out during a conversation she has with Lauren while completing the assessment that she does not have hot water at her house and does not bathe at home. She only bathes when she goes to the YMCA, and since the weather has been inclement she has not been going to the Y to bathe. Moreover, when she does go to the Y, she reports having difficulty juggling all the things she needs "to do my bathing." She states, "I can't hold the soap and wash and I have a hard time reaching everything I need to wash."

When discussed her issues bathing at home she stated that while she does have water, her hot water heater is out of order and she does not have the funds to replace it at this time. She also said that she stores household items in her shower and, since she does not have hot water, does not plan on using it anyway. The same issues around reaching body parts and organizing bathing equipment exist at home as well. She is able to dress herself, including putting on her shoes and socks, and has no problems with dental care. She does have a problem brushing the back of her hair and states that when she cannot get to the gym she uses dry shampoo. The Klein Bell assessment also reveals that she has some difficulty with toileting, including wiping herself when she urinates and has a bowel movement.

While Lauren has decreased strength and ROM throughout her body, she is able to manipulate items and has functional fine motor coordination. She is not able to stand for long periods of time due to balance and strength problems, and she needs rails around a chair to be able to go from a sitting position to a standing position.

Next we will present a variety of low- to high-tech options available to help Lauren with her bathing and toileting needs, and then we will present the conclusion to the case study with the solutions that she ultimately used. As mentioned above, while there are many options to increase one's independence in the area of bathing, barriers exist to their use (Naik and Gill 2005).

Bathing

Applying soap

At the no-tech end of the spectrum are devices that can be used by someone who may have limited strength and ROM or other issues. These include the bathing mitt or soap on a rope. These no-tech devices can easily be made. Pump-style soap dispensers are available as well. Soap and other liquid dispensers can be mounted in a shower or close to a sink, so the user does not need to manipulate or hold a piece of soap (see Figure Figure 22.1).

There are also long-handled devices for those who have limited ROM, such as the long-handled sponge (see Figure 22.2).

Stationary washing devices may be placed on the floor or wall of a bathroom or shower to help a person wash body parts they cannot reach (see Figure 22.3).

Some medium-tech devices that might be used for washing are battery-operated soap dispensers and battery-operated scrub brushes. These may be useful for those with limited strength and ROM.

At the high-tech end of the spectrum, work is beginning on robots that will be able to bathe people. Cody the robotic nurse assistant developed at the Georgia Tech Healthcare robotics lab is an example of

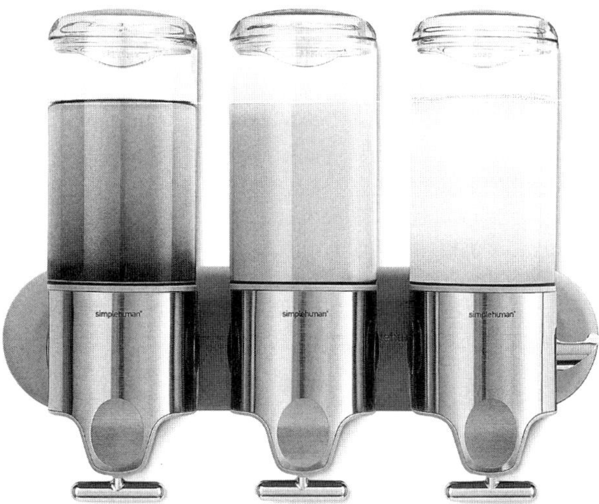

Figure 22.1 Pump-style soap dispenser. Source: Courtesy of Simplehuman.

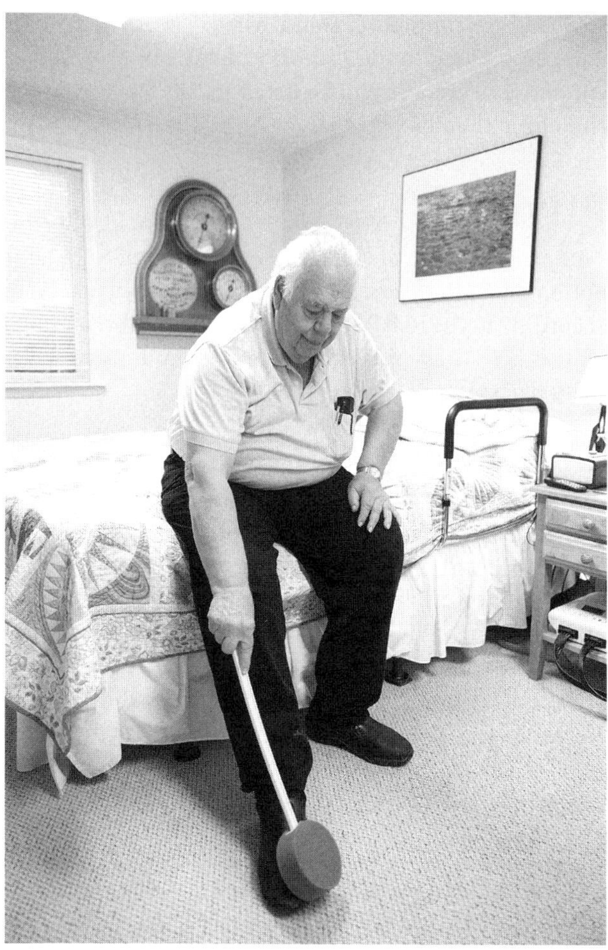

Figure 22.2 The soaper sponge. Source: Reproduced with permission of North Coast Medical, Inc.

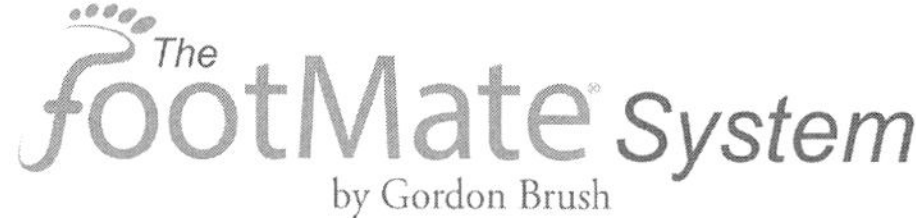

your feet will
LOVE YOU!...

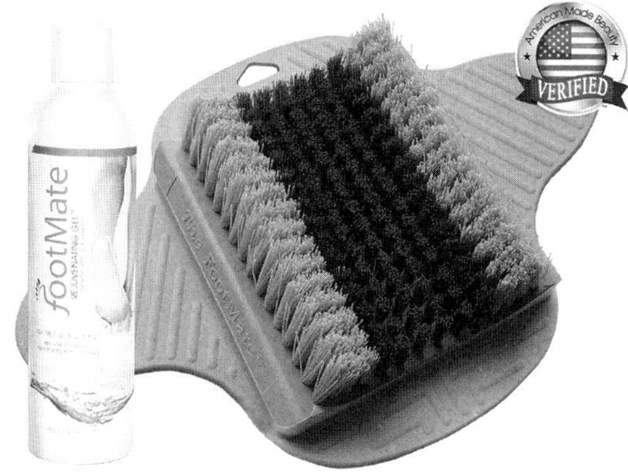

Figure 22.3 The footmate system. Source: Courtesy of Gordon Brush Mfg Co.

what may be possible in the future for bathing options (Bogue 2013; Park 2016). Other robotic options for bathing are under development or available for research as well (Bedaf et al. 2015).

Water for bathing

Next we will consider water delivery for bathing. As mentioned above, there are many different environments in which one can bathe, such as at a sink, in a shower or tub, or even in a pond.

There are many types of faucets for sinks and showers. There are the basic ones that you turn on and off yourself. Lever or paddle style handles are more accessible than the standard ones and have been recommended as universally designed features to make life easier. One-handed faucets reduce the need to use two hands to regulate water temperature and can be useful for making faucets more accessible. There are also devices that can turn a two-handled faucet into a one-handed device (Figure 22.4).

Spray hoses can be added to faucets to increase their reach for someone who has limited ROM (see Figure 22.5). These can be used in both the sink and the shower where there are many options for extending the reach of the showerhead.

There are a variety of shower spray configurations that may be helpful for someone who needs to remain seated and has limited ROM. Shower spray tiles can be placed throughout the shower or shower panels with jets

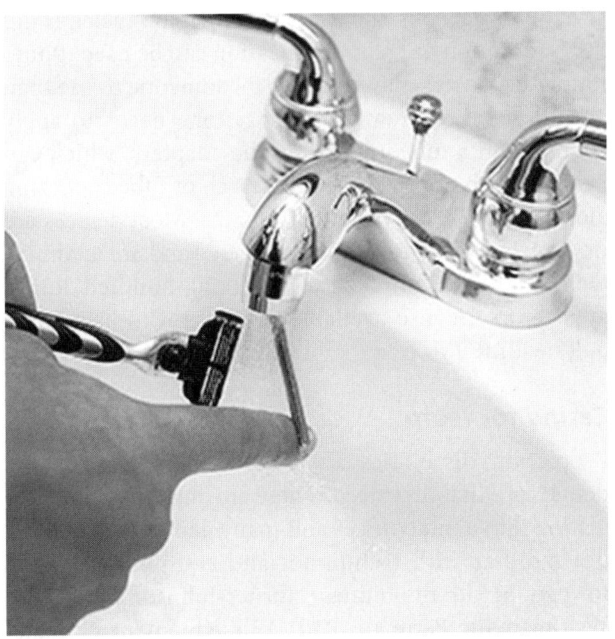

Figure 22.4 INSTANT-OFF. Source: Reproduced with permission of INSTANT-OFF.

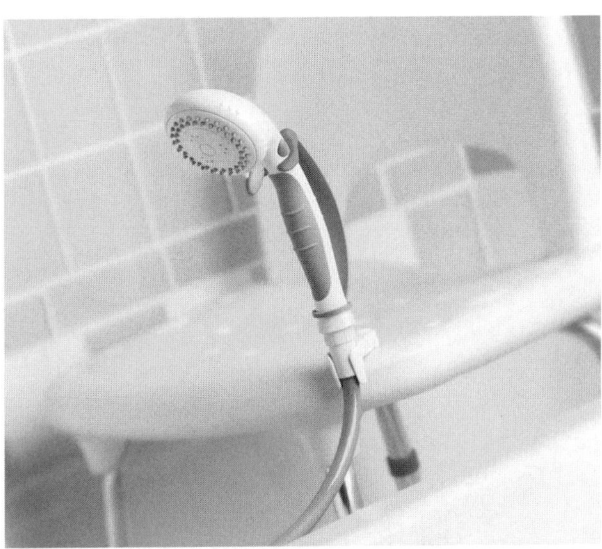

Figure 22.5 Handheld shower head with pause control. Source: Reproduced with permission of North Coast Medical, Inc.

are also available. There are also adjustable-height sinks for those with balance or ROM problems.

Tubs and showers

Grab bars and tub rails are low-tech devices that can help someone get in and out of the tub or shower. There are many styles and types available, and research exists that reports preferences and effectiveness of grab bar placement for a variety of users (Guitard et al. 2011). Additionally, some researchers have found that adding auditory cues to supplement grab bar use can increase their utility in certain populations (Guitard et al. 2012).

Non-skid surfaces on the bottom of showers and bathtubs and on bathroom floors are helpful in creating a safer environment for bathing (Korp et al. 2012). Additionally, shower and bath chairs, along with additional transfer supports, can help someone with a variety of problems to get in and of and remain in a bath or shower. Some shower chairs are presented in Chapter 16, so we will not discuss them here. Do remember, given the numerous chairs that are available, that the choice of a shower chair involves matching a person with the correct chair. Balance, trunk stability, ROM, and many other factors need to be considered when choosing a shower chair for a bathtub or shower situation (Gill et al. 2007).

At the next level of the tech spectrum are devices that can lower and raise a person into a tub, such as water- or air-operated lifts. There are also floor-mounted and ceiling lifts (Bonecutter 2014).

There are do-it-yourself (DIY) or commercially available portable temporary showers, which can be set up in a variety of locations in one's house for bathing. See Figure 22.6 for an example.

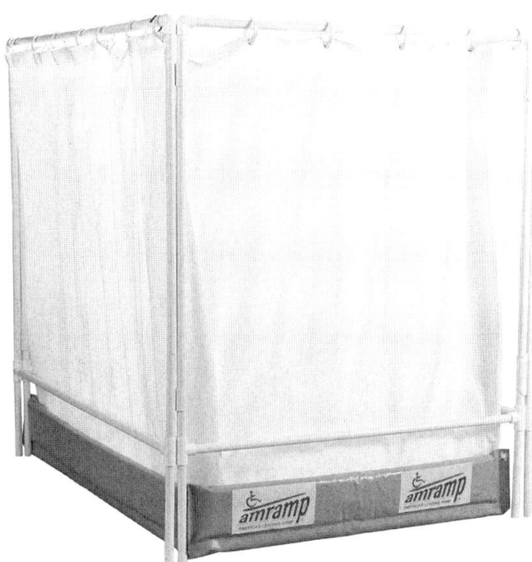

Figure 22.6 The Amramp shower. Source: Courtesy of Amramp.

Finally there are a variety of bathtubs on the market for accommodating people with a variety of needs. These include walk-in tubs or tubs with sides that move.

In Chapter 16 there are a number of examples of shower and tub seats. Please refer to that chapter for this information. Additionally, Chapter 8 has information on grab bars and alternative bathroom configurations for showers as well.

Drying

After washing, one must dry off. At the no-tech end of the spectrum there are various toweling options, including a large bath towel that can be used for someone who has ROM limitations. Loops or pockets can be attached to towels so a person with limited hand strength can use these adaptations to secure the towel rather than having to grasp onto the end of it. Towel mitts and towel capes are also options. If toweling is not an option, at the higher end of the tech spectrum body dryers are available. An example of a body dryer can be seen in Figure 22.7. One is the Apres Body dryer (http://www.wetroomsdirect.net/apres-body-dryer.html) and another is the Tornado Body dryer (http://www.tornadobodydryer.com/photosreviews.html).

We have discussed washing feet above and will discuss washing the perineal area when we discuss toileting options.

Caring for skin

Applying lotion or cream to one's body may also be challenging. There are many reasons that one may want to apply cream or lotion to one's body or face, from beauty regimens to prescription application. There are several no-tech options for making that job easier. Hand mitts for lotion or cream application can be used. Pump lotion dispensers may be easier for someone to use than a bottle with a screw top. Also, if one needs to apply cream from a tube, there are tube adapters, which can make the job easier. A Google search of tube squeezing aids reveals a great variety of options. Most devices are no-tech but some are motion activated and are medium-tech as they require batteries. Long-handled lotion applicators are also available for those who have difficulty with ROM.

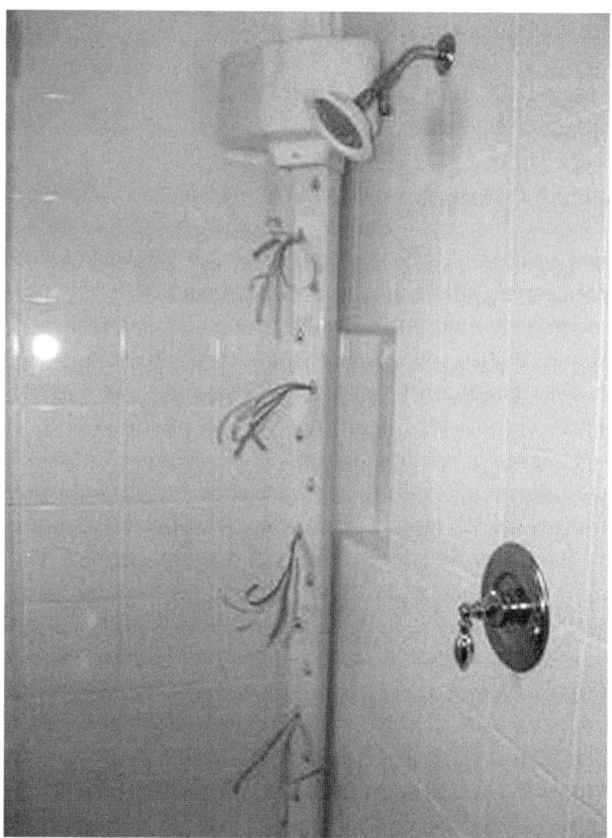

Figure 22.7 Tornado body dryer. Source: Reproduced with permission of Tornado Body Dryer.

Caring for teeth

People with disabilities face many barriers to getting the dental care that they need. There are physical barriers to getting into dental offices and many dental practices are not familiar with techniques and equipment needed for people with disabilities (Horner-Johnson et al. 2015; Waldman and Perlman 2010). While the issue of dental care for people with disabilities is beyond the scope of this chapter, some problems that people with disabilities may have when caring for their teeth include cognitive, sensory, and physical issues. Primarily we will provide some TEI solutions for those with physical disabilities here, but we will also present on a higher-tech solutions that may be useful for those with cognitive disabilities as well. Adapted handles can be attached to the brush handle to make it easier to hold. Tooth brushes with toothpaste beads already on them can be an option for those who may have difficulty getting toothpaste onto the brush. Alternative toothpaste dispensers can be helpful as well. Tube adapters, as mentioned above in the lotion application section, are options for toothpaste tubes as well. A higher-tech option is an electric toothbrush. There are also smart electric toothbrushes with apps that can provide information about how long you have brushed and how effectively you have brushed (https://oralb.com/en-us/products/genius-8000-electric-toothbrush-with-bluetooth). These are useful for those with a cognitive disability and have been used by caregivers to monitor and provide feedback to a person with a cognitive disability on how much more or less time to spend on this task (Dr. Amy Gerney, personal communication).

Finally, there are flossing options. For example, you can make a floss loop for one-handed flossing or there are flossing devices available.

Hair care options

Many options are available for hair care as well. Dry shampoo or alternative shampoo dispensers are available. If one has difficulty with ROM, there are long-handled options for brushing and combing hair, which can be fabricated or purchased. Different-sized handles can also be an option. A universal cuff can be used to hold a brush or comb if someone has issues with holding onto a brush handle. Hairdryer stands are commercially available, or one could make one's own stand out of a variety of materials. The Instructables (www.instructables.com/) and Pinterest (www.pinterest.com) websites are great places to find ideas for these sorts of DIY options.

Before we end this section, it is important to mention the role that robotics is beginning to fill in this area. We have mentioned some caregiving robots above. There are those that are dedicated to a specific function, such as a hair-washing robot and a bathing robot (Park et al. 2016), but there are also multipurpose robots under development, mentioned in the feeding section of this chapter, that can be used to brush your teeth, shave you, scratch your head, or provide other assistance in the area of ADL (Hawkins et al. 2014).

Caring for fingernails and toenails

Taking care of nails may be an issue for those who have disabilities (Evans et al. 2015). It becomes difficult to cut toenails as one ages due to loss of strength and ROM (Longevity Explorers n.d.). Poor toenail care may be partially responsible for falls in elders (Rokkaku and Kaneko 2012). In this section we will present some AT options for those who have decreased ROM and strength when it comes to nail care. Nailbrushes with suction cups that hold them in place may be useful for one-handed people or those with decreased strength. There are a variety of long-handled toenail clippers that can be used by those who cannot reach, and there are super strong clippers for people who have nails that are hard to cut. Another option would be to obtain a manicure and or pedicure. If these options do not work, referral to a podiatrist for foot care may be the best option. See Box 22.4 to revisit the case study on Lauren.

Box 22.4 Case study: Lauren revisited

Before we go on with other self-care options, let us return to our case study and apply some of the options from the above sections.

The first part of the self-care spectrum talked about with Lauren was "juggling all of the items I need to do my bathing." A net bag was decided upon so that Lauren could gather her tools in it and take it to the kitchen sink in her house or to the gym when she when to shower there.

Next, we trialed several options for the soaping and washing part of the task. First we trialed a long-handled brush, which worked well to reach parts of Lauren's body that she could not reach; however, attempting to apply the soap to it did not produce satisfactory results. The solution that Lauren liked the best was soaping up a long towel that had loops on the end of it for holding and then using that to wash her body. A similar long towel with loops on the ends for easy holding was used for drying her body as well. She had two sets of washing and drying towels, one that she used at home and one that she used at the gym. The ones for home were shorter than the gym ones because she washed at the kitchen sink rather than in the shower. When she washed in the kitchen sink she used an electric tea kettle to heat water, which she then added to the sink water. She also used a stool to sit on at the sink for balance. In the gym she used the accessible shower, which had a bench for sitting and a long-handed shower hose, which moved so she could remove it to wet and rinse herself. We will discuss her toileting solutions in the next section of the chapter.

Toileting

In this section of the chapter we will discuss TEI solutions for toileting. Other chapters have discussed accessible bathrooms, grab bars around toilets, and toilet heights and devices that can be used to elevate the toilet. Much of the literature regarding toileting problems for those with disabilities relates to positioning and lifting issues that interfere with independent toileting. In this section we will discuss options that may be used to help people maintain independence in toileting hygiene. For urinating and defecating there are number of medical products which are available, such as urinals, both male and female, diapers, catheters, and rectal stimulators, that are beyond the scope of this chapter but are useful items for people who have trouble with regulating urination and defecation. In this section we will discuss options for cleaning oneself after urinating or defecating. Table 22.3 lists the ICF breakdown of the activities of toileting.

At the no-tech end of the spectrum there are a variety of long-handled devices that can be used for someone who has ROM problems in this area (see Figure 22.8 for an example).

Table 22.3 From the ICF Self-Care Chapter – Washing Oneself and Caring for Body Parts.

d530 Toileting
d5300 Regulating urination
d5301 Regulating defecation
d5302 Menstrual care
d5308 Toileting, other specified
d5309 Toileting, unspecified

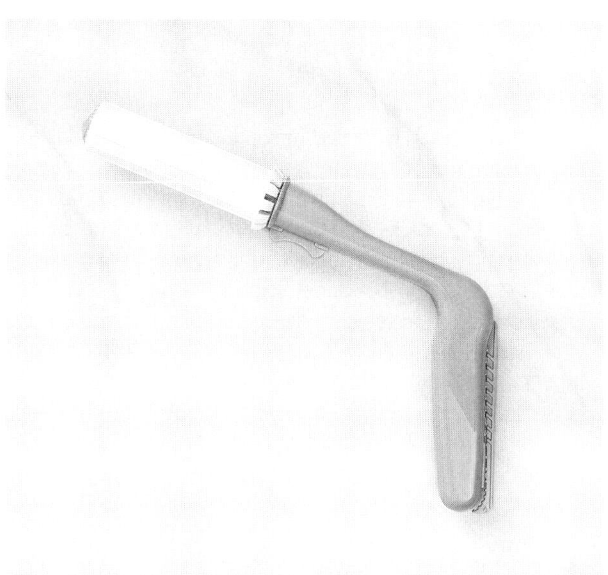

Figure 22.8 Self wipe bathroom aid. Source: Reproduced with permission of North Coast Medical, Inc.

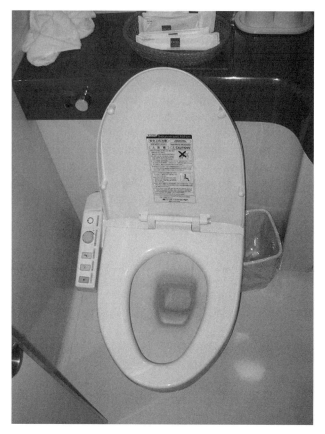

Figure 22.9 Lascar electronic bidet. Source: https://commons.wikimedia.org/wiki/File:Lascar_Electronic_Washlet_(Bidet_toilet)_(1298846095).jpg. Licensed under CC BY 2.0.

For persons with limited hand strength, for example, a strap or universal cuff can be adapted to a handle for toilet hygiene. Next there are handheld bidets, which can be attached to a sink and use a stream of water for toilet hygiene. There are also a variety of other bidet options which can be put on the toilet or built into the toilet or the toilet seat that provide water and even air for washing and drying the perineal area (Figure 22.9).

In a recent pilot study investigating 15 post-stroke clients who used technology assisted toilets (TATs) (defined as those which cleaned the user with a stream of water) results indicated that the TATs "provided adequate toileting hygiene and enhanced participants' quality of life compared with standard toileting" (Yachnin et al. 2015, p. e32).

For Lauren we devised a long-handled wiping device out of kitchen tongs that enabled her to wash and dry her perineal area more easily and efficiently than before she had this device. She wrapped a wash-cloth around the long-handled kitchen tongs and used them when doing her bathing at the sink or the gym.

Dressing

There are many issues that may interfere with one's ability to carry out the daily activity of dressing (Mann et al. 2005). Those with limited ROM may not be able to dress their lower extremities. Those with limited upper extremity ROM may have difficulty putting on jackets and shirts (Ardie Bennet, personal communication; Pendleton McHugh and Schultz-Krohn 2013) or fastening buttons and other dressing closures (Blennerhassett et al. 2008). Fine motor issues as well as sensory problems may also interfere with the ability to dress oneself; cognitive issues may also cause dressing problems (Sunderland et al. 2006). In this section we will present a variety of no-tech to high-tech TEI that are useful for people who have difficulty dressing.

For fastening zippers and buttons, a variety of no-tech option are available. Often buttons and zippers can be replaced with Velcro or small magnets to simplify the task. There are no-tech devices, which can help to open and close zippers and buttons.

A variety of products are available for people with decreased ROM. For example, one can use a dressing stick to don and doff shirts, jackets, and pants as well. Reachers can be helpful for obtaining clothes from closets or drawers and then getting shoes, socks, and pants to lower extremities for dressing (Chen et al. 1998). YouTube, Pinterest, Instructables, or similar online resources are useful when searching for great ideas to help clients with dressing options. Here is an example of one person's adaptations for donning pants that the author found while searching YouTube; it shows how a simple homemade adaptation can be used for donning and doffing pants: https://www.youtube.com/watch?v=r8FCsDWt_9Q.

There are also many devices to help people put on socks and shoes. A variety of body structure and function problems may make these activities difficult. Long-handled shoehorns and other shoe adaptations are available for donning shoes (see Figure 22.10).

For putting on socks, there are numerous sock donners, which can be used for socks or hose (see Figure 22.11 for an example of a sock donner).

Commercial companies make shoes with Velcro closures that can be useful to those who cannot tie shoelaces, and there are also adaptive shoelaces available to make fastening shoes easier (see Figure 22.12).

The Boa® closure system (https://www.theboasystem.com) is a relatively new closure system for shoe closure. Originally designed for athletic shoes, the Boa closure system uses a dial mechanism to tighten shoelaces. The laces are already in place and the dial can be used with one hand to tighten each shoe's laces.

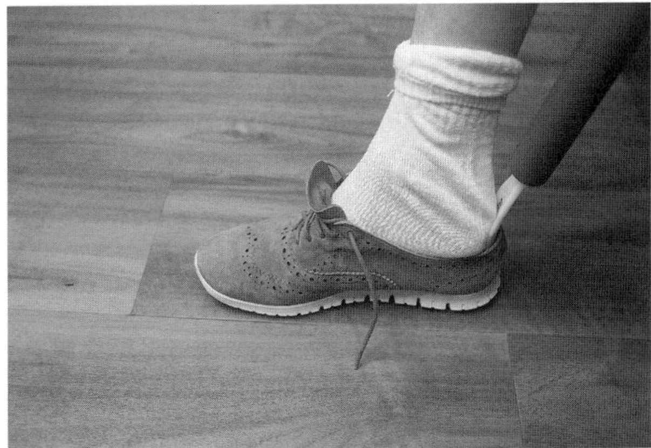

Figure 22.10 Long-handled shoe horn.

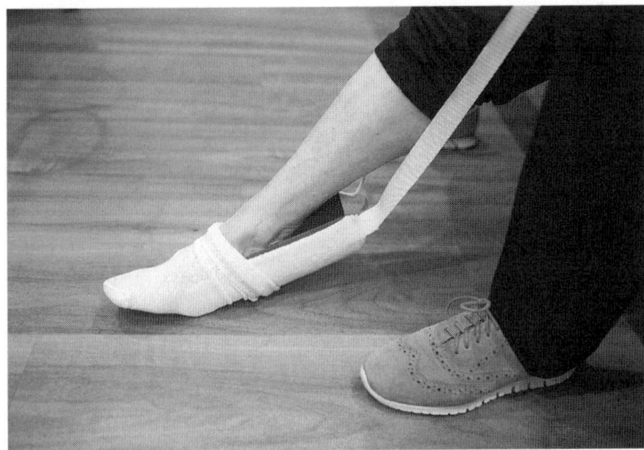

Figure 22.11 Sock donner.

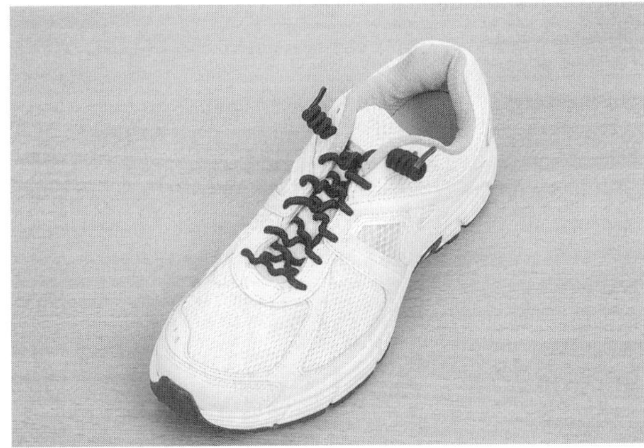

Figure 22.12 Coilers shoelaces. Source: Reproduced with permission of North Coast Medical, Inc.

Higher-tech options are now available for shoe tying. Shoes now come with self-tying features that are useful for those who have difficulty with this task. Nike was the first company to make self-tying sneakers, which are now available on the market.

Finally in this area there is research under way to develop robotic aids for dressing. For an example see The Robotic Assistance with Dressing project at Georgia Institute of Technology (http://www.cc.gatech.edu/~karenliu/Robotic_dressing.html) for papers and prototypes on work being done in this area.

Eating and drinking

In this section of the chapter we will discuss TEI for eating and drinking.

While there are many activities involved in these two ADLs, we will focus here on those described by the ICF definitions of these tasks.

Eating

First we will look at eating: "Carrying out the coordinated tasks and actions of eating food that has been served, bringing it to the mouth and consuming it in culturally acceptable ways, cutting or breaking food into pieces, opening bottles and cans, using eating implements, having meals, feasting or dining" (ICF Browser n.d.). There are a host of adaptations available to help people with a variety of body structure and function issues with the tasks of eating. There are devices that can serve a variety of people with different problems (Pendleton McHugh and Schultz-Krohn 2013; Rahman et al. 2012) as well as examples of products designed specifically to work for an individual (Louie et al. 2009) or adaptations that are relevant for cultural considerations, such as adapted chopsticks (Chang et al. 2006).

A variety of no-tech eating utensils are available to help those with ROM, tremor, and one-handed issues. For example, there are utensils such as the ones in Figure 22.13 that have built up handles, which are useful for those who have arthritis or other ROM issues (Pendleton McHugh and Schultz-Krohn 2013). One-handed rocker knives may be useful for those who only have the use of one hand for cutting tasks (see Figure 22.14).

Additionally, curved or jointed utensils are available for those with ROM issues. For those who have strength problems, there are a variety of adaptive devices that can be used to hold a utensil, such as universal cuffs. And for people who have tremors, some evidence exists that providing them with lightly weighted utensils can be useful for feeding (Hi et al. 2009).

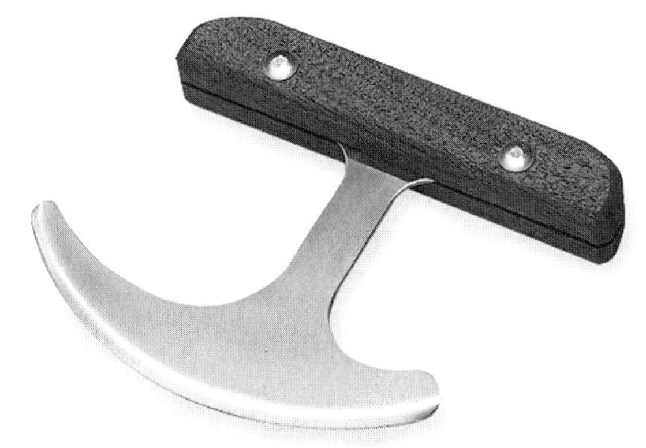

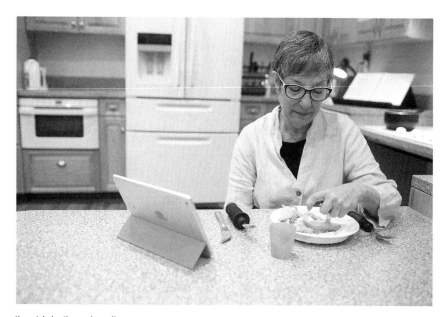

Figure 22.14 A Rocking T knife. Source: Reproduced with permission of North Coast Medical, Inc.

Figure 22.13 Utensils with built-up handles.

More high-tech utensils include Liftware (https://www.liftware.com), which has two products designed for those who have problems using utensils (see Figures 22.15 and 22.16). One device, the Liftware Steady, is useful for those with hand tremors, and the other, Liftware Level, is for those with limited hand and arm mobility. Both devices use computer technology to adjust the utensil to compensate for the problem the person might be having.

Mobile arm supports are devices that help an individual who has limited arm strength and/or ROM to engage in many activities, including self-feeding. These devices are often mounted on a table or a user's wheelchair or can be suspended from an overhead support. Some operate using springs or rubber bands to provide static balance, some are suspended from overhead supports, and some are powered by robotics (Herder et al. 2006). Some are commercially available and some of the robotic options are being researched or are under development. Research reports that these devices increase function and confidence in feeding for users and have the potential to reduce the cost of care for those who need assistance with feeding (Atkins et al. 2008; Kumar and Phillips 2013).

The JAECO company (http://jaecoorthopedic.com), SAEBO (https://www.saebo.com), and ZoncoArm (http://www.zoncoarm.com/products.htm) have examples of these devices on their websites.

If you search for low-tech plate or bowl options you will find a huge selection of these items. It is important to include the client in the decision of which options to use, remembering how important the psychological impact of using these devices can be on function (Pullin 2011).

Examples of these options include plates with raised lips that are available for those who may have the use of only one hand or who have decreased strength. There are also mats that can prevent plates on the table from moving and plates with rubber material on the bottom, which serve the same purpose.

Next there are feeding devices that include both the utensil and the plate in a system, which once set up allow a person to eat unaided. The Winsford Feeder is an example of this type of system. This device is powered by

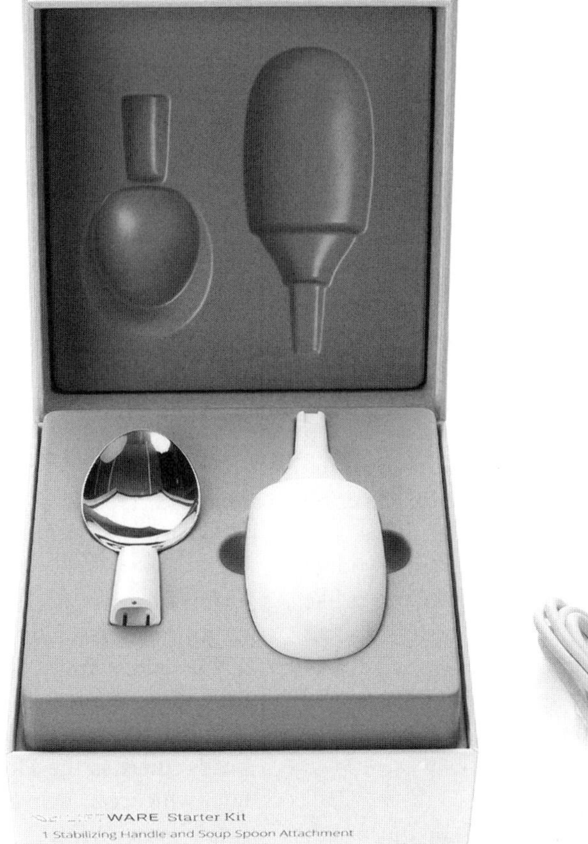

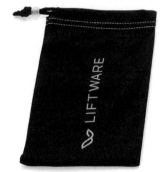

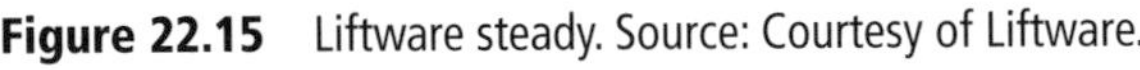
Figure 22.15 Liftware steady. Source: Courtesy of Liftware.

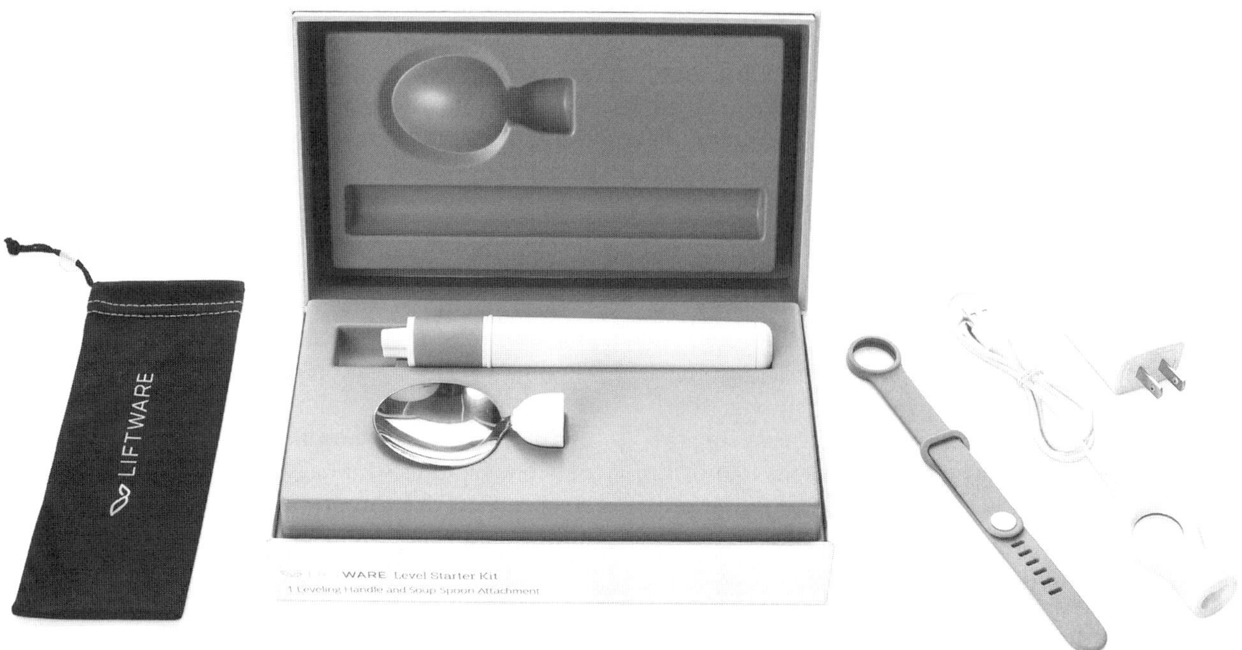

Figure 22.16 Liftware level. Source: Courtesy of Liftware.

electricity and, once the food has been placed into the plate, switch activation prompts the device, using a scoop, to move the food onto a spoon and place it at a level where the user can take it into his or her mouth. The bowl also rotates so that all of the food is available to be scooped. There is also a drink holder for a cup. Here is a YouTube video of the device in operation: https://www.youtube.com/watch?v=KZRFj1UZl-c. There are other similar feeding devices, such as the Neater Eater (http://www.neater.co.uk/neater-eater) and the Mealtime Partner Dining Device (http://www.mealtimepartners.com/dining/mealtime-partner-dining-device.htm). Finally, there are feeding robots. One example is Obi (https://meetobi.com). Once the food has been prepared by a caregiver according to Obi's directions and the arm has been "taught" where to deliver the food, the switch allows the user to choose between scooping the food and delivering it to their mouth. One or two switches can be used to manage this operation. Another robotic feeding product available on the market is the Bestic AB, which works like the Obi device, being switch activated (https://www.camanio.com/us/products/bestic). Robotic arms can also assist with feeding, as can general-purpose mobile manipulators, which are under development (Park et al. 2016).

Drinking

A variety of no-tech cups are available to help those with limited strength, ROM, tremors, and lip closure to drink liquids. Commercially available beverage holders with covers or covers and straws are often used for those who might have difficulty using an uncovered glass or cup. There are a variety of commercially available products for those who have difficulty with drinking. For those who have limited breath support or cannot lift their heads, there is the Flo-Trol vacuum activated drinking cup, which can deliver fluid with the push of a button (see Figure 22.17).

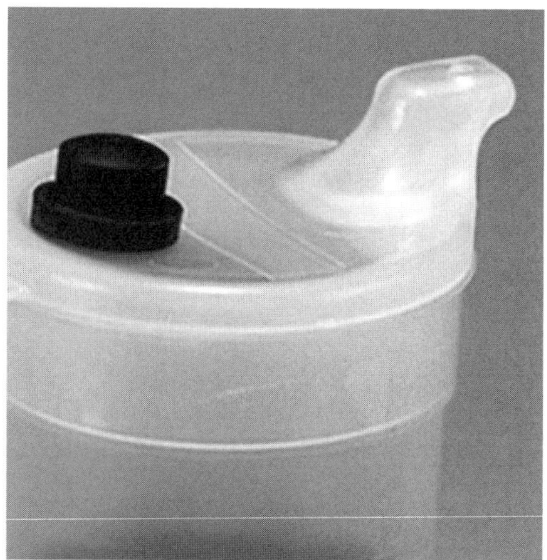

Figure 22.17 Flo-Trol vacuum activated cup. Source: Reproduced with permission of North Coast Medical, Inc.

Drink holders are also used for those who may have difficulty holding a cup or need to have a drink available to them during the day. These can be easily made or are commercially available as well. Cups are also available with two handles for those who need extra support. Be creative when thinking of options for hydration. Searching Google, Instructables, or other similar websites will give you great ideas.

Hands-free hydration systems are also commercially available or can easily be fabricated and then positioned for those who cannot pick up a glass or drink holder. These systems are designed for runners or bikers and can look like small backpacks with long straws. Finally, robotic mobile manipulators can also provide hydration (https://www.kinovarobotics.com/en/products/mobile-manipulators).

Taking care of one's health

In this section of the chapter we will present some options for taking care of one's health. We have talked about some of these options above, such as ways to apply lotion for skin care and options for maintaining dental health. The topic of medication management and health management is huge, and there has been an enormous growth in online, tele-health, and app options available to help people manage their health and adhere to medication regimes (Huckvale et al. 2012; Totten et al. 2016; Tran et al. 2012). Much of the evidence to support the efficacy of using apps to help with healthcare management remains inconclusive at this point (Huckvale et al. 2015; Kumar et al. 2015; Marcano et al. 2013); however, this is an area to pay attention to in the future.

As it is beyond the scope of this book to present all options available for this topic, we will focus here primarily on TEI for the physical aspect of medication management and healthcare management, such as monitoring vital signs and blood glucose. We will discuss options that are available to help people with physical disabilities to be able to manipulate their medicine and monitor vital signs. Given the complexity of this topic, a variety of strategies regarding medication management are also presented in chapters 13 and 19. We also encourage the reader to refer to the chapters regarding TEI for cognition and sensory issues. A variety of strategies exist to help people who have difficulty managing their medication due to ROM, strength, tremor, and other physical issues. Literature reports that many people will devise their own solutions to help with medication management. For example, those who have difficulty getting tops off pill bottles may put the tablets into a plastic cup next to the bottle for ease of access (Sanders and Van Oss 2013). It is often difficult for those with fine motor, strength, or sensory problems to open pill bottles. Some low-tech options to help with this include using a non-skid material such as rubber bands, shelf liner, or Dycem™ to open the bottles. Or there are devices that can secure the pill bottles so a person can use one hand to open it.

There are also a variety of low-tech pillboxes and containers, which can be used to hold pills for those who have difficulty opening bottles. Mid-tech devices include medication dispensing machines that may be useful for those who have difficulty with medication management (Medgaget 2013). High-tech options under development include robots, which may be able to deliver medication to people in their homes (Wilson 2016).

For managing liquid medications, people with tremors can use syringes or adaptive spoon-type devices to dispense liquids. Research reports that AT for dispensing eye drops is minimally effective in helping those with arthritis (Tuntland et al. 2009). Pill cutters and splitters are also available for those who need to divide their pills. A wide variety of medication management devices are available for those who have difficulty with this task. Please refer to the Toolbox at the end of the chapter for further resources for medication management devices.

There are also tools available to help people with physical problems who need to monitor their vital signs or check their blood glucose levels. There are a variety of no-tech to high-tech thermometers available for those who want to check their body temperature. Options include thermometer strips, which can be placed on the body, digital thermometers, and infrared thermometers. The latter two require operating a small button to turn the device on and off. There are also talking digital and infrared thermometers, which can speak the results as well. A variety of blood pressure cuffs that can be placed on the arm or wrist and operated with one hand are also available. Talking blood pressure monitors are available as well. Finally, we will present options for monitoring blood glucose levels. No-tech options may be difficult to use for those with physical disabilities such as arthritis or diabetes (Sokol-McKay 2016). Different-sized glucose strips as well as monitors with preloaded strips are available for this task. There are talking glucose monitors as well (Williams 2008).

In summary, numerous options are available to help those with physical disabilities manage their health care and medication management and these options will only become more ubiquitous as health care becomes connected and cloud-based. We did not list the variety of apps that are available for monitoring body functions above, given that the evidence regarding their efficacy is inconclusive (Belisario et al. 2013); however, this technology is certainly going to change the face of health care and is here to stay (Hussain et al. 2015). An example of ongoing research in this area of practice can be seen at http://www.apple.com/researchkit.

The Internet of Things (IoT) will provide systems that will collect patient data and make it available to healthcare providers to monitor and coordinate patient care (Niewolnhy 2013; Rose 2014). Examples of these types of options include the Fitbit (https://www.fitabase.com/research-library), Microsoft Health (https://www.microsoft.com/en-us/enterprise/health), and smart clothing and other smart wearables (Kosir 2015). Finally, robots that can take blood and deliver medication are under development (Medical Futurist 2016; Pillo 2016). From no-tech to high-tech, a variety of options are available to help with the ADL of healthcare management.

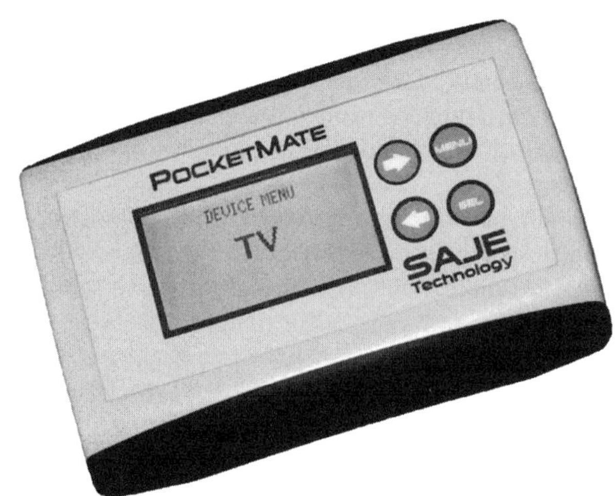

Figure 22.18 PocketMate. Source: Courtesy of SAJE Technology.

Electronic aids to daily living (EADLs)

In this final section of the chapter, we present some information on EADLs. Little (2010) reports that earliest mention of EADLs dated in the 1950s. Since that time, technological expansion has seen a huge growth in this area, with home automation and smart homes becoming an everyday option as of this writing (Barrineau 2017). EADLs can be used to help people with physical disabilities engage in "environmental regulation; information acquisition; safety and security and communication" activities (Little 2010, p. 33). Examples of these activities include turning on lights, controlling beds, opening doors and windows, and operating entertainment equipment such as televisions and game consoles and communication devices such as telephones and call systems. Devices and activities that typically require upper extremity function and fine motor control can be accessed using switches, touch screens, voice activation, or other devices such as computers, augmentative communication devices, wheelchair controls, or tablets and smartphones (Lange 2015; Little 2010). Device control can be provided through a variety of methods (Lange 2015; Little 2010), including direct control where the control is wired into the device, infrared (IR) transmission, radio frequency (RF), power line carriers including X-10, Zigbee, and Z-wave transmission, and Wi-Fi transmission and Bluetooth.

Please refer to Little (2010) for a more detailed description of these various modes of control. EADLs can be stand-alone systems such as the PocketMate (see Figure 22.18) and Bedmate devices available through SAJE Technology, or they may be included in other devices such as augmentative communication devices (http://www.tobiidynavox.com/windows-control/benefits-of-windows-control/environmental-control) or in a variety of Apple, Google, and Amazon products (Crist 2015). Research reveals that those with spinal cord injuries who use EADLs report increased quality of life, feelings of competence, and decreased reliance on caregivers (Rigby et al. 2011; Verdonck et al. 2011). While many of the EADLs described above are products designed specifically for those who have disabilities, the growth of smart homes, home automation, and robotics have expanded the options available for EADLs, and these options will continue to grow.

The Amazon Echo is an example of an everyday technology that can be used as an EADL. It can provide access to many of the features listed above, such as environmental regulation, information acquisition, safety and security, and communication. The Amazon Echo can be paired with other devices such as the WeMo® switch, which can control your lights or fans or other on/off devices. A search on YouTube (for example https://www.youtube.com/watch?v=RLxXKgXBYW8) will provide the user with a lot of information on how to set up Amazon Echo with WeMo products. Google has a similar product, called Google Home (https://madeby.google.com/home), and Apple has the Apple HomeKit (http://www.apple.com/ios/home). All of these devices combine voice activation, apps, and Wi-Fi to allow hands-free control of the devices in your home. We can expect much more of these types of systems to be on the market as the technology progresses.

In addition to these devices, there are other home automation systems available, such as the Insteon HomeKit or the Phillips HomeKit, which enable one to set up a smart home. While there are numerous definitions and configurations of smart homes (Gentry 2009), Alam et al. (2012) state that smart homes include three things: "1. Internal network – wire, cable, wireless; 2. Intelligent control –gateway to manage the featured systems; and 3. Home automation – products within the home and links to services and systems outside the home" (p. 2). As this technology continues to advance, the opportunity for these products to enhance the capabilities of those who have disabilities grows. Some excellent sources to keep up with developments in these products are http://www.smarthome.com and https://www.cnet.com/smart-home. There is no doubt that this technology will continue to develop and have implications for people who have disabilities.

In this chapter we have presented a variety of no-tech to high-tech options to help with ADL management, particularly for those who experience physical body structure and function barriers to carrying out daily living tasks (see the Toolbox at the end of the chapter). The use of Vicente's Human-Tech Ladder has presented the variety of factors that can impact the provision of TEI for those with problems at the physical level who need assistance in carrying out ADLs. Making sure to start the process of matching a person with the technology that they need using a conceptual practice model to guide a systematic evaluation is critical to the success of these interventions.

References

Abledata.com (n.d.). Products by category. Retrieved from http://www.abledata.com/products-by-category.

Agree, E.M. and Freedman, V.A. (2003). A comparison of assistive technology and personal care in alleviating disability and unmet need. *The Gerontologist* 43 (3): 335–344. https://doi.org/10.1093/geront/43.3.335.

Ahluwalia, S.C., Gill, T.M., Baker, D.I., and Fried, T.R. (2010). Perspectives of older persons on bathing and bathing disability: a qualitative study. *Journal of the American Geriatrics Society* 58 (3): 450–456. https://doi.org/10.1111/j.1532-5415.2010.02722.x.

Alam, M.R., Reaz, M.B.I., and Ali, M.A.M. (2012). A review of smart homes – past, present, and future. *IEEE Transactions on Systems, Man and Cybernetics Part C: Applications and Reviews* 42 (6): 1190–1203.

American Occupational Therapy Association (2014). Occupational therapy practice framework: domain and process (3rd ed.). *American Journal of Occupational Therapy* 68 (Suppl. 1): S1–S48.

Arthritis Foundation (n.d.). Ease of Use. Retrieved fromhttp://www.arthritis.org/living-with-arthritis/tools-resources/ease-of-use.

Asher, I.E. (ed.) (2014). *Occupational Therapy Aassessment Tools: An Annotated Index*. Bethesda, MD: American Occupational Therapy Association.

Atkins, M.S., Baumgarten, J.M., Yasuda, Y.L. et al. (2008). Mobile arm supports: evidence-based benefits and criteria for use. *The Journal of Spinal Cord Medicine* 31 (4): 388–393.

Baker, J.G., Granger, C.V., and Fiedler, R.C. (1997). A brief outpatient functional assessment measure: validity using Rasch measures. *American Journal of Physical Medicine and Rehabilitation* 76: 8–13.

Barrineau, T. (2017). CES 2017: home automation makes its mark. *Door and Window Market Magazine*. Retrieved from https://www.dwmmag.com/ces-2017-home-automation-makes-its-mark/.

Bedaf, S., Gelderblom, G.J., and de Witte, L. (2015). Overview and categorization of robots supporting independent living of elderly people: what activities do they support and how far have they developed. *Assistive Technology* 27 (2): 88–100. https://doi.org/10.1080/10400435.2014.978916.

Belisario, M., Huckvale, J.S., Greenfield, K. et al. (2013). Smartphone and tablet self management apps for asthma. *Cochrane Database of Systematic Reviews* (11): CD010013. https://doi.org/10.1002/14651858.CD010013.pub2.

Blennerhassett, J.M., Carey, L.M., and Matyas, T.A. (2008). Clinical measures of handgrip limitation relate to impaired pinch grip force control after stroke. *Journal of Hand Therapy* 21 (3): 245–253. http://dx.doi.org.ezproxy.ithaca.edu:2048/10.1197/j.jht.2007.10.021.

Bogue, R. (2013). Robots to aid the disabled and the elderly. *The Industrial Robot* 40 (6): 519–524. http://dx.doi.org.ezproxy.ithaca.edu:2048/10.1108/IR-07-2013-372.

Bonecutter, R. (2014). Getting in & out of the bathtub: benches, lifts, and transfer chairs. Retrieved from http://homeability.com/bathtub-transfer-chairs-lifts-benches.

Carlson, D., Erlich, N., Berland B. and Bailey, N. (2002). Highlights from the NIDRR/RESNA/University of Michigan Survey of Assistive Technology and Information Technology Use and Need by Persons with Disabilities in the United States. ISDS meeting minutes. Austin, TX: National Center for the Dissemination of Disability Research.

Chang, B.-C., Huang, B.-S., Chou, C.-L., and Wang, S.-J. (2006). A new type of chopsticks for patients with impaired hand function. *Archives of Physical Medicine and Rehabilitation* 87: 1013–1015.

Chen, L.-K.P., Mann, W.C., Tomita, M.R., and Burford, T.E. (1998). An evaluation of reachers for use by older persons with disabilities. *Assistive Technology* 10 (2): 113–125. https://doi.org/10.1080/10400435.1998.10131969.

Crist, R. (2015). A smart home divided: can it stand? Retrieved from https://www.cnet.com/news/a-smart-home-divided-can-it-stand.

Cynkin, S. and Robinson, A.M. (1990). *Occupational Therapy and Activities Health: Toward Health Through Activities*. Boston, MA: Little Brown and Company.

Erikson, A., Karlsson, G., Soderstrom, M., and Tham, K. (2004). A training apartment with electronic aids to daily living: lived experiences of persons with brain damage. *American Journal of Occupational Therapy* 58 (3): 261–271.

Evans, A., Menz, H., Bourke, J. et al. (2015). Foot care and people with intellectual disability. *International Journal of Child Health and Human Development* 8 (4): 471–491.

Farlex Partner Medical Dictionary (2012). Activities of daily living. Retrieved from http://medical-dictionary.thefreedictionary.com/activities+of+daily+living.

Federici, S., Meloni, F., and Corradi, F. (2012). Measuring individual function. In: *Assistive Technology Assessment Handbook* (ed. S. Federici and M. Scherer), 25–48. New York: CRC Press.

Gentry, T. (2009). Smart homes for people with neurological disability: state of the art. *NeuroRehabilitation* 25: 209–217.

Gill, T.M., Han, L., and Allore, H.G. (2007). Predisposing factors and precipitants for bathing disability in older persons. *Journal of the American Geriatrics Society* 55 (4): 534–540. https://doi.org/10.1111/j.1532-5415.2007.01099.x.

Guide for the Uniform Data Set for Medical Rehabilitation (1997). Adult FIM™ instrument, version 5.1. Buffalo, NY: State University of New York at Buffalo.

Guitard, P., Sveistrup, H., Edwards, N., and Lockett, D. (2011). Use of different bath grab bar configurations following a balance perturbation. *Assistive Technology* 23 (4): 205–215.

Guitard, P., Sveistrup, H., Fahim, A., and Leonard, C. (2012). Smart grab bars: a potential initiative to encourage bath grab bar use in community dwelling older adults. *Assistive Technology* 25 (3): 139–148.

Hannam, D. (1997). More than a cup of tea: meaning construction in an everyday occupation. *Journal of Occupational Science* 4 (2): 69–73. https://doi.org/10.1080/14427591.1997.9686423.

Hawkins, K.P., Grice, P.M., Chen, T.L. et al. (2014). Assistive mobile manipulation for self-care tasks around the head. Retrieved from https://smartech.gatech.edu/handle/1853/51633.

HealthyPeople.gov (2016). Disability and health objectives: systems and policies: DH-10. Retrieved from https://www.healthypeople.gov/2020/topics-objectives/topic/disability-and-health/objectives.

Herder, J., Vrijlandt, N., Antonides, T. et al. (2006). Principle and design of a mobile arm support for people with muscular weakness. *Journal of Rehabilitation Research and Development* 43 (5): 591–604.

Hi, M., Hwang, W.J., Tsai, P.L., and Hsu, Y.W. (2009). Effect of eating utensil weight on functional arm movement in people with Parkinson's disease: a controlled clinical trial. *Clinical Rehabilitation* 23 (12): 1086–1092. https://doi.org/10.1177/0269215509342334.

Hoenig, H., Taylor, D.H., and Sloan, F.A. (2003). Does assistive technology substitute for personal assistance among the disabled elderly? *American Journal of Public Health* 93 (2): 330–337.

Horner-Johnson, W., Dobbertin, K., and Beilstein-Wedel, E. (2015). Disparities in dental care associated with disability and race and ethnicity. *The Journal of the American Dental Association* 146 (6): 366–374.

Huckvale, K., Car, M., Morrison, C., and Car, J. (2012). Apps for asthma self-management: a systematic assessment of content and tools. *BMC Medicine* 10: 144. https://doi.org/10.1186/1741-7015-10-144.

Huckvale, K., Adomaviciute, S., Prieto, J.S. et al. (2015). Smartphone apps for calculating insulin dose: a systematic assessment. *BMC Medicine* 13: p106. https://doi.org/10.1186/s12916-015-0314-7.

Hussain, M., Al-Haiqi, A., Zaidan, A.A. et al. (2015). Computer methods and programs in biomedicine: the landscape of research on smartphone medical apps: coherent taxonomy, motivations, open challenges and recommendations. *Computer Methods and Programs in Biomedicine* 122 (3): 393–408. https://doi.org/10.1016/j.cmpb.2015.08.015.

ICF Browser (n.d.). Retrieved from http://apps.who.int/classifications/icfbrowser.

Katz, S., Ford, A.B., Moskowitz, R.W. et al. (1963). Studies of illness in the aged. The Index of ADL: a standardized measure of biological and psychosocial function. *Journal of the American Medical Association* 21 (185): 914–919.

Klein, R.M. and Bell, B. (1982). Self-care skills: behavioral measurement with the Klein-Bell ADL Scale. *Archives of Physical Medicine and Rehabilitation* 63: 335–338.

Korp, K.E., Taylor, J.M., and Nelson, D.L. (2012). Bathing area safety and lower extremity function in community-dwelling older adults. *Occupational Therapy Journal of Research* 32 (2): 22–29.

Kosir, S. (2015). A look at smart clothing for 2015. Retrieved from https://www.wearable-technologies.com/2015/03/a-look-at-smartclothing-for-2015.

Kumar, A. and Phillips, M.F. (2013). Use of powered mobile arm supports by people with neuromuscular conditions. *Journal of Rehabilitation Research and Development* 50 (1): 61–70.

Kumar, N., Khunger, M., Gupta, A., and Garg, N. (2015). A content analysis of smartphone-based applications for hypertension management. *Journal of the American Society of Hypertension* 9 (2): 130–136. https://doi.org/10.1016/j.jash.2014.12.001.

Lange, M.L. (2015). Basic electronic aids to daily living. Retrieved from http://www.atilange.com/ESW/Files/BASIC_ELECTRONIC_AIDS_TO_DAILY_LIVING.pdf.

Little, R. (2010). Electronic aids for daily living. *Physical medicine and rehabilitation clinics of North America* 21 (1): 33–42.

Longevity Explorers (n.d.). Toenail clippers for elderly people. Retrieved from https://www.techenhancedlife.com/explorers/toenail-clippers-elderly-people.

Louie, S.W.S., Lai, F.H.Y., Poon, C.M.Y., and Wong, S.K.M. (2009). Use of a tailor-made feeding device to improve the self-feeding skills of a woman with congenital upper limb deficiency. *British Journal of Occupational Therapy* 72 (9): 401–404.

Mahoney, F.I. and Barthel, D.W. (1965). Functional evaluation: the Barthel Index: a simple index of independence useful in scoring improvement in the rehabilitation of the chronically ill. *Maryland State Medical Journal* 14: 61–65.

Maia, F.B., Teixeira, E.R., Silva, G.V., and Gomes, M.K. (2016). The use of assistive technology to promote care of the self and social inclusion in patients with sequels of leprosy. *PLoS Neglected Tropical Diseases* 10 (4): e0004644. https://doi.org/10.1371/journal.pntd.0004644.

Mann, W.C., Ottenbacher, K.J., Fraas, L. et al. (1999). Effectiveness of assistive technology and environmental interventions in maintaining independence and reducing home care costs for frail elderly. *Archives of Family Medicine* 8 (3): 210–217.

Mann, W.C., Kimble, C., Justiss, M.D. et al. (2005). Problems with dressing in the frail elderly. *American Journal of Occupational Therapy* 59 (4): 398–408.

Marcano, B.J.S., Huckvale, K., Greenfield, G. et al. (2013). Smartphone and tablet self management apps for asthma. *Cochrane Database of Systematic Reviews* (11): CD010013. https://doi.org/10.1002/14651858.CD010013.pub2.

Medgaget (2013). e-pill station helps disabled folks take their pills. Retrieved from http://www.medgadget.com/2013/06/e-pill-station-helps-disabled-folks-take-their-pills.html.

Medical Futurist (2016). Robotics in healthcare – get ready. Retrieved from http://medicalfuturist.com/robotics-healthcare.

Module 9: Assistive technology to enhance independent living (n.d.). Retrieved from http://www.continuetolearn.uiowa.edu/nas1/07c187/Module%209/module_9_p1.html.

Naik, A. and Gill, T. (2005). Underutilization of environmental adaptations for bathing in community-living older persons. *Journal of the American Geriatrics Society* 53 (9): 1497–1503.

National Center for Health Statistics (2016). Health, United States, 2015: with special feature on racial and ethnic health disparities. Hyattsville, MD: US Department of Health and Human Services. Retrieved from https://www.cdc.gov/nchs/data/hus/hus15.pdf.

National Multiple Sclerosis Society (n.d.). Increasing accessibility. Retrieved from http://www.nationalmssociety.org/Living-Well-With-MS/Mobility-and-Accessibility/Increasing-Accessibility.

Niewolnhy, D. (2013). How the Internet of Things is revolutionizing healthcare. Retrieved from https://cache.freescale.com/files/corporate/doc/white_paper/IOTREVHEALCARWP.pdf.

Norman, D. (1990). *The Design of Everyday Things*. New York: Doubleday.

Oddo, C. (2010). Electronic aids to daily living. In: *International Encyclopedia of Rehabilitation* (ed. J.H. Stone and M. Blouin). Buffalo, NY: Center for International Rehabilitation Research

Information and Exchange Retrieved from http://sphhp.buffalo.edu/content/sphhp/rehabilitation-science/research-and-facilities/funded-research-archive/center-for-international-rehab-research-info-exchange/_jcr_content/par/download/file.res/pdf.zip.

Park, D. (2016). Robotic nurse assistant. Retrieved from http://pwp.gatech.edu/hrl/robotic-nurse-assistant.

Park, D., Kim, Y.K., Erickson, Z.M. and Kemp C.C. (2016). Towards assistive feeding with a general-purpose mobile manipulator. Retrieved from https://smartech.gatech.edu/bitstream/handle/1853/55813/icraws2016_fi.pdf.

Pendleton McHugh, H. and Schultz-Krohn, W. (eds.) (2013). *Pedretti's Occupational Therapy: Practice Skills for Physical Dysfunction*. St. Louis, MO: Elsevier.

Pillo (2016). Retrieved from https://pillohealth.com.

Pullin, G. (2011). *Design Meets Disability*. Boston, MA: MIT Press.

QIAT Leadership Team (2015). *Quality Indicators for Assistive Technology: A Comprehensive Guide to Assistive Technology Services*. Wakefield, MA: CAST Professional Publishing.

Radomski, M. and Trombly, C. (2014). *Occupational Therapy for Physical Dysfunction*. Philadelphia, PA: Wolters Kluwer Health; Lippincott Williams & Williams.

Rahman, T., Basante, J., and Alexander, M. (2012). Robotics and assistive technology to improve function in neuromuscular diseases. *Acta Mechanica Slovaca* 17 (4): 32–39.

RESNA (n.d.-a). RESNA code of ethics. Retrieved from http://www.resna.org/sites/default/files/legacy/certification/RESNA_Code_of_Ethics.pdf.

RESNA (n.d.-b). RESNA standards of practice for assistive technology professionals. Retrieved from http://www.resna.org/sites/default/files/legacy/certification/Standards_of_Practice_final_10_10_08.pdf.

Rigby, P., Ryan, S.E., and Campbell, K.A. (2011). Electronic aids to daily living and quality of life for persons with tetraplegia. *Disability and Rehabilitation: Assistive Technology* 6 (3): 260–267. https://doi.org/10.3109/17483107.2010.522678.

Rokkaku, R. and Kaneko, S. (2012). The impact of foot and nail condition on falling, in the context of the elderly in acute hospital settings. The Journal of Aging Research & Clinical Practice Retrieved from http://www.jarcp.com/996-the-impact-of-foot-and-nail-condition-on-falling-in-the-context-of-the-elderly-in-acute-hospital-settings.html.

Rose, D. (2014). *Enchanted Objects: Design, Human Desire and the Internet of Things*. New York: Scribner.

Sanders, M.J. and Van Oss, T. (2013). Using daily routines to promote medication adherence in older adults. *American Journal of Occupational Therapy* 67: 91–99. https://doi.org/10.5014/ajot.2013.005033.

Sandqvist, G., Eklund, M., Akesson, A., and Nordenskio, U. (2004). Daily activities and hand function in women with scleroderma. *Scandinavian Journal of Rheumatology* 33: 102–107.

Scherer, M. (2005). *Living in the State of Stuck: How Assistive Technology Impacts the Lives of People with Disabilities*. Cambridge, MA: Brookline Books.

Sokol-McKay, D. (2016). Managing diabetes with physical limitations. Diabetes Self-Management. Retrieved from http://www.diabetesselfmanagement.com/about-diabetes/general-diabetes-information/managing-diabetes-with-physical-limitations.

Spillman, B.C. (2004). Changes in elderly disability rates and the implications for health care utilization and cost. *The Milbank Quarterly* 82 (1): 157–194. https://doi.org/10.1111/j.0887-378X.2004.00305.x.

Sunderland, A., Walker, C.M., and Walker, M.F. (2006). Action errors and dressing disability after stroke: an ecological approach to neuropsychological assessment and intervention. *Neuropsychological Rehabilitation* 16 (6): 666–683.

Totten, A.M., Womack, D.M., Eden, K.B. et al. (2016). Telehealth: mapping the evidence for patient outcomes from systematic Reviews. Technical Brief No. 26. Retrieved from https://effectivehealthcare.ahrq.gov/topics/telehealth/technical-brief.

Tran, J., Tran, R., and White, J.R. Jr. (2012). Smartphone-based glucose monitors and applications in the management of diabetes: an overview of 10 salient "apps" and a novel smartphone-connected blood glucose monitor. *Clinical Diabetes* 30 (4): 173–178.

Tuntland, H., Kjeken, I., Nordheim, L.V. et al. (2009). Assistive technology for rheumatoid arthritis. *Cochrane Database of Systematic Reviews* (4): CD006729. https://doi.org/10.1002/14651858.CD006729.pub2.

Verdonck, M.C., Chard, G., and Nolan, M. (2011). Electronic aids to daily living: be able to do what you want? *Disability and Rehabilitation: Assistive Technology* 6 (3): 268–281. https://doi.org/10.3109/17483107.2010.525291.

Waldman, H.B. and Perlman, S.P. (2010). Disability and rehabilitation: do we ever think about needed dental care? A case study: the USA. *Disability and Rehabilitation* 32 (11): 947–951.

Wielandt, T., McKenna, K., Tooth, L., and Strong, J. (2006). Factors that predict the post-discharge use of recommended assistive technology (AT). *Disability and Rehabilitation: Assistive Technology* 1: 29–40.

Williams, A. (2008). Talking meters. Diabetes Self-Management. Retrieved from http://www.diabetesselfmanagement.com/diabetes-resources/tools-tech/talking-meters.

Wilson, J. (2016). Robot assistance in medication management tasks. Retrieved from https://hrilab.tufts.edu/publications/wilson2016hrip.pdf.

World Health Organization (WHO) (2015). Global disability action plan 2014–2021: better health for all people with disability. Retrieved from http://apps.who.int/iris/bitstream/10665/199544/1/9789241509619_eng.pdf?ua=1.

World Health Organization (WHO) (2017). Global Cooperation on Assistive Technology (GATE). Retrieved from http://www.who.int/phi/implementation/assistive_technology/phi_gate/en.

World Health Organization (WHO) & The World Bank (2011). *World Report on Disability*. Geneva, Switzerland: World Health Organization.

Yachnin, D., Jutai, J., Gharib, G., and Finestone, H. (2015). Can technology-assisted toilets improve quality of life for rehabilitating stroke patients? a pilot cohort study. *Archives of Physical Medicine and Rehabilitation* 96 (10): e32.

Toolbox: Assessment of ADL and medication management

Assessment of ADL
This is not a comprehensive list of resources but will get you started finding ADL assessment tools.

Source	Tool
Rehabilitation Measures Database http://www.rehabmeasures.org/default.aspx	You can search this database for a variety of ADL assessment tools
Spinal Cord Research Evidence Outcome measures https://scireproject.com/outcome-measures/list-sci/self-care-daily-living	Several ADL assessment tools are available here
Asher (2014)	This text has information on a variety of standardized ADL assessment tools

Medication management

Source	Description
http://www.epill.com/	Comprehensive website with medication management products
https://www.alzstore.com/SearchResults.asp?Search=medication+dispenser&Submit=GO	Here are several automated medication dispensers
http://www.forgettingthepill.com	Variety of medication management products

An incredible number of apps are available for medication management as well.

23

Implications for future practice and research in technology and environmental interventions

Steve Jacobs

Outline

Learning outcomes

After reading this chapter, you should be able to:

1. Identify the differences between the medical and social models of disability.
2. Understand the history of technology development in the twentieth century.
3. Understand the implications of technology on the meaning of place.
4. Understand to the concept of cloud computing and its implications for the future of technology.
5. Describe at least four projects that will impact the future of technology and environmental interventions.

Assistive Technologies and Environmental Interventions in Healthcare: An Integrated Approach, First Edition.
Edited by Lynn Gitlow and Kathleen Flecky.

Companion website: www.wiley.com/go/gitlow/assitivetechnologies

Active learning prompts

Before you read this chapter:

1. Compare and contrast the definitions of assistive technology and universal design.
2. View this YouTube video entitled, "Apps4Android's Tactile, Virtual Keyboard, Screen Protectors": https://www.youtube.com/watch?v=Cg8uSajkgGg Would you consider this product an example of assistive technology or a universally designed screen protector?
3. View this YouTube Video entitled, "InftyReader Automatically Converting a BMP Math Image to MathML": https://www.youtube.com/watch?v=eXPdugnzkow InftyReader is an Optical Character Recognition (OCR) application that *automatically* recognizes and translates image-based science, technology, engineering, and math (STEM) textbook content into LaTeX, MathML, and XHTML in support of individuals who are blind. What do you think of this technology?

Key terms

Medical model of disability
Social model of disability
Physical places of public accommodation
Virtual places of public accommodation
Universal design
Global Public Inclusive Infrastructure
The Leverage Model
The Technical Assistance Model
The Enforcement Model
The Corporate Social Innovation Model

Introduction

In the first chapter of this book the editors describe the difference between the medical and social models of disability. We learned that the "medical model" views a disability as a "people problem" caused by disease, trauma, or other health conditions, that it promotes the belief that a disability "necessarily" negatively impacts a person's independence and quality of life, and causes an individual to be "disadvantaged."

We also learned that the "social model" of a disability views a person with disability from *within the context* of the social and environmental factors that impact their disability and that disabilities are the result of not fully integrating individuals with disabilities into the fabric of society. Further, it views the management of people with disabilities as a collective responsibility of society and views the solution as making the modifications necessary to enable people with disabilities to enjoy full participation in all of life's activities. In this chapter, the author discusses the interactions between these differing definitions of disability along with interactions between humans and technology which lay the foundation of what the future holds in store in technology development. The interactions reflect the levels of Vicente's Human-Tech Ladder[1] presented in Chapter 1, which was used as a guide to structure the text and illuminate the numerous factors that must be considered when making a successful human-tech interaction, including the political and organizational levels and then moving down the ladder.

Technology's impact on the definition of a "public accommodation": Political and organizational levels of vicente's human-tech ladder

The 1980s was a decade of technical innovation. Products and services such as the IBM personal computer, fax machine, cable television, and the cell phone worked their way into the fabric of people's lives. In the late 1980s, members of Congress used these technologies to interact with each other, and their constituents, to craft the Americans with Disabilities Act of 1990 (ADA).[2] The purpose of the ADA was "to provide a clear and comprehensive national mandate for the elimination of discrimination against individuals with disabilities"[3] and to "bring persons with disabilities into the economic and social mainstream of American life."[4] Title III of the ADA, "Public Accommodations," requires that all new construction and modifications of places of public accommodations (i.e. restaurants, hotels, grocery stores, retail stores, and privately owned transportation systems) be accessible to individuals with disabilities, and if readily achievable, barriers to existing facilities and services must be removed.

The law defines the term Place of public accommodation as a facility, operated by a private entity, whose operations affect commerce and fall within at least one of 12 categories.[5] An "Entity" is defined as a person or organization possessing separate and distinct legal rights, such as an individual, partnership, or corporation. An entity can, among other things, own property, engage in business, enter into contracts, pay taxes, sue, and be sued.[6]

Had technology not changed from the way it was in 1990, people with disabilities would not be facing many of the barriers they do today.

But it did, and they do.

In 1990, members of Congress had no way of knowing that in five short years technology would dramatically change the fabric of the American way of life and unintentionally wreak havoc with Congress's definition of a "place of public accommodation." This is an excellent example of how organizational and political factors influence human-tech interactions. Technological change altered notions of organizations and political action was required to adjust this new phase of an organization to ensure that all citizens could benefit from this technological transformation.

Here's what happened

- In 1990, the first World Wide Web server and browser were created by Tim Berners-Lee. He named his browser "WorldWideWeb."[7]
- In 1991, Berners-Lee released a code library (with his assistant Jean-François Groff) that allowed others to create their own Web browsers.[8]
- In 1992, Intershop, a German company, began development of an online retailing infrastructure that came to fruition in 1994.[9]
- In August 1994, Santa Cruz Operation (SCO) and Pizza Hut announced PizzaNet, "a pilot program that enables computer users, for the first time, to electronically order pizza delivery from their local Pizza Hut restaurant via the worldwide Internet."[10]
- Two months later, in October 1994, the first online banking service in the United States was introduced. The service was developed by Stanford Federal Credit Union, which was a financial institution.[11]
- In the same year Amazon was founded.[12]
- eBay was founded in 1995.[13]

In light of all these events, the definition of the term public accommodation did not change … from a legal standpoint.

What did change was that technology began to evolve *physical places* of public accommodation into *virtual places* of public accommodation (the Internet).

Consumers spent $517.36 billion online with US merchants in 2018, up 15.0% from $449.88 billion spent the year prior, according to a new *Internet Retailer* analysis of industry data and historical US Commerce Department figures. That's a slight slowdown from 2017, when online sales grew 15.6% year over year, according to Commerce Department figures.[14]

The US Census Bureau's unadjusted e-commerce report for Q3 2013 estimates sales at an even higher level of $61.4B ($67B adjusted).

Rather than travel to places of public accommodation to

- acquire knowledge (libraries, schools, and universities)
- visit with each other (restaurants, community centers, churches)
- go shopping (brick-and-mortar retail establishments)
- watch a movie (brick-and-mortar theaters)

billions of consumers are opting to use the Internet to enjoy these same activities, and not on a small scale. For example, here are the top 10 most popular sites:

1. Google.com (Billions of people generate 3.5 billion searches every single day.)
2. Youtube.com (Five billion videos are watched on YouTube every day.)
3. Facebook.com (More than 1.4 billion active users access Facebook daily across the globe to communicate with family and friends.)
4. Baidu.com (With a 70% search market share, Baidu is the largest Chinese-language search engine and is used by millions of people every day.)
5. Wikipedia.org (More people use Wikipedia worldwide than any other knowledge-based resource on the web.)
6. QQ.com (QQ.com holds the Guinness World Record for the highest number of simultaneous online users on an instant messaging program with just over 210 million users. Active monthly users exceed 800 million.)
7. Taobao (Taobao is an online shopping website for China. It offers clothing and electronics for all ages and users can buy or sell on the site. Taobao is the world's largest ecommerce website, and has more than one billion product listings.)
8. Yahoo.com (Yahoo is a web portal and search engine. It offers mail, news, maps, videos and many more web services. Yahoo doesn't hand out its statistics freely, but a recent estimate put the number of visitors per month at about 1 billion.)

9. TMall (TMall is an online retail site in China. It's a spin-off of the Taobao site, which is operated by the Alibaba Group. It is the world's second largest ecommerce website, and has more than 500 million monthly active users.)
10. Amazon.com (Amazon is the No. 1 shopping website in the United States, with more than 600 million products available for sale. Globally, the site sells more than 3 billion products across 11 marketplaces.)[15]

Here's a question for you

Knowing what you know today, if you were drafting a 2020 version of the ADA with the same spirit and intent as was the case in 1990, would you exclude Internet-based "virtual places" from being included as part of the definition of places of public accommodation? I certainly wouldn't. As you can see, the nature of organization or place has been transformed by the Internet and its creation of virtual spaces. The first Agenda the Trump Administration issued, which went online July 20, 2017, placed the Department of Justice's rulemakings under Titles II and III of the ADA for websites, medical equipment, and furniture of public accommodations and state and local governments on this 2017 Inactive Actions list, with no further information. This means that there will be no regulations regarding public accommodations, or state and local government websites, for the foreseeable future. In other words, the placement of the ADA website accessibility regulations on the inactive list means an absolute U-turn from past positions of the Department of Justice.[16] Obviously, the uncertain legal landscape regulations will not only lead to more website accessibility lawsuits but also put judges in a murky position as they are trying to plug the hole with a mélange of decisions that often conflict with one another. In the absence of website regulations, lawsuits and demand letters filed and sent on behalf of individuals with disabilities alleging that the websites of thousands of public accommodations are not accessible are already on the rise. According to court papers, in New York, for instance, 14 retailers, including big names like Shake Shack, Nordstrom, and Katz's Delicatessen, have been sued in the first 13 days of July 2017.[17,18,19]

The states with the most website lawsuits in federal court as of August 15, 2017 were as follows: Arizona (7), California (65), Florida (385), Illinois (5), Massachusetts (17), New York (170), Ohio (4), Pennsylvania (85), Texas (4), Washington (5). There are at least this many lawsuits. These are a significant portion of the increase in total ADA Title III lawsuits filed in federal courts in 2017, which, as of April, was already over 2600 filings – an 18% increase over the number of federal cases filed in the same time period in 2016.[20] As you can see, the impact of organizational change from having a physical to virtual presence has certainly impacted the capacity of people with disabilities to participate in their communities.

Assistive technology vs. "Universally-designed" technology

An assistive technology (AT) device is "any item, piece of equipment, or product system, whether acquired commercially, modified, or customized, that is used to increase, maintain, or improve functional capabilities of individuals with disabilities."[21] Given this definition's focus on the capabilities of an individual, the author views it as a medical model definition where the outcome of technology intervention is at the level of the individual.

The term universal design is used to describe the design of products and environments to be usable by all people, to the greatest extent possible, without the need for adaptation or specialized design.[22] The intent of universal design is to simplify life for everyone. In the case of this chapter, it is to develop technology-based products and services that are accessible to as many people as possible at little or no extra cost. Universal design focuses on fixing "design problems," *not* "people problems." The outcome of technology use in this perspective is at a societal rather than individual level.

Unfortunately, not all companies/organizations embrace this practice … nor will this ever be the case. What *compels* most companies to take actions to accommodate the access needs of consumers with disabilities? It's supply-push market forces. They include:

*C*ompassion
*O*rganizational beliefs
*M*oral values
*P*ersonal beliefs
*E*thics
*L*egal mandates
*S*ocial pressure.

The unfortunate thing about these market forces is that they may not exist, for whatever reason, in the minds of organizations' decision-makers. On the other hand, demand-pull market forces rule the day. Demand-pull processes focus on making as much money as possible, as quickly as possible. In situations where both types of market forces balance each other out, everyone can be a winner.

A prime example of a push-pull project is the Global Public Inclusive Infrastructure (GPII).

Global public inclusive infrastructure

GPII's objective is to ensure that everyone who faces accessibility barriers due to disability, literacy, digital literacy, or aging, regardless of economic resources, can access and use the Internet and all its information resources.[23]

GPII is a paradigm shift. According to GPII architects, "The GPII will, for the first time, introduce automatic personalization of user interfaces and user context adaptation based on user preferences. Each information and communications technology (ICT) device will be able to instantly change to fit users as they encounter the device, rather than requiring users to figure out how to adapt, configure or install access features they need."[24] Does this approach strike a familiar note? If not, take a second look at the definition of the "social model of disability" presented earlier in this chapter and you will see the similarities. The GPII philosophy exemplifies the spirit of accommodating people with disabilities as a collective responsibility of society and embraces making whatever modifications are necessary to enable people with disabilities to enjoy full participation in all of life's technology-based activities.

The GPII will eventually allow people who cannot use standard interfaces and content to be able to use broadband connected ICT anywhere they encounter them. The GPII would then provide cloud-based services designed to invoke the interface adaptations they need, automatically, on any device, anywhere, anytime – so they can use the same devices in the same places for all the same purposes as everyone else. Here's a link to a video describing GPII: https://gpii.net/content/global-public-inclusive-infrastructure-gpii-video.

There are many mainstream technologies that, in their current form, are being used to accommodate the access needs of individuals with disabilities. For example:

1. Optical character recognition (OCR): OCR technology is used to convert printed text texts into electronic formats in support of individuals with print disabilities. In the mainstream, it is used for the same purpose.
2. Handwriting recognition: smartphone gestures are used to accommodate the access needs of individuals who are blind (and everyone else) who need an easy way to command their smartphones to do things. Gesture understanding technology is an offshoot of handwriting recognition technology. In the mainstream it is used to take notes by using your finger or a stylus to write on touch-screen displays.
3. Voice typing/speech dictation: software is used by individuals with mobility (and other) disabilities to "type" in a hands-free environment. In the mainstream it is used by millions of people to do the same thing.

Optical character recognition (OCR)

Some readers may be aware that OCR technology got its start as an AT and then evolved into mainstream technology. Here's the history of OCR technology and a description of how the technology is not being used in a manner that many developers thought impossible:

1972: Ray Kurzweil, the American inventor and futurist, happened to sit next to a blind gentleman on a plane flight. The gentleman explained to Ray that the only real barrier he faced was the inability to read ordinary printed material. Immediately, Ray realized that this gentleman just identified the "problem" his company's new invention was looking for. He could apply his company's "omni-font" (any font) OCR technology to overcome this disadvantage of blindness. By the end of 1975, his company had developed and released the Kurzweil Reading Machine (KRM). The KRM read ordinary books, magazines, and other printed documents out loud so that blind individuals could read anything they desired (http://www.kurzweiltech.com/kcp.html).

1980: Ray Kurzweil sold his company to Xerox.

1984: Caere Corporation developed the first OCR-based passport scanner for the US State Department.

1987: American retailers Sears, Kmart, and J.C. Penney start using OCR-based technology to scan price tags.

1989: ABBYY, a Russian OCR developer, started selling products designed to simplify converting paper files into digital data. This product is what really kicked off the evolution of OCR technology into the mainstream.

1996: Under the leadership of Masakazu Suzuki, Professor emeritus, Kyushu University, a team of mathematics professors and grad students began thinking differently about OCR technology. Their goal was elevate the capabilities of mainstream OCR technology "up to the next level." The software their team developed, and which has been maturing over the past 20 years, using a combination of *three different* OCR engines, is nothing short of a *miracle*. The Windows-based applications they developed are called InftyReader and ChattyInfty (http://inftyreader.org).

InftyReader automatically translates *images* containing both math content and text into each of three fully-accessible markup languages. These languages include LaTeX, MathML, and MS Word XML. Here's a bit more about each of these formats.

Latex

Blind and visually impaired students in the fields of mathematics, science, and engineering often encounter difficulties when they need to present mathematical material to sighted instructors and classmates. This is because in most classrooms, the teaching of mathematics, the physical sciences, and engineering rely heavily on visual representations. LaTeX was initially invented as a typesetting language for mathematical notation. It is text-based and non-graphical by design. By typing standard text on a keyboard, one can represent all mathematical symbols, from the most basic to the most advanced. LaTeX can be used to draw diagrams. Thanks to LaTeX, it is much easier for blind individuals to excel in science, technology, engineering, and math (STEM) fields! LaTeX can convert text-based code into a PDF file for the student to print or email to a teacher or professor. LaTeX can even be used to produce Nemeth Braille, which can be printed or displayed on a braille display.[25]

MathML and MS word XML

MathML and MS Word XML are XML-based encodings for describing mathematical expressions. MathML was created to provide a better and more efficient way of describing mathematical equations in web pages. MathML can also be used to publish accessible, digital, STEM documents. Their software (ChattyInfty) can then be used to read and/or automatically convert MathML content into fully accessible eBook formats including DAISY and EPUB3.

If you'd like to experiment with InftyReader and ChattyInfty on your own, you can do so for free by accessing the following tutorial: http://www.inftyreader.org/?p=1055.

Otherwise, here are some figures that show what InftyReader accomplishes.

It all starts by submitting a STEM-based PDF document/textbook to InftyReader (See Figure 23.1).

Here's a link to download the PDF we processed: http://math.slu.edu/~clair/mcmc/FTC-solutions.pdf.

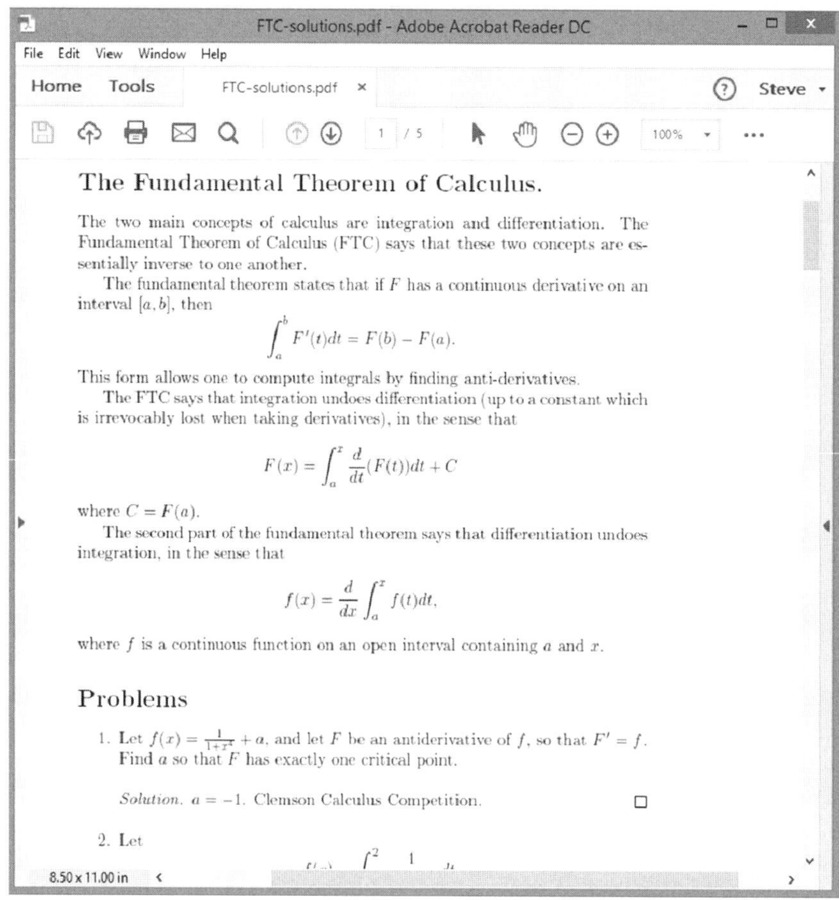

The Fundamental Theorem of Calculus.

The two main concepts of calculus are integration and differentiation. The Fundamental Theorem of Calculus (FTC) says that these two concepts are essentially inverse to one another.

The fundamental theorem states that if F has a continuous derivative on an interval $[a,b]$, then

$$\int_a^b F'(t)dt = F(b) - F(a).$$

This form allows one to compute integrals by finding anti-derivatives.

The FTC says that integration undoes differentiation (up to a constant which is irrevocably lost when taking derivatives), in the sense that

$$F(x) = \int_a^x \frac{d}{dt}(F(t))dt + C$$

where $C = F(a)$.

The second part of the fundamental theorem says that differentiation undoes integration, in the sense that

$$f(x) = \frac{d}{dx}\int_a^x f(t)dt,$$

where f is a continuous function on an open interval containing a and x.

Problems

1. Let $f(x) = \frac{1}{1+x^2} + a$, and let F be an antiderivative of f, so that $F' = f$. Find a so that F has exactly one critical point.

Solution. $a = -1$. Clemson Calculus Competition. □

2. Let

Figure 23.1 Sample page of the PDF file.

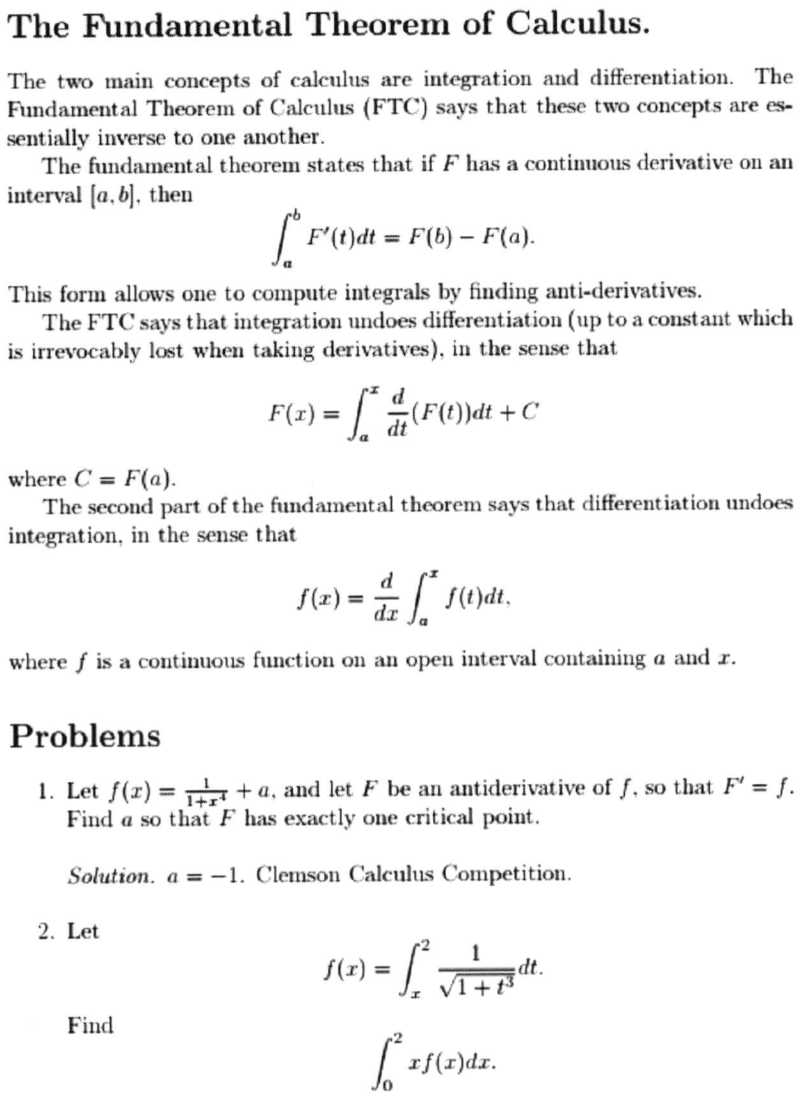

The Fundamental Theorem of Calculus.

The two main concepts of calculus are integration and differentiation. The Fundamental Theorem of Calculus (FTC) says that these two concepts are essentially inverse to one another.

The fundamental theorem states that if F has a continuous derivative on an interval $[a, b]$, then

$$\int_a^b F'(t)dt = F(b) - F(a).$$

This form allows one to compute integrals by finding anti-derivatives.

The FTC says that integration undoes differentiation (up to a constant which is irrevocably lost when taking derivatives), in the sense that

$$F(x) = \int_a^x \frac{d}{dt}(F(t))dt + C$$

where $C = F(a)$.

The second part of the fundamental theorem says that differentiation undoes integration, in the sense that

$$f(x) = \frac{d}{dx}\int_a^x f(t)dt,$$

where f is a continuous function on an open interval containing a and x.

Problems

1. Let $f(x) = \frac{1}{1+x^4} + a$, and let F be an antiderivative of f, so that $F' = f$. Find a so that F has exactly one critical point.

   Solution. $a = -1$. Clemson Calculus Competition.

2. Let

   $$f(x) = \int_x^2 \frac{1}{\sqrt{1+t^3}}dt.$$

   Find

   $$\int_0^2 xf(x)dx.$$

Figure 23.2 Black and white image of the PDF page displayed in Figure 23.1.

Here's what the results looked like when InftyReader was used to convert a page of the PDF file into a black and white TIF image (see Figure 23.2) (the first step in the conversion process for all formats):

Here's a link to download this image: http://www.inftyreader.org/inftyreader-examples/fundamental-5.50-pdf.jpg.

Here's what the results look like when InftyReader was used to produce the MathML representation of the PDF page displayed in Figure 23.1 (see Figure 23.3):

Here's a link to download this MathML file: http://www.inftyreader.org/inftyreader-examples/FTC-solutions.xhtml.

Here's what the results looked like when InftyReader was used to produce the LaTeX representation of the PDF page displayed in Figure 23.1 (see Figure 23.4):

Here's a link to download this LaTeX file: http://www.inftyreader.org/inftyreader-examples/FTC-solutions.tex.

Here's what the results looked like when InftyReader was used to produce the MS Word XML representation of the PDF page displayed in figure 23.1 (see Figure 23.5)

Here's a link to download this MS Word XML file: http://www.inftyreader.org/inftyreader-examples/FTC-solutions.xml.

More resources

- YouTube Video of InftyReader's OCR in action: https://www.youtube.com/watch?v=eXPdugnzkow.
- InftyReader homepage: http://inftyreader.org.
- PowerPoint presentation: http://inftyreader.org/Overview-of-InftyReader-ChattyInfty-InftyEditor-120917.pptx.

```
<?xml version="1.0" encoding="utf-8"?>
<!DOCTYPE html PUBLIC "-//W3C//DTD XHTML 1.1 plus MathML 2.0//EN"
"http://www.w3.org/Math/DTD/MathML2/xhtml-math11-f.dtd" [
                    <!ENTITY mathml "http://www.w3.org/1998/Math/MathML">
                              ]>
<html xmlns="http://www.w3.org/1999/xhtml"><head><title>No
Title</title><style type="text/css">.center{text-align:center;}
</style></head><body>
<p>The Fundamental Theorem of Calculus.</p>
<p>The two main concepts of calculus are integration and differentiation. The
Fundamental Theorem of Calculus (FTC) says that these two concepts are es-
sentially inverse to one another.</p>
<p>The fundamental theorem states that if <math
xmlns="http://www.w3.org/1998/Math/MathML"><mi
mathvariant="italic">F</mi></math> has a continuous derivative on an interval
<math xmlns="http://www.w3.org/1998/Math/MathML"><mo
mathvariant="normal">[</mo><mi mathvariant="italic">a</mi><mo
mathvariant="normal">,</mo><mi mathvariant="normal"> </mi><mi
mathvariant="italic">b</mi><mo mathvariant="normal">]</mo></math>,
then</p>
<p class="center"><math
xmlns="http://www.w3.org/1998/Math/MathML"><msubsup><mstyle
displaystyle="true"
mathvariant="normal"><mo>&int;</mo></mstyle><mrow><mi
mathvariant="italic">a</mi></mrow><mrow><mi
mathvariant="italic">b</mi></mrow></msubsup><mi
mathvariant="italic">F</mi><mo mathvariant="normal">&prime;</mo><mi
mathvariant="normal">(</mi><mi mathvariant="italic">t</mi><mi
mathvariant="normal">)</mi><mi mathvariant="italic">d</mi><mi
mathvariant="italic">t</mi><mi mathvariant="normal">=</mi><mi
mathvariant="italic">F</mi><mi mathvariant="normal">(</mi><mi
mathvariant="italic">b</mi><mi mathvariant="normal">)</mi><mo
mathvariant="normal">-</mo><mi mathvariant="italic">F</mi><mi
mathvariant="normal">(</mi><mi mathvariant="italic">a</mi><mi
```

Figure 23.3 MathML representation of the PDF page displayed in Figure 23.1.

```
\documentclass[a4paper,12pt]{book}
\usepackage{latexsym}
\usepackage{amsmath}
\usepackage{amssymb}
\usepackage{bm}
\usepackage{graphicx}
\usepackage{wrapfig}
\usepackage{fancybox}
\pagestyle{empty}

\begin{document}

The Fundamental Theorem of Calculus.

The two main concepts of calculus are integration and differentiation. The
Fundamental Theorem of Calculus (FTC) says that these two concepts are es-
sentially inverse to one another.

The fundamental theorem states that if $F$ has a continuous derivative on an
interval $[a,\ b]$, then
$$
\int_{a}^{b}F'(t)dt=F(b)-F(a)\ .
$$
This form allows one to compute integrals by finding anti-derivatives.

The FTC says that integration undoes differentiation (up to a constant which is
irrevocably lost when taking derivatives), in the sense that
$$
F(x)=\int_{a}^{x}\frac{d}{dt}(F(t))dt+C
$$
```

Figure 23.4 Latex representation of the PDF page displayed in Figure 23.1.

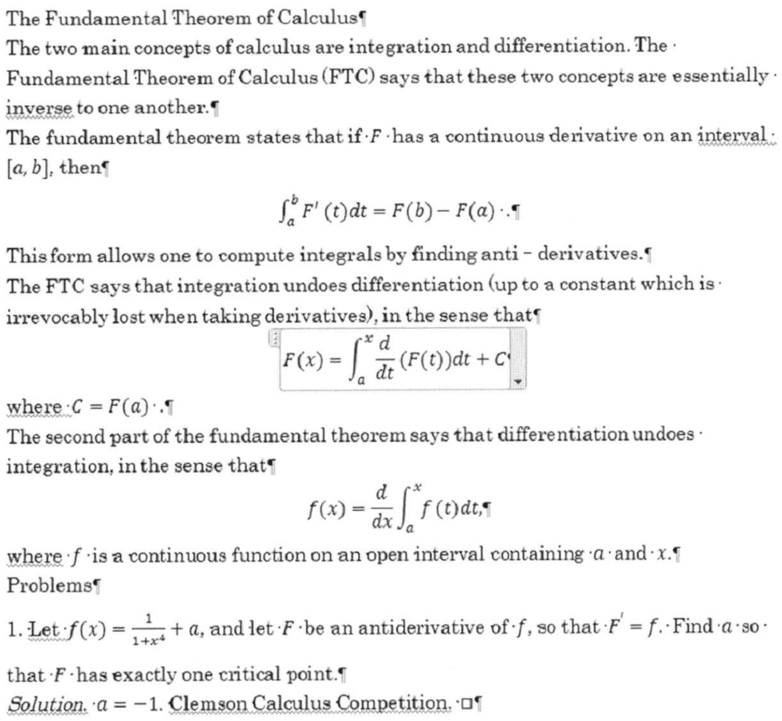

The Fundamental Theorem of Calculus¶
The two main concepts of calculus are integration and differentiation. The Fundamental Theorem of Calculus (FTC) says that these two concepts are essentially inverse to one another.¶
The fundamental theorem states that if F has a continuous derivative on an interval $[a, b]$, then¶

$$\int_a^b F'(t)dt = F(b) - F(a)\,.$$

This form allows one to compute integrals by finding anti - derivatives.¶
The FTC says that integration undoes differentiation (up to a constant which is irrevocably lost when taking derivatives), in the sense that¶

$$F(x) = \int_a^x \frac{d}{dt}(F(t))dt + C$$

where $C = F(a)$.¶
The second part of the fundamental theorem says that differentiation undoes integration, in the sense that¶

$$f(x) = \frac{d}{dx}\int_a^x f(t)dt,$$

where f is a continuous function on an open interval containing a and x.¶
Problems¶
1. Let $f(x) = \frac{1}{1+x^4} + a$, and let F be an antiderivative of f, so that $F' = f$. Find a so that F has exactly one critical point.¶
Solution. $a = -1$. Clemson Calculus Competition. □¶

Figure 23.5 MathML representation of the PDF page displayed in Figure 23.1.

Using InftyReader to make STEM content accessible to students with print disabilities is important for two reasons. First, to disprove commonly held beliefs that:

- Providing students with print disabilities access to math content is too difficult and time-consuming;
- Most students with print disabilities find math too complex; and,
- Because of these reasons, making math content accessible is not worth the time and effort.

Second, images of mathematical equations appearing on web pages and in eBooks/PDF documents, for the most part:

- Are not accessible by students using AT;
- Do not provide for alternative output modalities, such as Braille or synthetic speech;
- Cannot be altered, easily, to accommodate the learning needs of students with low vision (color and contrast changes); and,
- Require authors to redraw images when even small changes are made.

Handwriting recognition technology

Handwriting recognition technology enables a computer to receive and interpret handwritten input from documents, images, photographs, and touch-screens. Here's a short timeline of events leading to the handwriting technology we use today:

1980s: Retailers begin to use handwriting recognition systems to enable people to sign credit card receipts using an electronic pen and tablet.

1989: The first portable handwriting recognition computer is developed. It was called GRiDPad from GRiD Systems.

1996: The first handwritten address interpretation (HWAI) system was deployed by the United States Postal Service (USPS). Since field-testing began in 1996, HWAI has been implemented at all USPS mail processing centers.

Today: Handwriting recognition technology is popular on most smartphones.

So what's the new use?

In 2015, IDEAL Group harnessed the power of handwriting recognition to more easily create fully accessible STEM content in support of individuals with print disabilities. Their innovation is an Android application called IDEAL Math Writer. IDEAL Math Writer works as follows:

Users handwrite math equations on an Android tablet. The application recognizes the handwritten math formulas/equations in real time.

After recognizing a handwritten math equation/formula, IDEAL Math Writer *automatically* generates the following different representations of what was handwritten:

- LaTeX markup
- MathML markup
- High-quality image
- Alt-text description
- Expandable MathJax renderings.

IDEAL Math Writer recognizes more than 200 handwritten math symbols and characters.

Here, in Figures 23.6–23.10, are screenshots of a handwritten equation and the representations that IDEAL Math Writer renders automatically and saves to your private web account for copying to other applications and documents:

Here is the automatically generated text that can be edit-copied, edit-pasted as the image's alt-text description:

> upper S equals StartRoot StartFraction sigma-summation left-parenthesis x minus ModifyingAbove x With minus right-parenthesis squared Over n minus 1 EndFraction EndRoot

More resources

- General overview: http://apps4android.org/mathwriter.
- Promotional video: https://www.youtube.com/watch?v=Zp7jHEjOocE&feature=youtu.be.

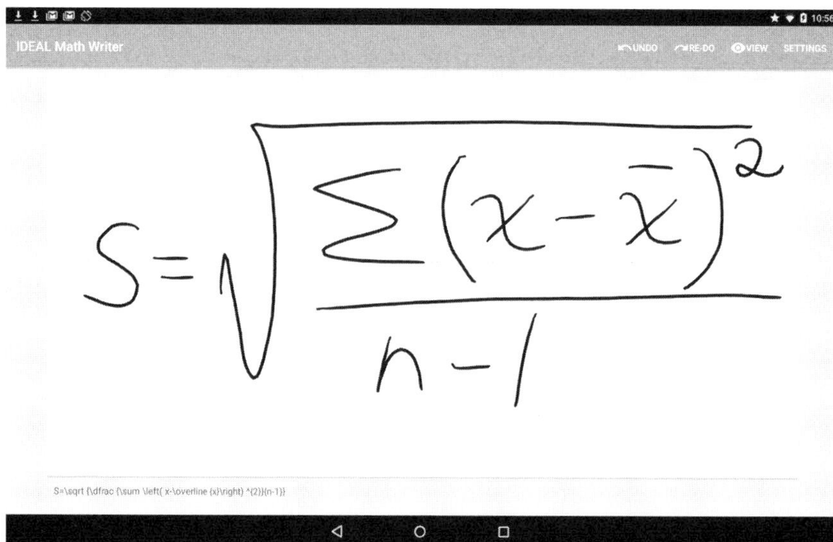

Figure 23.6 Handwritten equation.

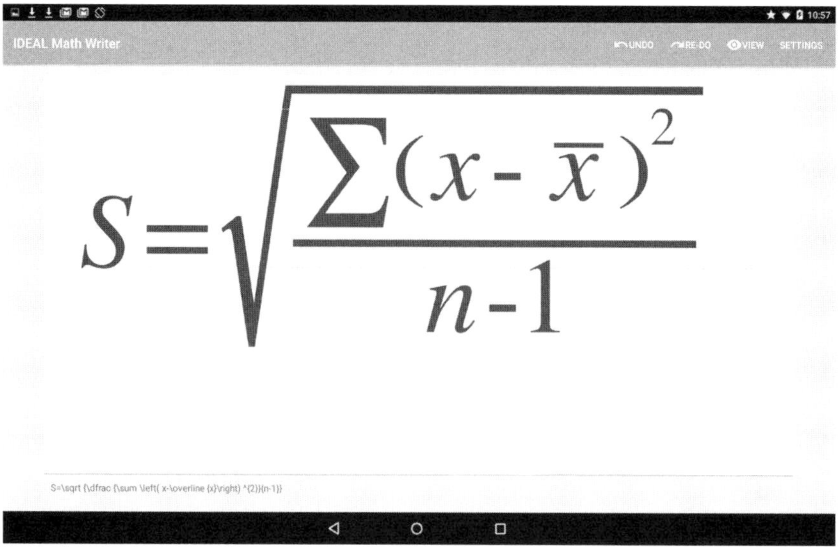

Figure 23.7 Equation automatically rendered into a high-quality image.

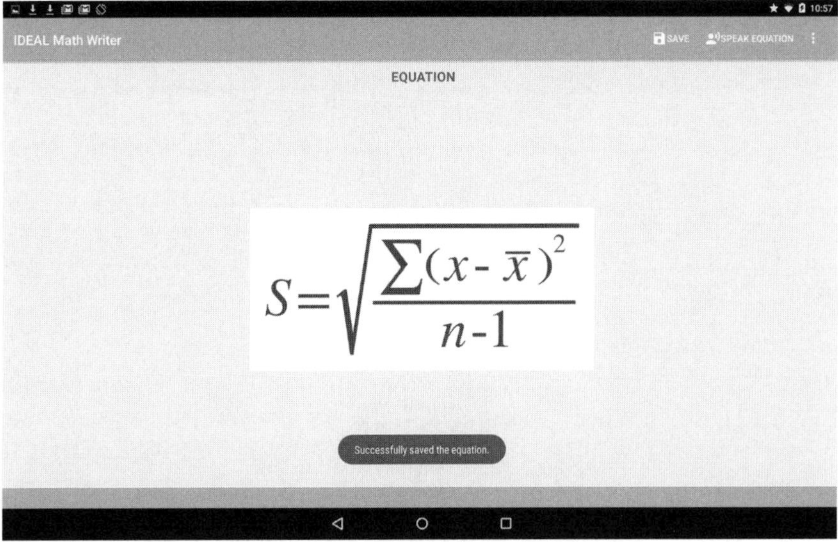

Figure 23.8 Actual image.

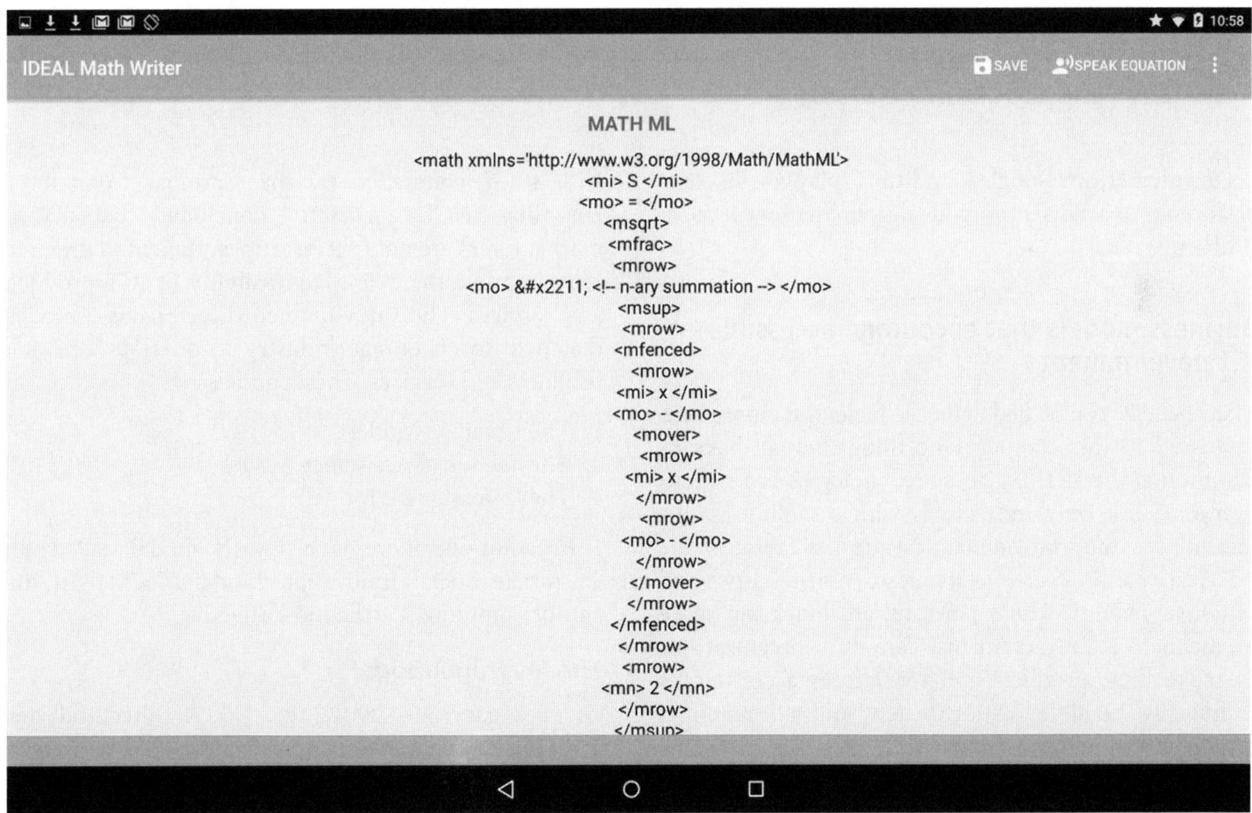

Figure 23.9 MathML representation.

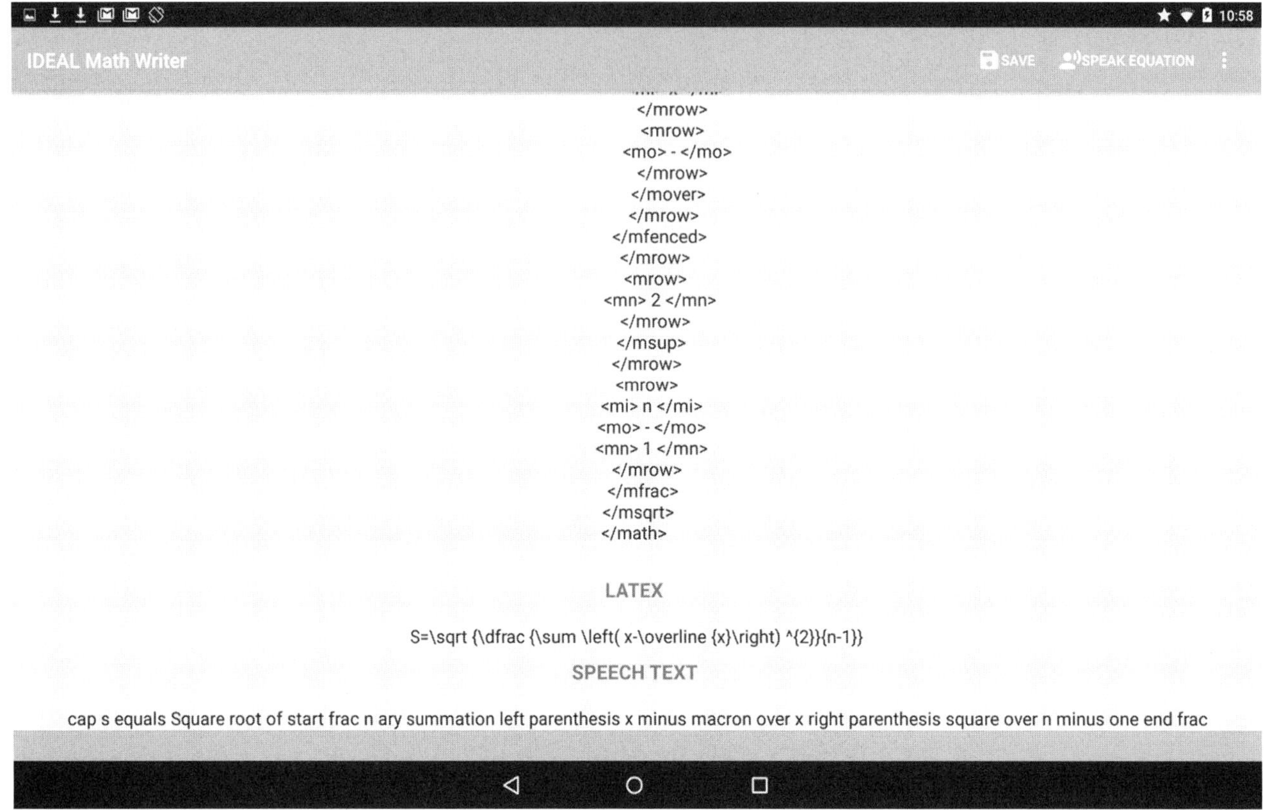

Figure 23.10 LaTeX and speech representation.

- Download from Google Play: https://play.google.com/store/apps/details?id=org.idealgroup.mathwritevo2&hl=en.

Business models that encourage accessible ICT development

Many benefits can be tied to the technological innovations discussed in this chapter. One thing they all have in common is the fact that these technologies can benefit everyone, not only individuals with disabilities. This fact injects important dynamics into the fabric of the AT ecosystem: cost-effectiveness, profitability, and self-sustainability. These powerful attributes can serve as magnets to attract mainstream ICT organizations to make their products and services as accessible as technically possible. Unfortunately, not all potential assistive "technological innovations" offer these benefits to industry.

I thought it appropriate to end this chapter by describing four business models designed to encourage ICT companies to more closely embrace accessible design practices. By considering all levels of the Human-Tech Ladder, the future holds promise to increasingly fold people with disabilities into the social fabric in all contexts.

A study conducted by the National Council on Disability (NCD) in 2001[26] concluded that natural market forces are not (necessarily) sufficient to dramatically improve the overall accessibility of ICT products and services. The study defined three business models that help to encourage industry to develop accessible products and services. These models are:

1. The Leverage Model
2. The Technical Assistance Model
3. The Enforcement Model.

In addition, there is a fourth model called the Corporate Social Innovation Model (CSIM). In this author's opinion, it is the most effective.

The leverage model

On February 20, 2001, the US Architectural and Transportation Barriers Compliance Board (Access Board) issued accessibility standards for electronic and information technology (E&IT), covered by Section 508 of the Rehabilitation Act Amendments of 1998. The author of this chapter was fortunate to have been one of the original authors of these standards. Section 508[27] requires that when federal agencies develop, procure, maintain, or use E&IT, they shall ensure that federal employees with disabilities have access to and use of that E&IT in a way that is comparable to the access to and use of information and data by federal employees who are not individuals with disabilities, unless doing so would pose an undue burden on the agency.

Section 508 also requires that individuals with disabilities who are members of the public seeking information or services from a federal agency have access to and use of information and data that is comparable to that provided to members of the public who are not individuals with disabilities, unless doing so would pose an undue burden on the agency.

On February 23, 2014, the Access Board submitted a proposed rule to update the Section 508 Standards and the Telecommunications Act Accessibility Guidelines to the Office of Management and Budget (OMB). On March 23, 2018 the Standards and Guidelines were updated.[28]

One of the expected benefits of publishing E&IT standards was to motivate government agencies, as well as companies providing E&IT services to government agencies, to make their products and services accessible to individuals with disabilities.

Every day, millions of Americans rely on Federal information technology (IT) to engage with Federal services and information. The President proposes spending nearly $45.8 billion on IT investments at major civilian agencies, which will be used to acquire, develop, and implement modern technologies that enhance digital service delivery.[29] Based on the law, any E&IT accessed by the general public needs to be fully accessible.

The technical assistance model

First enacted in 1988, then amended and extended in 1994 for a five-year period, and a three-year period in 1998, the Assistive Technology Act (Tech Act)[30] was the first major federal statute to deal with AT in its own right. The Tech Act created state technology assistance programs that operate in all 56 states and territories. It also established national technical assistance programs, including United Cerebral Palsy's (UCP's) AT Funding and Systems Change Project and the Rehabilitation Engineering and Technical Assistance Society of North America's (RESNA's) Technical Assistance Project. One of the major goals of the Tech Act was to bring about changes in the way public and private institutions operate, so that they provide greater ICT access to individuals with disabilities.

Technical assistance has played a major role in enhancing the accessibility of ICT products and services. Technical assistance can be provided in many ways, including the following:

- Increase the availability of/access to, and provision of training about, AT devices and services.
- Increase the ability of individuals with disabilities to acquire assistive technology devices as they transition from school to college, school to work, etc.
- Increase the capacity of public agencies and private entities to provide and pay for AT devices and services on a statewide bases for individuals with disabilities of all ages.
- Increase the awareness of practices, procedures, and organizational structures that provide consumers with AT devices and services.
- Increase awareness and knowledge of the benefits of AT devices and services among targeted individuals and entities and the general population.

While this model has been successful in increasing awareness and access to information about AT, it still focuses on a medical model approach to TEI.

The enforcement model

No disability civil rights law is absolute in its requirements. Where excessive cost or other factors make a proposed action or remedy an "undue burden," or render it "not readily achievable," the laws will not insist that it be done. In such cases, alternatives need to be found, but each of these is subject to the same tests. Accordingly, any suggestion that enforcement is now a primary tool on which we rely for accessibility must be qualified from the outset.

Within this framework, the ADA, Sections 255 and 508 of the Rehabilitation Act, and Twenty-First Century Communications and Video Accessibility Act (CVAA) – the four principal civil rights statutes – all create definite and measurable expectations of what private sector business must do in its multiple roles as employer, public-accommodations provider, and product developer or supplier. Coming from government, the disability community, and other segments of society, these expectations combine to create what may fairly be termed "a climate of enforcement." While this model has resulted in minimum requirements that organizations need to comply with to enable people with disabilities to access goods and services, it falls short of providing a societal solution that embraces principles of universal design.

The final model presented here provides organizations a way of meeting societal needs as well as sustaining the organization too. It is presented here as a model to guide technology development for the future. It is the model used by the organizations whose innovations are described in this chapter and promotes product development that aligns with a social model of disability.

The corporate social innovation model (CSIM)

Many people believe that corporations should have some "responsibility" to society for making ICT products and services more accessible. However, "giving something" to society is not necessarily self-sustaining or cost-effective if done for reasons of charity.[31] Corporations only have the ability to "give something" to society when they are making money.

This decade has seen dramatic changes take place in the way major ICT manufacturers view social responsibility as it relates to accommodating the ICT access needs of individuals with disabilities. These efforts exemplify the true spirit of the CSIM. Corporate Social Innovation (CSI) enables companies have their cake and eat it too. CSI enables companies to give something to society and at the same time generate additional revenue and gain competitive advantage in the marketplace.

Overview of the CSIM's technical assistance components

> Give a man a fish and you feed him for a day. Teach a man to fish and you feed him for a lifetime.—
> Chinese Proverb

In order for the CSIM to survive, it is important that its technical assistance components (services) be robust. It is for that reason they are listed below:

Fully integrated accessibility framework: This includes built-in accessibility support, including common, reusable programming components that enable developers to easily create applications that are fully accessible.

Robust operating platform: These include Mac, iOS, Windows, Windows Mobile, and Android.

Developer tools and resources:

- Software development kit (SDK) – An SDK is typically a set of development tools that allows for the creation of applications for a certain software package, software framework, hardware platform, computer system, operating system, or similar platform.
- Technical documentation – this is documentation that describes handling, functionality, and architecture of a technical product or a product under development or use and is critical to the success of any developer.
- Technical articles – articles are used to show examples to developers of how other users have created and maintained accessible tools.
- Tutorials and sample code – developers can share and distribute code and accessible tutorials in order to aid other developers in creating accessible tools.
- Developer forums – developer forums are online discussion sites. From a developer's standpoint, forums are web applications that support developers communicating with each other to discuss common topics and resolve technical issues.
- Discount device purchase programs (DDPP) – DDPPs are programs that provide developers with the hardware device(s) they need to develop applications for that hardware device(s). The device(s) are often offered at a discount.

Software distribution services

App Store services – software distribution services enable developers to sell what they develop by listing it for sale in an App Store. App Stores give customers the ability to purchase and downloaded developers' applications directly from the Internet. In the case of the examples cited in this chapter, software distribution services also include the following components:

- Order fulfillment
- Billing system
- Payment system
- Accounting system
- Automated profit distribution system
- User feedback reports
- Number of downloads
- Active installs
- Star ratings
- User comments
- Application error reports
- Application promotion services
- List of most popular apps
- Company blogs
- Showcase overviews of highly popular applications.

Accessibility value chain concept

According to Jim Tobias, President of Inclusive Technologies, all technology ecosystems (the real pattern of relationships in which it survives or fails) are called a value a "value chain." The concept of a value chain originated with Michael Porter, in his book *Competitive Advantage: Creating and Sustaining Superior Performance* (1985).[32] A value chain is the recognition that the value of a product is created not only by a single entity, like a manufacturer, but depends significantly on many other players: component vendors, distributors, retailers, trainers, and end users. Value chains can be used to analyze the total social benefit of products and services, and to clarify the relationships between and among links in the chain.

How does the value chain concept relate to accessibility? In some cases, a mainstream product provides an accessibility feature that the user needs to find and activate to use that feature. In other cases, the mainstream product does not have the necessary accessibility feature, so the user connects a piece of AT, and the AT product provides the necessary accessibility feature, working in conjunction with the mainstream product. In both cases, accessibility may still not be achieved if the content or service accessed or enabled by that product is not appropriately formatted or enhanced.

A good example of a value chain is the W3C's Web Accessibility Initiative (WAI). Their leadership recognized early on that authoring tools, content, and user agents must all be in alignment for accessibility to be available to the user. This is not only a "technology stack," but a set of relationships and professional norms.

Another example can be cited in the wireless environment. Even if handsets are accessible, consumers with disabilities have a hard time locating models that will work for them, largely because they rely on getting information in phone stores, like everyone else. The retail staff there are often ill-equipped to advise and inform on any specialized needs, disability or not. So the efforts of handset designers are always being jeopardized.

People in the value chain who train, guide, or advise the user, or manage the user's IT, are providers of critical value. This is especially true of institutional settings like schools, workplaces, and job placement centers. Organizational decision-makers and technology administrators are key links in the accessibility value chain, yet they are rarely well informed about accessibility features and AT compatibility for a variety of factors, including the fact that staying well informed in general about current features and capabilities of any new technology is increasingly difficult.

In conclusion, the author of this chapter has presented business models and examples of innovative technology that support achieving the many benefits of accessible E&IT design, which are to:

- Enable E&IT to benefit people with disabilities;
- Land lucrative government contracts;
- Reduce legal exposure;
- Obtain accessibility certifications;
- Improve your knowledge in the area of accessible design; and,
- Develop accessible websites.

Notes

1 Vicente, K. (2006). *The Human Factor: Revolutionizing the Way We Live with Technology*. New York: Routledge.

2 See Pub. L. No. 101-336, § 2(a)(1), 104 Stat. 327, 328 (codified at 42 U.S.C. §§ 12101–12213, § 12101(a)(1) (1994)), finding that currently 43 million Americans have one or more disabilities and "this number is increasing as the population as a whole is growing older".

3 42 U.S.C. § 12101(b)(1) (1994).

4 H.R. REP. NO. 101-485, pt. 2, at 22 (1989), reprinted in 1990 U.S.C.C.A.N. 303, 304. The genesis of this seminal legislation was the recognition that, despite the extraordinary efforts of advocates for the disabled, many disabled Americans lived their lives in intolerable isolation and dependence. See id. at 32, reprinted in 1990 U.S.C.C.A.N 303, 313.

5 42 USC § 12181 – Definitions: (7) Public accommodation. Legal Information Institute (LII). Cornell University Law School (n.d.). Retrieved from http://www.law.cornell.edu/uscode/text/42/12181.

6 LLCS-corporations-partnerships – Definition: Entity. Legal Information Institute (LII). Cornell University Law School (n.d.). Retrieved from http://www.law.cornell.edu/wex/entity.

7 The WorldWideWeb browser. Tim Berners-Lee: WorldWideWeb, the First Web Client (n.d.). Retrieved from http://www.w3.org/People/Berners-Lee/WorldWideWeb.html.

8 Before Netscape: the forgotten web browsers of the early 1990s (n.d.). Ars Technica. Retrieved from http://arstechnica.com/business/2011/10/before-netscape-forgotten-web-browsers-of-the-early-1990s.

9 E-Commerce Software and Services. Intershop, (n.d.). Retrieved from http://www.intershop.com.

10 PizzaNet – commercially licensed and bundled internet operating system (n.d.). Adafruit Industries Blog. Retrieved from http://www.adafruit.com/blog/2012/09/09/pizzanet-commercially-licensed-and-bundled-internet-operating-system.

11 Scholasticus, K. (n.d.). History of internet banking. Retrieved from https://wealthhow.com/history-of-internet-banking.

12 Amazon (company). Wikipedia.org (n.d.). Retrieved from https://en.wikipedia.org/wiki/Amazon_(company).

13 Our history, Ebay Inc. (n.d.). Retrieved from https://www.ebayinc.com/our-company/our-history/.

14 Ali, F. (2019). US ecommerce sales grow 15.0% in 2018. *Internet Retailer* (28 February). Retrieved from https://www.digitalcommerce360.com/article/us-ecommerce-sales.

15 Collins, J. (2019). The top 10 most popular sites of 2019. *Lifewire* (2 January). Retrieved from https://www.lifewire.com/most-popular-sites-3483140.

16 Tamturk, V. (2017). Trump moved web accessibility regulation to "Inactive list." CMSC Media (8 August). Retrieved from https://www.cms-connected.com/News-Archive/August-2017/President-Trump-Moved-the-Web-Accessibility-Regulation-to-Inactive-List

17 Ibid.

18 Vu, M.N. (2107). DOJ places website rulemaking on the "Inactive" List. Department of Justice website (21 July). Retrieved from https://www.adatitleiii.com/2017/07/doj-places-website-rulemaking-on-the-inactive-list.

19 https://www.reginfo.gov/public/jsp/eAgenda/InactiveRINs_2017_Agenda_Update.pdf.

20 Launey, K.M. and Aristizabal, M. (2017). Website accessibility lawsuit filings still going strong. ADA Title III (22 August). Retrieved from https://www.adatitleiii.com/2017/08/website-accessibility-lawsuit-filings-still-going-strong/.

21 29 USC § 3002 – Definitions: (4) Assistive technology device. Legal Information Institute (LII). Cornell University Law School (n.d.). Retrieved from http://www.law.cornell.edu/uscode/text/29/3002.

22 Mace, R. The Center for Universal Design – about UD. *The Center for Universal Design*. College of Design, North Carolina State University (n.d.). Retrieved from http://www.ncsu.edu/ncsu/design/cud/about_ud/about_ud.htm.

23 About the Global Public Inclusive Infrastructure (GPII) (n.d.). Retrieved from https://gpii.net/about.

24 Ibid.

25 For further information on this technology please refer to Maneki, A. and Jeans, A. (n.d.). LaTeX: what is it and why do we need it? Retrieved from https://nfb.org/images/nfb/publications/fr/fr31/2/fr310212.htm.

26 *The Accessible Future* (2001). Washington, DC: National Council on Disability. Retrieved from https://ncd.gov/publications/2001/June_2001.

27 *Electronic and Information Technology Accessibility Standards (Section 508)* (2000). Washington, DC: US Access Board. https://www.access-board.gov/guidelines-and-standards/communications-and-it/about-the-ict-refresh/final-rule/text-of-the-standards-and-guidelines#appendix-a.

28 Information and Communication Technology (ICT) Final Standards and Guidelines (2018). Retrieved from https://www.access-board.gov/guidelines-and-standards/communications-and-it/about-the-ict-refresh/final-rule.

29 The White House Budget Office (2017, October 1). Section 16: Information Technology. Retrieved from https://www.whitehouse.gov/wp-content/uploads/2018/02/ap_16_it-fy2019.pdf

30 *Assistive Technology Act of 1998 (Tech Act)* (2010). Washington, DC: United Cerebral Palsy. Retrieved from https://www.biausa.org/public-affairs/public-policy/assistive-technology-act.

31 Jacobs, S. (2010). The Corporate Social Innovation Model: enabling positive societal change through the distribution and use of accessible ICT products and services. Retrieved from http://apps4android.org/Corporate_Social_Innovation_Whitepaper.doc.

32 Porter, M. (1985) *Competitive Advantage: Creating and Sustaining Superior Performance*. New York: Free Press.

Index

Page locators in **bold** indicate tables. Page locators in *italics* indicate figures. This index uses letter-by-letter alphabetization.

Assistive Technologies and Environmental Interventions in Healthcare: An Integrated Approach, First Edition.
Edited by Lynn Gitlow and Kathleen Flecky.

Companion website: www.wiley.com/go/gitlow/assitivetechnologies